The Wisdom of Menopause

The Wisdom of Menopause

Creating Physical and Emotional Health
During the Change

Revised and Updated

Christiane Northrup, M.D.

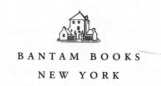

BANTAM BOOKS

NEW YORK

Many of the stories that appear in this book are composites; individual names and identifying characteristics have been changed. Nevertheless, they reflect authentic situations in the lives of the thousands of perimenopausal women I've seen in my practice over the years. If you think you recognize yourself in these pages, the similarities are strictly coincidental unless I have received your specific written permission to use your story.

Published in the United States by Bantam Books, an imprint of The Random House Publishing Group, a division of Random House, Inc., New York.

BANTAM BOOKS and colophon are registered trademarks of Random House, Inc.

Some of the material in *The Wisdom of Menopause* was originally published in *Health Wisdom for Women*, Phillips Publishing International.

LIBRARY OF CONGRESS CATALOGING-IN-PUBLICATION DATA
Names: Northrup, Christiane, author.
Title: The wisdom of menopause: creating physical and emotional health during the change / Christiane Northrup, M.D.
Description: Revised and updated. | New York: Bantam Dell, [2021] |
Includes bibliographical references and index. |
Identifiers: LCCN 2020038842 | ISBN 9780525486138 (trade paperback)
Subjects: LCSH: Menopause. | Menopause—Psychological aspects. | Menopause—Religious aspects.
Classification: LCC RG186 .N67 2021 | DDC 618.1/75—dc23
LC record available at https://lccn.loc.gov/2020038842

Printed in the United States of America.

2 4 6 8 9 7 5 3 1

This book is dedicated to the pioneering spirit embodied in the women of the baby boom generation

Contents

List of Figures

Acknowledgments

I would first like to acknowledge all those whose skills and insights helped me birth the first edition of this book during my own perimenopause back in the early 2000s, especially the late Joel Hargrove, M.D., and the masterly and legendary editor Toni Burbank.

For this updated version, I gratefully thank:

Katy Koontz, first and foremost, for living out her scribe archetype with skill, speed, and panache. She has been a godsend during this and so many other writing projects.

Marnie Cochran of Random House for always believing in my work and for skillfully midwifing it through the publication process.

Ned Leavitt for being a soul-mate agent and stalwart supporter of this work.

Ken Weinrib, my media lawyer, for being a true counselor who seeks solutions.

Joe Gajda, the CEO of Amata Life, for your guidance, skill, and humor, which have made running this business an adventure and a pleasure.

Peter Dunn, my accountant, for your skill, good humor, and steadfast attention to all things financial.

Scott Leighton for both his medical illustrations and his wonderful energy.

Hope Matthews, my Pilates teacher, for her genius as an intuitive movement healer and fascia expert. Her skill and guidance have proven to me that much that we think of as "aging" is nothing but dense fascia.

Chris Renfrow for his incredible knowledge of Traditional Chinese Medicine and how it plays out in the fascial structure.

Reid Tracy, Margarete Nielsen, and the entire staff of Hay House for helping me stay in touch with my global online community through my website, speaking engagements, and other media.

The late Louise Hay and Wayne Dyer—you two way-showers continue to inspire me from the Other Side. I am grateful for the path you created.

Belinda Womack—your spiritual guidance has been invaluable. I cherish you and the 12 Archangels.

Doris E. Cohen, Ph.D. I honor the work that we did together for so many years. Thank you.

Mike Brewer for keeping my home and grounds maintained and lovely.

Steve Meehan, whose genius with plants and gardening continue to inspire and uplift me and my home.

Pat McCabe for keeping the homefires burning and bringing beauty, whimsy, love, and organizational skill to my home.

Paulina Carr for her cheerful willingness to do whatever needs to be done. And also her ability to stick with it until she gets an answer.

Janet Lambert for her superior bookkeeping skills and general all-around great attitude.

Coulson Duerksen, my blog and website editor, for your skill, your courage, your compassionate heart, and your all-round solidarity.

Josephine Wilkins, for your intuitive skills, your friendship, your humor, and your support thorugh the enormous soul growth of the past few years.

Robert Fritchie of the World Service Institute. Your friendship and continual support are a gift in my life, and your teaching about the power of Divine Love has been life changing.

The late Ron Deprez, Ph.D., for supporting my way of thinking and giving me the courage to stand ever stronger in my truth. And for loving me.

My daughters, Ann and Kate, for shining your lights so beautifully out into the world and expanding women's wisdom in your own unique ways.

My granddaughters, Ruby and Penelope. You two old souls are precious to me beyond anything I could have imagined. Thank you for joining us here on Earth at this time.

Michael Watts, my son-in-law, for being such a stand-up man who protects and serves his family so well.

Edna and Wilbur Northrup, my parents, for providing precisely the training I needed to do the work I have done on this planet.

My siblings John, Billy, and Penny—and your spouses, Anne, Lori, and Phil, as well as your children. I am blessed beyond words by all of you, and by the solid support, laughter, health, freedom, and fun that we all enjoy. I know how rare and special this is.

Diane Grover for being the rock at the center of my whole life, my CEO of Everything. Thank you for keeping everything organized, clear, fun, meaningful, and on track—for over forty years. Diane is the woman behind the woman—and also the woman beside the woman. She is a first-chakra genius for whom I am enormously grateful every day. Together we are a miracle team.

Charlie Grover, Diane's husband, whose good humor and willingness to provide backup and down-to-earth commentary are precious.

Because of all of you, I feel and see the light of women's wisdom shining ever more brilliantly across this beautiful planet of ours.

Christiane Northrup, M.D.

The Wisdom of
Menopause

Introduction
The Journey Begins

In the year or two before I actually started to skip periods, I began to experience an increasingly common feeling of irritability whenever my work was interrupted or I had to contend with a coworker or employee who was not as committed to accomplishing the job as I was. Looking back, I recall that when I was in my thirties and my children were younger, their interruptions when I was in the middle of writing an article or talking on the phone were only mildly irritating to me. My love and concern for their welfare usually overrode any anger or frustration I might have felt.

But as I entered perimenopause—the years leading up to the final menstrual period (menopause)—I found myself unable to tolerate distractions such as my seventeen-year-old asking me, "When is dinner?" when she could clearly see I was busy. Why, I wondered, was it always my responsibility to turn on the stove and begin to think about my family's food needs, even when I wasn't hungry and was deeply engrossed in a project? Why couldn't my husband get the dinner preparations started? Why, for that matter, couldn't my teenage daughters get the job done? Why did my family seem to be almost totally paralyzed when it came to preparing a meal? Why did they all wait in the kitchen, as though unable to set the table or pour a glass of water, until I came into the room and my mere presence announced, "Mom's here. Now we get to eat"?

The same thing occurred when it was time to get into the car and take off on vacation. Only when I myself made a definitive move toward the door did my family mobilize. It felt as though my presence caused them to lose their own personal initiative to take charge of a situation, be it dinner or a family trip. Still, during my childbearing years I accepted this, mostly good-naturedly, as part and parcel of my role as wife and mother. And in so doing, I unwittingly perpetuated it, partly because it felt so good to be indispensable.

During perimenopause, I lost patience with this behavior on all levels, whether at home or at work. I could feel a fiery volcano within me, ready to burst, and a voice within me roaring, "Enough! You're all able-bodied, capable individuals. Everyone here knows how to drive a car and boil water. Why is my energy still the organizing principle around here?" My indignation grew as I mumbled to myself, "If I were a man of the same age and education level as I am, we'd consider him 'at the prime of life and at the pinnacle of his career.' There is no way he would be interrupted like this. If I were a man, everyone around me would be wondering how to help me, instead of the other way around!"

Little did I know that these bursts of irritability over petty family dynamics were the first faint knocks on the door marked Menopausal Wisdom, signaling that I needed to renegotiate some of my habitual relationship patterns and the ingrained beliefs that created and supported them. Nor did I know that by the time I began to actually skip periods and experience hot flashes, my life as I had known it for the previous quarter century would be on the threshold of total transformation. As my cyclic nature rewired itself, I put all my significant relationships and beliefs under a microscope, began to heal the unfinished business from my past, experienced the first pangs of the empty nest, and established an entirely new and exciting relationship with my creativity and vocation.

All of the changes I was about to undergo were spurred, supported, and encouraged by the complex and intricate brain and body changes that are an unheralded—but inevitable and often overwhelming—part of the menopausal transition. There is much, much more to this midlife transformation than "raging hormones." Research into the physiological changes taking place in the perimenopausal woman is revealing that, in addition to the hormonal shift that means an end to childbearing, our bodies—and, specifically, our nervous systems—are being, quite literally, rewired. It's as simple as this: our brains are changing, along with our bodies. A woman's thoughts, her ability to focus, and the amount of fuel going to the intuitive centers in the temporal lobes of her brain all are plugged into, and affected by, the circuits being rewired. After working with thousands of women who have gone through this process, as well as experiencing it myself, I can say with great assurance that menopause is an exciting developmental stage—one that, when participated in consciously, holds enormous promise for transforming and healing our bodies, minds, and spirits at the deepest levels.

If you are a midlife woman right now, you are part of a growing population that is at least 43 million strong in the United States alone. This group is no longer invisible and silent, but a force to be reckoned with—educated, vocal, sophisticated in our knowledge of medical science, and determined to take control of our own health. Think about it: more than 43 million women, all undergoing the same sort of circuitry update at the same time. According to the U.S. census, women between the ages of forty-five and sixty-four now make up more than a quarter of the population. By virtue of our sheer numbers, as well as our social and economic influence, we are powerful—and potentially dangerous to any institution built upon the status quo. Baby boom women (those born between 1946 and 1964) and Generation X women (those born between 1965 and 1980) are the most affluent and influential group in the world. It's clear that the world is changing, willingly or otherwise. And it is abundantly clear that those who have embraced the wisdom available at menopause are the ones who are changing it for the better.

It's no accident that the current movement of psychospiritual healing is composed largely of women in their thirties, forties, fifties, sixties, and seventies. We are awakening en masse and beginning to deliver a much-needed message of health, hope, and healing to the world.

My personal experience, now shared by millions of others, tells me that the perimenopausal lifting of the hormonal veil—the monthly cycle of reproductive hormones that tends to keep us focused on the needs and feelings of others—can be both liberating and unsettling. The midlife rate of marital separation, divorce, and vocational change confirms this. I, for one, had always envisioned myself married to the same man for life, the two of us growing old together. This ideal had always been one of my most cherished dreams. At midlife I, like thousands of others, had to give up my fantasies of how I thought my life would be. I had to face, head-on, the old adage about how hard it is to lose what you never really had. It means giving up all your illusions, and it is very difficult. But for me the issue was larger than where and with whom I would grow old. It was a warning, coming from deep within my spirit, that said, "Grow . . . or die." Those were my choices. I chose to grow.

MIDLIFE: REDEFINING CREATIVITY AND HOME

For most women, identity and self-esteem are generated by our associations and relationships. This is true even for women who hold high-powered jobs and for women who have chosen not to marry. Men, by contrast, usually get most of their identity and self-esteem from the outer world—the job, the income, the accomplishments, the accolades. For both genders, this pattern often changes at midlife.

Women begin to direct more of their energies toward the world outside of home and family, which may suddenly appear as a great, inviting, untapped resource for exploration, creative expression, and self-esteem. Meanwhile, men of the same age—who may be undergoing a midlife crisis of their own—are often feeling world-weary; they're ready to retire, curl up, and escape the battles of the workplace. They may feel their priorities shifting inward, toward home, hearth, and family.

It's an ironic transposition: the man (or the individual who tends to carry the most *yang* energy, which we call masculine) is beginning to look to relationships for his "juice"; the woman is feeling biologically primed to explore the outer world. In married couples, this often produces profound role shifts. In the best of all worlds, the man retires or cuts back on work, becoming the chief cook and bottle washer at home, and providing emotional and practical support for his wife's new interests. She, in turn, goes out into the world to start a business, get an education, or do whatever her heart dictates. If their relationship is adaptable and resilient, they adjust to their new roles. Some are so energized by their newfound freedom and passion that they fall in love all over again. If a woman's partner is not willing to grow, however, he (or she) may become jealous of her success and independence, and put pressure on her to continue to care for him as she has always done. He may even get physically sick, often in the form of heart disease and/or clinically dangerous high blood pressure. It's important to note that this is not a conscious or willful act; he's simply responding to the promptings of our lopsided culture.

A woman often finds herself in the difficult position, then, of having to choose between returning to the role of caretaker to nurture her husband or family at the expense of her own needs and pursuing her own creative passions. It's an old story, common to women in many cultures, not just our own. The woman in menopause, who is becoming the queen of herself, finds herself at a crossroads of life, torn between the old way she has always known and a new way she has just begun to dream of. A voice from the old way (in many cases it's her husband's voice or even that of a parent) begs her to stay in place—"Grow old with me, the best is yet to be." But from the new path another voice beckons, imploring her to explore aspects of herself that have been dormant during her years of caring for others and focusing on their needs. She's preparing to give birth to herself, and as many women already know, the birth process cannot be halted without consequences.

Caring for others and pursuing unexplored personal passions are not necessarily mutually exclusive choices, but our culture makes them seem so, always supporting the former at the expense of the latter. This is part of what makes the midlife transformation so much of a challenge—as I know only too well.

BLAZING A NEW TRAIL

Throughout most of human history, the vast majority of women died before menopause. The average life expectancy for a woman in 1900 was only forty. For those who survived, menopause was experienced as a signpost of an imminent and inevitable physical decline. But today, with a woman's life expectancy at eighty-one years, it is reasonable to expect that she will not only live thirty to forty years beyond menopause, but be vibrant, sharp, and influential as well. The menopause you will experience is not your mother's (or grandmother's) menopause.

Here's the truth: most Americans don't get old at age sixty-five, either physically or mentally. The groundbreaking research of Lydia Bronte, Ph.D., former director of the Aging Society Project (funded by the Carnegie Corporation) and author of *The Longevity Factor* (HarperCollins, 1993), reveals that many people will have three different careers over their life span. Bronte says they'll likely have their first career in their thirties and forties, another in their fifties and early sixties, and still another in their seventies. Almost half of the people who Dr. Bronte studied had a major peak of creativity beginning at about age fifty and, in many cases, lasting for twenty-five to thirty years. That means that the new middle age is from fifty to eighty!

Women of the World War II generation, in contrast, whose female role models tended to be like June Cleaver on *Leave It to Beaver*, had an entirely different social and political environment in which to make their transition. Menopause (like menstruation, for that matter) was not discussed in public. Today this is no longer true. As we break this silence we are also breaking cultural barriers, so that we can enter this new life phase with eyes wide open—in the company of at least 43 million kinswomen, all undergoing the same transformation at the same time. In fact, about 6,000 women in the United States reach menopause every day.[1] And, as you'll soon discover, the changes taking place in midlife women are akin to the power plant on a high-speed train, whisking the evolution of our entire society along on fast-forward, to places that have yet to be mapped. Whether you climb aboard this fast-moving train or step aside and let it pass will play a major role in how far you go and how you feel along the way.

Ultimately, I found this journey bracing, exciting, and health-enhancing. And as I look back now, I also see that the choices I made then quite literally saved my life. I'm certainly not alone. A 1998 Gallup survey, presented at the annual meeting of the North American Menopause Society, showed that more than half of American women between the ages of fifty and sixty-five felt happiest and most fulfilled at this stage of life. Compared to when they were in their twenties, thirties, and forties, they felt their lives had improved in many ways, including family life, interests, friendships, and their relationship with their spouse or partner. That mindset is growing. A 2010 survey of women between the ages of thirty-five and forty-nine, sponsored by the National Association of Nurse Practitioners in Women's Health (NPWH) in partnership with Teva Women's Health, reported that more than three-quarters of the women saw midlife as an opportunity for reinvention and believed their best years were yet ahead of them. In other words, the once-conventional view of menopause as a scary transition heralding "the beginning of the end" is dying out itself.

When I wrote the first edition of this book back in 2001, I truly wanted to believe that I too would find myself becoming happier and more fulfilled as time went on. I had faith in the process even though my heart was broken and the life I had known for twenty-five years was dying. Now, twenty-plus years later, I see clearly how every moment of that perimenopausal labor pain was a necessary part of my rebirth into the happy, healthy, fulfilled woman I have become today.

So no matter what is happening in your life right now, take heart. Please join me—and the millions of others who have come before and will come after—as we transform and improve our lives, and ultimately our culture, through understanding, applying, and living the wisdom—and joy—of menopause and beyond.

1

Menopause Puts Your Life
Under a Microscope

It is no secret that relationship crises seem to go hand in hand with menopause. Usually this is attributed to the crazy-making effects of the hormonal shifts occurring in a woman's body at this time of transition. What is rarely acknowledged or understood is that as these hormone-driven changes affect the brain, they give a woman a sharper eye for inequity and injustice, and a voice that insists on speaking up about them. In other words, they uncover hidden wisdom—and the courage to voice it. As the vision-obscuring veil created by the hormones of reproduction and one's cultural programming begins to lift, a woman's youthful fire and spirit are often rekindled, together with long-sublimated desires and creative drives. Midlife fuels those drives with a volcanic energy that demands an outlet.

If it does not find an outlet—if the woman remains silent for the sake of keeping the peace at home or work, or if she holds herself back from pursuing her creative urges and desires—the result is equivalent to plugging the vent on a pressure cooker: something has to give. Very often what gives is the woman's health, and the result will be one or more of the "big three" diseases of postmenopausal women: heart disease, depression, and breast cancer. On the other hand, for those of us who choose to honor the body's wisdom and to express what lies within us, it's a good idea to get ready for some boat rocking, which may put long-established relationships in up-heaval. Marriage is not immune to this effect.

"NOT ME, MY MARRIAGE IS FINE"

Every marriage or partnership, even a very good one, must undergo change in order to keep up with the hormone-driven rewiring of a woman's brain during the years leading up to and including meno-pause. Not all marriages are able to survive these changes. Mine wasn't, and nobody was more surprised about that than I. If this makes you want to hide your head in the sand, believe me, I do un-derstand. But for the sake of being true to yourself and protecting your emotional and physical health in the second half of your life—likely a full forty years or more—then I submit to you that forging ahead and taking a good hard look at all aspects of your relationship (including some previously untouchable corners of your marriage) may be the only choice that will work in your best interest in the long run, physically, emotionally, and spiritually.

From the standpoint of physical health, for example, there is plenty of evidence to suggest that the increase in life-threatening ill-nesses after midlife, which cannot be accounted for simply because of growing older, is partly rooted in the stresses and unresolved rela-tionship problems that simmered beneath the surface during the childbearing years of a woman's life, then bubbled up and boiled over at perimenopause, only to be damped down in the name of maintaining the status quo. The health of your significant other is also at stake. Remaining in a relationship that was tailor-made for a couple of twentysomethings without making the necessary adjust-ments for who you both have become at midlife can be just as big a health risk for him as it is for you.

This is not to say that your only options are divorce or heart at-tack. Rather, in order to bring your relationship into alignment with your rewired brain, you and your significant other must be willing to take the time and spend the energy to resolve old issues and set new ground rules for the years that lie ahead. If you can do this, then your relationship will help you to thrive in the second half of your life. If one or both of you cannot or will not, then both health and happi-ness may be at risk if you stay together. One of the most common midlife wake-up calls for women (and many men, for that matter) is the realization that you have been pouring your life energy into a dead-end job or relationship that will never change—no matter how much you care or how much you give. Like the line in the popular song "Say Something," which Christina Aguilera helped make famous, you finally have to face the truth about some of the characters who have been draining your bank account or life energy account without ever replenishing it. They are not going to change no matter how much faith, hope, and commitment you possess. For those who have almost unlimited faith in the power of hope and love, this realization is simultaneously devastating and liberating. And the pattern is so common that I wrote a separate book on the subject, entitled *Dodging Energy Vampires: An Empath's Guide to Evading Relationships That Drain You and Restoring Your Health and Power* (Hay House, 2018). More on that later.

Preparing for Transformation

At midlife, more psychic energy becomes available to us than at any time since adolescence. If we strive to work in active partnership with that organic energy, trusting it to help us uncover the unconscious and self-destructive beliefs about ourselves and our unhealed hurts that have held us back from what we could become, then we will find that we have access to everything we need to reinvent ourselves as healthier, more resilient women, ready to move joyfully into the second half of our lives.

This process of transformation can only succeed, however, if we become proactive in two ways. First, we must be willing to take full responsibility for the problems in our lives. This is the most difficult step you will ever take, and the most liberating one. It takes great courage to admit our own contributions to the things that have gone wrong for us and to stop seeing ourselves simply as victims of someone or something outside of ourselves. Even if it's true, such as in cases of sexual abuse or domestic violence, we must not allow ourselves to stay in this victim role overly long, because continuing this stance and arguing for it long after the initial trauma is over is ultimately devoid of any power to help us change, heal, grow, and move on to a more fulfilling and joyful life. And trust me, each of us has far more power to create a joy-filled life than we've been led to believe.

The second requirement for transformation is more difficult by far: we must be willing to feel the pain of loss and grieve those parts of our lives that we are leaving behind. And that includes our fantasies of how our lives could have been different *if only*. Facing and feeling such loss is rarely easy, and that is why so many of us resist change in general and at midlife in particular. A part of us rationalizes, "Why rock the boat? I'm halfway finished with my life. Wouldn't it just be easier to accept what I have rather than risk the unknown?"

The end of any significant relationship, be it a marriage, a job, or any major phase of our lives, even one that has made us unhappy or held us back from our full growth and fulfillment, feels like a death—pure and simple. To move past it, we have to feel the sadness of that loss and grieve fully for what might have been and now will never be. And we must speak the truth of it out loud without trying to make it sound noble or uplifting. We must be willing to break the silence that keeps so many women stuck in dead-end situations.

And then we must pick ourselves up and move toward the unknown. All our deepest fears are likely to surface as we find ourselves facing the uncertainty of the future. During my own perimenopausal life changes, I would learn this in spades—much to my surprise.

By the time I was approaching menopause, I had worked with scores of women who had gone through midlife "cleansings"; I had guided and counseled them as their children left home, their parents got sick, their marriages ended, their husbands fell ill or died, they themselves became ill, their jobs ended—in short, as they went through all the storms and crises of midlife. But I never thought I would face a crisis in *my* marriage. I had always felt somewhat smug, secure in my belief that I was married to the man of my dreams, the one with whom I would stay "till death do us part."

Delirious Happiness and Shaking Knees

I will always remember the happiness of meeting and marrying my husband, a decision we made merely three months after we met. He was my surgical intern when I was a medical student at Dartmouth. He looked like a Greek god, and I was deeply flattered by his attention, especially since I wasn't at all sure I had what it took to attract such a handsome man with an Ivy League, country-club background. Something deep within me was moved by him beyond all reason, beyond anything I'd ever felt before with any other boyfriend. For the first five years of our marriage my knees shook whenever I saw him. There wasn't a force on this planet that could have talked me out of marrying him. I remember wanting to shout my love from the tops of tall buildings—an exuberance of feeling that was very uncharacteristic of the quiet, studious valedictorian of my small graduating class at the Ellicottville Central School.

He, however, was considerably less eager to display his feelings. I couldn't help but notice during the years we were both immersed in our surgical training that my husband seemed uncomfortable relating to me when we were at work, and often appeared cold and distant when I'd try to show affection in that setting. This puzzled and hurt me, since I was always proud to introduce him to my patients when we happened to see each other outside of the operating room. But I told myself that this was because of the way he had been raised, and that with enough love and attention from me, he would become more responsive, more emotionally available.

THE CHILDBEARING YEARS: BALANCING PERSONAL AND PROFESSIONAL LIVES

My husband's life didn't change much when we had our two daughters. Mine, however, became a struggle—one that millions of women will recognize from their own experiences—as I tried to find satisfying and effective ways to mother my children, remain the doctor I wanted to be, and at the same time be a good wife to my husband. Nonetheless, these were happy years, for both of us adored our daughters from the beginning and enjoyed the many activities we shared with them—the weekend walks, the family vacations, the simple daily contact with two beautiful, developing young beings.

I did sometimes resent the disparity between what I contributed to the upkeep of our family life and what my husband did. Once, when the children were still young, I asked him if he'd consider working fewer hours so that I wouldn't have to give up delivering babies, an aspect of my practice that I dearly loved. He replied, "You've never seen a part-time orthopedic surgeon, have you?" I admitted that I hadn't, but suggested that this didn't mean it couldn't happen with a little imagination on his part. It was not to be, however. It was I who, like so many other women, became the master shape-shifter, adjusting my own needs to those of everyone else in the family.

In the early years of our family life, I was also becoming increasingly aware that the inequities that bothered me in my marriage were a reflection of inequities that existed in the culture around us. I saw many people like my husband and me—people who had started their marriages on equal ground financially and educationally, even people who, like us, did the same work—and always, once the children arrived, it was the wife who made the sacrifices in leisure time, professional accomplishment, and personal fulfillment. (I am, however, seeing evidence that this is changing in the marriages of my daughters' generation.)

Change Yourself, Change the World

During those often exhausting years, I began to put into action some of the ideas I'd been developing about women's health—while always being careful not to say much about those ideas at home, where I knew they would not be welcomed by my husband. Inspired by my own experiences as well as those of my patients, and buoyed by the conviction that my ideas could make a difference in people's lives, I joined three other women in the venture of establishing a healthcare center we called Women to Women. Though the idea of a health center run by women for women is unremarkable now, it was virtually unheard of at that time. Our central mission was to help women appreciate the unity of mind, body, and spirit, to enable them to see the connection between their emotional health and their physical well-being. I wanted to empower women, to give them a safe place in which to tell their personal stories so that they could discover new, more health-enhancing ways of living their lives.

I knew that sometimes this would involve challenging the status quo, because the inequities of the culture take a terrible toll on women's bodies as well as their spirits. But as I practiced this new, holistic form of medicine, which was quite revolutionary for its day, I realized that the fact that I had a normal, happy family life, as well as a husband with conventional medical ideas who practiced in the same community, provided a kind of cover for me. It made me appear "safe" at a time when my ideas were considered unproven at best, dangerous at worst.

My three partners in Women to Women and I bought an old Victorian house that we could convert into a center for our new practice. We all agreed that we wanted to keep our husbands out of our new venture, lest their participation undermine our enthusiastic but still tender confidence in ourselves as businesswomen.

Of course, in my case, at least, that didn't necessarily mean that I didn't want my husband's support. I clearly remember a day at the beginning of the building and site renovation. Two bulldozers sat on the lawn, workers were everywhere, and the existing building had been torn apart. At that moment the whole project suddenly became real for me, and I realized that my colleagues and I were now responsible for paying for all of this. This was an overwhelming thought.

When I came home that evening, I uncharacteristically reached out to my husband for help in calming my fears. "I'm scared," I told him. "I'm not sure I can do this." He replied, "I hate it when you're disempowered like this." I quickly realized that he wasn't about to coddle me emotionally.

His response to my uncharacteristic and risky moment of emotional vulnerability simply reinforced the coping style I'd developed in childhood, a stoicism that was a necessity in a household where emotional neediness was frowned upon and we were told to "keep a stiff upper lip." Another favorite saying in my family was "Don't ask for a lighter pack, ask for a stronger back." So, as usual, I pulled myself up by my own bootstraps, dug into my inner resources, and pretended that I wasn't afraid. Though there can be a dark side to this kind of upbringing, I am very grateful for the inner core of strength and self-reliance it nurtured within me.

As it turned out, Women to Women became a great success back then. Our work struck a resonant chord with our patients, and the center grew steadily by word of mouth. As excited as I was about what I was doing, I could never interest my husband in any of the ideas about alternative medicine that were at the core of my new clinical practice. We did, however, have enough other areas of mutual interest so that I didn't think his attitude toward my work mattered. In fact, I was rather proud of myself for being able to sustain a loving relationship with a card-carrying member of the American Medical Association.

Marrying My Mother

Looking back, I see that in marrying my husband I had made a secret and mostly unconscious vow that I would do whatever it took to make this marriage work and be the woman I thought he wanted—as long as I could also pursue the work that I loved. (Back then, like most women, I didn't know that the secret to happiness for both ourselves and our loved ones requires that we first and foremost become who we really are—not who we think we should be!) Unbeknownst to me, I was re-creating with my husband many aspects of the unfinished business I had carried over from my relationship with my mother, a fact that would only begin to dawn on me some twenty-two years later, as I entered perimenopause.

Until then, in my marriage I would continue to play the role of the eager-to-please child I had once been, while my husband would fill the role of my remote, emotionally unavailable mother. As the quiet, sensitive child in a family of outgoing, athletic siblings who loved to spend every moment of life charging full speed ahead up mountains and down ski slopes, I had always been the type who tended to disappear, going off by myself into a quiet room where I could listen to music, read fairy tales, sit dreamily by a fire, or gaze out onto the ocean. My mother was much more tuned in to the other members of our large, bustling family, and she and I were a temperamental mismatch, with completely different innate interests. Although my father supported my studious side, he, like most men of his era, left the hands-on parenting to my mother.

Longing for my mother's approval, I tried to win her love by being good. So I worked and studied hard, never got into trouble, and made myself into my mother's little helper, cooking, cleaning, creating centerpieces for holiday dinners—whatever I could think of that would prove my worth, other than athletic pursuits. Intuiting that my mother was in some pain—though it would be many years before I understood the nature of that pain—I tried to be a comfort as well as a help to her, just as I would later try in my marriage to heal what I perceived were my husband's childhood wounds, to give him enough love to make it possible to overcome his early fears and hurts.

Meanwhile, I looked to my teachers for the applause I couldn't get at home. My search for acknowledgment made me a classic overachiever at school, a pattern that would continue all the way through medical school and into my marriage.

Eventually, just as I had turned to my schoolteachers for the support and approval I didn't get at home, I would one day turn to people other than my husband to meet my emotional needs. But until I began the process of self-knowledge that culminated in the dismantling of my marriage, I simply accepted the fact that, like my mother, my husband could not really see or appreciate me for who I was. In fact, I never expected him to. I was operating under the assumption that I was fundamentally unworthy of being cherished by such a special person.

Had I felt more worthy of love, I never would have chosen someone like my husband. Several of the boyfriends I was involved with before I met him did admire and value me. But when your working belief about yourself is that you have to earn love—earn it both by overachieving in your own life and by rescuing someone from the pain of their own life (or at least from what you believe is their pain)—then you will attract a person who reflects those beliefs back to you. Inevitably the young men who were supportive of me were not the ones I wanted. I wanted precisely the kind of emotional un-availability that felt most like home to me—and I got it. My colleague Doris Cohen, Ph.D., a clinical psychologist and the author of *Repetition: Past Lives, Life, and Rebirth* (Hay House, 2008), points out that re-creating the unfinished emotional business of our past is not neurotic. It's the way we heal. And at perimenopause, our need for healing the past arises with great urgency.

With the wisdom of hindsight, I realize now that my husband was a true soul mate—tailor-made to force me to heal my unhealed past. And so I do not blame him for what happened between us. It was only when I was able to be true to my soul—to change from the inside out, in the most fundamental of ways—that we ceased to be life partners. In retrospect, he was one of the biggest gifts of my life, contributing more to my personal growth than I ever would have dreamed possible.

After my divorce, I found myself face-to-face with my unfinished business with my mother—a very common theme—and eventually worked through that. (See my book *Mother-Daughter Wisdom* [Bantam Books, 2005]—a book that should have been called "Mothers and Daughters: The Bond That Wounds, the Bond That Heals"—and also *Dodging Energy Vampires* [Hay House, 2018] for all the details.)

WHY RELATIONSHIPS MUST CHANGE AT MIDLIFE

When we look at the typical dynamics of intimate family relationships in this culture, it's reasonably safe to say that the vast majority of the nurturing, supportive, subordinate roles fall to women, as does most of the self-sacrifice. Yes, it has become somewhat more common for women to achieve high-ranking positions in corporate, political, and scientific arenas. Women now make up almost 47 percent of the workforce,[1] as opposed to a third fifty years ago, and slightly more than 42 percent of women are their family's primary breadwinner. But even so, whenever career concessions must be made for the sake of the family, it's still likely to be the woman who steps down or cuts back. Married mothers in the United States spend almost *twice* as much time on housework and childcare as married fathers do.[2] That's why we have the term "mommy track."

It's true that a woman's biology tends to encourage her involvement with her family at the expense of other interests during the childbearing phase of her life. And, quite frankly, what is more important than raising healthy children? But it's also true that the culture's atmosphere of gender inequity exploits this tendency to an extreme. Consider this: women everywhere are underrepresented in business and in the media. For example, women occupy only 10 percent of top management positions in S&P 1500 companies.[3] They make up only 12.5 percent of chief financial officers[4] and 5 percent of chief executive officers[5] in Fortune 500 companies. As Julie Burton writes in her foreword to *The Status of Women in the U.S. Media 2015,* a report from the Women's Media Center, "In print news, women report 37 percent of stories; on the Internet, women write 42 percent of the news; and on the wires, women garner only 38 percent of the bylines."[6]

This can lead to an incredible surge of pent-up resentment when the hormonal veil lifts and a woman suddenly sees with clarity what has happened in her life.

The emotional changes that come about in the years leading up to and during menopause can feel earthshaking and even terrifying, particularly for those of us who are accustomed to thinking we're in control. It's one thing to resist change from some external force. It's quite another when the change is coming from within, and everything you cling to that's comfortable in its familiarity, including your very identity, is metamorphosing from the inside out. There are only two ways to avoid this abrupt, jolting level of change: defy social and cultural dictates throughout your childbearing years, so that by the time you approach menopause you will already have put into effect many of the changes that cry out to be made at midlife, *or* defy your body's wisdom at perimenopause and ignore its call for truth, creative expression, and personal fulfillment. The latter course can have disastrous consequences for your own health as well as the health of your significant other, not to mention your relationship, which would then be based on something other than mutual respect and love. And you'd never find the treasure that perimenopause is desperately trying to bring to your attention—a life based on true freedom and joy!

During perimenopause, we are hormonally primed to remember and act upon our dreams. There is no more powerful example of this than the story of Tererai Trent, Ph.D., author of *The Awakened Woman: Remembering and Reigniting Our Sacred Dreams* (Atria/ Enliven, 2017). Dr. Trent grew up in rural Zimbabwe and was married (to an abusive man) before the age of fourteen for the bride price of a cow, went on to birth four children by the age of eighteen, and then managed—against all odds—to tap into her inner power and eventually get not only a high school diploma but also a Ph.D. in the United States. She provides us with invaluable advice when she writes: "Taking a good hard look at these social and statistical narratives is informative, but we cannot stop there, for they tell only one side of the story. When we remain frozen in statistics or stuck as supporting characters in someone else's story, we remain silent and forgotten. In this we risk being forever kept in a secondary role—we risk seeing the problem and not the potential. If power isn't willingly given up [and in patriarchy, it never is], then we must claim it in words and deeds."[7]

We must rewrite our stories and become the heroine in our own lives.

How Your Brain Is Hardwired for Relationships

Nothing in our lives affects us more profoundly, both physically and emotionally, than our relationships with others. The neural pathways that enable us—that actually compel us—to relate to other human beings are laid down in our brains in early childhood. The experiences we have at this critical stage will influence the circuitry that develops and stays with us for life. If, for example, our needs as infants are met by a loving caretaker who responds to our cries by feeding or changing or stroking or rocking us when we are hungry or cold or wet or scared, then we will feel good about ourselves, and trusting of the outside world. Our needs have been validated, our emotional cravings met, with our relationship with another human being serving as confirmation of our worthiness. And certainly the biochemistry of motherhood supports this outcome. The hormones associated with birth and nursing in a happy, healthy, well-supported mother predispose her to fall in love with her baby and to fill the child with a sense of being loved and accepted unconditionally.

Sometimes, however, our parents did not themselves experience this kind of unconditional love, or they may simply have been born with the inability to feel empathy. Either way, they are incapable of meeting our needs. George K. Simon Jr., Ph.D., an expert on character disorders and author of *In Sheep's Clothing: Understanding and Dealing with Manipulative People* (A. J. Christopher, 1996), points out the fallacy of believing that only people who have been hurt in childhood hurt other people. It simply isn't true. And the deeply ingrained belief that all people are good at heart is one of the things that needs to be faced and transformed at midlife, especially if one of your parents had this type of personality. Some people truly are just in it for themselves and are simply not capable of actual love. What they're after is status, money, sex, fame, and attention. This is known as narcissistic supply. If an early caregiver was this type of person, then your cries may have gone unheeded or, worse, been met with active disapproval or resentment, and you'll end up with the belief that something is fundamentally wrong with you and that you have to make up for it with acts of service to others. You may also feel that the universe is not a safe place. Your relationships with others will seem undependable, even threatening.

The feelings we develop about ourselves and others as children become etched into the circuitry of our brains and bodies, where they will continue, albeit subconsciously, to affect our relationship choices and responses throughout life. They are part of our basic emotional portfolio, easily accessible and freely expressible, sometimes excessively so. On the other hand, those feelings that were not reinforced by early experience tend to wither away, to become unavailable to us until we make a conscious effort to access our innate power to change our circuitry.

Your ability to live successfully, however you might define success, depends to a great degree on how you relate to other people. If that part of your life is unsatisfactory, the only way you can revise the old relational circuits that determine your current relationships is to expose them and update them. Once you have a better understanding of the environment in which you were born and raised, it becomes possible—though never easy—to change some of the choices you usually make automatically, as a consequence of that old wiring.

But change can occur only when you understand how important it is to change. You must ask yourself why you feel the emotions you feel, choose the mates you choose, act the way you act. The answer is in those early life experiences that served as the architects of your neural circuits and live on today in your very cells. Thankfully, science has now proved beyond any doubt that each of us has the ability to change our thoughts and our brains throughout life—a quality known as neuroplasticity.

During and after adolescence we almost invariably find ourselves attracted to mates who enable us to revisit and perhaps heal the unfinished emotional business of childhood. In our culture, romantic love is where we express our deepest longings. Thus each romantic relationship we enter into can serve as a microscope into our emotional circuitry. More than any other aspect of our lives, our intimate relationships bring to light the old wounds still begging for closure. And many women have been taught to put their needs last in relationships because we feel unworthy. This is particularly true for those who are empaths. Empaths are innately sensitive to the emotions of others and even to the energy in a room. They often can't tell where they end and another person begins. If someone is angry, they feel it—and often feel that it is their job to fix it. If someone is sad, they feel that too, and once again, they may well assume the role of "uplifter" of the situation. Those who are empathic often don't even know what they want until they give themselves permission to remember!

CHARACTERISTICS OF EMPATHS

Empaths are highly sensitive people. Some are simply highly sensitive to their environment and to other people's feelings, while others are what I call "old-soul empaths" who take empathy to a different level. These "old-soul empaths" are highly resourceful, conscientiousness, self-directed, optimistic, and loyal. They tend to be very agreeable and have a can-do attitude, being very willing to help and serve others. They're known for being the kind of person who gets things done, as well as the person everyone goes to for help or advice with tricky problems. They are compassionate and patient, and they naturally see the best in everything and everyone, believing that all people are good at heart. In my experience, 75 percent of these "old-soul empaths" are women and 25 percent are men.

All are extremely sensitive to energy. Even if they're not aware of it, empaths pick up energy from other people, sensing their pain (even if that pain isn't readily apparent), and actually taking that energy on themselves. This porousness can easily affect their emotional and physical health, especially if they are not aware how porous they actually are. For example, empaths may feel nauseated or exhausted in certain situations or around certain people. They also tend to put on weight more easily, usually around their midsections (in part because the weight adds a layer of protection). Because of this porousness, empaths tend to avoid crowds. They also avoid scary or violent movies or television shows because watching them is simply too painful.

Empaths may find that any kind of electrical technology around them—including watches, computers, and cellphones—tends to malfunction on a fairly consistent basis. They are also extremely sensitive to smells and may not be able to tolerate scents from artificial chemical ingredients.

In retrospect, I can see that this was true of my feelings toward the man who became my husband. I was acting out with him a family drama that was still ongoing for me. And although I can't speak on his behalf, in all likelihood I served a similar purpose for him. It took the hormonal and developmental changes of the climacteric to help me see that the role I played in my marriage was based on old beliefs about myself and my worth, beliefs that no longer served me well and were no longer valid.

Menopause to the Rescue

It may not feel like a rescue at the time, but the clarity of vision and increasing intolerance for injustice, inequity, and lack of fulfillment that accompany the perimenopausal changes are a gift. Our hormones are giving us an opportunity to see, once and for all, what we need to change in order to live honestly, fully, joyfully, and healthfully in the second half of our lives. This is the time when many women stop doing what I call "stuffing"—stifling their own needs in order to tend to everybody else's. Our culture expects women to put others first, and all during the childbearing years most of us do, no matter the cost to ourselves. But at midlife we get the chance to make changes, to create lives that fit who *we* are—or, more accurately, who we have become.

If, however, a woman cannot face the changes she needs to make in her life, her body may find a way to point them out to her, lit up in neon and impossible to ignore. It is at this stage that many women reach a crisis in the form of some kind of physical problem, a life-altering or even sometimes life-threatening illness. Scientist and author Gregg Braden, who has traveled extensively and studied indigenous people all over the world, added an additional piece to my understanding when I interviewed him on my radio show. He said he routinely finds healthy women the world over as old as 120 who are agile and able to take care of their daily needs. He told me that the cultures he has studied believe that the human body can tolerate unresolved hurts without physical harm until about age fifty. After that, if not resolved, this unfinished business forms the basis for physical illness.

One very common physical problem in the years leading up to menopause, for example, is fibroid tumors in the uterus. Forty percent of all perimenopausal women in our culture are diagnosed with one or more fibroid tumors, and many of them will undergo midlife hysterectomies to deal with the problem. In conventional medicine, we doctors are content to explain that fibroids occur so frequently in women in their forties because of changing hormone levels, with too much estrogen being produced compared to progesterone.

Though this is true as far as it goes, it is not the whole truth. I know this both personally and professionally, through the experience I had with a fibroid tumor that was first diagnosed when I was forty-one. Bodily symptoms are not just physical in nature; often they contain a message for us about our lives—if we can learn to decipher it. Sometimes, as happened with me, the message becomes clear in stages, with its full meaning available only in retrospect. But what I learned firsthand over the course of the eight years during which I was processing the experience of my fibroid is that we attract precisely the illness or problem that best facilitates our access to our inner wisdom—a phenomenon that is both awe-inspiring and sometimes terrifying. Though this is true throughout our lives, it hits us harder and more directly during perimenopause and menopause, as though nature is trying to awaken us one last time before we leave our reproductive years, the era when our inner wisdom, mediated in part by our hormones, is loudest and most intense.

I had a fibroid as my wake-up call. Another woman might have had a flare-up of migraine headaches, thyroid problems, PMS, breast symptoms, high blood pressure, or any of the several other conditions so common at perimenopause. Your body's message to you will be in the language that best breaks through your particular barriers and speaks most specifically to the issues you need to change in your life. The wisdom of this system is very precise.

MY PERSONAL FIBROID STORY:
THE FINAL CHAPTER

My fibroid was initially diagnosed several years before my first book, *Women's Bodies, Women's Wisdom,* was published. By then I had been working on the book for over three long years, and for a while there it felt literally like a stuck creation. In my darkest moments I sometimes doubted that the book would ever be published. I assumed at the time that my fibroid was related to my frustration at how long it was taking me to finish the book and get it out into the world. Fibroids can often represent blocked creativity, or creativity that hasn't been birthed yet, usually because it is being funneled into dead-end relationships, jobs, or projects. (Blocked creative energy can also express itself in other locations, such as the ovaries, fallopian tubes, lower intestines, lower back, bladder, and hips, as well as the uterus—all of which are part of the second female energy center, or what Eastern medical practitioners call the second-chakra area.)

When *Women's Bodies, Women's Wisdom* was finally published, it was well received, much to my surprise. I had secretly feared that I'd be vilified by my beloved profession for writing the truth as I saw it about the profound connection between women's lives and their health. Though the book wasn't exactly embraced with open arms by my fellow OB-GYNs, it wasn't rejected, either. And the women for whom I had written it received it with great enthusiasm. (I'm also delighted that I'm often approached by women whose mothers gave them a copy of *Women's Bodies, Women's Wisdom* when they were going off to college. Those same women are now entering perimenopause!)

Back then, I was happy and relieved about the response I got, and my fibroid remained quiescent. It didn't go away, but it didn't get much larger, either. It remained as a kind of semi-dormant whisper from my inner wisdom. I knew the fact that it was there was not a fluke. It meant something. So I vowed to remain open to its message.

Over the next few years I continued to heed my inner voice—as far as I was able to understand it. I tried to change relationships that weren't working for me, I found new ones that were more reciprocal, more of a partnership, and I tried to follow my creative instincts wherever they led me. Thus, after more than a decade of what had been deeply fulfilling work with my colleagues at Women to Women, I found that my heart was increasingly drawn to writing and teaching. Because I was eager for my message to reach a larger audience than ever before, I began to reduce my involvement in the center.

I gave up my surgical practice and gradually, ever so gradually, cut back on direct patient care, too. Though I was very excited by the new direction my life was taking, I was conflicted about losing this close connection with my patients. I loved having a regular practice in which I saw the same women year after year, helping them in times of illness, celebrating with them as they learned the skills of creating health. But the pile of charts requiring my attention at the end of each day was increasingly giving me a knot in my stomach.

Meanwhile, the monthly newsletter that I had started in 1994 was doing well, and I was spending a great deal of time researching and writing it each month. I also began traveling around the country teaching and lecturing. All during this time of change I was trying to understand what my fibroid was attempting to teach me—especially when, after having been stable for almost four years, it began to grow larger, until finally it was the size of a soccer ball. Although I didn't feel that my life was acutely out of balance in any way, I was aware that the various changes I was making were accompanied by a lot of guilt, and that guilt about doing something we love is always a clue that points to blocked energy. But since I was feeling so fulfilled in my work life (despite feeling guilty that I was having too much fun), I did not understand what the blockage could be.

On Thanksgiving Day two years after *Women's Bodies, Women's Wisdom* was published, while trying to find something to wear for dinner that would conceal the now visible swelling in my belly, I finally realized that I was tired of trying to dress around my fibroid, tired of the discomfort it caused me whenever I lay down on my abdomen. I decided that it was time to give up my attempts to shrink it through visualization, homeopathy, diet, and acupuncture. I was ready to ask for help and have my fibroid surgically removed.

After scheduling the surgery, I started to take a GnRH agonist, a medication that decreases estrogen levels and therefore shrinks fibroids. This creates an artificial menopause, with many of the same side effects experienced by women in real menopause, such as memory change, hot flashes, and bone loss. Nonetheless, I decided that the benefits I would get from shrinking the tumor—the smaller the tumor, the smaller the incision, and the lower the risk of excessive blood loss—were worth the inconvenience, especially since I was only going to be taking the drug for two months.

Little did I know that the benefits would extend far beyond the shrinking of the tumor. Looking back on this period now, I see that the two months of artificial menopause brought on by the drug jump-started the changes in my brain—and my life—that set the stage for a complete cleansing and reorganization of some of my closest relationships, including, ultimately, my marriage.

Fired Up and Having My Say

One evening, a couple of weeks after I started taking the GnRH agonist, all of the family, including our household manager and former nanny, whom I shall refer to as Lida, was gathered before the television set watching an episode of the show *ER*. At the end, one of the nurses was telling a visitor that he should come in and talk to his friend, a man who had been so badly burned that he was near death.

Observing that the nurse was not telling the visitor the truth about how serious his friend's condition was, Lida said to me, "Do they teach you to be like that in your medical training?" "Be like what?" I asked her. "Do they teach you to withhold the whole truth when the situation is very dire?" she clarified. After thinking about her question for a minute, I replied that there was indeed an unspoken belief among our teachers in medical school that patients (and family and friends) were not really able to handle the truth, and that this belief resulted in many things being left unsaid—a fact that was beautifully illustrated in what we had seen on television.

My husband stood just then, drawing himself up to his full, quite impressive height, and proclaimed, "Of course they don't teach you that. I don't know what you're talking about!" Something within me snapped. After years and years of down-regulating my personal truth to make myself acceptable to my husband and to every authority figure like him in medical school, I simply couldn't keep still another moment. I told him that I felt that I—and everybody else—had been socialized in a thousand nonverbal ways to talk with my patients in a certain way, and that this way left out a lot of the truth of their experience and mine. Of course there was no Don't Talk to Patients 101 course, I said, but I'd learned by example that a hand on the doorknob, the sight of a doctor racing from bed to bed on rounds, conveyed a world of information to patients about what they could and couldn't expect in the way of communication and contact with their physician.

As the conversation heated up, my husband and I retired to the bedroom to spare the others our anger. And for the next forty minutes I felt myself grow taller and taller with my own truth. I told my husband what I believed—about medical practice, about our relationship, about the inequity in the way we'd been living all these years—and I offered no excuses for what I said, nor any attempt to make it easier to hear. This was one of those amazing volcanic eruptions that occur from time to time when the lid finally blows on the container overstuffed with things we know but can't talk about because we are female and have been taught that in order to survive, we must keep quiet so that authorities (mostly men) will like us. Everything we've tried to ignore and struggled to keep beneath the surface bursts forth in all its unedited glory. At the end, my husband did not look as tall as he had at the beginning, and he was speaking softly and apologizing to me. That was the turning point in our marriage. There was no going back.

What had happened in that moment when I suddenly opted to

speak out instead of remaining silent was a direct result of my artificial menopause. Usually menopause comes on gradually, of course. But when it happens more or less instantly because of medication, as it did for me, or because of surgery or radiation, as it does for other women, the sudden hormonal changes can result in insights about our lives that are as dramatic and unexpected as the hot flashes that often plague us at this time. Though my own premature menopause was not permanent and the hot flashes ended as soon as I stopped taking the medication that caused them, the inner change brought about by that brief menopausal interlude *was* permanent. It brought to the surface all the hidden conflicts in myself and my marriage. Fibroids don't jump out of the closet and land on your uterus. They represent blocked creativity—usually from funneling creative energy into a dead-end job or relationship. I had been trying for years to make my marriage work. And my body was telling me that it was time to stop.

THE JOY OF CO-CREATIVE PARTNERSHIP

Although until that time I had been in a marriage that had silenced my voice at home, it had not stopped me from becoming increasingly vocal in my work, and I was now being heard by people far beyond my immediate circle. My career star was definitely on the rise. I had co-founded a very well-known women's center, become president of the American Holistic Medical Association, and written a book that had brought me enormous validation for my work and my ideas. My faith in my own work—work that I absolutely adored—was growing all the time. And so were nourishing relationships outside of my home and marriage. I was starting to connect with true colleagues and good women friends.

I was also proud of the fact that I was contributing more and more to the family finances, and as usual had looked to my husband for approval—but that was not to be. Every time I presented a royalty check or other evidence of my worth, he'd say, "It's already spent." I couldn't win there. But I was winning in many other arenas.

More Validation: My Message Goes to Television

Early in 1997, I began working on my first two public television specials. Soon after GnRH had jump-started my brain, I met Jack Wilson and Bill Heitz, two producers from Chicago whose wives had suggested they track me down and put my work on television. Co-creating what eventually turned out to be four successful public television specials with Jack and Bill also boosted my self-confidence. Now I had the experience of being truly seen and highly valued by two people who had believed in me even when I was a complete novice as a television personality.

This was an enormously exciting time for me. However, by this point I was out of the office more often than I was in it. My dream of teaching and writing, of bringing my message to an ever-wider audience, had become a full-time reality—and then some. Reluctantly I cut the cord with Women to Women completely, selling my share of both the business and the building to my partners. The work I was doing no longer fit the model that we had started together. I knew it was time to go out on my own.

THE FORCES THAT CHANGE THE GOOSE
ALSO CHANGE THE GANDER

As I was making and experiencing all these changes in my life, my husband was going through changes of his own. His midlife reevaluation started with questioning his career goals. The era of managed care was forcing him to change the way he practiced, and he found himself increasingly unhappy in his work. He was also becoming very anxious about money, a fear that my own success seemed only to intensify, rather than to soothe. I couldn't understand why he worried so much about our finances. After all, I reasoned, I was making good money, and we were in this together.

One reason for his anxiety was that he was thinking about retiring when our younger daughter graduated from high school—which was just two short years away. In contrast, I felt as though I was just hitting my stride, and I had no intention of retiring, then or ever. During the retirement-planning sessions my husband scheduled with our accountant, I felt as though we were in two different worlds. There didn't appear to be any computer programs designed to take into account two sets of goals as different as the ones my husband and I described in these meetings.

Like many other men at midlife, my husband seemed to deal with his anxiety about change by trying to exert more and more control over our financial resources—resources that were increasingly from my earnings. Or perhaps he had always exerted that kind of control and I was just now waking up to it. For, like many women of my generation, I had always been convinced that my husband was better at money management than I was, so I had turned it over to him. He did all the planning and paid all the bills, spending hours at his computer each week doing so. As he went through his midlife crisis, this task seemed to fill him with ever-more dread and worry every time he did it, with the result that he tried to micromanage my own expenditures. A part of me was convinced that we were indeed overspending, and I was always on the verge of succumbing to the same fears that plagued him.

But no matter how hard I tried, I could never live within the budget he considered appropriate to our circumstances. I found myself hiding purchases from him, lest he blow up at me. Of course, the conflict between the ideals I had been promoting all these years to my patients and the reality I was living was not lost on me. But my fear of my husband's anger was very real. I let myself be controlled by it, and silenced by it, for years. Even then I was still in some ways the person who wanted more than anything to please and to appease as a way to earn love.

REAL MENOPAUSE HITS

Two weeks after leaving the center I had co-founded nearly fifteen years before, my "official" hot flashes began. They were much less intense than the drug-induced hot flashes I had experienced earlier—flashes so extreme that I routinely removed my winter coat and stripped down to a tank top in the middle of a Maine winter! Nonetheless, they were eloquent enough to make me realize that I was finally entering menopause for real.

It was December 18, 1998—the end of a year and, as it turned out, the end of an era. The separation I had just negotiated from Women to Women was only a warm-up for what was about to happen on the home front—though on the surface things looked fine, even festive. The day my hot flashes started was also the day I, my husband, and our daughters embarked on a long-awaited family ski trip to Austria, where we would spend Christmas with my mother and my siblings. This was something I had dreamed for years about doing.

The trip was wonderful in many ways, and I was very happy to be with my extended family in such a magical place, but I felt the strain in my marriage as never before. When I looked at other couples around us, men and women who were clearly engaged with and enjoying each other, I felt very alone. I found that I was avoiding my husband on that trip, skiing mostly with my daughters, my sister, and my mother. I simply didn't want to use my energy to try to soothe my husband and keep him comfortable, as I had always done before. The coming of my hot flashes had signaled another stage in my own midlife reevaluation—a commitment to setting healthier boundaries, to taking better care of myself, to speaking the truth.

In case I had any doubts, my body reinforced my decision to honor my own needs. I broke out in adult acne, a sign that something had "gotten under the skin" and was now about to erupt. When I turned to the Motherpeace tarot cards I used to help me access my intuition, I kept drawing the Shaman of Swords card, whose message is about saying what you know to be true. The universe was speaking to me in many guises. I was now ready to hear.

MY MARRIAGE GOES BANKRUPT

Soon after the New Year, at the beginning of 1999, a series of overdraft notices that arrived from our bank seemed to me to symbolize the degree to which my husband and I had failed to create a viable partnership. Our household account had insufficient funds. So did our marriage. When I suggested that I needed my own space for a while and wanted us to consider separate bedrooms during this period, my husband left in a fit of rage. He did not return. Almost overnight I was handed the opportunity—and the responsibility—to assume complete financial dominion over both my business and my household.

Up until the moment my husband left, it had never occurred to me in all my years of marriage that I would ever end up divorced. My fantasy was always that my husband would change or that I would change or that something would change so that the two of us could become the team I thought we were capable of being. For years psychics and astrologers had been telling me we were meant to be together. This couldn't be happening.

And yet despite what seemed to be in the stars, and despite our three years of couples therapy, I had reached the end of the road. I could no longer allow myself to be in what I perceived was an unbalanced relationship. I needed to come into my own. I was no longer willing to be controlled by another person, emotionally, financially, or physically. I had come too far.

Finally I was ready to do the last part of the self-healing that I'd spent half a century preparing for. Menopause had spurred me to make the ideals I'd been promoting in my work a reality. I knew I now had two choices: to mute my voice so that I could stay in my marriage, or to find the courage I needed to take steps toward divorce. But what a hard choice it was.

Perhaps one reason it was so hard was that the 1950s was the period in which my brain had been wired for relationships. If my marriage had broken up in that era, it would have been widely agreed that I had wrecked our relationship with my ambition. Why couldn't I have just put my husband's needs before my own? Why did I insist on being fully supported and fully met in my marriage relationship? Why did I insist on pushing my husband past where he felt comfortable going? I did it because I had no other choice. Something within me, some voice from my very soul, was urging me on, and I had to trust it. Back then, I didn't know anything about the personality disorder known as narcissism. It wasn't on society's radar yet.

Nonetheless, I was frightened of what it would be like to live without my longtime mate. And then one day I remembered something one of my daughters had said to me several months before: that things were so unpleasant in our house, she doubted she would come home for vacations once she had left for college. That gave me courage to move forward.

Healing Through Pain

Even though I could see, in retrospect, that I had started the process of letting go of my marriage several years before, I was still not prepared for the deep sense of loss I felt when it ended. Initially I felt as though one of my limbs were missing. For weeks I awoke before dawn, feeling an acute ache in my throat and in my heart as soon as the realization hit me, once again, that my husband was not next to me in bed.

Once out of the house, I found I could sometimes get along okay for days at a time. Then I'd go somewhere and have to fill out one of those forms that are ubiquitous in our lives, and I'd think about how the day was going to come when I would have to check the box that said "divorced." I dreaded that day.

I remembered how hard it was for my mother after her marriage ended. But hers was a happy marriage, cut short when my father died suddenly on the tennis court at the age of sixty-eight. That had been a terrible blow for her. Still, in the early months of my separation, I remember thinking that my own pain was in some ways even worse, because it made me question the most central fact of my life for the past twenty-four years. Even though I knew that 50 percent of all marriages ended in divorce, I felt like an incredible failure. I was afraid I was becoming the kind of woman I'd always heard no one wants to invite anywhere lest she steal another woman's husband: a woman alone at midlife, unclaimed, unwanted, and dangerous to the status quo.

Loss is a recurrent theme at midlife. Even women who don't go through divorce at this time often face other losses—the death of parents or spouse, estrangement from a child, being let go from a job, changes in physical appearance, or the realization that the reproductive years are over. For a woman who has never borne a child and had always hoped that that was in her future, the end of her fertility can be a terrible loss. But no matter what the circumstances, nearly every woman has to give up *some* dream about what she thought her life would be like.

And when that realization hits, it is very painful. Gradually I allowed myself to feel all my grief and pain, secure in the knowledge that it would not destroy me. I knew that only then could I move forward with my life.

Healing Through Anger

I would be lying to you, and perpetuating a grave disservice to midlife women, if I allowed you to believe that my feelings at this time were solely about grief and loss. There was also another feeling brimming up from my depths, and this emotion saved me from the paralysis that I might otherwise have felt.

It was the emotion of anger that gave me the energy to proceed with the onerous task of dismantling twenty-four years of married life—and building another kind of life. I used the volcanic energy of my anger to guide me toward identifying my needs and then getting them met. Having experienced my husband's departure as an abandonment of me and our daughters, I was determined to do whatever I had to in order to make our lives whole again.

At first I wasn't sure I could do it. My anger was tempered by a liberal dose of fear. But every time I teetered on the brink of despair or terror, some piece of evidence would arrive in the mail that compelled me to see the truth: overdraft notices from the bank, credit card bills, and lawyers' letters were showing up with great regularity. Like it or not, I was on my own, financially and in every other way. I was going to have to give up my sentimental fantasies that our marriage could still be saved. My focus would have to be on ensuring my own and my daughters' well-being.

I also had another source of energy during this hard time. My brother had gone through a divorce himself some years before. He seemed to know instinctively when to call me and what to say to give me encouragement. His clear-sightedness proved to be invaluable to me.

Healing Through Acceptance

I began a daily prayer practice to give me the courage to continue the process of letting go of my marriage and my identity as a married woman. This involved taking a walk every morning and stopping halfway through to look out over the harbor. There I would think about all that I had to be grateful for in my life—which was a lot.

Then I would say a prayer of thanks out loud, sending the words down the river to its source. Each day as I stood there I watched the ice on the river receding, the tides changing. Spring would come soon, I knew, and with it the healing energy of rebirth and renewal. I was grateful for winter and the time it gave me to grieve, grateful for having spring to look forward to.

On the weekend just before our twenty-fourth wedding anniversary, about three months after our separation, I felt especially bereft, my feelings of loss temporarily obliterating all my intellectual and emotional reasons for proceeding with the divorce. A friend of mine had called that morning and told me how sad she felt about our split, since she could feel that there was still so much love between my husband and me. She told me she would spend part of the weekend burning prayer sticks for us in the ashram where she worships.

Monday, the day of our anniversary, I felt filled with longing. I spent the whole day wanting to call my husband. Then, as I was sitting down to dinner with the girls, the doorbell rang. It was the florist, delivering a dozen white roses accompanied by a card that read, "Thanks for almost twenty-four years together. And our two daughters." I wept and said to the girls, "Never doubt that your father and

I have always loved each other." As I review this episode now, years later, I see it for what it was. My husband was providing me with the kind of gesture that I longed for—but it was too little too late. And, as I now know, this is very characteristic of a narcissist. Looking back, I see that I was in love with an illusion. That illusion had me on a treadmill, trying to earn more, be more, and do more—just to prove myself worthy of his love. Of course, I didn't know this at the time.

ARMADILLO MEDICINE:
THE POWER OF VULNERABILITY

During the weeks just after my separation, a newspaper reporter interviewed me for a story she was doing about my work. "I have only one more question," she said at the end. "Has Chris Northrup ever really suffered?"

I was shocked. At that very moment I was feeling the loss of the most significant relationship of my life, and feeling it in every cell of my body. How could she assume my life was easy? But I said nothing. It was too soon to discuss my situation publicly. The wounds were too new, too raw.

Earlier that same month a good friend had said to me, "You're not vulnerable enough, so no one feels drawn to take care of you. I, on the other hand, have had so many health problems that everyone feels drawn to take care of me. I attract 'mothers' wherever I go."

This made me furious. It hadn't felt safe to allow myself to be vulnerable with my husband, or before that with my mother. Somewhere along the line I had lost the ability. Besides, it hadn't been an ability I admired. I'd watched far too many women milk the victim role, playing on the sympathy of others to get their needs met. I had never wanted to be such a woman. But I knew that our culture identified so deeply with victims that it doubted the humanity of those who didn't assume that role. That was really what the newspaper reporter had been saying to me with her question.

For two nights in a row after my conversation with my friend, I sought guidance in a set of animal "medicine cards" that worked something like a tarot pack. Each time I drew, I picked the card known as Armadillo (in the reversed position), whose message is this:

> You may think the only way to win in your present situation is
> to hide or to pretend that you are armor-coated and invincible,

but this is not the way to grow. It is better to open up and find the value and strength of your vulnerability. You will experience something wonderful if you do. Vulnerability is the key to enjoying the gifts of physical life. In allowing yourself to feel, a myriad of expressions are made available. For instance, a true compliment is an admiration flow of energy. If you are afraid of being hurt and are hiding from anything, you will never feel the joy of admiration from others.[8]

This message was right on target for me. And once again I was reminded of how well I had learned from my stoic mother to hide my vulnerability. It was now time to change this pattern, as part of letting go of my past.

At midlife, some women seek new satisfactions in the world beyond that of home and family life. They may need to don some armor. But other women need to let the armor down a bit. That was the case for me. And it's also true for many men, who traditionally spend the years leading up to midlife focused on achieving success in the workplace. The point is that at midlife, more than at any other time, the aspects of your personality that kept you alive and functional for the first half of your life may actually put you at risk in the second half. All of us must find the courage to make the changes that will enable us to live our lives in an empowered fashion.

CELEBRATING THE PAST WHILE CREATING A NEW FUTURE

Our household became much more relaxed once my husband left. The tension was gone. I adopted a couple of kittens from our local animal shelter and found that they brought me and my daughters a great deal of comfort and enjoyment. We had never had pets before, because a dog had always seemed like too much trouble, and my husband was allergic to cats.

Surprisingly, I also found that I was sleeping better than I had in years, waking up easily every morning without the alarm clock. This had never happened before. Looking back now, I can finally appreciate how much energy I had been using in the effort to keep my marriage going.

As the weeks went by, I began the slow process of feeling what it was like to have myself to myself. And on some very deep level I began to feel, ever so gradually, that I was recharging my inner batteries from a source deep within me. As with all grieving and letting go, there were ups and downs to this process. One week, for example, I found myself crying while watching the Thursday night TV shows I used to watch with my husband and daughters as a weekly ritual. But then one week later I was able to spend the evening alone, away from the TV, reveling in the beautiful light on the river outside my home. I was alone, but I was not lonely. I knew I was going to make it. I was happy.

The kind of marriage I had worked well for me for many years, and I am very grateful for having been able to experience all the joys and pleasures of family life with my husband and our two children. Those joys were very real, as I was reminded the day my husband came to claim his share of the paintings that were hanging on our walls. After he removed them, I was left with that awful feeling of loss that newly bare walls give you at such times. To get me past this latest milestone in grief, two friends and I spent an afternoon creating an entire wall of family photos in the dining room—providing concrete and comforting evidence of the good times in my past. A year later I replaced the photos of my husband with those of my daughters and me. Later still, when I remodeled that room, I changed the space yet again. I have learned that letting go is a process, not an event.

I have also learned that part of the process is acknowledging the past value of the relationship you are leaving behind, and doing this not just silently, to yourself, but, when appropriate, to the person who was part of that relationship.

I did this myself five months after our separation, when my husband and I were nearing a settlement. As we were leaving one of our mediation sessions, I asked him to meet with me privately, and then I poured out everything that was in my heart. I apologized for trying to change him. I said how glad I was that neither of us had used an affair to get out of the marriage. I thanked him for the safe haven of the family we had created together, and for the wonderful children who would not have existed without our relationship. I told him I was grateful for the support and structure he had provided for me when I was out blazing new trails in women's health. I also told him that I loved him.

My feelings were so poignant during that outpouring of gratitude that I could easily see why estranged couples might want to keep their anger and resentment alive. (I can also see why women so willingly go back to those who have given very little during the relationship.) Staying angry means they wouldn't have to feel all the pain of what they think they are losing. But I could also see how damaging this could be to their children, themselves, and everyone else involved, and I was glad I had found the courage to express what was in my heart—and then let it go.

I let go of so much that year, including my feelings of failure. Margaret Mead, the renowned anthropologist, once pointed out that in the past, most marriages continued "till death do us part" because after twenty-five years of marriage, one or both members of the couple had died! In other words, at the same age that most of us are going through the changes of menopause, our ancestors were falling ill and dying—or were already dead. "Till death do us part" was much easier to accomplish when lives were shorter. Mead's observation helped me feel less of a failure for being unable to preserve my marriage.

My health remained good throughout the difficult and painful year of my divorce. I allowed my tears to flow freely, my anger to erupt and dissipate. I also called on spiritual guidance unceasingly, and this, together with my new emotional openness, helped me negotiate a period characterized by significant hormonal change with minimal symptoms. If I were advising a woman in my situation today, I would, of course, suggest that she learn all about the empath/narcissist relationship—which is what I was actually going through.

In addition to spiritual and emotional work, I also used a variety of natural approaches to hormonal balance, as I will discuss in chapter 6. As I write this now, more than two decades later, I look back with amusement and compassion on the woman I was then—so frightened about the future and so worried that I had wrecked my children's lives. A woman who didn't know what she was really dealing with: the empath/narcissist dyad. I see now that my divorce actually saved my life and also ushered in a whole new world for me to enjoy with my daughters. In many ways, I feel it also saved their lives—which is what happens when someone has the courage to walk away from domination and control and begin to live life on her own terms.

From the age of fifty onward, I, like so many other women, began re-creating the second half of my life on my own terms. If you are reading this book, there is no doubt that you are embarking on that same adventure. As women do this individually and collectively, we must keep in mind that physical and emotional health is our natural state, even during this time of transition. And although the life ahead of many is uncharted territory, fraught with all the uncertainty that accompanies change, I have now been on the other side for quite a while. And I can guarantee you that this second stage of your existence is set up to be the most liberating and fulfilling time if you heed your inner wisdom and follow its dictates.

Have no regrets, whatever you decide. Take advantage of the clarity of vision that is the gift of menopause, and use that gift to let the second half of your life be truly your own.

2

The Brain Catches Fire
at Menopause

Awoman once told me that when her mother was approaching the age of menopause, her father sat the whole family down and said, "Kids, your mother may be going through some changes now, and I want you to be prepared. Your uncle Ralph told me that when your aunt Carol went through the change, she threw a leg of lamb right out the window!" Although this story fits beautifully into the stereotype of the "crazy" menopausal woman, it should not be overlooked that throwing the leg of lamb out the window was undoubtedly Aunt Carol's outward expression of the process going on within her soul: the reclaiming of self. Perhaps it was her way of saying how tired she was of waiting on her family, of signaling to them that she was past the cook/chauffeur/dishwasher stage of life. For many women, if not most, part of this reclamation process includes getting in touch with anger that arises because of unmet and unacknowledged needs. Anger often triggers blowing up at loved ones for the first time, but the events that evoke anger are never new. What is new is our willingness and newfound energy to let that anger be acknowledged and expressed, both to ourselves and to others. This can be the first step toward much-needed change in our lives . . . change that is often long overdue. With time, we must also learn how to skillfully articulate our needs as the first step to getting them met.

This can happen only when we stop feeling guilty or ashamed for having needs in the first place!

Regardless of where you currently stand in your menstrual or perimenopausal transition, chances are you've inherited a few beliefs about your cycle that boil down to a variation of the following: "The issues that arise premenstrually have nothing to do with my actual life. They are strictly hormonal. My hormones exist in a universe that is completely separate from the rest of my life." I found a superb example of this culturally sanctioned unconsciousness about premenstrual syndrome (PMS) in a popular women's magazine:

> I love PMS! It gives me so much perspective! It makes me cry in the supermarket aisle because they're out of Kalamata olives— a deliberate plot by the Stop & Shop stock boy to sabotage the new recipe I'm dying to try on my one day off! It makes me pick fights with my husband over incredibly important stuff—like the fact that he's forgotten to put out my morning coffee cup alongside his, which is incredibly symbolic of something deeper, don't you think? . . . And then, POOF! My period arrives and I wake up to a world that looks rosy. Gone is the pressure to get a divorce, send my kids to reform school, and move to another country. In fact, compared to how I felt the previous week, I feel pretty good indeed.[1]

The writer goes on to explain that her PMS has only intensified as she has gotten older and that her OB-GYN has suggested that she go back on the pill, or try Prozac before her period. In other words, she needs to get "fixed." But she's ignoring potentially important messages from her body. PMS and the escalation of symptoms that is so common during perimenopause are really our inner guidance system trying to get us to pay attention to the adjustments we need to make in our lives, adjustments that become particularly urgent during perimenopause.

If we don't pay attention to the issues that come up for us every month during the years when our periods are regular, our symptoms will escalate as we get older. Every premenstrual issue that this writer blames on PMS is potentially related to a larger and deeper need that is not being met. The issues she raises may appear superficial or even silly at first glance. But if she were to be completely honest with herself, she would realize that the lack of a specific kind of olives at the grocery store and the fact that her husband doesn't put out her coffee cup in the morning may be doorways to deeper needs that she has been ignoring: the need for more time off, a longing for the sensual satisfaction of cooking, a longing to be cherished daily by her husband. When these needs aren't acknowledged, the body ends up screaming louder and louder to get our attention.

By reducing her body's signals to physical symptoms, the writer has bought into the dualistic belief system that pervades Western medicine. Her attitude—one that is all too common—is that troublesome hormones are a woman's cross to bear, but with a variety of remedies or drugs, and a sense of humor, they can be kept to a low roar, so they're at least tolerable. Instead of seeing an opportunity for insight here, she has diminished and dismissed her inner guidance.

OUR BRAINS CATCH FIRE AT MENOPAUSE

Our brains actually begin to change at perimenopause. Like the rising heat in our bodies, our brains also become fired up! Sparked by the hormonal changes that are typical during the menopausal transition, a switch goes on that signals changes in our temporal lobes, the brain region associated with enhanced intuition. How this ultimately affects us depends to a large degree on how willing we are to make the changes in our lives that our hormones are urging us to make over the ten years or so of perimenopause.

There is ample scientific evidence of the brain changes that begin to take place at perimenopause. Differences in relative levels of estrogen and progesterone affect the temporal lobe and limbic areas of our brains, and we may find ourselves becoming irritable, anxious, emotionally volatile. Though our culture leads us to believe that our mood swings are simply the result of raging hormones and do not have anything to do with our lives, there is solid evidence that repeated episodes of stress (due to relationship, children, and job situations you feel angry about or powerless over, for example) are actually behind many of the hormonal changes in the brain and body. This means that if your life situation—whether at work or with children, your husband, your parents, or whatever—doesn't change, then unresolved emotional stress can exacerbate a perimenopausal hormone imbalance. In a normal premenopausal hormonal state it's much easier to overlook those aspects of your life that don't really work, just as you can overlook them more easily in the first half of your menstrual cycle—the time when you're more apt to feel upbeat and happy and able to shove difficult material under the rug. But that doesn't mean the problems aren't there.

LEARNING TO RECOGNIZE AND HEED OUR WAKE-UP CALLS

Whether you are in early perimenopause at thirty-five or standing at the threshold of menopause, your body's inner wisdom will attempt to catch your attention through four kinds of escalating physical and emotional wake-up calls.

FIGURE 1: THE FIRST TWO WAKE-UP CALLS: PMS AND SAD

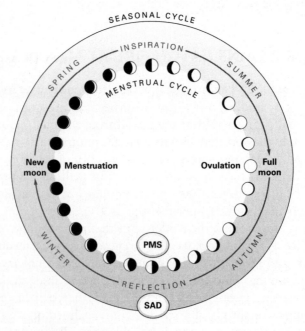

PMS is to the monthly cycle as SAD is to the annual cycle. Both conditions respond to the same treatment while asking us to deepen our connection to our cyclic wisdom.

Our First Wake-Up Call: PMS

What happens if, during our childbearing years, we ignore our cyclic
~~ disconnect from the body's wisdom, and attempt to function
/ were linear beings, with the same drives, the same
e same aptitudes day after day? Very often PMS hap-
; physical and emotional discomfort, PMS is one way a

woman's body elbows her every month to remind her of the growing backlog of unresolved issues accumulating within her. Everything from unbalanced nutrition to unresolved relationships can disrupt the normal hormonal milieu, wreaking physical and emotional havoc during the childbearing years. Ignoring these early, relatively gentle nudges month after month sets her up for sharper and more urgent messages. Inconvenient as they are, these pains are our allies, begging us to look up and see what's not working in our lives. Often we don't, however. Most of us are too busy, and the discomfort isn't that bad, after all. It's easier to just ignore it or medicate it in some way. But the body is insistent!

A Poignant Wake-Up Call: Postpartum Depression

It is well documented that women who have significant PMS are also more apt to suffer from postpartum depression in the first weeks after giving birth. Or sometimes those who suffer from postpartum depression will go on to develop PMS when their menstrual cycles resume. Because new mothers often feel far too vulnerable to complain, postpartum depression is underdiagnosed and undertreated in our culture, even though between 10 and 15 percent of all women experience some form of mood disorder following childbirth, ranging from major depression to anxiety disorders such as panic attacks. As with all illness, there are genetic, environmental, and nutritional factors that are associated with postpartum depression. But it is also true that postpartum depression is often a sign from a mother's inner wisdom that she isn't getting the support and help she needs at this time, and that certain areas of her life, especially her relationships with one or both parents or with her partner, require some attention. If these issues aren't resolved, they are very likely to resurface during the hormonal shifts of perimenopause.

An Annual Wake-Up Call: SAD

If the monthly messages go unheeded, a woman's body may send a louder wake-up call on a yearly basis, in the form of seasonal affective disorder, or SAD. It begins with an intensification of the symptoms of PMS during the autumn and winter of the year, when the days are shortest and darkness dominates. Eventually it can evolv into full-blown depression and despair during the time of year when daylight is abbreviated. It is well known that providing two hours of full-spectrum artificial light in the evening, to trick the body into thinking the days are longer, can reverse the weight gain, depression, carbohydrate craving, social withdrawal, fatigue, and irritability of SAD. (Studies have also shown that light therapy helps depression in pregnancy.)[2] But without continued use of the artificial lights, the symptoms return the following autumn . . . unless the wake-up call is heeded. The link between PMS and SAD is a profound example of how women's wisdom is simultaneously encoded into both our monthly cycles and the annual cycle of the seasons.

Perimenopause: The Mother of All Wake-Up Calls

For many women perimenopause can be, as one of my patients described it, "PMS times ten"—and this is particularly the case for those who, for one reason or another, hit the snooze button instead of heeding their monthly and seasonal wake-up calls. This is not to discount the direct physical effects of changing hormone levels. However, given the effects of stress on hormone levels and blood sugar metabolism, it is clear that any uncomfortable symptoms that reveal themselves during times of hormonal shift will be magnified and prolonged if a woman is carrying a heavy load of emotional baggage. According to a 2010 study from the Netherlands of perimenopausal women, those who felt more negative emotions, specifically anger and sadness, also experienced an increase in pain.[3] The more anger and sadness the women in the study felt, the more physical pain they experienced throughout the day. (The effect was especially strong in women who have fibromyalgia.) These symptoms are the body's wisdom, pleading yet again that unresolved life issues be attended to. Throughout a woman's childbearing years, a kind of "debt account" is established where existing and future issues accumulate, compounding interest with each passing month that the debt goes unpaid.

   Thus the average woman, blessed with approximately 480 menstrual periods and 40 seasonal cycles to bring her to the threshold of _____ gets about 500 progress reports. How is her physical _____ ition? How are her emotions? What's happening in _____ s and her career? Is she scheduling pleasure into her _____ rpose or putting herself last? There have been approximately 500 opportunities to resolve those issues . . . or sweep them under the rug. At perimenopause the process escalates. The earnest, straightforward inner self, which has tried for years to get our attention, makes one final hormonally mediated attempt to get us to deal with our accumulated needs, wants, and desires. This is likely to turn into a period of great emotional turmoil, as each woman struggles to make a new life, one that can accommodate her emerging self. Externally and internally, this period is a mirror image of adolescence, a time when our bodies and brains were also going through major hormonal shifts that gave us the energy to attempt to individuate from our families and become the people we were meant to be. At menopause we pick up where we left off in adolescence. It is now time to finish the job.

It should be no surprise, then, that research has documented that those women who experience uncomfortable—even severe—symptoms of PMS are often the same women who have a tumultuous perimenopause, with physical and emotional symptoms that become increasingly impossible to ignore.[4]

As a woman makes the transition to the second half of her life, she finds herself in a struggle not only with her own aversion to conflict and confrontation, but also with the culture's view of how women "should" be. The body's inner wisdom gets a huge opportunity to break through culturally erected barriers, while shining a light on aspects of a woman's life that need work. To resolve the situation, then, it is up to the individual woman to meet her body's wisdom halfway.

IS IT ME OR IS IT MY HORMONES? DEBUNKING THE MYTH OF RAGING HORMONES

The fluctuating hormone levels that most women experience during perimenopause and during menopause do not, in and of themselves, cause the distressing emotional and psychological symptoms (such as anger and depression) that so many women suffer with PMS and at midlife. But if there is an underlying susceptibility to distress in the first place, there is no doubt that hormonal swings will help bring that distress to the surface.

Though hormone levels and mood do tend to fluctuate widely during our reproductive years, and even more widely still during oⁱ perimenopausal years, research has failed to show any appreciable differences between the hormone levels of those women who suffer from PMS-like symptoms and those who don't. What has been well documented, however, is that the *brains* of women who suffer the most from PMS-like symptoms are more susceptible to the effects of fluctuating hormone levels.[5] In other words, it is not the hormone levels per se that are the problem. Rather, it is the particular combination of a woman's hormone levels and her preexisting brain chemistry along with her life situation that results in her symptoms. It is estimated that 27 percent of all women who experience agitation and depression during their periods, and 36 percent of all women who become depressed premenstrually, will be very sensitive to the hormonal changes that occur at menopause.[6]

Though we tend to blame perimenopausal symptoms on hormonal shifts in the body, their origins are far more complex. Several women in my practice, for example, have experienced symptoms such as hot flashes and mood swings in their later forties—despite having been on full hormone replacement for over twenty years because they had undergone hysterectomies and removal of their ovaries while still in their twenties. Clearly, changes in reproductive hormones alone do not account for these symptoms. They are signals from our mind and body that we have reached a new developmental stage—an opportunity for healing and growth.

ANATOMY OF MENOPAUSAL WISDOM

Menopause combines the wisdom of the prior stages and brings it to a new level.

Body Process	Encoded Wisdom
MENSTRUAL CYCLE	Cyclic intuitive wisdom and emotional recycling and processing
PREGNANCY/ FERTILITY	Capacity to conceive an idea or a life with another, hold it, nurture it, and allow it to be born
	Passage into the wisdom years Capacity to be open to constant intuitive knowing Reseeding the community

Moving Inward

Until midlife, it is characteristic for a woman's energies to be focused on caring for others. She is encouraged to do so, in part, by the hormones that drive her menstrual cycles—the hormones that foster her instincts for nurturing, her devotion to cohesion and harmony within her world. But for two or three days each month, just before or during our periods, there is a hormonal interlude when the veil between our conscious and unconscious selves is thinner and the voice of our souls beckons to us, subtly reminding us of our own passions, our own needs, which cannot and should not always be subsumed to the needs of those we love.

This fluctuation between inner and outer worlds and the way it is influenced by our hormones was revealed in a fascinating study done in the 1930s by a psychoanalyst and a physician. Therese Benedek, M.D., studied the psychotherapy records of patients, while Boris Rubenstein, M.D., studied the ovarian hormonal cycles of the same women. By looking only at a woman's emotional state, Dr. Benedek was able to identify where she was in her menstrual cycle with incredible accuracy. The two doctors found that just before ovulation, when estrogen levels were at their highest, women's emotions and behavior were directed toward the outer world. At ovulation, women were more relaxed and content and quite receptive to being cared for and loved by others. During the postovulatory and premenstrual phase, when progesterone is at its highest (and PMS symptoms are also at their peak), women were more likely to be focused on themselves and more involved in inward-directed activity.[7]

I like to think of the first half of our cycles as the time when we are both biologically and psychologically preparing to give birth to someone or something outside of ourselves. In the second half of our cycles, we prepare to give birth to nothing less than ourselves. It is at this time that the more intuitive parts of our brain become activated, giving us feedback and guidance about the state of our inner lives. One of my e-news subscribers, Lucinda, describes the process eloquently.

LUCINDA: Healing PMS

PMS has been an issue for me that has severely limited my life, dis torted my children's experience of their mother, and made my h band's life with me very scary. He insisted for years that an must take over my body when my hormones fluctuated in preparation for my menstrual cycle! Migraines were part of this pattern, too. I insisted that it was the "true ugly me" that surfaced at a weakened time! One minute I would be rational and peacefully attending to my life tasks, the next I would be argumentative until war broke out!

Then I would cry and feel like the worst person on the planet. This didn't happen every month, but when it did it was on schedule, around the seventeenth day of my cycle. The consequence of this pattern was that I feared I was crazy, and I could not count on myself for normal planning of life events, making me an unreliable family member. While I longed for intimacy, I was too scary a person to approach. I was caught in the busy schedule of a working wife and mother and couldn't figure out this problem in my life. I limped along, trying to appear normal to the outside world but becoming more and more exhausted.

As the years passed I was introduced to new theories about the mind-body connection and information about the benefits of physically releasing emotional distress, past as well as present, through crying, yawning, sweating, shaking, and so on. These things remained a concept for a long time. I knew the information in my head, but I had not assimilated it into my being for use. I was still fighting the monthly disability of PMS and internally asking why—why did I, who was creative, intelligent, and loving, have this condition that was ruining my life?

Insight came one day as I was getting a migraine and knew what would follow. I consciously asked myself what would happen if, instead of fighting the feeling and judging myself as a defective person, I instead allowed myself to fully feel what was happening in my body. I surrendered my control and focused on just being present with my body for the first time ever.

I felt vulnerable. The shift in my hormones left me feeling vulnerable. That was not a state of being I could tolerate. I was a warrior, not a maiden. I cried, acknowledging my defenselessness. I experienced my feminine side for the first time. In fear, I had raged against it in the past. No wonder I felt like a victim. I was battering my own feminine side—my internal goddess.

with the feeling. I didn't die. I needed her softness and raine faded. I eased up on my self-judgment and rt of myself long hidden—even from my own view. symptoms that had accompanied my PMS lessened. creased energy to do some other things for myself. I nutritionist and slowly am improving my diet. I use a good massage therapist. I continue to feel and release my past and present feelings. I have fun at whatever I am doing because I see it as important, as my own creative expression. I talk before crisis occurs.

I have continued to be challenged by my body's response to my poor choices. I am grateful for its ability to do so, and now when I wonder, it is more a question of what than of why: what am I doing that denies my feminine inner wisdom and goes against my true spiritual identity?

As I sit present with that question, the answer bubbles up from within. We do come with an instruction kit, if we will just quiet ourselves to receive the information and learn some new skills.

Moving from an Alternating to a Direct Current of Wisdom

At midlife, the hormonal milieu that was present for only a few days each month during most of your reproductive years, the milieu that was designed to spur you on to reexamine and redirect your life just a little at a time, now gets stuck in the on position for weeks or months at a time. We go from an alternating current of inner wisdom to a direct current that remains on all the time after menopause is complete. During perimenopause, our brains gradually make the change from one way of being to the other.

Biologically, at this stage of life you are programmed to withdraw from the outside world for a period of time and revisit your past. You need to be free of the distractions that come when you are focusing your mothering efforts solely on others. Perimenopause is a time when you are meant to mother yourself.

It may be no accident that the word *menopause* invites the association "pause from men." We don't really need to withdraw from men per se. We need, rather, to put our focus on ourselves instead of spending so much time and effort pleasing them—or pleasing the more *yang* member of a partnership, regardless of gender, such as a female boss or even your mother. In truth, you are being urged, biologically, to pause from everyone—from humankind in general—in order to do important work on yourself. As a result of this, one of the most common threads running through women's descriptions of how they feel during the menopausal transition is the longing for time alone, for a refuge that provides peace, quiet, and freedom from distractions and demands.

It's a wistful dream, seemingly out of reach in this bus·

of multidirectional tugs-of-war. But those who have the yearning know deep within that their uncomfortable menopausal symptoms would simply dissolve if only they had the luxury of shutting out the world so they could tune in to the growth process occurring within

FIGURE 2: CURRENTS OF WISDOM

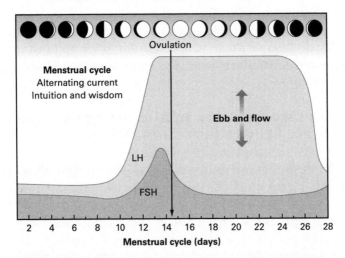

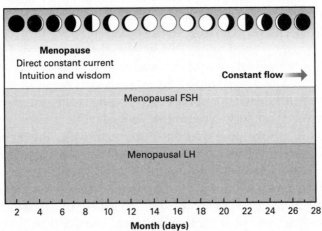

¬d LH stimulate ovulation and are released cyclically each
the years before menopause. They then undergo a
which ovulation gradually ceases and FSH and LH
increase. I believe that these high levels have to do
om "AC current" to "DC current." The intuitive wis-
nce available most clearly during only certain parts of
cycle is now potentially available all the time.

themselves. This wistful dream is real. It comes from your soul. You can trust it and believe in it—and to remain healthy, you must do its bidding.

Even if this dream seems out of reach, the simple truth is that every woman *can* find refuge within her existing environment. Even if you can't charter a plane to a deserted island, odds are that if you acknowledge and validate your need for solitude, then you can clear some time and find a private corner to retreat to daily. You can insulate yourself from noise, telephones, the internet, and interaction with others. I encourage every woman to find a way to do this on whatever level is possible, even just for fifteen minutes a day. When we commit to taking this first step, we have the chance to develop a newfound sense of ourselves and our life's purpose, which gives us an exhilarating sense of what is possible for us during the second half of our lives.

THE MULTIPLE ROLES OF YOUR "REPRODUCTIVE" HORMONES

It has long been known that our female hormones are not involved solely with reproduction. They are connected with our moods and with the way our brains work. Boys and girls have the same rate of depression up until puberty. After that, when ovarian hormones surge and cycling begins, depression increases in females, with the highest incidence reached between ages twenty-two and forty-five. The lifetime incidence of depression in males is only one in ten, while in females it is one in four. After menopause, the rates of depression in men and women reach gender parity once again. Cross-cultural studies have shown that women have a higher lifetime incidence of depression in other societies as well.

I believe that this gender-wide susceptibility to depression is in part related to the subservient roles that most women (or those in the more feminine role) in most cultures have been forced to play for millennia. That said, it is also true that the menstrual cycle, pregnancy, the postpartum period, and the perimenopausal period are all associated with depression in many women. And those who are susceptible to PMS are also the most susceptible to postpartum depression and perimenopausal mood problems. Part of the reason for this has to do with the complex interaction between the hypothalamus, the pituitary gland, the ovaries, and the multiple hormones that are produced in and interact within these key areas. These key hormones are:

~ *GnRH* (gonadotropin-releasing hormone), which is produced in the hypothalamus

~ *FSH* (follicle-stimulating hormone) and *LH* (luteinizing hormone), which are produced in the pituitary and stimulate, in turn, the rise of estrogen and progesterone during the monthly menstrual cycle

~ *Estrogen,* produced in the ovaries, body fat, and other areas

~ *Progesterone,* which is produced primarily in the ovaries and together with estrogen, prepares the lining of the uterus for implantation and growth of an embryo

~ *Testosterone,* which we tend to think of as a male hormone, although it plays a vital role for women as well, though at much lower levels. DHEA, the precursor for testosterone, is made in the adrenal glands and then converted into testosterone in concert with the ovaries. There is a distinct testosterone surge at ovulation, which heightens sex drive.

The hypothalamus regulates the production of all of these hormones and is in turn regulated by them—and by many others. It has receptors on it not only for progesterone, estrogen, and androgens (e.g., DHEA, testosterone), but also for norepinephrine, dopamine, and serotonin, neurotransmitters that regulate mood and that are affected in turn by our thoughts, beliefs, diet, and environment.

If estrogen, progesterone, and androgens had no other role in the body besides driving reproduction, your levels of these hormones would drop to zero after menopause. But they don't. Similarly, if GnRH, FSH, and LH suddenly were without purpose after menopause, one might expect that there would cease to be any of these hormones circulating in your system after that time. In fact, quite the contrary is true.

During perimenopause, GnRH levels begin to rise in the brain, causing FSH and LH to surge to their highest levels ever. A popular explanation is that this is the body's attempt to "kick-start" the ovaries into resuming their original function, which might make sense if it weren't for one eloquent fact: those elevated FSH and LH levels *stay* elevated, permanently, well after it is physiologically obvious that the ovaries (which are, essentially, out of eggs) have no intention of jumping back onto the reproductive bandwagon. It would seem that your body, in its wisdom, has ulterior motives for continuing to produce the so-called reproductive hormones, and reproduction no longer is the point. In fact, evidence is mounting that at least one of the roles for this off-the-charts production of FSH and LH, and of the GnRH that precipitates this rise, is to drive the changes taking place in the midlife woman's brain.

For biological reasons, females of the human species are often easier to control—intellectually, psychologically, and socially—during their childbearing years than they are before puberty (from birth to age eleven) or after menopause. Interestingly, hormone levels after menopause are identical to those in girls before puberty. When we are creating a home and building a family (whether biologically or otherwise), our primary concern is to maintain balance and peace. We seem to know instinctively that when we're raising a family, it's better for all if we compromise and maintain whatever support we have, even if it's less than ideal, rather than risk going it alone. Though this may mean we lose sight of our individual goals, our ability to "go along with the program" is in fact protective. A medical study done in Sweden, for example, demonstrated that single mothers had an almost 70 percent higher risk of premature death than did mothers with partners. And, surprisingly, this increase in the rate of premature death was the same regardless of socioeconomic or health factors. In other words, even single mothers with adequate economic resources who were physically and psychologically healthy were at greater risk.[8] This needn't be the case, of course. Many single mothers have created thriving support systems, so it's important to take this and all such studies with a grain of salt. One always has the capacity to be an outlier, statistically speaking.

This process of sublimating our truest selves begins early, in adolescence. The "activist" mindset of the prepubescent girl, her child-like forthrightness and honesty, and her tendency to jump in when there is conflict all become hormonally sublimated—aided and abetted by a patriarchal culture. Though an adolescent girl may be concerned with social injustice, she is likely to be even more preoccupied with her body image and attractiveness to potential mates (of whichever gender she prefers). Put another way, while a woman is being biologically primed for childbearing, child-rearing, and nurturing of others—all vital and species-enhancing roles—the conflicts in the world at large become somewhat blurred to her. Her concern with personal injustices and childhood traumas may also fade or be suppressed. She is likely to give minor offenses no more than cursory attention, for to lick her own wounds, analyze old hurts, or confront long-standing abuses would demand precious energy. She needs to fulfill her primary role, which, biologically speaking, is to reproduce and nurture.

FIGURE 3: THE HYPOTHALAMUS-PITUITARY-OVARY CONNECTION

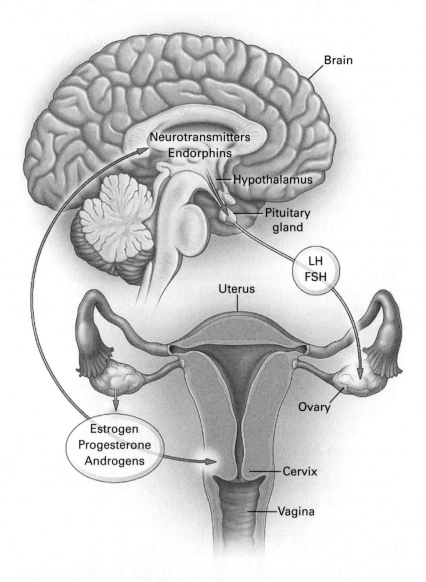

The brain and the reproductive organs are intimately connected by a complex series of feedback loops.

She is rewarded handsomely for complying with this biological agenda. Reproductive hormones are directly responsible for stimulating opioid centers in the brain. These areas actually produce narcotic-like chemicals that swirl into the bloodstream and provide a feel-good sensation, a natural high. Estrogen, for example, is richly provided during the high-fertility phase of the menstrual cycle, when a woman is most "electric" to men and most receptive to their advances. Hormones such as prolactin and oxytocin also flood the system while she is in mothering mode, breast-feeding her baby or nurturing her loved ones. Those strong feelings of attraction, that deep sense of satisfaction, that mantle of loving warmth and purpose that a woman feels when nurturing—all are due in part to natural, narcotic-like chemicals produced by the brain in response to reproductive hormones. Since it feels wonderful, she is encouraged to continue. This is one of the reasons why women are extraordinary caretakers. Conversely, the stress hormones epinephrine and cortisol can, over time, lower levels of oxytocin and prolactin—which is one of the reasons why mothers who have undergone the stress of losing a child can end up divorced. Their bonding circuits can get so caught up in grief and loss that there's not enough left over to maintain their primary relationship, unless both members have the resilience to know this and work through it together.

FIGURE 4: REWARD ACROSS THE LIFE CYCLE

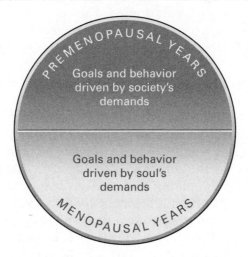

Women who are lesbians or transgender are not exempted from this built-in incentive system, because it is stamped into their circuits within the first few days of life as a female embryo. I am unclear about what happens with a transgender individual, and I'm also very aware that gender is, in part, a social construction. That said, whether the nurturing behavior is related to pregnancy and child-rearing or to other forms of caregiving, the biological feedback is unavoidable, powerful, and very, very positive. Research has clearly shown that when women are under stress—especially as a group—we produce the bonding hormone oxytocin, which promotes sup-porting others. UCLA professor of psychology Shelley Taylor, Ph.D., author of *The Tending Instinct* (Times Books, 2002), calls this the "tend-and-befriend" response to stress, versus the more male "fight-or-flight" response.[9]

How Menopausal Hormonal Changes Facilitate Your Brain Rewiring

As a woman enters menopause, she steps out of the primarily child-bearing, caretaking role that was hormonally scripted for her. This is not to say that the postmenopausal woman is no longer an effective nurturer. Rather, she becomes freer to choose where she will direct her creative energies, freer to "color outside the lines." Many of the issues that had become blurry to her when the hormones of puberty kicked in may suddenly resurface with vivid clarity as those hor-mones recede. This is why so many midlife women recall and decide to confront and resolve past abuses. The concern with social injus-tices, the political interests, and the personal passions that were sub-limated in the childbearing years now surface in sharp focus, ready to be examined and acted upon. Some women funnel this heightened energy into new businesses and new careers. Some discover and cul-tivate artistic talents they never knew they had. Some women note a surge in their sexual desire, to heights never before experienced in their lives. Some report changes in sexual preference. However they channel it, there's a wonderful sense of living from the inside out!

Tererai Trent is the author of *The Awakened Woman: A Guide for Remembering & Igniting Your Sacred Dreams* (Simon & Schus-ter, 2017). I met Tererai in Phoenix a couple of years ago when we both presented at an international women's conference there. Her story of growing up poor in a village in Rhodesia (now known as Zimbabwe), having her first child at the age of fourteen, and eventually—against massive odds—fulfilling her dream of getting a Ph.D. in the United States moved me deeply. Tererai is a magnificent woman who is full of joy and goodwill—the very embodiment of midlife wisdom. In her book, she writes of the "Great Hunger," which is a powerful way to describe what happens to many during the menopausal transition. This Great Hunger has a voice so powerful that those who try to silence it do so at their peril. If we don't understand it, this energy can very easily be turned inward and fuel sickness or depression.

In her book, Tererai writes, "The Great Hunger—the greatest of all pangs—is the hunger for a life of meaning. The Great Hunger is liberating and energizing; it enables us to move beyond immediate gratification and toward fulfillment. The Great Hunger inspires us, leading us to discover new ways to grow, give, and help others. If you tap into the Great Hunger, you will awaken your sacred dream. With the awakened consciousness of a sacred dreamer, you will come to know yourself as part of the larger circle of women, the sacred sisterhood. Your whole life will be a ritual in the service of this great purpose, this togetherness."[10]

EMBRACING THE MESSAGE BEHIND OUR MENOPAUSAL ANGER

The GnRH pulses associated with menopause prime the brain for new perceptions—and, subsequently, for new behavior. It is very common for women to become more irritable, even downright angry, about things that were more easily overlooked before. Long before we begin to feel hot flashes from changing hormonal levels, our brains undergo changes in the hypothalamus, the place where GnRH is produced. This same brain region is key for experiencing, and ultimately expressing, emotions such as anger.[11] It is well known that hormones modulate both aggression and anger. Our midlife bodies and brains fully support our ability to experience and express anger with a clarity not possible prior to midlife.

GnRH is just one of several hormones that supports the changes occurring in the brain. Estrogen and progesterone molecules bind themselves to areas such as the amygdala and hippocampus, which are important for memory, hunger, sexual desire, and anger. Changing levels of these and other hormones may well help to bring up old memories, accompanied by strong emotions, especially anger. This is not to say that anger is caused by hormonal change. Rather, it means that the hormonal changes simply facilitate remembering and clearing up unfinished business.

Many women are disturbed or frightened when they feel this anger arising. Maybe you don't feel angry. Maybe you're "just" irritable, grouchy, aggravated, envious, overwhelmed, or depressed, or you "just" have high cholesterol or high blood pressure. Believe me, all these emotions and physical conditions are associated with the same thing: anger. Anger in women has a bad rap in general unless that anger arises in the service of others. This probably accounts for the fact that although anger has been studied exhaustively in men, the gender in which it is acceptable, the only kind of female anger that has received a great deal of study is maternal anger, the function of which is to protect a child who is threatened. It is also culturally acceptable for women to express their personal anger by fighting for social justice, which too often becomes a platform for releasing personal anger. Though we're socialized to believe that our anger arises from observing the injustice done to others, the political is always personal: our anger is ultimately about ourselves, and its energy is always urging us toward self-actualization.

That doesn't mean we should abandon social protest, reform, and a quest for justice if we feel passionately about these areas. It simply means that we must be mindful of our personal motivation for participating in these arenas, not allowing them to distract us from self-transformation and self-healing—processes that always render us even more effective as agents for social change.

We need to claim our anger. Especially during midlife, it can play an important role in improving the quality of our lives and our health. It is a powerful signal from our inner wisdom—one we should learn to listen to and act on. Anger always arises from a genuine need that isn't being met. In fact, in his groundbreaking work on nonviolent communication, the late Marshall Rosenberg, Ph.D., who established the Center for Nonviolent Communication, pointed out that all human behavior is an attempt to get a need met. (I recommend that you go to the center's website, www.cnvc.org, for an extensive inventory of needs, which include food, safety, touch, and love. The site also contains an inventory of emotions that signal those unmet needs.)

Here are some situations from which anger arises, and the messages behind the anger:

~ Being unable to count on promises or commitments made to us (need for reassurance, honesty, and integrity in relationships)

~ Losing power, status, or respect (need for respect or recognition)

~ Being insulted, undermined, or diminished (need for respect or recognition)

~ Being threatened with physical or emotional pain (need for comfort, safety, intimacy, or healing touch)

~ Having an important or pleasurable event postponed or canceled to suit someone else's convenience (need for support, integrity, fun, joy, pleasure, or grieving)

~ Not obtaining something we feel should legitimately be ours (need for fairness or recognition)[12]

If, before menopause, a woman hasn't learned to identify her anger and the needs that it signifies (and this describes many women), perimenopause is her best remaining opportunity to do so. At perimenopause, the rewiring of her brain makes her vision clearer and her motivations easier to identify. Using anger as a catalyst for positive change and growth is always liberating.

In the early stages of perimenopause, the irritability you feel may be subtle. Irritability is a low-voltage form of anger that doesn't usually lead to lasting change—or any change. Irritability is like keeping a pot on simmer but always adding more water or turning down the heat just before it boils. If we do not attend to the unmet needs that lead to irritation, nature will turn up the flame on the burner in an attempt to mobilize us.

GLADYS: *Never Bringing the Pot to a Boil*

Gladys was a poster child for menopausal irritability. In my office she complained often about her husband, her children, and her job. She had chronic sinusitis, a condition often linked to emotional irritability, anger, and sadness just beneath the surface. Whenever I asked Gladys when she was going to take steps to actually change the aspects of her life that so constantly irritated her, she'd always recover herself immediately, give me a big smile, and say, "But, dear, my husband is really a wonderful man. And my children are really very loving. I really can't complain about any parts of my life." Gladys went to her internist and was put on Prozac, but she never felt as though it, or anything else, ever really helped her. Over the years I cared for her, Gladys's health never improved. Gladys's situation is very, very common.

Killing the Messenger: Medicating Our Anger and Irritability to Maintain the Status Quo

In our culture, unfortunately, the usual approach to perimenopausal symptoms such as mood changes and irritability is to prescribe something to soothe us and make us feel better. We seldom ask ourselves—and certainly our doctors rarely ask—"What is out of balance that needs to be changed?" If we look to hormone replacement therapy for relief without addressing the underlying issues, then even appropriate doses of hormones may not help much.

The women who are most vulnerable to the effects of hormonal swings and have the most difficulty finding relief from hormone replacement regimens and other medication are those who have had problems with mood during menarche, postpartum, and during perimenopause.[13] If the emotional issues in their lives are not attended to, if their midlife losses are not fully grieved and released (if, in other words, they don't listen to the need fueling their anger and take action), they may end up with full-blown depression—which is sometimes described as anger turned inward. Depression, in turn, is a very well-documented independent risk factor for heart disease, cancer, and osteoporosis.

Emotional turmoil affects the brain and all its functions. Continuing in the same upsetting situation virtually guarantees that a woman's hormones will stay unbalanced. The longer she allows negative situations to persist, the more out of whack her hormones will become, and the more physically uncomfortable she will feel. A prescription for estrogen may stop this cycle temporarily, but the body will eventually demand that its message be heard.

DORIS: Bypassing Anger

Many women downplay their pain by comparing themselves to someone else who is much worse off. If unresolved, this pattern can be a setup for health problems, especially at midlife. Here's an example from my practice.

Doris was suffering from high blood pressure and slightly elevated cholesterol, both of which were getting worse as she approached the end of her menopausal transition at age fifty-two. Doris told me that her socialite mother had devoted herself to her husband and his career in an unbalanced way that led to rather significant emotional neglect of her children, who were cared for by nannies and household help. Doris had unwittingly created the same pattern with her husband, who was so caught up in his work that he simply wasn't available to her emotionally. But she would not permit herself to state her needs for emotional support to either her husband or her mother. Doris, like so many women whose lives appear relatively privileged, said to me, "I feel so selfish and foolish for feeling sorry for myself. I really have nothing to complain about. After all, there are all these women who've been raped or been victimized by incest, or whose husbands have left them penniless at midlife. I have so much to be grateful for."

I call Doris's approach the intellectual bypass—intellectual because the logical part of our brains can always come up with good reasons why we have nothing to complain about. And on the surface this may well be true. However, there's a deeper problem. Comparing our pain to that of someone else invariably takes us away from our own emotions and the messages from our souls that are crying to be heard and acted upon. Attending to our emotions is a crucial part of remaining healthy because the part of the brain that allows us to feel emotions has far richer and more complex connections with our internal organs, such as the heart and cardiovascular system, than does the area associated with logical, rational thought.[14] Comparisons keep us stuck in our intellect and out of touch with our bodies. It's not enough to simply think about our feelings or talk about them. Remember, the word *emotion* contains the word *motion* within it! Our feelings are meant to move us toward greater fulfillment.

Healing doesn't take place until we surrender to our feelings and allow them to wash over us. Doris won't be able to create full cardiovascular health until she allows herself to feel how painful it is to have a husband who is emotionally unavailable to her, a situation that mirrors so many aspects of her childhood. When she finally surrenders to the grief and rage that have been bottled up for years, first during her childhood and again during her marriage, she will be on her way to creating not only cardiovascular health, but the gift of a healed life as well. She will find that hiding behind her grief and rage are desires, legitimate needs, and dreams that have been patiently waiting for years to find expression.

EMOTIONS, HORMONES, AND YOUR HEALTH

Your emotions, desires, and dreams are your inner guidance system. They alone will let you know whether you are living in an environment of biochemical health or in an environment of biochemical distress. Understanding how your thoughts and your emotions affect every single hormone and cell in your body, and knowing how to change them in a way that is health-enhancing, gives you access to the most powerful and empowering health-creating secret on earth.

Natural foods, supplements, herbs, meditation, acupuncture, and so on are all powerful tools for building and protecting your health. But regardless of what supplements you take and what kind of exercise you do, when all is said and done it is your attitude, your beliefs, and your daily thought patterns that have the most profound effect on your health. How many times have you heard someone say, "I don't understand it—she always ate right and exercised. How come she, of all people, got sick?" On the other end of the spectrum is the person who smokes cigarettes and drinks too much alcohol, yet lives without any apparent illness well into healthy old age. The answer lies at least in part in the individual's attitudes and emotions. You have, within you, the power to create a life of joy, abundance, and health, or you have the same ability to create a life filled with stress, fatigue, and disease. With very few exceptions, the choice is yours.

Specific Emotional Patterns Are Associated with Specific Illnesses in Specific Parts of the Body

It has now been scientifically documented that specific patterns of emotional vulnerability can adversely affect specific organs or systems of the body. Conversely, emotional resilience in these same areas shores up health.

Dozens of medical studies on breast cancer alone show that feelings of powerlessness in important relationships and an inability to express the full range of emotions raise the risk of developing breast cancer and lower survival rates from it. Similarly, dozens of studies have suggested that difficulties in handling negative emotions, especially hostility and resentment, are linked to sudden death from heart attack.[15] Beyond these are literally hundreds of studies showing that lack of social support, loss of or separation from one's family, or difficulties balancing a feeling of belonging with a sense of independence can affect the immune system and increase susceptibility to infection and autoimmune diseases.

Clinical practitioners have known for hundreds of years that the connection between emotions and states of health is direct and powerful. Amazingly, our outward-focused, cause-and-effect, data-driven culture simply ignored the evidence. Even as late as the 1970s, the pioneering work of scientists such as Walter B. Cannon and Hans Selye, who did groundbreaking research on stress and the mind-body connection, was not accepted in the mainstream. It was scientifically accurate and compelling, but our culture simply wasn't ready for it.

We midlife women *are* ready, and we have the perfect opportunity right now to live this knowledge for ourselves, while also sparking the fire of change in the culture at large. We needn't wait for the medical profession or culture to change. In fact, we ourselves are in the perfect position to change it!

Our state of health and happiness depends more upon our perception of life events around us than upon the events themselves. This is a truth that our culture does not teach. Instead, we are taught from an early age that our health is largely the result of our genetic heritage, whether or not we've been vaccinated, how many supplements we take, and how much exercise we get. There is no doubt that these factors can contribute to our state of health. But their influence pales in comparison to the power of our beliefs and attitudes.

How Your Thoughts and Perceptions Become Biochemical Realities in Your Body

Your autonomic nervous system is the system that helps transform your thoughts and emotions into the physical environment that, over time, becomes your actual physical body. This part of the nervous system, which also governs the day-to-day activity of all your internal organs, is divided into two parts: the *parasympathetic* nervous system and the *sympathetic* nervous system. These two systems innervate every organ of your body, including your eyes, tear ducts, salivary glands, blood vessels, sweat glands, heart, larynx, trachea, bronchi, lungs, stomach, adrenals, kidneys, pancreas, intestines, bladder, and external genitalia.

In general terms, the parasympathetic nervous system (PNS) is the brake in your body. It promotes functions associated with growth and restoration, rest and relaxation, and deals primarily with conservation of bodily energy by causing your vital organs to "rest" when they are not "on duty." It has been called the "rest and digest" system.

In contrast to the PNS, the sympathetic nervous system (SNS) is the gas. It revs up your metabolism to deal with challenges from outside the body. Stimulation of the SNS quickly mobilizes your body's reserves so that you can protect and defend yourself. This is where the fabled fight-or-flight mechanism kicks in and your stress hormone levels (cortisol and adrenaline) skyrocket: your pupils dilate, the rate and force of your heart's contractions increase, and your blood vessels constrict, so your blood pressure rises. Blood is borrowed from the intestinal reservoir and shunted to your major muscles, lungs, heart, and brain, preparing you for battle. Bowel and bladder functions shut down temporarily, conserving energy needed to power your muscles, whether you choose to stay and fight or run away. (This is the exact opposite of the PNS's function, which is to constrict the pupils, slow the heart, make the bowels move, and relax the bladder and rectal sphincters.)

Since the parasympathetic nervous system deals primarily with restoration and conservation of bodily energy and the resting of vital organs, any activity or thought pattern that engages the PNS puts deposits into your health bank. Conversely, SNS action makes withdrawals from that bank.

It is at this point that perception becomes so important. What is experienced in the body as a challenge from outside—a stressor—will vary from person to person, influenced by each individual's past history, childhood, family background, learned beliefs, diet, job, and activities at the moment. Many midlife women live in a state of constant anxiety overload, much of which is a side effect of the culture around us and the beliefs we have about ourselves and our worth. We want to be good women. We want to do what is right. But the culture around us is changing so fast, and the information overload that it generates is so huge, that we easily become overwhelmed and confused, dancing faster and faster just to keep up. Not knowing what to choose and what to avoid, we give our bodies mixed signals. We may step on the gas and the brake at the same time. Or we may let the gas get stuck in the on position, living in a constant state of fight-or-flight—and making far too many withdrawals from the health bank.

Biologically speaking, we may be undergoing an evolutionary process that will enable our species to handle all this stress more gracefully and healthfully. Frankly, I believe that the multimodal brain of the midlife woman is leading the way. We've always had to be able to do at least three tasks at once. And now, at midlife and beyond, when the dictates of our souls make themselves known more fully than ever, we wake up to discover that our brains and bodies are being retooled to facilitate this beautifully.

Stress and Your Temperament

Scientific studies have found a link between temperament, personality, and the ability to deal with stressors. Have you noticed that some people, regardless of what happens to them in their lives, seem to be happy, while some are down even when life seems to be on the upswing? Or that others are anxious or fearful even when they're safe and secure? To a degree, we are born with one of these temperaments, and there is evidence of measurable *biological* differences that go along with each temperament. For example, Stephen Porges, M.D., has found that each individual has—from birth—his/her own characteristic balance between the PNS and SNS, resulting in what is known as "vagal tone."[16] Your individual balance is visible on a type of EKG (electrocardiogram) and illustrates how your heart rate coordinates with your breathing rate, yielding valuable information about your metabolic balance and inherent resilience to stress. Porges has found that, even in premature babies, those who have higher vagal tone, meaning that their parasympathetic nervous system is more activated, are less stressed by external events in the nursery (such as being handled and having IVs started) than are babies with low vagal tone. He has also observed that the personality characteristics that go along with high vagal tone are happiness, resilience, and trustingness, while those associated with low tone are melancholy, anxiety, fearfulness, and feeling down—tendencies that follow each individual throughout life. These differences are also reflected in genetic differences in the body's ability to metabolize adrenaline!

This explains much about our individual responses to life situations. For instance, it has been clearly shown that one patient may feel great stress while undergoing a relatively simple medical procedure, while a much more difficult procedure might cause little stress in another patient. However, it is also true that the same person may respond minimally to an experience at one time and then have a massive physiological response to the same experience at another time. This is why attempts to rate stressors are not very useful. A study by Charles B. Nemeroff, M.D., Ph.D., at Emory University School of Medicine found that women who were sexually or physically abused in childhood, compared to those without this history, show very exaggerated physiological responses in later life to stresses such as giving a speech or solving arithmetic problems in front of others. They are also at greater risk for depression, anxiety disorders, and other emotional illnesses later in life.[17] Given the large number of women with a history of abuse of some kind, it is not surprising that so many women have mood and other problems during perimenopause.

One of the worst things people can do is beat themselves up for their inherent temperament or pattern of response to stress. That's why I don't want to suggest that there is some gold standard for emotions. This would be no different from telling women they should strive for an ideal weight, height, dress size, and so on. Besides, each temperament appears to predispose people to certain types of genius. If you spent your life wishing you had a "healthier" kind of temperament, for example, you would not be embracing your full genius or taking full advantage of your natural gifts.

How Menopausal Emotions Affect Our Health

Imbalances between the sympathetic and parasympathetic nervous systems, combined with the changing hormonal milieu of menopause, can increase our body's susceptibility to symptoms or disease. The thymus (which creates your immune system's T cells), the lymph nodes (which create your immune system's B cells), and the bone marrow (which creates your red and white blood cells) are all innervated by the autonomic nervous system. Therefore, each area that creates immune system cells has both a gas pedal (sympathetic tone) and a brake pedal (parasympathetic tone).

Why is this important? Because it is via this system that your body records and processes your emotions and the hormones and neurochemicals they promote. As I've noted, if you have a backlog of unprocessed emotions from past trauma or unmet needs, they are going to surface around the time of menopause. As a result, your susceptibility to illness may increase. Over time, if the fear-driven fight-or-flight response is triggered again and again, you may fall victim to diabetes, hypertension, or possibly even an autoimmune disease such as lupus or rheumatoid arthritis. Where you are affected will be determined by the weakest link in your body, the place where your genetic structure plus your childhood programming and beliefs have made you most vulnerable.

The bottom line is that whatever goes on in your mind has well-documented effects on every cell in your body via either parasympathetic or sympathetic nervous system activity.[18] Every thought and every perception you have change the homeostasis of your body. Will it be the brakes or the accelerator, a health account deposit or a health account withdrawal? This, in a nutshell, is how your autonomic nervous system translates how you view your world into the state of your health. Happily, you have the power to change your automatic responses—with practice.

How Thoughts Affect Hormone Levels at Menopause

The "language" spoken by your autonomic nervous system is translated to the rest of your body by hormones. The primary messengers of the sympathetic nervous system are hormones called norepinephrine and epinephrine, which are often referred to together as adrenaline. They are produced in the brain and in the adrenal glands. Every time adrenaline levels go up, levels of another adrenal hormone, cortisol, also go up. (For more about cortisol levels in menopause, see chapter 4.)

If you persist in the perception that events and demands in your life are stressful and uncontrollable, you are adopting the mindset that continually whips your adrenals into producing more and more cortisol. Over time, your adrenals may become exhausted, losing their ability to keep up with the demand for increasing amounts of this hormone. This is often coupled with suboptimal nutrition, impaired digestion, and poor assimilation of nutrients, all of which go hand in hand with a stressful life. Insomnia is also very common in this situation. The resulting immune system incompetence increases susceptibility not only to infectious diseases, but also to autoimmune disorders and all cancers.

The overstimulated sympathetic nervous system also causes an imbalance in a group of hormones known as eicosanoids, resulting in impairment of the cells' ability to metabolize fatty acids. This is associated with weight gain, as the body tends to break down muscle and replace it with stored fat and excess fluid. Imbalanced eicosanoids are also associated with tissue inflammation, which is now known to be the cause of nearly all chronic degenerative diseases, such as heart disease, diabetes, and cancer. Tissue inflammation also increases the discomfort felt in a host of chronic diseases such as lupus and rheumatoid arthritis, and has been shown to increase the speed of tumor growth in individuals already harboring cancer.

In a healthy, normal body, cortisol levels are highest upon awakening in the morning. During the night, the parasympathetic nervous system has done its job of providing rest and renewal to your organs. In other words, a deposit has been made into the "health bank." The morning's increased cortisol levels help you get out of bed and get ready for the day ahead. As you wind down in the evening, cortisol levels normally decrease, reaching their lowest at about midnight, easing you into a rejuvenative, restful night. For many stressed-out women, however, the rise-and-fall pattern of cortisol secretion begins to invert itself. Levels are lower in the morning, affording little or no "gas in the tank" to start the day, and they're higher at midnight, making it virtually impossible to wind down and rest.

It does not end there. In addition to causing a deranged output of cortisol, overstimulation of the sympathetic nervous system also causes decreased production of progesterone, one of your body's natural calming agents. The result is that women who are chronically stressed also tend toward hormonal imbalance between estrogen, progesterone, and testosterone (which is important in women as well as in men).

Soothing Your Emotions Before They Become Disease

First of all, there is nothing to be gained by categorizing emotions as "good" or "bad." Instead, think of them as guidance. Every one of them signals a specific need. For some women, anger is simply a sign that they need rest or recognition. For others, anger signals the need for nourishment. So-called negative emotions exist for a reason; identify the reason, feel the emotion fully, release it, and then you are well on your way toward better health. Easier said than done, I know, but nothing is more important. The bottom line is that emotions that feel good are guiding you toward health, while the ones that feel bad are trying to get your attention so that you can change your perception, get a need met, and subsequently change your behavior. It truly is as simple as that.

Emotions can also become toxic if they are allowed to persist unresolved, rather than being worked through fully and released. Consider, for example, the woman who lost a child and fifteen years later, now well into menopause, still hasn't moved anything into that child's room, keeping it exactly as it was the day the child died. The emotions that drive her to enshrine that room—the unresolved grief, the refusal to move forward in life, the denial—are toxic. They not only have robbed her of fifteen years of life, but also are setting her up for physical illness, especially given the intensity with which our unresolved baggage from the past arises at menopause.

The ill health and pain you may experience at midlife are caused not by difficult emotions per se, but rather by a willingness to let those emotions and the needs behind them persist unresolved—or by a misperception of what they mean in your life. Unresolved, "stuck" emotions keep setting up the same body biochemistry over and over again. The effect of negative emotions on our bodies can be likened to water in a river. Our bodies stay clean and fresh as long as our emotions keep flowing, triggering changes in our perception and behavior. The minute that water stagnates, all manner of decay and germs start to flourish.

One of my menopausal patients arrived at a wonderful insight. She began to realize that whenever she feels happy, she also begins to feel nervous, because it is her perception that whenever good things happen in her life, she has to leave behind past aspects of her life that have supported her. Getting a promotion at work, for example, had always been tainted with pangs of regret, because she knew that moving up changed the dynamics of her old relationships. The people she had been friends with before didn't accept her in the same way anymore. I have certainly had the same experience in my own life. The silver lining in that cloud, however, is that by allowing yourself to continually move toward ever-increasing success and joy, you attract new friends and circumstances that support you fully for who you are becoming. The key for this woman is to focus on all the good that has come from allowing herself to become happier and more successful.

Psychologist Gay Hendricks, Ph.D., in his brilliant book *The Big Leap: Conquer Your Hidden Fear and Take Life to the Next Level* (HarperCollins, 2009), points out that we've all been programmed (sometimes starting in utero) with an inner thermostat for how much love, abundance, and success we are comfortable allowing into our lives. And when we get close to going beyond our upper limit of these good things, we unconsciously get back into our comfort zone by starting an argument, getting sick, having an accident, or sabotaging ourselves in some other way. Since midlife is designed to help us burst through the upper limits of the first half of our lives, it's essential that we recognize our upper-limit problems and see them for what they are. This is the first step toward going beyond them.

Our beliefs, after all, have a very powerful effect on us. The work of Ellen Langer, Ph.D., of Harvard illustrates this beautifully. In one of her trademark mindfulness studies on how beliefs affect the body, she looked at two groups of hotel room attendants. One group was told that their work was actually vigorous exercise. The control group carried on as usual. At the end of the study, the group who were told they were exercising at work had lost weight and had lower blood pressure. Nothing was different between the two groups except their belief about the meaning of their work![19]

Again, however, beware the oversimplification that "happiness" is good and "sadness" is bad. Both emotions are necessary to function as a normal human being. Without sadness, the experience of happiness would lose its sweetness. Health is enhanced by allowing all emotions to wash in and out like the tides of the sea. Just as the tides are essential for cleansing the ocean, our emotions cleanse our minds and bodies. At midlife, sadness and regrets from our pasts may take on a heightened role for a time, helping us to truly clean out the silted-up river bottoms of our emotional lives, thus pushing our upper limits higher and setting the stage for more fulfillment and joy to come in.

Are We Responsible for Our Health?

Critics of the mind-body connection say that focusing on the emotional dimension of illness makes people feel worse when they are already vulnerable, as though they are guilty of causing their own disease. I agree that there is the potential to carry this philosophy too far and blame ourselves for ill health. However, the value of the mind-body connection is too great to discard. The simple truth is that the people who heal fastest and remain healthiest the longest are those who feel that their lives are fulfilling and joyful. Even when they're sick, they feel that their life has meaning and that they have some locus of control. Here's an example: I once came down with pneumonia due, in part, to a particularly rigorous travel schedule that included getting on a plane when I knew I needed to sleep and rest to get over a cold. I had scheduled a meeting in New York for which people were traveling from as far away as Thailand, so I didn't want to cancel. But when I finally got home four days later, I ended up in bed for four days, and then had a cough that lasted for weeks. All I could do for days was take baths, read books, and sleep—all most unusual for me. My body was simply doing what it needed to do to get me off my feet to rest. During this time, my colleague Deena Spear, a vibrational healer, told me that my illness was a sort of "energy upgrade" or transformation and that my body needed rest in order for this to happen. I can't prove that, but what she said felt right and it was far more empowering than believing I had caught some random bug that was going around. I cleared my schedule of everything that could be cleared for the next several months.

Those who think, "I catch everything that is going around no matter what I do," or "The world is doing it to me. . . . There's nothing I can do about it. . . . I can't get a break. . . . The world is out to get me. . . . This is just the way the world is," et cetera, are disempowered by their thoughts and perceptions. This directly contributes to an imbalance in the autonomic nervous system and associated hormonal systems. Twenty-five years of medical practice have shown me so clearly that emotions are the primary energy at work, tipping the scales one way or the other, toward illness or toward health, and that the victim mentality from adverse childhood programming is at the root of many illnesses. Cellular biologist Bruce Lipton, Ph.D., has documented the most recent and groundbreaking research on the profound impact of our beliefs on our states of health in his book *The Biology of Belief* (Hay House, 2008, updated and expanded in 2016). In almost every case, beliefs are more powerful than genes. In fact, belief and perception control how genes are expressed!

Despite what we learn daily about healthy exercise practices, healthy diets, and good medical care, the bottom line is that the most significant way of contributing to our own good health is through the quality of our thought processes. This power is a valuable gift, in light of the absolute lack of control we have over other aspects of life. Think about being on a turbulent flight in bad weather. You have no control over the winds, or the skills or the mental state of the pilot flying the plane. But you do have the power to minimize your discomfort. You can decide to read a book, strike up a conversation with the person next to you, take your antioxidants, wrap up in a warm blanket, sleep, listen to music, or watch the movie. Alternatively, you can listen to every engine noise and allow yourself to be debilitated by worry the entire flight. It's your choice.

Ultimately, you are the only one who can make significant deposits into your health bank account. This is not the job of your doctor, your nutritionist, your lover, or your parents. There is no supplement, no healthcare provider, and no exotic herb that can possibly do for you what you can do for yourself.

The key is compassion for yourself. Dr. Hendricks has noted that any area of pain, blame, or shame in our lives is there because we have not loved that part of ourselves enough. No matter what you're feeling, the only way to get a difficult feeling to go away is simply to love yourself for it. If you think you're stupid, then love yourself for feeling that way. It's a paradox, but it works. To heal, you must be the first one to shine the light of compassion on any areas within you that you feel are unacceptable (and we've all got them). The hormonal shifts you experience around the time of menopause can facilitate this.

HOW OUR MIDLIFE BRAINS AND BODIES ARE SET UP TO HEAL OUR PASTS

Though memories are distributed throughout the body and the brain, certain areas of the brain, notably the amygdala and hippocampus, are especially important for the encoding and retrieving of memories. Interestingly, these areas of the brain are particularly rich in receptors for estrogen, progesterone, and GnRH, the hormones that fluctuate the most during the perimenopausal years. Given the heightened activity of these hormones in these areas, it makes sense that memory activation and retrieval would be enhanced during the years immediately surrounding menopause.[20] Hurts and losses we've managed to forget or minimize for many years, even decades, may suddenly become overwhelming—even if we think we should be "over" all that pain from the past.

FIGURE 5: WHY TRAUMATIC MEMORIES MAY BE
RELIVED AT MIDLIFE

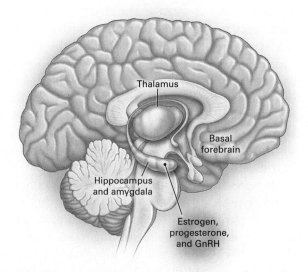

The brain's memory centers are rich in receptors for the hormones that fluctuate in perimenopause.

RACHEL: *Sudden Anxiety Strikes*

Rachel was a strong, self-assured woman with a challenging job and a no-nonsense attitude. But around the time she turned fifty-one, all sorts of physical and emotional health issues started springing up. First, she began experiencing nausea and weight loss. Then her doctor found and removed a benign uterine polyp. But after her dentist pulled an abscessed tooth in what seemed like a fairly routine procedure, Rachel felt as though she'd gone off the deep end. She experienced such extreme anxiety, fear, and panic that she needed to receive treatment for post-traumatic stress disorder. Although she had no previous history of anxiety or depression, Rachel had completely lost her zest for life and felt powerless over the emotions she was experiencing.

I assured Rachel that she was perfectly sane and that what she was describing was a classic midlife example of how the past roars back to be healed. Though Rachel was willing to seek additional professional mental health counseling, if necessary, I first recommended the following: I suggested she pick a number from one to ten, choosing the first one that came into her head. Then I told her to think back to what was happening in her life when she was that age. A part of her childhood self may well have been traumatized, I told her, and was still running her central nervous system. Now that she had the life experience and skills to deal with this long-repressed event, Rachel needed to call on her fully functional adult self to take care of the situation and "grow up" the unhealed little girl inside her who was begging for attention and help. Whatever the trauma had been, Rachel was finally ready to feel it so she could heal it—and let it go forever.

I recommended that she follow the steps outlined in the magic garden exercise in the book *Repetition: Past Lives, Life, and Rebirth* (Hay House, 2008) by clinical psychotherapist Doris Cohen, Ph.D., or that she contact Dr. Cohen through her website (www.healingrep etition.com) to schedule a session with her. I also suggested she learn about the Divine Love healing process from the World Service Institute (www.worldserviceinstitute.org).

CHRISTINE: *Midlife Brings Self-Healing*

On the tenth anniversary of the day she was raped, Christine wrote, she awoke with a greater rush of energy than ever before. These torrents of feeling had become increasingly powerful as she advanced through perimenopause, like exaggerations of the hormonal crests and troughs of the monthly cycles she described as "like PMS times ten." Uncomfortable physical symptoms increasingly accompanied these waves, as her body begged for attention to the wounds left by her sexual assault.

> Headaches, body aches, queasiness, insomnia, anxiety attacks, diarrhea, toothaches, and many other symptoms manifested themselves along the way to my recovery again and again. Over time, I learned to quiet myself and fully experience what I was feeling as each of these "illnesses" struck me. Each time, strong emotions came up and were eventually released, sometimes within minutes—and the symptoms disappeared.

Christine's openness to the messages being sent by her body helped facilitate her healing.

> The most incredible insight that became clear to me during the process of discharge, release, and healing that occurred time and time again was that I am my own healer. It was amazing to me how interrelated my emotions were with the various symptoms I was experiencing.

SUSAN: *Standing Up for Herself at Menopause*

At forty-five, Susan wrote, "Menopause for me is the courage and push I've needed all of my life." Both of Susan's parents were weekend alcoholics, and while they "partied," she and her brother took care of their younger sisters. She left home at eighteen to marry.

> Naturally I married an alcoholic, but I didn't know it until years later. The relationship was very controlling and abusive—mentally, emotionally, and physically. He controlled my every decision, from when I could see my family to where I worked, what furniture to buy, what cars I drove, and the decision to not have children. I convinced myself that we had a wonderful, close relationship. We became my parents, partying and drinking on weekends just like they did—I drank to keep my husband company and to be "part of" something. I also started smoking up to two packs a day. When I became pregnant at age thirty, he convinced me to get an abortion, saying he was under too much pressure, promising we'd try again the following year. Instead, he had

an affair. I hung in there, and eventually he ended it and came back to me. I took this to be proof positive that he truly loved me.

Four years later Susan sought couples therapy, but at the last minute her husband refused to go. Rather than cancel, she went alone. Through her counselor, she started attending meetings of Adult Children of Alcoholics and Al-Anon, where she learned that she was not alone. This marked the beginning of a new life for her.

For Susan, the first major milestone was talking about her abortion. Next she quit smoking. "That opened up a whole new world for me. I no longer had to stuff my feelings and light up a cigarette. I had a mouthpiece. I had something to say, and oh, I said a *lot*—I had diarrhea of the mouth. And such honesty!" Then she quit drinking. "My husband didn't like this new me at all. I no longer was a party girl, at his beck and call."

As Susan changed, she felt herself being torn in two, because the life around her, the life her husband had laid out for her, was not changing at all. "I became a married woman living a single life. We no longer went anywhere or did anything with each other." There were a series of attempts at marriage counseling, separation, reconciliation, and alcoholism therapy for him, all to no avail. Then came the ultimate boost—menopause! Susan wrote: "I became perimenopausal at forty-two. I really feel this gave me the courage and the push and the honesty to look at my life with an eye for what I wanted and needed." She started doing "so many things I've been wanting to do and never did." Eventually she filed for divorce and started the life she'd always wanted to have, 3,000 miles away from her native New York. "I had such an easy transition," she marveled. "I walked away from my whole life there—husband, job, friends, and all but the few things I packed when I left—but I guess I did my grieving while I lived in the marriage. My life is so full today."

The primary defense against unpleasant memories and emotions is avoidance. This subterfuge often works reasonably well until the perimenopausal transition, when the hormonal shift of focus and accompanying changes in brain activity conspire to call buried traumas and unresolved issues into the light, expressing them through physical symptoms that cannot be ignored. Whatever causes a woman's lingering wounds, perimenopause can be seen as a built-in support system that sets her up to do deep healing and reclaiming of the treasure within. Although it may not be seen this way at first, it is a gift.

In addition to providing the clarity and courage to face past abuses or pain, menopause can help a woman step back, acknowledge the necessity to change, and do whatever is needed to separate herself from long-term destructive life patterns. Even the most deeply ingrained patterns can be changed with the support of menopause-induced shifts in the brain, energy, and focus. Sometimes the most effective way to make these changes is to begin adding pleasurable activities that you've always wanted to do, such as manicures, pedicures, or dancing lessons.

Caution: Reinforcing Past Trauma

The disturbing memories and the depression that so often arise at menopause are much less scary and disabling if we see them for what they are. They are evidence that we are now strong enough, deep within, to allow the pain and secrets of the past to rise to the surface and be cleared out once and for all. The midlife investigation and release of the painful patterns from the past is necessary if you are to truly heal. Trust your brain and body to give you the information you need to handle when you're prepared to handle it. You don't need to dwell on it. Think of it as an emotional "catch-and-release" program.

It is valuable to have someone else witness and validate your pain. Many people have found that it was not just the painful experience itself that was so wounding to them as children, but also the fact that there was no one to whom they could safely turn, no one who could understand or validate their reality at the time.

You may choose to work with a therapist, and you may also consider a course of medication to deal with the sleep problems, anxiety, or panic that may arise. However, note that many anti-anxiety drugs are highly addictive. Far too many women have been put on psych meds such as Xanax, Valium, or Zoloft during their menopausal transition, only to find themselves dependent on them for the rest of their lives. If you're willing to work in therapy and make the requisite changes in your life, you most likely can stay off medication entirely. I highly recommend the monthlong Vital Mind Reset Program created by my colleague Kelly Brogan, M.D., a holistic psychiatrist and functional medical doctor who specializes in a holistic approach to mental conditions (see www.kellybroganmd.com). Because psych meds are so addictive and difficult to discontinue, think very carefully before beginning one. There are far more effective and safer alternatives. (See chapter 10, "Nurturing Your Brain," for more information on this subject.)

While I cannot outline the course of recovery in detail here, I do want to caution you about one pitfall: some forms of therapy actually reinforce negative patterns both in your brain and in your body. These include "reliving" the trauma repeatedly and digging for buried memories. Here's why: significant stress of any kind, including the reexperiencing of past painful memories, is associated with high levels of cortisol. This is the very hormonal milieu that increases the likelihood of laying down memories of all kinds, especially traumatic ones, which are mediated through an area of the brain known as the amygdala.[21]

If you are a highly sensitive or suggestible individual, receptive to mental imagery, and you have a lot of cortisol in your bloodstream (as when you're stressed), it is very possible for you to incorporate new traumatic "memories" into your brain and body that have no basis in your past experiences. Instead, they may be the product of your current environment, combined with the suggestions and imagery you picked up from a well-meaning therapist. For example, if a therapist asks you, "Did your father rape you when you were three?" and you are in a susceptible biological state, your brain may simply incorporate the question as fact—"My father raped me when I was three"— whether or not that actually happened. This scenario may then be encoded as a new trauma memory—one that you'll have to cope with on top of the original memories that have arisen on their own.

Ultimately, make it your goal to move on to forgiveness of yourself and those involved in causing you pain in the past. Forgiveness doesn't mean that what happened to you was acceptable. It simply means that you are no longer willing to allow a past injury to keep you from living fully and healthfully in the present.

FINDING A LARGER MEANING

In some cultures, such as that of Hindu India, midlife is a time associated with the serious pursuit of the spiritual dimensions of life. For years, I have witnessed something comparable: the vast majority of attendees at conferences on the connection between the body and soul have been midlife women. (I'm happy to report that more and more men are now coming to these events as well—a change I've witnessed in the last decade.) With our child-rearing or career building either behind us or well established, our creative energies are freed. Our search for life's meaning begins to take on new urgency, and we begin to experience ourselves as potential vessels for Spirit. I've long believed that each of our lives is directed by a force that I think of as God. This force is much bigger than our own intellects,

THE SEVEN EMOTIONAL-ENERGY CENTERS
The Physical Effect of Mental and Emotional Patterns

Emotional Center	Organs	Mental, Emotional Issues
7	Can involve any system	Ability to sense or trust in life's purpose Connection to God or universal source of energy Ability to balance responsibility for life events with acceptance of things we cannot control
6	Brain Eyes Ears Nose Pineal gland	Perception: clarity vs. ambiguity Thought: left brain vs. right brain; rational vs. nonrational Morality: conservative vs. liberal; social rules vs. individual conscience Repression vs. lack of inhibition
5	Thyroid Trachea Neck vertebrae Throat, mouth, teeth, and gums	Communication: expression vs. comprehension (speaking vs. listening) Timing: pushing forward vs. waiting; feeling rushed or like there's not enough time Will: my will or Thy will
4	Heart, lungs Blood vessels Shoulders Ribs, breasts Diaphragm Upper esophagus	Emotional expression: capacity to feel fully, express joy and love, resolve anger, hostility, and grief; experience forgiveness Relationships: capacity to form mutual reciprocal partnerships with balance; nurturing self vs. nurturing others; intimacy with others vs. capacity to be alone

Emotional Center	Organs	Mental, Emotional Issues
3	Abdomen Upper intestines Liver, gallbladder Lower esophagus Stomach Kidney, pancreas Adrenal gland Spleen Middle spine	Self-esteem, self-confidence, and self-acceptance Personal power; competence and skills in the outer world Overresponsibility vs. irresponsibility Addictions to sugar, alcohol, drugs, and tobacco Aggression vs. defensiveness Competitiveness vs. noncompetitiveness; winning vs. losing
2	Uterus, ovaries Vagina, cervix Large intestine Lower vertebrae Pelvis Appendix Bladder	Personal power: sex, money, and relationships Fertility and generativity: individual creativity vs. co-creation with others Boundaries in relationships: dependency vs. independence; giving vs. taking; assertiveness vs. passivity (being pissed off)
1	Muscles, bones Spine Blood Immune system	Safety/security in the world; knowing when to trust or mistrust Knowing when to feel fear and when not to Balance between independence and dependence

Sources: C. N. Shealy and *C. M. Myss,* The Creation of Health: Merging Traditional Medicine with Intuitive Diagnosis *(Walpole, NH: Stillpoint Publications, 1988); James L. Oschman,* Energy Medicine: The Scientific Basis *(New York: Elsevier Limited, 2000); Richard Gerber, M.D.,* Vibrational Medicine *(Rochester, VT: Bear & Company, 2001); Barbara Ann Brennan,* Hands of Light: A Guide to Healing Through the Human Energy Field *(New York: Pleiades Books, 1987).*

and it always moves us toward our highest possible purpose, working directly through the unique expression that each of us represents. My lifelong interest in metaphysics and astrology has provided me with very clear evidence for this truth.

Barbara Hand Clow, an author who specializes in using astrology to give us more access to our power, explains that all of us must go through several key life passages in order to reach our full wisdom. Each passage is associated with very specific and predictable shifts that, if negotiated consciously, open us to our full potential. In her 1996 book *Liquid Light of Sex: Kundalini Rising at Mid-Life Crisis,* Clow writes, "We *form* at age 30, we *transform* at age 40, and we *transmute* at age 50."[22]

Around age forty, the universal energy known as *kundalini* (which is depicted as a snake in many ancient healing traditions) begins to rise naturally and gradually from the base of our spines, activating each energy center (or chakra) of our bodies as it does so. Sometimes the resulting sexual energy that is released at this time can be quite intense, driving some women to have affairs or to channel this energy into painting, building a new home, or some other creative pursuit.

This energy activation may also manifest in bodily symptoms. The degree of unfinished business we have in each of these energy centers will determine the type and severity of symptoms we will experience in that area. Yogic traditions refer to psychic knots known as *granthis* that block the passage of life force (*kundalini*) until they are dissipated through awareness and other practices. For example, I personally experienced several bouts of rather severe chest pain in the year when I started to skip periods and have hot flashes, an indication of grief and despair, emotions of which I hadn't been fully conscious. In retrospect, I can now see that I had unmet needs for touch, affection, and a new "family" during that time, a time when I divorced and my youngest went off to college. Many other women find themselves feeling heart palpitations, anxiety, pelvic pain, or indigestion at midlife.

When we reframe our symptoms and see them as our inner guidance knocking on the door of each emotional center, asking us to allow more light, wisdom, and fulfillment into that particular area, then we don't feel victimized by our bodies. Instead, we have the opportunity to feel empowered by the life energy that is coursing through us at midlife. For example, my divorce culminated during what is astrologically known as my Chiron return, the peak time for me to transmute and connect more powerfully than ever with my spirit and my life purpose. Simultaneously I had been under the influence of an astrological configuration known as a *yod,* which means "the finger of God." The purpose of this was to move me out of my old life so that I had the time and motivation to create new, healthier relationships—which I eventually formed. Though this knowledge did not entirely free me from the suffering I went through, I took great comfort in knowing that there was a larger purpose and meaning in the events that coincided with perimenopause—that my experience amounted to something more than a painful divorce and the onset of hot flashes.

FIGURE 6: EMOTIONAL ANATOMY

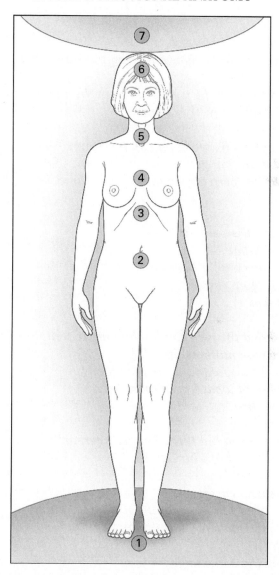

The connection between emotions and physical anatomy comes together in the seven emotional centers. These correspond roughly to traditional energy maps of the body that delineate seven energetic centers or chakras.

Finally, I'd like to share a poem by Wendy Beth Rosen, an early-childhood and elementary teacher and education consultant, that captures her experience of the menopausal transition and perfectly describes some of the ideas outlined in this chapter.

Letting Go

I could have set my watch
By the synchronized signs and symptoms and rhythm
Of my life blood.
I traveled through the weeks and months and years of my life
In a beautiful, perfectly round
Orbit.
And then one day, seemingly all too soon,
It all began to change.
The beautiful, perfectly round orbit became
An ellipse.
Wobbly.
Asymmetrical in, and of, time.
But still, my path.
And then one day, it became
A rhythm of no rhythm.
My beat was . . .
Gone.
And I swirled through time feeling unmoored
From my own mothership.
What am I now, without my life blood?
The symbol of what I hold most dear,
Being a mother,
Has left me.
So many women bid this adieu with fervor,
Happy to be rid of The Curse.
Not me.
It was never a curse.
(Okay, except maybe when I got it on vacation,
And definitely when I got it on my honeymoon!)
But still,
It was always a blessing.
And I am deeply grieving the loss of it.
Even through all the symptoms and changes and hormonal chaos
I have not wanted to let it go.
I have kept myself in a holding pattern.

The irony of resisting the flow of life
Is not lost on me.
The FLOW!
My beautiful flow.
I will miss you.
To this dear, sacred core of a space so deep within me
That is home to my essence and my being, and
First home of my dearest loves,
I give you permission, now,
To let go.
Let go of the remnants of my final little bursts of hormonal effort
That are just a little stuck, still,
In between places in me,
In between places in my life.
This little bit of life blood,
Not wanting to leave,
Not able to leave,
Without help,
Cannot, should not, remain stagnant in me.
I have to move with it, too,
And move through this change
So that I don't remain stagnant.
This space now holds the promise, and the seeds
Of my own birth,
Where a new flow of creative energy
Will nurture
New life
Within me,
Born of deepest gratitude.

  —WENDY BETH ROSEN

3

Coming Home to Yourself: From Dependence to Healthy Autonomy

The need and desire to assume more dominion over our lives becomes a burning issue at midlife. Suddenly we find ourselves questioning the meaning and value of many of the relationships that we'd never dared to look at too closely before. Although we all want to maintain the relationships that support us at the deepest levels, we often discover that our old ways of feeling or behaving with those closest to us—whether parents, children, spouses, friends, or bosses—need updating. And any time we update our lives, we have to grieve for the old life that has been lost. Having the courage both to embrace the necessary changes of midlife and to feel the loss that is associated with those changes is a crucial part of creating a firm foundation for health in the second half of our lives.

THE EMPTY-NEST SYNDROME

You don't have to be a mother to experience the empty nest, that aching sense of personal loss, loneliness, and limbo that so often results when your life undergoes significant change. No matter how secure and settled a woman may feel prior to midlife, the transformative passage into the second half of life almost invariably involves an exodus of some kind. Whether it's the final breakup with a husband from whom you have long been estranged, career changes or reversals, the departure of children who have come of age and left home to start lives of their own—lives that no longer include you as an everyday presence or necessity—or all of the above, when your once-bustling home becomes quiet and/or your daily routine suddenly changes and leaves you feeling at loose ends, the experience is not unlike the unexpected death of a loved one. And even if you saw it coming and thought you were prepared for it—even if, in fact, you are the one doing the leaving—it's painful. This is because it's impossible to fully prepare for the kind of upheaval that is so profound, it holds the potential to completely transform you from the inside out.

One of my friends, a woman who has managed to maintain a high-powered corporate career while also raising two children, recently told me, "When my youngest left for college this fall, I was very busy consulting with a wealthy, creative upscale company, which sent me on frequent trips overseas. Though my days were full of excitement, newness, and adventure, I nevertheless found myself bursting into tears at stoplights while driving. I sometimes feel as though a part of my heart has been ripped out of my chest. After all those years of purposeful and fierce mothering, always managing to put my children first in spite of my career, I have been surprised at how very physical and painful this loss feels. And there was no way I saw it coming."

I can relate completely. As a sneak preview into my own empty-nest scenario, my younger child left home the summer before her senior year of high school for a month at camp, just two weeks after my firstborn left for another summer program in preparation for starting college in the fall. With my husband gone and the divorce nearly complete, this marked the first time in my life since college and medical school that I had been truly alone in my house. For a while it felt okay. My house was cleaner than it had been in years (not that this was ever a goal of mine), and the freedom from other people's chaos was a pleasant side effect as I began the process of re-creating the house on my terms. I ate whatever and whenever I wanted, worked whenever I felt like it, lit candles, and watched movies late into the night. I slowly began to enjoy the opportunity to be still and contemplate my life without interruption. After all, I told myself, I wasn't really alone. My daughters would be home soon enough.

But I had a head-on collision with grief and loneliness a month later. I'd picked up my younger daughter at camp, and together we had driven to Dartmouth for a tour, since she was beginning to contemplate her college options. As my medical school alma mater, not to mention the place where I first met my husband, Dartmouth held many fond memories for me. I remembered vividly the exhilaration I'd felt on arriving twenty-eight years before, when I was completely smitten by the place. Now I was standing on that same campus, a fifty-year-old, newly divorced mom watching the second of her two children make plans for her own life. I was facing not only the loss of my husband and my daughters, but also the loss of all the dreams I'd had for my future. During the three-hour drive home, my daughter slept the whole way, and I realized with surprise that I felt even more lonely than I had when she was gone.

Back at home the next morning, I awoke feeling acutely grief-stricken, and I said to myself, "Ah, this is the empty-nest feeling I've heard about, the feeling that says, 'You're not at home in your new world, and your old world no longer fits you.'" I was in limbo, aching for what was and for what might have been. Intellectually I knew this was a growth phase, a kind of labor pain that would yield wonderful things if I could just allow myself to go through it. (It helped to know that I didn't really have a choice.) Rather than smooth it over and find mind-numbing ways to spare myself the anguish, I let myself feel it. I was lonely, disappointed, heartbroken, and scared, and I sat on my bed and cried for everything about my life that was dying.

But there is good news, too. Anyone who has undergone the emotional upheaval of midlife changes can tell you that though the painful feelings associated with the empty nest arise again and again, over time they come less often, their stay is briefer, and their pain penetrates less deeply with each revisit. So our job is simply to be present with them. My own experience, and that of all the women who have shared their empty-nest experiences with me, indicates that the ultimate reward for fully participating in the emotions that wash over us at this time is that the struggle is over sooner than it would be if we tried to resist or deny them. Whether or not a woman realizes it going in, that hollow, unsettling, empty-nest experience is a blessing in disguise. Think of it as a kind of labor pain. What you are trying to give birth to is your new life, which your hormones, your brain, and your body have already welcomed and embraced, even though you may not yet be consciously aware of it. To create a renewed life, it is necessary to go into the abyss, into the emptiness you may have spent a lifetime using relationships and busyness to avoid. Having looked into the abyss myself, I can understand why a woman entering it might find the prospect of a positive outcome very difficult to believe in. But now that I have come out on the other side, I can assure you that letting go of the past, albeit painful, is well worth it. I am now happier and freer than I've ever been in my life, and many other postmenopausal women feel exactly the same way!

To make this an easier, more joyful transition, give at least as much attention to what you want to create for yourself as you give to what you are letting go of. Start doing some of those things that you've been pushing aside for years. Maybe you want to earn a degree, travel to places you've always dreamed about, get into shape, redecorate your house, or dive into a new interest, such as horseback riding, dance lessons, yoga, meditation, writing, cooking classes, or singing. I myself took up Argentine tango about ten years ago because I'd always wanted to learn partner dancing. It changed my life in many ways and provided me with an entirely new community of friends. If an interest doesn't automatically come to mind, remember what you loved when you were eleven—chances are that will give you some clues to a long-buried passion or vocation waiting to be rediscovered.

HOW TO FIND YOUR SOUL'S TRUE CALLING

It is never enough to pursue paths that lead only to personal gain. In order for an endeavor to be deeply fulfilling and sustainable over the long haul, it must somehow touch and uplift a greater community. The inimitable Tererai Trent, Ph.D., suggests in her book *The Awakened Woman: Remembering and Reigniting Our Sacred Dreams* (Enliven Books, 2017) that when women are trying to find their purpose in life, they ask themselves, "What breaks my heart?" because that which breaks your heart always contains vital information that points to your soul's purpose and fulfillment. As I read this, I was reminded that I nearly fell to the floor weeping the first time I ever saw a baby born, back in medical school. I was so deeply moved that I became an OB-GYN physician. And even though I no longer deliver babies, I have found that the process of conception, gestation, labor, and birth, along with the postpartum period, is a physical metaphor for the way creation comes into form. So it has been as satisfying to "midwife" women through midlife and beyond as it was to deliver physical babies. I have been fortunate enough to have discovered something early in life that touched my heart deeply and that has allowed me to serve a larger community. That didn't change at midlife. What did change were my most intimate one-on-one relationships. It matters little whether your soul task at midlife is a new vocation or a new approach to relationships. Either way, your future fulfillment and happiness depend on heeding the call of your soul. What might this look like? Many women find satisfaction in rescuing stray or injured animals. Others dream of planting beautiful gardens. Still others go back to college and earn long-postponed degrees. Others work with children or immigrants. And many start new businesses.

The important thing isn't what you do—it's that you're willing to explore your dreams and desires. Remember, this is the time to reinvent yourself as more than someone's mother or wife or employee. And your children or other loved ones will end up loving you for this because the alternative is to collapse your life into theirs (longing for the "good old days"), eventually becoming more of a burden than a source of unconditional love and continuing inspiration. (For lots of ideas about how to rebirth yourself at this stage of life, see my books *The Secret Pleasures of Menopause* [Hay House, 2008] and *The Secret Pleasures of Menopause Playbook* [Hay House, 2009].)

PATRICIA: *Delaying the Inevitable*

Many women do everything in their power to try to resist change and transformation, often retreating into the kind of nurturing and caretaking they've participated in for their whole lives. They spend precious energy trying to keep vital life changes at bay, in essence paddling upstream rather than letting the current carry them into new, uncharted waters. Often their fear of going forward is so great that it leads to a step backward instead.

After raising five children, Patricia came to a crossroads that took her completely by surprise.

My husband always ruled the roost, made all the decisions— what groceries to buy, which children helped with which chores, what color to paint my kitchen—and over the years I learned to deal with it by clamming up and withdrawing into the world I'd created with my kids. When our youngest left home, it hit me like a ton of bricks: it was just me and him. I'd frankly never even thought about that before. We got along okay, but mainly because he did his thing and I did mine. Whenever our purposes crossed, I was submissive and compliant—it had become my habit, and it was easier. Now that the kids were all out of the house, I suddenly realized that this could be my time for *me*. But my husband had never allowed it before; I knew he wouldn't allow it now.

Marriage counseling and divorce were taboo subjects in her husband's family, and Patricia realized that she was unwilling to make further concessions in order to "color within the lines" of the way he'd sketched their lives. Instead she decided to avoid the unacceptable future by trying to re-create the past. At the age of forty-seven, she talked him into adopting a baby girl.

I didn't realize it consciously at the time, but looking back, I guess I knew the baby would spare me from having to put our marriage under lights. I wanted to set the clock back. Going forward was too scary. In some ways it did the trick—it kept me occupied. But even though raising children was my joy in my younger years, I realized—too late—that I'd changed. Devoting my life to children was my past life. Now, in my mid-fifties, I know it's not at all what I want to do at this stage in my life. I'm so tired all the time that I feel sedated, and it's not that it's such hard work physically—it's that my heart isn't in it. I feel tugged, like some force is trying to pull me away from here. I feel like I age ten years for every two. But I'm committed to this little girl now, who deserves all I can give her. I hope I can last until she's grown.

BOOMERANG BABIES

Variations on Patricia's theme are becoming more and more common, thanks to the higher-than-ever numbers of adult children who, for one reason or another, boomerang back home—often with kids of their own for Grandma to raise while they try to get their feet under them. If a woman is to claim the second half of her life for herself, to explore her own creative potential and choose the endeavors onto which she focuses her life energy, then she must find a way to stand firm against forces that could induce her to shoulder someone else's long-term responsibilities—forces such as guilt and the compulsion to shield her children from the consequences of their own choices. When decisions and outside circumstances conspire to keep the nest full, there is the strong potential for a woman's new life to become a tired rerun of the old one—with chronic degenerative disease as an accompaniment.

ANITA: *Finally Cutting the Cord*

When Anita and Ralph's newlywed (and pregnant) daughter and her husband rented an apartment in their complex, Anita was thrilled. But over the ensuing months something began to feel wrong.

> At first I thought I was in heaven. Jenny was over here all the time, sometimes to do laundry (claiming she was perpetually having trouble with her machine and Jim didn't have time to fix it), sometimes to bum a cup of sugar, sometimes just to "hang." I thought it was great—it was as if I'd never lost my daughter. Instead of an empty nest, I had the promise of keeping her and having a new little baby around, too. But then, gradually, I started peeling back the layers of what was bothering me. I thought back to when I was a newlywed, and although I adored my folks, I didn't spend nearly as much time with them as Jenny was spending with me. I began to watch for signs of trouble in her marriage, not realizing that I already had recognized a big one—Jenny hadn't really left home yet.
>
> A month later Jim got a promotion, which meant a transfer to the West Coast. I felt as though I'd been kicked in the stomach. Jenny is our only child, and she had been my whole life. It was to be a quick move—they had six weeks to tie up loose ends and get settled in California—but I noticed that in the midst of all the preparations for moving, Jenny started spending even more time with me.
>
> Two weeks later there was a big fight, and the next thing I knew there she was on our doorstep, ready to move "back home," with a look on her face that was both anguished and maybe a little triumphant at the same time. She told me later that she thought I'd be pleased—she knew how much I was going to miss her. That's partly why my response really surprised her.
>
> It was heart-wrenching for me. I hated to see my daughter

hurting, her face blotched from crying and her belly beginning to show evidence of her pregnancy. But somehow, fortunately, I woke up, and none too soon. I told her that moving back was not an option. I told her it was time to move forward, not back. I realized that I needed to cut the cord and start exploring my own life, and she needed to do the same—otherwise we'd both be stuck in a phase of life that we'd outgrown.

As a woman faces the prospect of an empty nest, daunting though it may be, the bottom line is this: separation is a necessary and, ultimately, blessed thing, clearing the way for her next developmental phase. To block that process can be akin to leaving a pot-bound plant, restricted and stunted, in a too-small container. A woman can choose to facilitate her growth, which may be initially painful, or she can choose to block that growth, a path that results in accelerated aging and loss of vitality—just as it would for that pot-bound plant. Staying in place, in other words, is not a viable option. Grow—or die.

POWERFUL FEELINGS, POWERFUL HEALING

In order to take a new path, you must leave the old path behind. This can be one of the most terrifying aspects of the midlife transformation—leaving behind what is familiar and embracing what is unknown. During the first summer after my divorce, for example, I watched my daughter and former husband pull out of the driveway one perfect summer day to go sailing together, a family activity that we had enjoyed for years. I felt left behind, wondering what had happened to my life. In fact, I felt as though, other than my work, I no longer had a real life. When we are standing at a crossroads in our lives, doubts inevitably arise. "Am I capable of pulling this off? Do I have the talent? The strength? Can I make it out there?" Or, as in my case, "What's the use of having made it out there if I have no one to come home to?" Plucked from the milieu in which she has already proven herself and cast adrift in unfamiliar surroundings, a woman would have to be extraordinary not to be afraid. Her self-doubt may be magnified by the fact that as she faces loss, very often the path that will lead to her new life is not clear.

It is vital to a woman's comfort level to understand that the direction of her new path, and her willingness to try it, will come . . . in time. Those directions are, after all, already inside her. The steps that separate her old life from the new one were not meant to be easy, any more than the birth process is meant to be easy (although it sometimes is). As difficult as it is to accept, especially in our quick-fix culture, the struggle that accompanies a woman's midlife transformation appears to be an integral part of the learning process, without which she would not have the incentive to set one foot in front of the other. Your empty nest, your altered living space, your disrupted life focus, that directionless feeling—all must first be acknowledged and experienced, with the attendant emotions, in order for the healing process to begin. In the interim, while we experience the upheaval and wait for the new path to become clear, we have to hang out in the "underworld" for a while, allowing our fears and grief and confusion to be fully experienced. Then, and only then, will the fog begin to lift, revealing hints of new doors, new directions, and a new focus for that shining new life.

Well and good, you might say. But how does one go about fully experiencing powerful emotions without dwelling on them excessively or becoming engulfed in self-pity?

Identifying Your Emotions in Your Writing

There is a writing technique that has been proven effective in helping a woman acknowledge, identify, and express those feelings with focused attention, then release them proactively, on a moment-to-moment basis as they come up, unbidden. It is a skill that requires practice, but the rewards are immediate—and they only get better as your skill level grows. Here's what's involved.

Make a commitment to honor and respect your body by being willing to learn from the emotions that affect it, even if that simply means bringing your loving awareness to it. In other words, be willing to be there for your body and your emotions, just as you would for a child or anyone else you love. If you feel suddenly overwhelmed with sadness or anger, for example, choose to stop and identify that feeling, rather than simply react to it. Acknowledge it. Say to yourself, "I feel sad" or "I feel angry."

Gaze upon your sadness without trying to fix it. The essence of being a good listener—to yourself or to a dear friend—is simply allowing emotion to be expressed freely and honestly. Over time, your caring focus can change pain to compassion. Make the effort to notice your emotions and be with them rather than try to change them, shrug them off, or stuff them into a private corner. Then, once you've focused on them, take the time to write them down.

When I feel strong emotions that stop me in my tracks, I'm almost always helped by writing about the experience as soon as I can find a moment.[1] I sit down, light a candle, put on some adagio baroque music, take three breaths, and come up writing, recording my thoughts like a good secretary. When a particular thought has a certain buzz or energy associated with it, I urge myself to go deeper, asking what I mean by "sad," "angry," "irritated," or whatever. Within ten to fifteen minutes, I've generally figured out what the emotion is trying to teach me as well as what old, outmoded beliefs and thoughts the emotion was based on. And, more than that, I find that the writing moves my energy to a whole new place. Then I'm in a position to shift my focus to something more pleasurable.

Tell Your Story: Listen for Your Needs

As you write about what's going on in your life, listen for your needs. As mentioned in chapter 2, the Center for Nonviolent Communication's website (www.cnvc.org) has an extensive list of needs—such as rest, recognition, and support—that will help you identify yours. Almost no one I know had her needs validated as a child or as an adult. In fact, we've been shamed and blamed for even having them, let alone expecting to get them met. I personally found it life-changing to list my needs and then learn how to skillfully ask for them to be met by the appropriate person. For example, with a co-worker, I had a need for timely completion of agreed-upon tasks. So I said to her, "I have a need for promptness and meeting completion dates on time. Would you be willing to help me meet my need by arriving at our meetings on time?" The most important part of asking others to help us meet our needs is the understanding that they may or may not be able to do that. And if they can't, understand that the very act of asking is the first and most crucial step toward fulfilling the need. After that, the universe itself will often conspire to create circumstances in which you get your needs met.

Identifying Your Emotions in Your Body

A related form of awareness involves tuning in to bodily sensations. When you feel the muscles in your temple tighten, for example, simply observe them, and notice how they relax because of your focused attention. Step back and try to recognize the many ways in which each emotion manifests in your body—the slump of your shoulders, the lump in your throat, the tension in your jaw muscles, the trembling weakness in your legs, the hollowness in the pit of your stomach, the congestion in your nasal passages as tears flow. Apply the healing power of your awareness to all of these sensations, the emotional and the physical. Your mindfulness first validates the emotions and the messages behind them, then eventually clears away any blockage to your ability to be healthy and fully present in your life. Eckhart Tolle teaches that each of us has a "pain body," an accumulation of hurts and pain from our past. It is our egos that keep us identified with our pain bodies. Judging ourselves or getting tense about our pain merely strengthens it. The only way to dissolve a pain body is to soften around it with consciousness and mindfulness. The grace and beauty of this approach is that it allows your suffering to have its time, so it can then flow through and out of you, which it will do. In so doing, you are setting the stage for your own healing . . . and for your own ability to move on. You can also move difficult emotions through more efficiently by crying, moving, and breathing fully. Holding our breath or breathing shallowly always stops us from feeling. And to heal anything, we have to feel it. So breathe mindfully whenever possible. I have the word *breathe* posted in strategic places throughout my home and office.

CARING FOR OURSELVES, CARING FOR OTHERS: FINDING THE BALANCE

We are all knit together by continuity of care, which is one of the feminine values that the world needs more of, not less. Yet it is also true that women's lives are sometimes unnecessarily sacrificed to this virtue.

Midlife women are often referred to as being in a "sandwich" because so many are caught between caring for their still-dependent children while increasingly being called upon to take care of elderly parents or other relatives. This is a time when a woman's programming and her desire to be a good daughter, a good mother, and a good wife—roles that bring her the love and approval of others—run headlong into the increasingly urgent need to care for herself and the needs of her soul. The resulting competition between those two strong but apparently conflicting desires can wreak havoc with our health if we don't examine them carefully and set priorities. The late

Marshall Rosenberg, Ph.D., warned us of the dangers of emotional slavery—a condition that results when we feel responsible for the emotional well-being of others at the expense of ourselves. A psychic once told me that I was here to serve but that I was not supposed to be the main course—a hard-won lesson!

I've watched hundreds of women run themselves ragged at mid-life trying to care for a parent with Alzheimer's, hold down a full-time job, and also run a home and family. This three-ring-circus approach to life too often contributes to health problems such as increased blood pressure and cholesterol, anxiety attacks, heart palpitations, severe hot flashes, and insomnia. In fact, research has documented that people who care for parents with chronic disease have more medical conditions requiring treatment than those who don't have this responsibility.[2]

SHARON: Too Good for Her Own Good

Sharon first came to see me when she was fifty-one years old, complaining of hot flashes and an inability to fall asleep. When I asked her what her exercise and eating habits were like, she shrugged and said, "Who has time to exercise or eat well?" Though Sharon was about thirty pounds overweight and said she wanted to lose weight, she simply couldn't see how she was going to make the time to improve her lifestyle in any way. As I discovered, Sharon was the eldest of five siblings and the only daughter. When her mother died, she was left to care for her father, a man who, at age seventy-two, had been somewhat abusive and distant to his children for most of Sharon's life. His health had mildly deteriorated after Sharon's mother died. Though Sharon's father didn't require skilled nursing care, he did need someone to come in and cook his meals, do the laundry, and keep the house clean—tasks that had always been done by his wife.

Sharon automatically added these tasks to her own day even though her father lived about thirty minutes away from her and even though she was holding down a full-time job as a nurse, was married, and had two teenage sons still living at home. The first thing I asked Sharon was, "Where are your brothers?" She told me that two were living out of state, but two lived in the same town as their father. The obvious next question was, "Are your brothers pitching in with your father's care?" Sharon said that she couldn't really rely on them to help out. After all, they had jobs, wives, and children of their own. "Besides," she added, "they aren't very good at cooking and cleaning. Also, my father really wants me to be the one to come into his house to help out."

I pointed out to Sharon that if she didn't get some help with her caregiving and also add some pleasure to her life, chances were she was going to end up with a health problem herself. Then she wouldn't be able to help her dad at all! I've seen this self-sacrifice many times in my practice and in my life. I also validated her fear that her brothers might be quite resistant to her need for their help and that they would be likely to resent her for a while. Her willingness to take on the whole job herself had made it quite comfortable for her brothers, a perk they weren't likely to give up easily. And her willingness to sacrifice herself for their approval brought her love, gratitude, and a sense of purpose.

Though Sharon felt victimized by her situation, it had never occurred to her to ask her brothers for help. Nor did she like hearing that suggestion from me. But when I raised the possibility that her weight problem and increased blood pressure were related to her current workload, she could see that something had to give. The first thing I advised was that Sharon take a long, hard look at her beliefs about caregiving.

Sharon, like her mother before her, truly believed that "if I don't do it, it won't get done." She had grown up in a household full of boys, none of whom cooked, cleaned, or washed dishes. She and her mother, a woman whom the family described as "a saint," did all the household work. Not surprisingly, Sharon married a man who didn't share in the household tasks, either. And her brothers all married women who were happy to stay home, like their mother, and care for their homes and children.

Unfortunately, this sort of martyrdom had already claimed Sharon's mother, who was only sixty-eight when she died of a heart attack. If Sharon wanted to escape the same fate as her mother, she was going to have to revise her beliefs and behaviors about sacrifice and caregiving. She would have to ask herself, "Am I willing to exercise, meditate, get more sleep, and [fill in the blank] to add more quality and years to my life, or do I prefer to be dead for twenty-four hours a day—and then be unable to help anyone?"

Changing this kind of pattern is rarely easy, however, because when a caregiver like Sharon finally takes a stand, a kind of emotional domino effect gets put into action. When I saw Sharon several months later, she had spoken with her brothers about chipping in toward their father's care. One was so angry with her, he didn't speak to her for a month. But another was a bit more understanding. Eventually, a split developed in the family over the stand she took. Her brothers eventually assumed about 40 percent of their father's care, while he was forced to do more for himself. (Imagine that!) Sharon has lost some weight as well as lowered her blood pressure. Though she feels bad about the rift she "caused" in her family, she is encouraged by the positive changes that have taken place in her health. She knows that she is on the right track and that she is changing her legacy of self-sacrifice and martyrdom.

Breaking the Chain of Self-Sacrifice

Every one of us makes choices every day. For every choice we make, there will be consequences. The more honest we are with ourselves about the motivation that drives our choices, the healthier we will be. This is as true for caregiving as it is for any other area of our lives, perhaps even more so. The following steps are designed to help you consciously care for yourself while caring for others if and when the need arises.

STEP ONE: Acknowledge that women have inherited a cultural and personal legacy of self-sacrifice that has been passed down to us for generations. If you routinely sacrifice yourself for others, relax. You're normal. We've been socialized to value our contribution to our family or social group—our social worth—more than we value ourselves and our relationship with our soul. For at least the past 5,000 years, a woman's worth has been largely determined by how well and how much she serves those who have more power and clout than she has. If you doubt this, remember that American women won the right to vote only in 1920, a mere hundred years ago—barely a blip on the screen when you consider how many millennia men have been in control. Before that, women's opinions and lives didn't even receive official recognition in the government. We haven't had much time in which to shed the automatic caretaking roles that have won us so much praise and support for millennia, let alone replace them with new beliefs and behaviors associated with taking our lives as seriously as we take those of others, particularly men. Despite this legacy, thousands of women all over the world are now taking themselves and their own fulfillment seriously. We are in the midst of a very fast-moving—and often delightful—evolution in this area!

STEP TWO: Learn the difference between care and overcare. True care of others, from a place of unconditional love, enhances our health, in part because it's associated with oxytocin, the bonding hormone. That's one reason why volunteering and community service feel good and are associated with improved health. Overcare and burnout result from not including ourselves on the list of people who require care. Burnout destroys our health and runs our batteries down. Overcare is often motivated by guilt and unfinished business, for which we hope to somehow compensate through the caregiving role. The way to tell the difference between the two is to be aware of how caring for another makes you feel. You must also be 100 percent honest about what you're getting out of excessive caregiving.

One of my friends told me, "When I do things to make my family happy, I feel good and loved. The more I do, like baking, cooking, and keeping the house picked up, the more compliments I get. Though this can be exhausting, and though I keep saying that I need to get a life for myself other than work and cleaning up after everyone, I'm secretly afraid that if I take a stand and delegate responsibility to other family members for some of the caregiving work, they will resent me and not love me as much. So the payoff of doing it all myself is that I get my parents' love and my husband's love." When I hear something like this, I have to wonder whether it really is pleasure that motivates the caregiving, as she believes, or whether it's fear. (About five years after my divorce, as I was coming home to myself, I seriously contemplated not putting up a Christmas tree—then relented at the last minute. I didn't really want one, but I thought my daughters would enjoy it when they were home. Turns out, they didn't care one way or another. So I didn't put one up for a number of years. And then I decided I would enjoy one once again—once I found a friend who enjoyed putting it up, decorating it, and taking it down so that I didn't have to do it! This small thing was a lesson for me in examining my own caring versus overcaring behaviors.)

Each of us needs to examine what we get from martyring ourselves. One of my patients, a woman whose mother was physically and verbally abusive, learned early on that the only way to avoid being hit was to make all the meals, scrub the floors, and clean the rest of the house. To this day whenever she meets new people, she feels compelled to cook, clean, and bring them gifts to earn their love. She recently told me that she'd had the following insight: "If you act like a saint, no one ever confronts you—no one beats up on you. You become a valued part of every group you're in."

Sainthood of this kind seems mainly an avoidance strategy. On the other hand, the desire to nurture others, including plants and animals, is a positive emotion that is built right into the biological programming of most women (and many men as well). Studies have shown, for instance, that when volunteers in nursing homes are taught how to give massages to the residents, the health of the volunteers is enhanced as well as that of the recipients. Who hasn't enjoyed the satisfaction gained from making a special school lunch that surprises and delights a child, or helping out a sick friend who needs a meal or someone to watch her children?

It feels good deep inside me to bring comfort to those who are suffering. In fact, my entire career is based on helping others feel better. Oftentimes, as I give health assistance to someone, I feel as though I'm in touch with a power that is greater than me but moves through me, helping me as it helps the other person. But many women, including myself, have learned over the years, sometimes through the wisdom of personal illness, that we cannot be available to another in a healthy way unless we're also getting our own needs met. And those needs must include time for pleasurable activities such as eating well and getting enough sleep. If you happen to be living with an individual who is self-centered and narcissistic, chances are very good that a large part of your midlife rebirth will involve freeing yourself from your guilt over caring for yourself.

STEP THREE: Learn the health benefits of benign self-interest. Here's a basic scientific truth: our health is best served by participating in those activities that are in our own highest and best interests and that bring us the most pleasure. This is not selfish. It is the very basis for a healthy life. There is not a single cell in our bodies that flourishes through sacrificing its own health for the health of the surrounding cells. It simply doesn't make sense. Instead, cells communicate with one another constantly. The health of one affects the health of them all. The more fully you are participating in the work and activities that bring you the most joy, the healthier you and your entire group become.

This lesson was brought home to me very clearly a couple of years ago when my mother was honored along with a number of other women for being a distinguished citizen of New York State. The entire family gathered in the state capital, Albany, for the ceremony. All of the honorees had provided their communities with a huge amount of service in the areas of home healthcare, breast cancer advocacy, and so on. And I could tell that my mother was feeling nervous about how her contribution would compare with those of the other women. Although she had served as mayor of her town for two terms, she had also completed the Appalachian Trail after the age of sixty and climbed the hundred highest peaks in New England, many of them on unmarked trails. She did this solely for her own pleasure. As it turns out, her contribution provided such inspiration for everyone in the room about what's possible as we get older that there was no question about its value to the community!

STEP FOUR: Understand that caring for parents or aging relatives inevitably brings up unfinished business from our family past. Claris, one of my menopausal patients whose diabetes was particularly difficult to bring under control while she was tending her dying father, told me that the very thought of not caring for her father, who had cancer, caused her to feel overcome with guilt. She said, "Daddy didn't want any strangers in the house, so I didn't feel as though I could hire a nurse or home health aide even though the money was available. To tell you the truth, his insistence that I be the only one to help him made me feel special." When Claris entered therapy after her father's death, she realized that she had never felt her father valued her as much as her brothers, so she tried to prove her worth through caregiving, something she did better than her brothers. She came to see that being constantly available for her father, even though other choices were available, was a way of trying to win the love and approval she had never felt from him in childhood. For some women, caring for a dying parent is an enormously fulfilling and satisfying experience. On the other hand, for those who have a particularly self-centered parent, the experience of caregiving can be draining and is a health risk. Don't attempt to do this without support.

STEP FIVE: Learn to delegate and ask for help. Caregiving at midlife is yet another opportunity to learn how to establish healthy boundaries, set limits, and get clear about the ways that other family members can assume some of the burden or pay for your help. If your husband isn't working or is working fewer hours than you are, for example, there's no reason why he can't pitch in. (You will have to learn the skill of asking for this help without anger and resentment in order to get what you want. And to do that, you first have to believe that you deserve and are worthy of help. You are!)

Many women are not in a financial position to hire outside help to provide care for family members. But in almost every case there is a caregiving solution that needn't fall squarely on only one woman's shoulders. It's time that everyone (including men, women, and older children) learned the basics of cooking and cleaning. Or, if no one else in the family can or will pitch in, another tactic would be to figure out what your caretaking time is worth, by finding out what it would cost to hire someone to come in and do the work you are doing. Then you could ask your siblings or other family members to pay you directly so that you can cut back on the hours you work elsewhere. That way you would have more time to replenish yourself each day, including time to exercise and eat well. It's no secret that the work of caregiving is grossly undervalued and undercompensated all over the planet. So please understand that including self-care in your caregiving is a radical and courageous act of power.

Like Sharon, you will no doubt have to recover from the family programming that leads you to believe that your role as a woman must include self-sacrifice and that to do anything less is to be selfish—something women are so afraid of being called. Sharon had to let her father know that he needed to learn how to receive care from someone other than her. And her father also needed to undo a lifetime of conditioning telling him that all his household tasks would automatically be taken care of. It is well documented that older people, including men, can learn and grow until the end of their lives. There's no reason a man can't learn how to boil an egg, broil a piece of chicken, or stick a load of clothes in a washing machine! Parents who truly love us want what is best for us, even if that means making some adjustments in their behavior and expectations.

STEP SIX: Plan ahead. Don't wait until a parent or relative is in need of care before discussing a potential plan with your siblings. That way you can avoid the emergency caregiving that seemingly "just happens" to us but in reality was set in motion by our beliefs and choices years before. One of my friends, an eldest daughter who has just turned forty and has no children, has already made it clear to her younger sister, who lives in the same town as their mother, that she has no intention of allowing the mother, a very dependent woman, to come live with her should something happen to their father. My friend is not being selfish. She's being realistic. She loves her mother but does not intend to sacrifice her life and career for her. Her unblinking approach concerning her mother's possible future care alerts other family members that they can't automatically rely on her to house her mother in the future should the need arise. This breaks the chain of eldest-daughter sacrifice before it even gets welded in the first place.

STEP SEVEN: Learn how to say no. The art of saying no with grace and ease is one of the most important skills you can ever develop. The beauty of midlife is that you've now paid your dues and have had enough life experience to know what is likely to drain you and what will replenish you. In her groundbreaking book *The Art of Extreme Self-Care* (Hay House, 2009), my colleague Cheryl Richardson writes, "Funny, but after years of practicing Extreme Self-Care, I've realized something ironic: if you want to live an authentic, meaningful life, you need to master the art of disappointing and upsetting others, hurting feelings, and living with the reality that some people just won't like you. It may not be easy, but it's essential if you want your life to reflect your deepest desires, values, and needs."[3] I couldn't agree more. Which is why I loved the chapter in her book entitled "Let Me Disappoint You"!

HITTING PAY DIRT: GETTING CLEAR ABOUT MONEY AT MIDLIFE

Whatever the changes that precipitate a woman's empty-nest experience, the only path that will allow the full expression of her creative potential in the second half of her life is the path that establishes her true independence, both financially and emotionally. Even if she currently has a husband who supports her or money coming in from her family, it's important for her to know that if the need arose, she could manage alone. Inability to support themselves financially is the number-one reason why women stay in less-than-ideal relationships in which they are not treated as autonomous individuals with equal decision-making power. Being able to care for ourselves financially opens up a whole new world of pleasurable possibilities.

Though I do not claim to be a financial expert, I do know this: how, what, where, when, and on whom a woman spends money, and where she gets that money, tells you more about her true values, beliefs, and priorities than any other aspect of her life. Our behavior around making, spending, and saving money lays bare our core beliefs about ourselves and our worth in the world, pure and simple.

The dynamics of money also hold up a mirror to our relationships, telling us how each partner's contribution is valued and whether we are in a truly co-creative partnership. That's why discussing who pays for what and who does what tasks in a relationship is such a loaded and often unpleasant topic.

Cultural Ambivalence About Women and Money

It's no huge surprise that these days many women make more money than their mates. The U.S. Bureau of Labor Statistics reported that in 2018, 29 percent of U.S. wives earned more than their husbands (in marriages where both partners worked), up from 16 percent in 1981.[4] Yet the data suggest that we are still not comfortable, as individuals or as a culture, with that pattern.

When a woman earns more than her husband, it doesn't wipe out the power differential. If anything, it seems to exacerbate it, due to the ambivalence couples feel about their status reversal. Research shows that in such cases, women actually spend more time on household chores than their mates, couples are less satisfied with their marriages, and they are more likely to divorce.[5] Julie Brines, Ph.D., a sociologist at the University of Washington who studies status-reversal couples, found that in marriages where women outearn men, women cede much of the decision-making power to their spouses. This is the opposite of what happens in traditional marriages, where the husband, who brings home the bacon, tends to call the shots. In other words, when women are the major wage earners, there's not a straightforward relationship between income and power. Instead, there's an effort to achieve balance, even though this so-called balance is anything but.

The implications of this research are clear: no matter how much of the financial burden we shoulder, we still feel responsible for keeping our husbands happy, for making them feel good about themselves— especially if they're not making as much money as we are.

The sad truth is that many of us are still unsure of our worth as women in relationship to men (or alpha-type females), which is perfectly understandable given our history. So we do even more than our share to keep the men in our lives happy, lest they leave us for someone who appreciates them more than we do. Secretly we're afraid that if we demand too much, we'll be left alone. We don't realize how much inner power we have to create the life of our dreams because we've been talked out of it! Or, alternatively, we realize at midlife that we are empaths with hardwired personality traits that lead us to believe our loyalty, skills, and conscientiousness will be enough to change the self-centered individuals we find we are living or working with.

And then there's that other deeply feminine desire: we want to be cherished and taken care of. We keep hoping (sometimes despite ample evidence to the contrary) that to have a husband (or wife) means that we will be taken care of. I grew up loving Tarzan movies. Recently I watched the classic *Tarzan and His Mate*, which I hadn't seen in years. This time I saw it through a new lens. The programming about gender roles was very clear: Jane provided the playfulness and the sex, while Tarzan protected Jane by fighting off wild things and doing a lot of heavy lifting to make sure she had a secure, comfortable home. Very compelling. Very appealing. And like most women, I want to get in on the good parts of this but without having to sacrifice myself to do so. I have finally figured out how to do this, but first I had to reprogram my subconscious beliefs and behaviors around relationships. This endeavor took me a number of years during and after perimenopause.

In my own family, as soon as my brothers turned eighteen my father sat them down and told them that they had to start supporting themselves. But he paid for my college tuition without question. I did put myself through medical school with student loans and scholarships, but when I got married, during my last month of med school, I gladly let my husband take care of all the details of buying our first home—a process that mystified and terrified me at the time. He used the last of his educational trust fund as a down payment, and I felt unbelievably lucky to be living this fairy-tale life! We paid off my medical school loans without difficulty.

My husband also made all the decisions about charitable donations and investments, though our incomes were basically equal. Donations went to the educational institutions and charities he favored. I never questioned this. I found the topic of money burdensome until I was forced to wake up at midlife. I'm not alone; many women find themselves in the same situation. Though we went through women's liberation in college, in the interest of creating a happy home and family life we were always willing to do "a little more" housework and childcare than our husbands. Now our generation is taking the next step and waking up financially.

When I first went through my divorce, I secretly hoped that my life would be miraculously fixed by meeting a financially savvy and successful new man to marry so that I could get squared away again. Yep, I admit it. I was hoping that Prince Charming would ride up on his white horse and save me. (I saw how thoroughly this old programming lived in me, despite my career success.) As time went on, however, and no Prince Charming rode up to my door, I was forced to learn how to save myself. I learned that saving myself was not only fun, it was exhilarating. As the scales fell from my eyes and I learned to trust and value myself, my desires, and my financial savvy more and more, I was finally able to withdraw my projections from men, too. They were human and flawed, just like me. No better. No worse. Through my dealings with bankers, brokers, insurance agents, and accountants, I learned that men didn't have any more financial or other "magic" than I had. In fact, the more I saw myself as the source of my own magic, the better my life became. And from this new perspective, flush with pleasure and delight at my new, more prosperous way of being in the world, I began to appreciate men more than ever! I found out that when you're clear with them about what you want and ask nicely—without any anger or neediness—they're often more than happy to provide it for you! One Christmas, for example, I told my oldest brother that I wanted a bonfire outside on the solstice. When I arrived at his house, he and my younger brother had prepared a pile of wooden pallets so substantial that I was sure my solstice bonfire could be seen from space! I was completely moved and gratified by this gesture of support. This past spring, a male friend came over to the house and replaced my car battery when the car wouldn't start. I realized that all I had to do was ask instead of being determined to figure it out myself. My old, stoic "I don't need anybody" attitude began melting away in the warm glow of self-acceptance, compassion, and vulnerability. But this magic all started only when I no longer looked to a man to "complete" me or make me happy. When I discovered that I had what it took to make myself happy and I gave up the futility of self-sacrifice as a way to get my needs met indirectly, my whole world changed. And so can yours.

MARY: *It's Never Enough*

Forty-six-year-old Mary had long been convinced her husband was better at finances than she was. He paid all the bills and did the taxes every year. But these activities always upset him. His mantra seemed to be "There's never enough. There's never enough." Increasingly Mary felt as though she couldn't ask her husband for money for anything but the barest of essentials, and it seemed the only way she could help the situation was to spend less. Finally, after much soul-searching, Mary decided to get recertified as a nurse, the profession she'd had when she had met and married her husband. Given the nursing shortage and the fact that they lived in a city with several large hospitals, Mary had no difficulty getting a job with a good salary and decent benefits. Within a year or so she began to make substantial contributions to the family income. This made her feel good, even though she hated the on-call part of her job. Despite her contribution, however, her husband continued to exercise iron control over all their financial decisions.

Mary suspected that one reason her husband was reluctant to share the financial decision making, as unhappy as it seemed to make him, was that he was going through his own midlife crisis at work. He seemed depressed about his career and the fact that he hadn't reached the success he thought he should have during his forties— a time he referred to as his "power years." He had started talking about retiring early, selling the house, and traveling around the country in an RV. Mary hoped that her husband was just going through a phase and would recover soon. She suggested that he get some individual counseling, but he became angry with her and said absolutely nothing was wrong with him and that he was not depressed.

Meanwhile, bringing home a paycheck had allowed Mary to become much more empowered in the world, if not at home. Nevertheless, she began to suffer from a host of health problems, including palpitations, severe hot flashes, and lower back pain. Her periods also became very irregular and very heavy. It was at this point that Mary came to see me, and I asked her what was going on in her life. When she told me, I gave her a series of recommendations to help her physical symptoms. (I will discuss these in later chapters.) I also suggested that she begin to assume a more proactive role in managing the family finances, which she agreed to do.

When she came back three months later, many of her menopausal symptoms were better. She reported that at first her husband had been resistant to her desire to know about their finances and help with spending decisions. However, soon after she initially raised the issue, he started to experience chest pain, which was diagnosed as angina. He realized that if his life continued in the way it had been going, he could die of a heart attack. This was his own midlife wake-up call, and it made him realize that he, too, needed to revamp some of his outmoded beliefs and behaviors.

In the meantime, Mary took steps on her own to increase her financial knowledge. Her new confidence forced changes in her marriage, of course. She told me that she and her husband had to completely rework their agreements about money and household chores. It wasn't easy. But as she identified her own needs, and also assumed a more playful attitude about the whole matter, things began to shift. She found that lightening up around the serious subject of money not only helped her, but also helped her husband, who had been taught that money was his burden alone. In time, Mary's husband realized that it was in both his and Mary's best interest if both of them knew everything about their mutual finances and agreed upon their spending habits.

Changing Your Cultural Legacy

Middle-class white women of my mother's generation were brought up to believe that they would be taken care of by their husbands. With the help of life insurance policies and the unprecedented economic growth that followed World War II, many of them were. The majority of my mother's friends, women now in their eighties and nineties, never worked after marriage and never had to return to work after they became widows. The women's movement brought to our collective consciousness the price that many of our mothers and grandmothers paid for being taken care of in this way, and my generation vowed that we wouldn't become our mothers. (My mother told me once how dismayed she was at the dismissive and abusive ways in which many of her friends' husbands treated their wives.) Though we've come a very long way when it comes to earning and handling money, the truth is that far too many women still lack basic money skills and are overly dependent upon husbands, employers, or family members to do their financial planning for them. It boils down to this: many women were raised to think that money was too complicated for them to manage and that someone else would take care of them financially if they were willing to do the caregiving. So they invested in the people (such as spouses or bosses) who they believed would provide for them and love them. A bumper sticker from the Women's Institute for Financial Education (www.wife.org) says it all: "A Husband Is Not a Financial Plan."

In fact, more than 11.6 million businesses in the United States are owned by women (including one in five businesses with revenue of $1 million or more), according to 2017 figures from the National Association of Women Business Owners (www.nawbo.org). These businesses generate $1.7 trillion in sales and employ nearly 9 million people. The Federal Reserve estimates that, whether through earnings or inheritance, women will control two-thirds of the wealth in the United States by 2030. According to the Women's Institute for Financial Education, the average woman will be on her own financially for one-third of her adult life, and 90 percent will be managing their own money for at least some of their lives.

The good news is that despite fears of becoming bag ladies (fears that are very common), we women are actually really good at handling and managing money. A study of more than five hundred Fortune 500 companies showed that those with the highest percentage of women on their board of directors reported a 53 percent higher return on equity, a 42 percent higher return on sales, and a 66 percent higher return on invested capital compared with those companies with the lowest percentage of women board members.[6] The key to becoming financially literate is to recognize money as simply the manifestation of life energy and to realize that we have the innate ability to deal with it effectively—with a little education. If our bodies have the skill and know-how to turn our life energy into an entirely new human being from our own flesh and blood, it ought to be a piece of cake to manage the life energy that money is simply a symbol of!

The news is good. Women, particularly midlife women, have now been identified as a lucrative new market for the financial industry. And, as already stated, we have an aptitude for managing money. Studies have shown, for example, that women's investment groups do better over the long haul than men's. Women tend to focus more on long-term financial goals than on short-term performance, in part because womanly values tend to support families and communities, not just a woman's own personal goals. This is why, in both our own country and in developing nations, the key to a sustainable economy is to invest in women-owned and women-run enterprises.[7]

The Value of Becoming Financially Savvy

Regardless of your current circumstances, it is crucial that you get very clear about your beliefs about money so that you can begin to assume dominion over your money in the same way you are daily assuming dominion over your health. Money is a very concrete form of energy—it is power in our society, allowing you to go where you want to go and stay where you want to stay. Having control over your money gives you a sense of freedom and safety. In study after study, higher socioeconomic status is consistently associated with better health. But I believe it is the sense of empowerment and control, not the absolute number of dollars involved, that makes the real difference.

Many women report that in the early stages of taking financial control, they feel fueled by both anger and fear. I was no exception. In those first few months after my separation, I found myself possessed by a new sense of purpose, driven by the need to get my life free, clear, and settled. I had to get myself out of debt, pay off the overdrafts, and get the household accounts reorganized. It was quite scary and burdensome at first, but it quickly became exhilarating as I came to the realization that I *could* do it all by myself. The truth is, I had never actually acknowledged the fact that I had doubted that ability before. I learned I could manage my household finances just as effectively as I had for many years managed my professional and business finances—all without my husband's income, advice, or support. This is not to minimize or disparage his contribution during all the years of our marriage. Rather, it is to acknowledge the personal empowerment that comes from becoming financially independent. As I look back now, I see how crucial this step was for my health and well-being. In shoring up my financial well-being, I also strengthened the health of my second chakra and entire pelvic region (the second chakra, remember, is greatly influenced by our relationships).

From Poverty Consciousness to Prosperity Consciousness

The rubber really met the road for me when I came to the realization that I was the one who was responsible for paying the mortgage and the vast majority of two private college tuitions. I had dabbled in reading about the universal laws of prosperity but had never really been "up against it" enough to apply them in my life. Not so anymore. Every day, as I ran on my treadmill, I read *Think and Grow Rich* (Briggs Publications, revised edition, 2003) by Napoleon Hill, about how desire and consciousness create the mindset that attracts prosperity; Suze Orman's *The Courage to Be Rich* (Riverhead Books, 1999); and also everything by Robert Kiyosaki, author of *Rich Dad, Poor Dad* (Doubleday, 1999). I played his brilliant game Cash Flow 101 over and over until I could easily get out of the "rat race" (living from paycheck to paycheck) and into the "fast track"—having residual income from businesses and investments that come in regularly whether you work or not. For the very first time in my life, I began to see myself as a business that was producing a product. I saw that my books, recordings, online courses, lectures, and e-newsletters were all "products" and all marketable.

I also saw how clearly my beliefs about money and prosperity were reflected in my bank accounts. At around this time, I met Suze Orman in the greenroom at the *Today* show. She told me that you can see people's ill health in their money and cash flow first because money has nowhere to hide an energy imbalance. You either have positive cash flow or you have debt. Simple. Sooner or later, if the behavior patterns and beliefs that create money problems are not addressed, they will manifest as health problems in the body. At the time, I was complaining to her about having to shoulder all the financial responsibility for my daughters. She said, "The only thing holding money back from you is anger and fear." I realized that she was right on the mark. My anger at my ex-husband, who by this time was remarried with a baby on the way, had left me full of resentment. And it was time to let it go instead of staying stuck in the prison I'd created for myself. Suze's remark was a wake-up call. Instead of seeing myself as a victim, I decided to be grateful for the opportunity to really learn how to support myself. I decided then and there to manifest more prosperity than I'd ever dreamed possible. I realized that what my ex-husband did or didn't do with his life or his money didn't have to affect me adversely at all—if I didn't allow it to. I realized that I could manifest the money I needed, and support myself and my kids even better than before. I read Catherine Ponder's *The Dynamic Laws of Prosperity* (De Vorss & Company, revised edition, 1985) and began to do affirmations about prosperity regularly. I still do them every day to ward off the ill effects of the poverty consciousness that pervades most people's way of thinking—and attracts its equivalent. Read the following and see how it makes you feel.

> I am now experiencing perfect health, abundant prosperity, and complete and utter happiness. This is true because the world is full of charming people who now lovingly help me in every way. I am now come into an innumerable company of angels. I am now living a delightful, interesting, and satisfying life of the most widely useful kind. Because of my own increased wealth, health, and happiness, I am now able to help others live a delightful, interesting, and satisfying life of the most widely useful kind. My good—our good—is universal.

Now imagine thinking thoughts like this day in and day out. It changes your life. As a result of my efforts in this area, my financial status is now light-years better than it ever was when I was married. And so are my mental and physical health. In fact, I've been so impressed with the result of this approach in my own life and in the lives of my daughters, family members, and close friends that I have started to include prosperity consciousness as a crucial part of creating health.

Getting Started

If you're already one of the many women who run their own businesses and also do the family finances, I urge you to update your prosperity consciousness so that you can do even better than you're doing now. It's crucial to understand the link between self-worth and net worth. Because money difficulties often run in families and are a reflection of self-worth issues, I strongly recommend the twelve-step Debtors Anonymous program (see www.debtorsanonymous.org) to those with persistent underearning behavior. I would also recommend the book *Money, A Love Story* (Hay House, 2013), as well as the online course that goes along with it, written by my daughter Kate Northrup—a book that was, in many ways, born out of the money legacy (and need for updating) that she learned from me and from her father.

Women who are currently being supported by a husband or other family member can put themselves on the road to financial competence by doing the following exercise for one month. Pretend you are divorced, widowed, or suddenly faced with supporting yourself. Continuously ask yourself questions such as these: "Where are the insurance papers? The deed to the house? The mortgage papers? The pension plan? The tax forms from past years? What is the appraised value of the house? What is my net worth? When was the last time I filled out a financial statement?" Having a firm grasp on this type of information can help ensure that you remain in your relationship for all the right reasons—because it fulfills you and makes your life better on many levels—rather than because you believe you would fall apart without it. You simply cannot be available for true partnership and exhilarating co-creation with another until you know how to pull your own weight and have faced your own dependency squarely—and then done something about it. Whether or not you are financially savvy, it's clear that the financial power structures that have kept so many enslaved for centuries are changing. Each of us, particularly women in the Western world, have the agency and inner power to survive and thrive on our own terms—more than at any other time in written history. Every business that is not sustainable and not based on providing real value is being phased out. You can benefit from this trend by thinking of yourself and your finances as a microcosm of this macrocosmic shift. Please realize that the healing you personally do around money and finance helps heal the global economy as well.

COMING HOME TO YOURSELF

When I wrote the first edition of this book, I was well into perimenopause, a time when I should have been in the throes of what many call "hormone hell." Yet I felt better than I had in years. The severe hot flashes I was experiencing in the last few months of my marriage virtually disappeared after my husband left—a phenomenon I've seen repeatedly in other women who've had the courage to leave dead-end relationships. Over and over I've watched perimenopausal symptoms resolve in women who've had the courage to negotiate the rapids of their midlife transitions consciously and in an empowered way in which they finally give their own needs high priority.

But I've also watched something even more profound occurring: the emergence of what can only be described as pure joy, the feeling that arises when a woman is truly coming home to herself. My own experience bears this out. I marveled at the power of my newfound nesting instinct and at how differently I chose to do things once I had set both feet across the threshold of my new life.

One of the most striking things I discovered after my husband left was an almost physical need to reclaim and redecorate my home, especially the family and guest rooms. One day, with catalogs, telephone, and credit card in hand, within less than an hour I bought a couch, a rug, end tables for the guest bedroom, and even curtains, something that at the age of forty-nine I had never done. My work in combination with my mothering had left no time or inclination to contemplate decor, let alone participate in choosing it. But that was my old life. Now, with my inner landscape rapidly changing, I felt a powerful compulsion to make my outer surroundings reflect the rejuvenation that was going on inside me.

I discovered that feng shui, the Chinese art of placement, helped me enormously in this process. I came to see that our homes reflect our lives, and that by consciously changing our living spaces according to the principles of feng shui, we can actually create improvements in our lives on all levels. By using a tool known as the *bagua* map, one can determine which areas of a room or an entire home correspond to specific aspects of life—for example, health and family, wealth and prosperity, helpful people and travel, love and marriage. This information allows you to enhance and change your physical space in order to enhance and change that particular area of your life. And as with all things in life, when you do this, things sometimes get worse before they get better—kind of like taking out the garbage as part of the process of spring cleaning. When my friend and colleague Terah Kathryn Collins, the author of *The Western Guide to Feng Shui* (Hay House, 1999), did a consultation with me, we both laughed when we realized that my husband had left within four months of the time I had enhanced the love-and-marriage area of our property with a beautiful arbor. She said, "I see this over and over. When you enhance an area of your life that isn't working, you first have to let go of the parts that are standing in the way of getting what you really want." I also put a lighted lamppost in the helpful-people-and-places area of the property. Within two months my life became filled with skillful people who help me on all levels of my life, both at home and at work. (See Resources for feng shui information.)

I wanted my home to be the kind of place where people felt comfortable and welcome. And I wanted to feel at home there, surrounded by colors and textures that drew me in. For the first time in my life, I knew exactly what my personal style was and exactly how I wanted my rooms to look and feel. As the furniture began to come in and the rooms took shape, I felt delighted with the results, going back to look at them over and over again. Slowly it began to dawn on me what I was really doing: I was creating a potential space for all the new energy that was beginning to stream into my life. Whereas before I had been grieving the empty nest, now I was re-creating my old nest into a revitalized place that reflected who I was becoming. It was a nest that would, of course, comfortably accommodate my children, their friends, and the new people who, I felt sure, would be coming into my life. And come they did. I eventually removed all the furniture from my traditional "living room," leaving bare wood floors for a dance floor. I put mirrors on the walls to create a dance studio atmosphere. I also hosted regular tango dance parties and enjoyable theatrical evenings with the many singers, dancers, and actors my daughters brought home for visits. In short, I created the kind of home and life that was a reflection of me—not some pantomime of the kind of home I thought was "proper" by someone else's standard.

PAMELA: A Home of Her Own

While for me the process of coming home to myself meant accepting the breakup of my marriage, Pamela found a different—and very unconventional—path. She wrote:

> I am forty-seven years old and have been in a relationship with Don for eight years, married for five. He's twelve years older, and his philosophy of life is pretty much "My way or the highway." Don's unilateral decisions aren't always supportive of me, and last year I decided that I needed to make choices that reflected my beliefs and prepared me for my future. He travels frequently for business and pleasure, and I spent a good deal of time alone in a house that didn't feel like home. I had even created a room of my own, but it wasn't enough.
>
> So I've bought a home of my own. The marriage has had to undergo a transformation now that we are not together on a daily basis, and it could have failed. Don lives where he wants to, and I live where I need to. I cannot describe the joy I feel at living in a place that supports me emotionally and spiritually. I am moved to nurture my home and garden just as it nourishes me. I am delighted by the simplest things. Friends who have visited agree that it is me.
>
> I am grateful that I earn a living and am capable of being financially independent of Don. And perhaps finally succeeding at my career gave me the confidence to create my dream home. After a lifetime of determining my worth through male approval, I am now living from my heart rather than from obligation.

VOCATIONAL AWAKENING AT MIDLIFE

For some women, the home—which had been the central focus before midlife—becomes secondary to a new passion, which reveals itself in the form of a vocational calling. Other women leave their previous work "home" to start their own businesses or change careers. Still others are simply forced by life circumstances onto a new path.

The breadth of a woman's interests and contacts outside the home during the childbearing and career-building years will have an impact on the ease with which she moves into her new life. Some experimentation may be required before a woman can discover where her passions lie, and it may take longer for some to find their niche than others. Those who continue to define themselves by the roles they no longer have—such as mother or wife or even daughter or sister—and who have long lived enclosed in those roles may be overwhelmed by fear and lapse into immobility. But the key to finding new passions is getting out and getting moving, even if you don't know where you are going. Sometimes it's simply a matter of stumbling from point A to point B with your eyes wide open to the possibilities.

SYLVIA: Discovering the Artist

Sylvia retired from teaching the same year her youngest son married and moved to California. It was difficult for her to simultaneously relinquish her role of mother and mentor to her own children as well as to the third-grade students she'd taught for the past twenty-five years. She kept in contact with me through the grieving process, and she admitted there were times she felt she'd never find herself.

"Everything about who I am is wrapped up in kids," she wrote. "On one hand, the extra free time made it more difficult, because I didn't know what to do with myself. The days were so long and bleak." But in retrospect that time was a luxury, because it allowed her to give focused attention to her feelings and let them out—loud and clear. "My husband continued to go to work, so I was able to cry out loud, wail, even roar in frustration. I made some pretty anguished, animal-like sounds alone in that house—just me and those powerful feelings, bouncing off the walls."

Then, a few weeks later, Sylvia started looking at her house as though it were real estate she was contemplating buying—it had lots of potential but needed adjustments to fit her new life. She knocked down walls and incorporated the kids' rooms into the main living space, creating a great room that could accommodate her monthly meetings with local career women who gathered for the camaraderie and to share new skills, projects, and philosophies. Sylvia did much of the remodeling work herself, despite never having hung wallboard or laid ceramic tile before. When it was Sylvia's turn to demonstrate a new skill to the group, she showed them the tilework she'd done in her bathroom. Sylvia started tiling bathrooms for her friends, using handmade tiles and innovative patterns. What started out as a project spanning several weekends has turned into a second profession: two years later, through word of mouth, she has landed clients as far away as New York, and she's hired and trained two women to help her keep up with the demand. "I love the travel—I've always been a homebody, and I never went anywhere without my husband. Now I traipse off to visit beautiful homes and work my magic to make those homes even more beautiful, while my husband stays here and runs the household. Several clients asked me to sign my name on a prominent tile in their finished bathroom, like an artist signs paintings. I feel exhilarated and free as a bird. I love this new life."

JUDITH: *Finding Her True Vocation*

For many women, the key to finding their niche at midlife is in identifying the passions they've always had but never pursued full-time. At fifty-four, after more than thirty years in the corporate world, Judith chose to take early retirement. Having looked back over her many years of doing volunteer work, she realized that caring for the elderly was a dream she wanted to pursue. Rather than make excuses for herself because of her age, she undertook a demanding graduate program to prepare for her new work. She wrote:

> I chose to leave my position as a business analyst and embark on a career change. I left with a mission statement: to dedicate my life work to the self-enlightenment, creative development, and joy of being an elder, and to provide services to elders that enhance their physical, mental, and spiritual growth. I interviewed with daycare directors and program managers while continuing my volunteer efforts by delivering hot meals to elderly shut-ins. This past June I completed the required coursework and internship for a master's degree in gerontological psychology.
>
> I have learned that although it can be extremely painful at times, it is only through the process of transition, with eyes and heart wide open, that an individual can truly succeed in personal growth. Now I feel the excitement and fear of taking my plan to fruition—actually doing what I have been studying and talking about doing! My daughter says, "Mom, who will hire you at your age?" My husband wishes me to succeed. I know I have unlimited inner resources and that new birth is emerging as I enter this new phase of my life.

Many midlife women discover that as they find new direction in life, they themselves become new, and so they attract new friends. One patient put it to me this way: "I became more interesting. I had more to offer on a personal level—I had more to talk about than kids and soccer practice and my husband's promotion. This new me is someone I really like!"

A ROAD MAP FOR NAVIGATING UNKNOWN TERRITORY

Taking those first steps on your journey home to yourself may be one of the hardest things you'll ever do. But as you venture onto this new path you will find that it loses its intimidating aspects and becomes instead a voyage of exploration and discovery. Here are a few signposts to help you along.

TAKE HEART: Though painful, your feelings of loneliness, like all feelings, will gradually lessen and change as time goes on, especially as you choose new and healthier ways of thinking and being in the world. Be present for your own experience while it's happening. The depth to which you allow yourself to feel pain is the depth to which you will also feel joy. And you have to trust that joy will come again, even though your life will never be exactly the same again. The news is good. I've been hearing about it for years. And I'm a living example myself.

One of my newsletter subscribers wrote:

I haven't felt this good since the whole nonsense started in my early teens. After a hideous perimenopausal epoch in my forties, I look forward to my fifty-second birthday with a big smile! All those years of chasing relationships to make my identity! I now live blissfully alone (except for Harriet the cat) and have an interesting relationship with an unusual man that does not define me. Even though my body will no longer put up with whatever I want to do to it, the aches and pains are treated with acceptance and equanimity. Life is filled with possibilities and delightful friendships, home and garden, dancing the Argentine tango, travel, lots else to do—but great respect for quiet, restful, self-indulgent times.

EMBRACE THE WISDOM OF ROUTINE AND DISCIPLINE: Either start or continue at least one activity that is scheduled regularly. I recently learned that the word *discipline* comes from the Latin word *disciplina,* which means "instruction" or "knowledge." At midlife when we are being asked to heed the dictates of our souls, the discipline we require is that of listening to our inner beings—and not letting ourselves be distracted so much by outside influences. And so it's not outside discipline to get you to "behave" that is important. It is the discipline of listening to your innermost self and setting up your life to make that a priority.

You cannot imagine how healing a regular routine is. In my case, this routine includes daily exercise and a twice-weekly Pilates class. Pilates is a demanding type of exercise that involves moving from and focusing one's attention on what is known as one's "center" or "powerhouse," the muscles of the deep pelvis, buttocks, and abdomen that form a band around the lower body. No matter what else is going on in my life, I make the time to go to the studio and work on the link between my muscles, my brain, and my emotions. The sameness of it and the discipline involved in this activity are very anchoring for me—a part of my life that hasn't changed or gone away. In fact, on the morning my husband left, I went to my class as usual. Though I had no idea what would happen to our marriage at the time, and though my heart was racing and I was scared, getting on the Pilates equipment and going through my usual routine was very calming and reassuring. Though a significant part of my world was falling apart, I could still concentrate on my breathing, the strength of my muscles—and the fact that the planet was going to keep spinning. Pilates has been a key discipline that has transformed my body, mind, and spirit, making all of me stronger and more flexible than ever before.

ENHANCE YOUR DAILY LIFE: In the first few months of my almost-empty nest—my younger daughter was still home but deeply involved in her own activities—I began the practice of lighting a fire every night and keeping the doors of the woodstove open so that I could enjoy watching the flames as I ate dinner. In all our years of marriage, my husband and I had rarely opened the doors of this stove because it lessens the amount of heat that is produced. But now I was much less interested in thermodynamics and instead simply wanted to bring the comfort of firelight into my home—especially at dinnertime, when the prospect of facing an evening alone loomed large before me. I also lit candles at dinner each night and played my favorite music. Six months later, when my second daughter left for her first semester away and I was truly faced with being alone every night, I was determined to use my time to tune in to and deepen my relationship with myself and my spirit. Mostly I wanted to heal the parts of myself that had led to my need to go through a divorce in the first place. And I wanted to get comfortable enough being alone in my home that I didn't need to jump into a new relationship right away just to avoid the pain of my husband's and daughters' absences. I knew that to do so might result in a relationship that simply repeated old, unhealed patterns. I've noticed that the people who allow themselves this time tend to end up with much healthier and happier relationships down the road.

KNOW THAT THE FEAR OF LOSS IS OFTEN WORSE THAN THE ACTUAL LOSS: I found that my dread of the empty nest was much worse than the actual experience. In fact, I was so busy with work that I enjoyed having only myself to take care of. I learned that I liked reading in bed as late as I wanted to, going to as many movies as I felt like, taking a bath at any hour of the day or night, and generally discovering what my own needs and desires actually were. Though I had originally planned to have my mother come visit and go skiing with me during my first empty-nest winter, the time flew by so quickly that we never got around to it. Nevertheless, it felt good to know that she was willing to come and provide support and recreation if I needed it.

REMEMBER THAT WE'RE STRONGER AND MORE RESILIENT THAN WE MAY THINK: On the day that would have been my twenty-fifth wedding anniversary, I awoke and just stayed in bed, allowing myself to experience my emotions for a few minutes. I hadn't made it to the quarter-century mark in my marriage, and I felt bad about that. I thought I might spend the whole day feeling sad. But to my surprise, I didn't. Diane, a woman who has worked with me for decades (she was my first office nurse and now runs everything in my business), gave me a funny card. On the cover there was a ridiculous photo of a muscular man dressed up in a tutu with a snake draped over his shoulder. When you opened the card, the greeting read, "Still looking for Mr. Right!" I laughed out loud and put the card in my journal. Later I went out to dinner to celebrate a friend's birthday. The day came and went, and I stayed calm and happy. The previous year my heart had been breaking on the day of my anniversary, and I'd dissolved into tears at dinner that night with my two daughters. One year later I was renewed and at peace. Now, years later, I've pretty much forgotten all about my wedding anniversary. It almost feels as though that prior life never even happened! But that is only because I've completely worked through all the lessons and growth challenges that were presented to me.

I won't pretend that going through a divorce and seeing both my daughters leave in the same year was easy. That first empty-nest year was the most difficult time of my life, as I experienced the crumbling of everything I had always thought I could count on. Paradoxically, that year also proved to be one of the most strengthening and exhilarating of my entire life. Looking back, I marvel at how far I've come. By turning my life over to Source energy and being willing to roll up my sleeves and rebuild my life, I've become infused with the vitality of hope, joy, and new beginnings. Every day I'm reminded that the energy that supports new life abounds. We just have to believe in it, surrender to it, and ask for help.

4

This Can't Be Menopause, Can It?
The Physical Foundation
of the Change

Many women are caught off guard by the first signs of the climacteric. They don't expect symptoms to occur until they've reached the end point—the absolute cessation of periods. But a woman's last period is usually preceded by a long period of transition, which may include symptoms such as hot flashes, mood swings, difficulty sleeping, irritability, and night sweats. In fact, so-called menopausal symptoms are worse during perimenopause and then usually cease within a year or so after the last period.

Doreen was a vital, youthful-looking woman of forty-six when she had her first hot flash. She'd noticed a certain irritability in the way she related to her husband, who had begun to tease her about being menopausal, but she adamantly denied the possibility. "I'm still having my periods like clockwork," she argued. "My mom was fifty-three when she hit menopause. I'm not old enough to be going through the change!"

It is true that the age at which a woman's mother had her last period is probably the best predictor of when it will happen to her. (Though there are certainly exceptions.) But if she doesn't understand that the first symptoms of the climacteric may reveal themselves well before that time—sometimes ten or more years earlier—she is likely to protest, as with Doreen, "This can't be menopause . . . can it?"

The quick answer is this: if you have reason to ask, then it probably is.

WHAT IS HAPPENING IN YOUR BODY: HORMONAL CHANGES

Menopause is officially defined as that point in time when our periods stop permanently. A woman undergoing natural menopause really has no way of knowing whether any given period is truly her last until a year has passed. As menopause approaches, cycles can become quite erratic, and it's not uncommon for several months to go by between periods. By the age of forty some of the initial hormonal changes associated with perimenopause (*peri* means "around" or "near") are well under way. Research has shown, for example, that by age forty many women have already undergone changes in bone density, and by age forty-four many have begun to experience periods that are either lighter and/or shorter in length than usual, or heavier and/or longer. About 80 percent of women begin skipping periods altogether.[1] In fact, only about 10 percent of women cease menstruating altogether with no prolonged period of cycle irregularity beforehand. In an extensive study of more than 2,700 women, most experienced a perimenopausal transition lasting between two and eight years.[2] And there are also exceptions to all of this—I've seen women who cycle regularly until their late fifties!

MOTHERHOOD OVER FORTY

Thanks to a variety of factors (including women delaying childbearing because of their careers), the number of older mothers today is skyrocketing. The birthrate for women in their forties has increased by 3 percent every year since 1982.[3] When a woman is going through menopause, her focus is turned inward, so attending to the needs of a five-year-old can be challenging when all she wants to do is go into a cave and meditate. (An excellent resource for older mothers is the book *Hot Flashes, Warm Bottles: First-Time Mothers over Forty* [Celestial Arts, 2001] by therapist Nancy London, herself a midlife mother, as well as *Midlife Motherhood: A Mother-to-Mother Guide to Pregnancy and Parenting* [St. Martin's Griffin, 2002] by Jann Blackstone-Ford. The blog "Motherhood Later . . . than Sooner" [motherhoodlater.com] provides good information as well.)

On the other hand, the research of Harvard professor Ellen Langer, Ph.D., documented in her book *Counterclockwise* (Ballantine, 2009), reveals that older mothers actually live longer. Dr. Langer explains that this is because they are primed to act and feel young by the cues they receive in their environment, because they're always around younger people. The flipside of this concept is also worth considering: when people expect us to act old and disabled, we *do*!

Unless you've gone into menopause abruptly because of surgery or medical treatment, perimenopause can be thought of as the other end of a process that began when you first started your periods. That first menstrual period is usually followed by five to seven years of relatively long cycles that are often irregular and frequently anovulatory. Eventually, in the late teens or early twenties, cycle length shortens and becomes more regular as a woman reaches her prime reproductive age, which lasts for the next twenty years or so. In our forties, our cycles begin to lengthen again. Though most of us have been led to believe that twenty-eight days is the normal cycle length, research has shown that only 12.4 percent of women actually have a twenty-eight-day cycle. The vast majority have cycles that last anywhere between twenty-four and thirty-five days, and 20 percent of all women experience irregular cycles.[4]

Two to eight years prior to menopause, most women begin skipping ovulations. During these years, the ovarian follicles, which ripen eggs each month, undergo an accelerated rate of loss, until the supply of follicles is finally depleted. Research suggests that, in this culture at least, the acceleration in follicle loss begins around age thirty-seven or thirty-eight. Inhibin, a substance produced by the ovaries, decreases, which results in rising levels of FSH, the follicle-stimulating hormone produced by the pituitary gland. (This doesn't mean you can't get pregnant. For further information about fertility during this time, see my book *Women's Bodies, Women's Wisdom,* chapter 11, "Our Fertility.")

Contrary to the standard belief, our estrogen levels often remain relatively stable or even increase during perimenopause. They don't wane until less than a year before the last menstrual period.[5] Until menopause, the primary estrogen a woman's body produces is estradiol. However, during perimenopause the body starts making more of a different kind of estrogen, called estrone, which is produced both in the ovaries and in body fat.

Testosterone levels usually do not fall appreciably during perimenopause. In fact, the postmenopausal ovaries of many women (but not all) secrete more testosterone than the premenopausal ovaries.

On the other hand, progesterone levels do begin to fall in perimenopause, often long before changes in estrogen or testosterone. As I will discuss below, this is the most significant perimenopausal issue for the majority of women.

The prevailing message appears to be this: although reproduction is no longer the goal, there continue to be important roles for these so-called reproductive hormones—vital, health-enhancing roles that have nothing to do with making babies. Evidence for this can be seen in the fact that steroid hormone receptors are found in almost every organ of our bodies. Estrogen and androgens (like testosterone) are important, for example, in maintaining strong and healthy bones as well as resilient vaginal and urethral tissue. And both estrogen and progesterone are important for maintaining a healthy collagen layer in the skin.

PERIMENOPAUSE IS A NORMAL PROCESS, NOT A DISEASE

The main thing to keep in mind about perimenopause is that it's a completely normal process, not a disease to be treated. But in order for her body to continue producing levels of hormones adequate to support health, a woman must be optimally healthy going in—physically, emotionally, spiritually, and situationally. In other words, her future well-being depends not only on the health of her physical body but also on her emotional, mental, and social support systems, all of which are a reflection of how she cares for herself today and how she has lived up to this point. Because perimenopause occurs at the midpoint of our lives, it is a very good time to take stock and make sure that we are doing everything possible to restore or build our health.

Despite all the media focus on supplemental hormones—which ones to take, what dose, natural versus synthetic, and so on—it is important to bear in mind this often-forgotten fact: a woman's body begins life fully equipped to produce all the hormones she needs throughout life. All of the so-called sex hormones (estrogen, progesterone, and the androgens) are manufactured from the same ubiquitous precursor molecule—cholesterol. In addition, our bodies also have the ability to convert one type of sex hormone into another. So, for example, estrogen can be converted into testosterone, and progesterone can be converted into estrogen. Whether or not these conversions actually take place depends upon our body's minute-to-minute needs, our emotional states, our nutritional states, and so on.

What all this means is that not every woman will need or want hormone supplementation. In many cultures hormone supplements are infrequently prescribed, yet women in those cultures rarely have uncomfortable perimenopausal symptoms. How can this be?

First of all, the ovaries only slow down; they do not shut down. Moreover, a woman's body is designed to produce estrogen, progesterone, and testosterone at other sites besides the ovaries, and it is ready and willing to increase or mediate the output from those auxiliary sites when the need arises at midlife. Research has shown, for example, that estrogen, progesterone, and androgen are produced in body fat, skin, the brain, the adrenal glands, and even peripheral nerves! But whether or not adequate production occurs depends on what else is going on in a woman's life.

If, for example, a woman is under significant stress—if she is overworked, if her diet fails to meet her body's needs, if she is physically ill, if she smokes and/or drinks, if she is avoiding spiritual issues that are beckoning her, or if she is involved in relationships in which the energy outflow is not matched by the energy coming back—then she may find that her ability to keep up with the demands on her endocrine system is diminished. It will remain so unless and until she is able to implement some changes in those areas of her life that need work. The result may be a tumultuous midlife transition, fraught with her own individual combination of symptoms—from headaches, hot flashes, bloating, and fading libido to mood swings and sleep disturbances.

Given the nature of our current culture, with its ever-accelerating

pace of life, about 75 percent of perimenopausal women have symptoms of menopause that are uncomfortable enough to cause them to
seek relief, whether through supplemental hormones, antidepressant
drugs, dietary change, exercise, or alternative therapies. If a woman
finds that she needs supplemental hormones in order to reestablish a
physical and emotional comfort zone, this should not be seen as a
personal failure. Rather, it is a wake-up call and an opportunity to
implement much-needed change. A woman in this situation might

FIGURE 7: HORMONE-PRODUCING BODY SITES

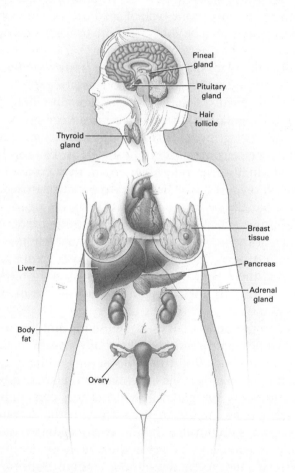

The healthy body is equipped to produce all the hormones a woman
needs throughout her life. This natural ability can be supported or
thwarted, depending on lifestyle patterns and the state of a woman's
health—physically, emotionally, spiritually, and situationally.

want to consider trying some tried-and-true herbal remedies that have enjoyed centuries of safe use, such as *Pueraria mirifica* or maca, or accepting what I like to call a dusting of supplemental hormones—just enough to provide her with the support she needs for comfort and health, and no more. At the same time she would also be wise to pay attention to the messages her body is sending. It is asking for more than just a prescription or a supplement.

The bottom line is this: before you take something to relieve menopausal symptoms, acknowledge and listen to your body's inner wisdom in creating those outward symptoms. They are uniquely yours. How your hormones behave during perimenopause and how your body and mind respond to hormonal changes is as personalized as your fingerprints.

THE THREE TYPES OF MENOPAUSE

Imagine that you are standing at the foot of a beautiful mountain. You can see the light shining from behind the peak, and you're eager to enjoy the view from the top. There are three ways to get there: you can take the gradually sloping, winding path, which may require you to climb over a few rocks now and then. You can take the short path up, which is much more difficult and will require more equipment and technical support. Or you can skip the climb altogether and have someone else take you up via helicopter—which sounds easy until you realize that your muscles and organs will not have had the time or the conditioning to cope with the cold and lack of oxygen at the summit.

~ NATURAL MENOPAUSE (the sloping, winding path) occurs gradually, usually between ages forty-five and fifty-five, in a woman who has at least one of her ovaries. Duration, in most cases, is five to ten years, though the entire process sometimes takes up to thirteen years. During this time, periods may stop for several months and then return, and they may increase or decrease in duration, intensity, and flow. All other things being equal, women who are going through a natural menopause may or may not need any treatment for the sake of physical comfort, because their overall health may be strong enough, and their transition may be occurring gradually enough, for their bodies to keep up with the changing demands. It will depend, in other words, on what else is going on in their bodies and in their lives. Though the medical literature is currently rife with the concept of a "critical window" of time following the final menstrual period when estrogen must be supplemented in order to prevent future dementia, there is no good reason for a healthy, vital woman to start taking a prescription with many side effects simply out of fear. (For a fuller discussion of the "critical window" concept, see chapter 5, "Hormone Therapy: An Individual Choice.")

~ PREMATURE MENOPAUSE (the short path) occurs somewhat faster as well as earlier, in women in their thirties or early forties who have at least one ovary. Approximately one in a hundred women completes the menopausal transition by age forty or younger. She may have an illness (such as a so-called autoimmune disease or nutritional deficiency) or some chronic stress (including excessive athletic conditioning) that has adversely affected hormone-related reproductive functions. Duration usually is shorter than natural menopause, one to three years. Because the transition is quicker, and because the early change is often linked to a preexisting physical condition, there is a strong likelihood a woman undergoing premature menopause will need supplemental hormones during the adjustment.[6]

~ ARTIFICIAL MENOPAUSE (the helicopter ride) can occur quite abruptly, induced by surgical removal or disruption of the reproductive tract (including removal of ovaries or surgical disruption of the blood supply to the ovaries), by radiation or chemotherapy, or by administration of certain drugs that induce or mimic menopause for medical reasons (such as to shrink uterine fibroids).

Even tubal ligation—at least in the past—has been shown to lower progesterone levels for at least a year following the procedure.[7] And many women who undergo hysterectomy *with* preservation of their ovaries experience symptoms of hormonal change—in addition, of course, to the loss of their periods.

Approximately one in every four American women will enter an abrupt, artificial menopause. Because there's no opportunity for gradual adjustment to the hormonal drop-off, the symptoms of artificial menopause can be severe and debilitating. Almost invariably, supplemental hormone therapy is elected in order to alleviate physical discomfort.

PATTI: *Artificial Menopause*

Six weeks after vague symptoms (night sweats, weight loss, and a persistent rash in her bikini area) had been misdiagnosed at an urgent-care center as "perimenopause and stress," Patti, a forty-one-year-old single mother and owner of a small business, was diagnosed with Hodgkin's disease, a type of lymphoma. Two six-week courses of chemotherapy left her feeling temporarily exhausted and without her curly blond hair . . . but cured. The one side effect that turned out not to be temporary was the loss of her periods.

She wrote, "A couple of weeks after the chemo was over, when I began to get some of my energy back, I started having night sweats again. This scared me, because I thought it was the cancer coming back, and I thought my mood swings were just due to the constant worry." Her internist ran hormone tests and confirmed that Patti had undergone menopause, and she prescribed the appropriate hormone replacement therapy in the form of a skin patch, which gave Patti's body gentle doses of hormone slowly, throughout the day and night. "I felt much better within just a few days, and I think in my condition—after all I'd been through—it really helped me recover quicker, because my body was pretty traumatized and my mind was frazzled."

PERIMENOPAUSE AND HORMONAL LEVELS

The conventional view of what happens at perimenopause is that estrogen levels plummet. This is a gross oversimplification and too often leads to treatment that can make mildly uncomfortable symptoms worse. In natural menopause, the first hormonal change that occurs is a gradual decline in levels of progesterone, while estrogen levels remain within the normal range or even increase. Because progesterone and estrogen are meant to counterbalance each other throughout the menstrual cycle, with one falling while the other rises and vice versa, an overall decline in progesterone allows estrogen levels to go unopposed—that is, without the usual counterbalance. The result is a relative *excess* of estrogen, a condition that is often called estrogen dominance—which is precisely the opposite of the conventional view.

If a woman begins to experience uncomfortable symptoms at this stage, it's because her body can sense—and attempts to adjust to—that relative estrogen excess. Estrogen excess is also exacerbated by high insulin and stress hormones. And, quite frankly, high insulin levels and what is called insulin resistance have reached epidemic proportions. There's a great deal of overlap in the symptoms of various hormone imbalances, and it's not uncommon for a woman experiencing symptoms of estrogen or stress hormone excess to be given a prescription for more estrogen or even antidepressants. Not surprisingly, her mild symptoms can worsen as a result.

As the transition goes on, progesterone continues to decline, and eventually estrogen levels may begin to swing widely. The estrogen highs occur because the ovaries have begun to allow entire groups of follicles to grow and mature during successive menstrual cycles, instead of only one at a time, as though attempting to hurriedly "spend" those remaining eggs. (This is the reason why the incidence of twin pregnancies increases with age.) The progesterone decline occurs because fewer and fewer of those maturing eggs actually complete the entire ovulation process.

Levels of the hormones FSH and LH, which the pituitary gland in the brain normally releases in precisely metered amounts to stimulate controlled follicular growth and ovulation, become erratic as our ovaries start to skip ovulations. Closer to menopause, hormonal levels start to stabilize. FSH and LH levels smooth out and climb to their new, higher cruising altitude, where they stay for the rest of our lives.

SYMPTOMS OF DECREASED PROGESTERONE AND ESTROGEN DOMINANCE

~ Decreased sex drive
~ Irregular or otherwise abnormal periods (most often, excessive vaginal bleeding)
~ Bloating (water retention)
~ Breast swelling and tenderness
~ Mood swings (most often irritability and depression)
~ Weight gain (particularly around the abdomen and hips)
~ Cold hands and feet
~ Headaches, especially premenstrually

IS THERE A TEST I CAN TAKE?

For years the diagnosis of menopause was simply based on your age and symptoms. Now it's becoming more mainstream to use laboratory confirmation of your hormone levels. Here's why: First, as illustrated by the story of Patti, there are illnesses that mimic perimenopause rather convincingly. (Hypothyroidism is another example; see page 136.) By having your entrance into the climacteric confirmed, you'll simultaneously be ruling out an unexpected medical problem. Second, by determining your levels of the relevant hormones—estrogen, progesterone, and testosterone, and possibly DHEA and thyroid hormone as well—you and your healthcare provider can better determine where you stand in the perimenopausal timeline and what approach to take to your symptoms, if any. One caveat about hormone testing: menopausal symptoms do not necessarily correlate well with hormone levels. For example, many women with low testosterone levels have normal libido. And some women with normal testosterone levels have low libido. Bottom line: it can be useful to get your hormone levels tested. But it's far more useful to tune in to how you're feeling rather than focus on a lab test, which gives, after all, just a single snapshot of an ever-changing process.

If you decide to seek laboratory confirmation, it is important that you understand what tests are available, and what they can (and cannot) reveal about your current status.

Hormone Levels: FSH and LH

The testing method employed by many medical practices is to test FSH and/or LH levels through either blood or saliva. This is based on the fact that at menopause and thereafter, a woman's FSH and LH levels rise to their highest ever. But there are problems with this method. First of all, it will tell you nothing about estrogen levels, because FSH is controlled by inhibin, not by estrogen. (This is one of the reasons why estrogen replacement doesn't decrease FSH levels after menopause.)[8] In addition, during the five or ten years of perimenopause—before menstruation ceases for good—FSH and LH levels can fluctuate widely. The ovaries may become inactive for a few days or weeks and then resume production of eggs. It is possible, for example, for a woman's FSH levels to reach postmenopausal levels (greater than 30 IU/1 for blood) while she is still having normal periods. Her LH levels, meanwhile, will remain in the normal premenopausal range. For that reason, a single high FSH/LH level can't be used to determine whether or not a woman is in menopause. Until a woman has had no periods for a year and has FSH/LH levels well within the postmenopausal range—FSH greater than 30 IU/1 and LH greater than 40 IU/1—it is even possible for her to get pregnant. This is why it's prudent to use contraception for a year after you think your periods have stopped.

Hormone Levels: Estrogen, Progesterone, and Testosterone

Another common blood test analyzes the total amount of estrogen, progesterone, and testosterone in the bloodstream. The largest drawback to this method is that most of the hormone so measured is inactive. The healthy woman's body produces upward of ten times more of these hormones than she can use, so specialized proteins hook themselves to more than 90 percent of the hormone molecules produced, inactivate them, and lock the "doors" that would otherwise allow them to leave the bloodstream and enter the tissues. The biologically active form of the hormone is the part that is unbound or free. This goes quickly into the tissues instead of hanging around in the bloodstream. Thus the standard blood test, which does not distinguish bound from free hormone, will give an irrelevant result, because it measures primarily inactive, unusable, protein-bound hormone.

Preferred Testing Methods

With the individualized approach to menopause that has become the new standard of care, many clinicians are finding that measuring hormone levels can provide helpful information for balancing hormones through either nutritional means or bioidentical hormone replacement. Blood tests are the usually agreed-upon standard for hormone testing. But the newer DUTCH test (dried urine test for comprehensive hormones), which measures urinary hormones over a twenty-four-hour period, gives a much broader picture of what is happening hormonally than do blood tests. In addition to sex hormones, the DUTCH test also measures cortisol to determine whether high levels of stress are involved with symptoms. The test is available from Precision Analytical (503-687-2050; dutchtest.com). Salivary testing is another good option for measuring levels of sex hormones, cortisol, DHEA, and melatonin. Laboratories that can do the saliva testing with a doctor's prescription include Genova Diagnostics (800-522-4762; www.gdx.net).

These newer tests are extremely useful because blood levels of hormones do not reflect the level of hormone in the actual tissues of the body, where the hormones have their effects. There is evidence that salivary or urinary levels are a more accurate reflection of this activity.[9] In addition, blood tests measure a single value taken at a specific time—even though hormones are secreted in spurts about every two hours. The difference between the highest point and the lowest point can be up to 500 percent![10] Salivary or urinary testing, on the other hand, can involve taking a total of four to eight samples throughout the day, about three hours apart, to account for this variability. Another advantage of these tests is that they can easily be done at home without the stress of having to go to a lab and have your blood drawn—an activity that in and of itself can alter hormone levels.

The challenge with such home testing, however, is that it is so far not covered by most insurance companies, so women who opt for it have to pay the entire expense out-of-pocket (which can be as high as several hundred dollars per test, depending on the specific testing profile you select). Furthermore, the chance for human error in taking the salivary sample is higher because both food residue and blood from bleeding gums or a sore in the mouth can contaminate the samples. That said, there are many clinicians, particularly naturopaths, who use salivary hormone levels with good results. And some research exists to show that salivary levels of testosterone in particular can indeed be useful.[11] So the bottom line is this: go with the type of testing that your healthcare provider is most comfortable with. At the end of the day, he or she is treating you, not a lab test!

The good news is that more and more research in the area of hormone metabolism is being done. New and improved FDA-approved assays are now available that measure not only biologically active levels of estrogen, progesterone, and testosterone, but also their breakdown products. A growing body of research is showing that hormone balance can affect bone turnover, lipid metabolism, and immune function, as well as hormone-dependent cancers, including breast and uterine. Since hormone levels can be easily modified by changes in lifestyle, including supplementation, diet, exercise, and possible hormone replacement, it is probably worthwhile to have a hormone profile done (either blood, urine, or saliva) if you're having a lot of symptoms, or if you are planning on using hormone replacement. It's important to work with a healthcare practitioner who is familiar with this kind of hormone testing. The specific tests I recommend include the Menopause Check Plus profile from Genova Diagnostics and the Dutch Complete and Dutch Plus tests from Precision Analytical.

How and When to Test

If you're having symptoms and are actively working with a program to improve hormone balance, I recommend checking your levels both before and after treatment. In an ideal world, it would be good if everyone could get a couple of different sets of hormone tests before embarking on therapy. But in the real world, it's hard enough for most women to schedule any testing at all before getting treatment. Just remember that regardless of what your tests say, your hormone levels can and do fluctuate widely during the month and even throughout the day. The best time of day to collect a sample is the early morning (especially for testosterone levels), and the best time of the month is between days 20 and 23 of your menstrual cycle, when progesterone levels are apt to be highest.

Because hormone levels so often normalize or improve with life-style changes, it's also empowering to see how well you're doing in follow-up testing. Just remember: how you feel is a much more accurate measure of your hormone balance than any test.

MENOPAUSE AND THYROID FUNCTION

The ovaries are the organs that we focus on most commonly at menopause, but the physical foundation of a woman's menopausal experience actually rests on the health of all her endocrine (hormone-producing) organs. This is especially true of the thyroid, which acts as a major coordinator of the entire endocrine system. Thyroid problems are very common during the perimenopausal and postmenopausal years. While many women with these problems are completely asymptomatic, others may have a wide variety of symptoms that often match those we associate with perimenopause. These include mood disturbances (most often seen in the form of depression and irritability), low energy level, weight gain, mental confusion, and sleep disturbances.

Thyroid problems are intimately intertwined with menopause, and not just because of the epidemiological fact that about 26 percent of women in or near perimenopause are diagnosed with hypothyroidism.[12] According to the late John R. Lee, M.D., a noted clinician and author, there appears to be a cause-and-effect relationship between hypothyroidism, in which there are inadequate levels of thyroid hormone, and estrogen dominance. When estrogen is not properly counterbalanced with progesterone, it can block the action of the thyroid hormone, so even when the thyroid is producing normal levels of the hormone, the hormone is rendered ineffective and the symptoms of hypothyroidism appear. In this case, laboratory tests may show normal thyroid hormone levels in a woman's system, because the thyroid gland itself is not malfunctioning.

It is no surprise, then, that this problem is compounded when a woman is prescribed supplemental estrogen, leading to an even greater imbalance. In that circumstance, a prescription for supplemental thyroid hormone will fail to correct the underlying problem: estrogen dominance. Estrogen dominance and also glycemic stress (see chapter 7, "Six Steps to Midlife Weight Control") are very often accompanied by high adrenaline levels. And this metabolic situation can exacerbate thyroid problems. Here's what happens. Adrenaline stimulates the sympathetic nervous system, as does glycemic stress. It can also stimulate the growth of EBV (Epstein-Barr virus), which is associated with thyroid problems (see below). Adrenaline and cortisol from the adrenals stimulate the heart rate and blood pressure, which can lead to palpitations. But it also causes estrogen to be metabolized into substances known as catechols—estrogens that themselves have adrenaline-like effects. The main thyroid hormone, thyroxine, stimulates the heart and the sympathetic nervous system. To adjust to the already too-high level of adrenaline in the system, the thyroid gland often shuts down a little to lower thyroxine stimulation—which is reflected in slightly high levels of thyroid-stimulating hormone (TSH).

Hypothyroidism can be confusing because there's a continuum between overt and subclinical hypothyroidism, with a great deal of overlap between the two. Depending upon which expert you talk with and which criteria are used for the diagnosis, as many as 25 percent of perimenopausal women have some kind of thyroid problem. Most of these are cases of subclinical hypothyroidism. With this condition, although symptoms may be present, tests of thyroid function are only slightly abnormal (TSH of 0.5–5.0, with normal levels of triiodothyronine, or T3, and thyroxine, or T4). According to the American Association of Clinical Endocrinologists, the upper limit for TSH should be only about 3.0, not the higher number of 5.0 or more (although many experts, including myself, are more comfortable setting the limit at 2.5).[13] Unfortunately, most labs still report 5.0 to 5.5 as the upper limit of normal. Hence, thousands of women who could use thyroid support, through taking thyroid hormone and/or iodine, are told that their tests are normal when they are not.

Thyroid Function, Hashimoto's Disease, and the Epstein-Barr Virus (EBV)

As a physician, I have always found thyroid testing and thyroid function very confusing, especially since tests so often fail to provide a clear diagnosis and treatment path. The conventional approach—to just give prescription synthetic thyroid hormone (e.g., thyroxine) instead of figuring out how to support optimal thyroid function—never made sense to me. When I learned about the association between certain types of Epstein-Barr viruses and thyroid function from the renowned Medical Medium, Anthony William, a fellow Mainer and author of *Medical Medium Thyroid Healing: The Truth Behind Hashimoto's, Graves, Insomnia, Hypothyroid, Thyroid Nodules & Epstein-Barr* (Hay House, 2017), a far clearer picture emerged.

William's explanation of what is really going on with thyroid function—at least at the physical level—makes perfect sense to me even though it is not yet accepted by mainstream medicine. Let's start with a brief overview of the Epstein-Barr virus (EBV). EBV is a member of the herpes family of viruses and is conventionally known as herpes type 4. The herpes group also includes the mononucleosis virus (which causes what's called the "kissing disease" because it is spread through bodily fluids, including saliva) as well as the viruses that cause genital herpes (herpes type 2) and oral herpes (type 1, which causes cold sores). The chickenpox and shingles viruses are herpes viruses too; in fact, the shingles virus is simply the chickenpox virus at another stage. EBV is also considered the causative agent of fibromyalgia and chronic fatigue syndrome. Williams points out that there are dozens and dozens of different types of Epstein-Barr viruses, many of which have yet to be identified. Some are more virulent than others. But here's the thing: while more than 90 percent of the population has been exposed to at least a couple of different types of EBV, most of these viruses remain dormant—a benign part of the body's overall bacterial and viral environment, known as the microbiome. When an individual is well nourished, rested, and under little stress, the EBV just remains a part of this microbiome—an enormous community of bacteria, viruses, and fungi that live peacefully on our skin, in our guts, and in our genital tracts, as well as in our ears, eyes, noses, and throats. As a matter of fact, our bodies are host to three times more bacteria and viruses than we have human cells! Some of the most important health discoveries of the last decade have demonstrated how important this microbiome is to healthy functioning of the body. So we naturally have viruses in us at all times—and most of the time they don't cause any trouble. The only time a virus, bacterium, or fungus becomes capable of causing disease is when a person's endocrine, immune, or central nervous system becomes compromised by some kind of stress, resulting in the unchecked growth of the microorganism in various organs and with various effects. And that is precisely what happens with EBV and the thyroid.

Here's how it works. Let's say you go to college and the stress of being away from home, staying up too late, drinking too much, eating poorly, and cramming for exams results in a compromised immune system and a case of mononucleosis. You become so fatigued that you might have to drop out for a semester and come home and rest. Eventually your body's immune system quells the viral infection in that stage and you go back to living a normal life. Meanwhile, the virus lies dormant in your system, not causing any particular problems. Williams points out that EBV actually goes through four stages. The first stage is when you're exposed and the virus is in the bloodstream. Stage two is when the virus springs to life and results in something like mononucleosis or chronic fatigue syndrome. Meanwhile, the virus seeks out a home in the infected person's organs (usually the spleen or liver), where it can lie dormant for many months or even years. The only symptom might be occasional tiredness or a scratchy throat.

In stage 3, the virus enters the thyroid. And this can result in either very subtle or very dramatic symptoms, depending upon the type of EBV involved (Williams says there are more than sixty) and how fast it's growing. Over time, if left unchecked, the virus drills deep into thyroid tissue, resulting in scarring and impeded function. In this weakened state, the thyroid becomes less able to do its job. This is called hypothyroidism or an underactive thyroid. But according to Williams, the symptoms of hypothyroidism—fatigue, weight gain, muscle weakness, mood changes, and hair loss—are merely symptoms of the virus itself, not of a lack of thyroid hormone.

What About Hashimoto's Thyroiditis?

Williams points out that when certain types of EBV invade the thyroid, the body's immune system goes after the viruses with full force. This results in inflammation of the thyroid tissue and the production of antithyroid antibodies. It has been assumed that these antibodies are the result of the immune system attacking the thyroid tissue itself—a so-called autoimmune disease. But Williams believes that the body never attacks itself—and that this misunderstanding is, by itself, disheartening. What is going on instead is a valiant attempt by the immune system to quell the EBV virus. And the end result can be thyroid nodules, hyperthyroidism, hypothyroidism, or even thyroid cancer.

Wilson's Syndrome and EBV

If your body temperature is persistently low and you have symptoms of hypothyroidism (low thyroid hormones) despite routine thyroid tests showing normal levels, you might have a condition called Wilson's syndrome (sometimes called Wilson's temperature syndrome). Although Wilson's syndrome isn't recognized by mainstream medicine, naturopathic medical schools are including it in their curricula, and it's gaining attention from an increasing number of alternative and complementary medicine practitioners around the country. Wilson's syndrome is most likely caused by EBV as well, so everything I've written about EBV above also applies to Wilson's syndrome.

Wilson's usually develops during a period of fairly significant emotional or physical stress, but its symptoms persist even after the stress has passed. Those symptoms include a wide range of seemingly unrelated problems, including fatigue, headaches, migraines, weight gain, irritability, depression, memory loss, anxiety, joint and muscle aches, constipation, irritable bowel syndrome, and many other debilitating conditions. The telltale sign that you do indeed have Wilson's is a consistently below-normal body temperature.

Here's why it develops. Normally, your body converts T4 (one of two thyroid hormones) into T3 (the other thyroid hormone). But when your body stays at a subnormal temperature, it loses the ability to make that conversion. The end result is that cell metabolism is blocked, which encourages weight gain, among many other symptoms. If a person with Wilson's syndrome is given a standard thyroid medication such as Synthroid, it doesn't work because these medications contain only T4, which people with Wilson's can't convert into T3.

To see if you may have Wilson's syndrome, check your temperature for five days first thing after you wake up in the morning, then take it again in three hours, and again after three more hours. Add all three numbers together and divide the result by three to obtain your daily average temperature. Follow this procedure for five days. (If you're not yet in menopause, do this only during the first two weeks of your cycle.) If your daily averages are below 98.3 degrees, you may have Wilson's.

The usual course of treatment involves taking a pill containing sustained-release triiodothyronine (SR-T3) every twelve hours. You'll continue to check your body temperature, and once it reaches 98.6 degrees and stays there for three weeks, your healthcare practitioner will gradually wean you off the medication until you no longer need it at all. One study of eleven people following this protocol conducted by the Friedman Clinic in Montpelier, Vermont, found improvement in all five symptoms that the study measured over periods ranging between three weeks and one year.[14] I would first recommend that you follow the Thyroid Healing Protocol recommended by Anthony William. If that doesn't work for you, then locate a healthcare practitioner who is familiar with Wilson's syndrome or with William's protocol. To find a doctor familiar with the diagnosis and treatment of Wilson's syndrome, visit www.wilsonssyndrome .com/patients/medical-providers. An individual trained in functional medicine could also be most helpful; to find one near you, visit the website for the Institute for Functional Medicine at www.functional medicine.org.

The Role of Iodine in Thyroid Disease

Some people with hypothyroidism are deficient in iodine, an essential element that your body needs to produce thyroid hormones. Iodine also has very powerful antiviral, antibacterial, and antifungal properties (which is why the iodine-containing antiseptic Betadine is painted on the skin before doctors make that first incision in the operating room). These properties make iodine an essential nutrient for fighting EBV infection.

If your T3 and T4 levels are normal but your TSH is elevated, you may indeed be suffering from iodine deficiency. (By the way, the numbers 3 and 4 in the names of the thyroid hormones refer to the number of iodine molecules in each type of hormone.) Other signs of iodine deficiency include apathy, depression, reduced mental function, and breast tenderness. Because the kidneys excrete unused iodine in the body, your healthcare provider can tell if you are iodine deficient by ordering a test that involves collecting your urine for twenty-four hours. An easier and quicker way to tell if you need more iodine is to paint a two-inch-square patch of skin on your abdomen, inner thigh, or inner arm with tincture of iodine. (You can use Lugol's solution for this, or even Betadine.) If you have optimal iodine levels, that yellow iodine stain should still be there twenty-four hours later. If it isn't, chances are good that your body needs more iodine. You'd be amazed at how quickly this transdermal dose of iodine is absorbed when you don't have enough in your system. (Iodine also helps balance excess estrogen. Some practitioners recommend painting iodine on breast cysts, which helps them go away. Whether taken orally or through the skin, iodine can be very helpful for hormone balance and detox.)

While iodine deficiency is just one reason for low thyroid levels, it's one that has received more attention over the last several decades. The first National Health and Nutrition Examination Survey (NHANES I), carried out between 1971 and 1974, found that 2.6 percent of U.S. citizens were iodine deficient. But by the time the third survey was conducted, between 1988 and 1994, that number had shot up to 11.7 percent. Currently at 13 percent, levels have stabilized since this earlier research.[15] Still, iodine remains an important consideration for those with thyroid issues.

Experts cite a number of reasons for the lower iodine levels. Environmental concerns such as deforestation and erosion are resulting in lower concentrations of iodine in our soil, which means there's less iodine in the food that's grown in that soil. People are also consuming fewer eggs (due to concerns about cholesterol) and fish (because of concerns about mercury), both sources of iodine. Perhaps most significant is the fact that Americans are using less iodized table salt, an important source of iodine, because they're concerned about hypertension. We're also cooking less and eating more processed foods, which generally contain a type of salt that has lower levels of iodine.

Even so, more liberal use of the salt shaker isn't necessarily the answer, because according to the World Health Organization, the amount of iodine added to salt isn't always consistent and levels can vary from package to package. Levels of iodine also decrease if salt is stored in open containers, especially in a humid environment. A better way to pump up low iodine levels is by eating sea vegetables (including nori, kombu, bladderwrack, wakame, and arame), which have the highest concentrations of iodine of any food available. You can find these vegetables in health food stores, in the Asian foods section of your grocery store or in Asian grocery stores, or on the internet. I use Maine Coast Sea Vegetables (www.seaveg.com), which are sustainably gathered and processed from the pristine waters of the Maine coast. And I sometimes also use Lugol's solution, a very rich source of iodine; start with 1 to 2 drops per day in water or juice.

Ironically, too much iodine in your body can shut down the production of thyroid hormone, also leading to lower levels, so don't overdo it. Start slow, adding 1 or 2 tablespoons of sea vegetables per week to your diet. At the same time, be sure to eat foods high in the trace element selenium (including meat, fish, cereals, and nuts). If you're already taking thyroid medication, your doctor will probably want to monitor your TSH levels every eight weeks or so in order to adjust your dose, if necessary.

WHAT EVERYONE SHOULD KNOW ABOUT IODINE

Iodide (a type of compound that includes iodine, and the form that is added to table salt) is a chemical known as a halide. Other halides include chloride, fluoride, and bromide. Over the last forty years or so, commercial breadmakers have substituted bromide for iodide, and fluoride has been added to the water supply. (Although the government at one point had to lower the recommended levels because children were already getting so much fluoride from toothpastes, in addition to tap water, that they were developing splotches on their teeth.) These halides, which can be highly toxic, can displace iodine from the cells. When you add iodine to your diet or start taking iodine supplements, it can sometimes displace chloride, fluoride, and bromide from the cells. The result is often a rash. This rash is then attributed to iodine, when in fact it's simply a detoxification reaction from the body getting rid of excess bromide or other toxic halides. The solution is to simply cut back on the amount of iodine you are using and then reintroduce it very, very slowly until your iodine skin patch test shows you have an adequate supply.

In those who are taking thyroid hormone, the introduction of iodine often increases the body's capacity to produce thyroid hormone on its own. It also helps fight EBV infection. Thus women taking thyroid medication who begin taking iodine may well develop shakiness, rapid heart rate, and nervousness—all resulting from renewed thyroid function. This can be remedied by cutting back on the thyroid dosage slowly and carefully. When adding iodine as a supplement, work with a practitioner who is familiar with the effects of iodine and thyroid hormone so that you can achieve optimal balance. Note that the entire topic of iodine supplementation is highly controversial.

Once adrenal stress, glycemic stress, iodine deficiency, EBV infection, and estrogen dominance are addressed through modalities such as supplementation, adequate rest, and natural light, thyroid levels often recover. In the meantime, it's often helpful to take a small dose of thyroid replacement that contains both types of thyroid hormones (T3 and T4). A good place to start that works for the majority of women and is nonprescription is Allergy Research Group's Thyroid Natural Glandular, available online at www.allergyresearchgroup .com, at www.iherb.com, or on Amazon. Armour Thyroid is also a commonly used preparation that includes both hormones. It is widely available at all pharmacies by prescription.

It's important to understand that taking supplemental thyroid hormone of any kind doesn't actually heal the underlying problem. Even if supplemental thyroid hormone does help alleviate the existing hypothyroidism, in a significant portion of these cases the symptom of depression persists, for a separate and rather surprising reason: depression itself can result in thyroid dysfunction. Of course, depression can be one of the symptoms of EBV infection. Therefore, a truly holistic approach that addresses all the underlying issues that contribute to thyroid dysfunction is essential. And that includes exploring the connection between thyroid function and self-expression.

Reclaiming Your Voice and Your Will

The thyroid gland is located in the fifth chakra, the part of the body related to our creative expression, timing, and will. Let's first explore creative expression. Though every one of us is creative by nature, we tend to think of creativity as being reserved for those whom society identifies as "artists." But calling oneself an artist and even making a living at it is only one way to express one's unique creativity. Others include creating order and beauty in a home, a room, at work, in a garden, or in the kitchen. I have a friend whose refrigerator is a work of art. And so is her handwriting! There are also endlessly creative ways to do business or raise a family. It's no secret that there are far more successful and well-known male artists, writers, composers, and musicians than female ones. This is because, up until very recently, women's creative expression, including the words we're longing to speak or sing, have been either undervalued or downright silenced. So many women are afraid that we won't be heard or that what we have to say will be discounted. And this has been the experience of millions of women the world over. In order to keep the peace and get along, too many of us learn to swallow our words or to edit out the parts that we fear others will criticize us for.

My own daughter just wrote this in a description of a podcast that she and her husband did with my colleague Kelly Brogan, M.D., the author of *Own Your Self* (Hay House, 2019)—a brilliant volume that explores the dangers of turning your health (and your will) over to the medical system and believing that those medical professionals know more than you do. Kate was aware that this information might touch a nerve with her community, and she was worried about it. Still, like most women finding their voice, she decided to plow ahead and risk being criticized.

She wrote in the episode description: "While I love sharing ideas that are against the grain, I rarely go full-on controversial. But today I am. To be honest, I'm squirming as I write this because my central nervous system has trouble with the inner explosion that happens when someone has been offended by something I've said or an idea I've shared. My husband, on the other hand, is built differently. He goes right for the truth in an at times shocking way and is far less (and sometimes not at all) concerned about what other people think." Kate is all about building community and helping people fit in— which far too often involves silencing ourselves in order to make others more comfortable. Her husband—like many, but not all, men—isn't nearly as concerned about keeping the peace. Having spent a lifetime as an outlier, trying to make controversial information more palatable, I know the territory well. By the time we hit midlife, most of us are sitting on decades of unspoken words that need to be expressed if we are to maintain our health—and that of our thyroids, throats, and necks!

Then there's the issue of timing. Our experience of time directly affects every cell of our bodies, including our thyroids. How often do we say, "I don't have time," "I'm running out of time," or "There's never enough time"? We are currently living in a culture in which each of us has to process more information in a day than our grandparents had to deal with in an entire year. Time, it seems, is speeding up, with more and more to do and less and less time in which to do it. When I wrote the first edition of *Women's Bodies, Women's Wisdom,* I didn't have a cellphone, and the internet was just getting started! The only way to stop this headlong race to nowhere is to change our relationship to time. Psychologist Gay Hendricks suggests that we adopt "Einstein time" and see ourselves as the place where time comes from. He also points out how subjective our experience of time really is. If your hand is on a hot stove, every second feels like an eternity. When you're making love, time flies. Hendricks points out that we never have enough time to waste it on the things we don't want to do. This is especially true at midlife, when we must find a way to participate in those activities that feed our souls—activities in which time seems to stand still for us.

And what about will? Midlife is a time when you must surrender your ego's will to your soul's Divine will. A friend of mine told me that her thyroid problems started when she began to view her job as a mother and business owner as a supreme test of her will. How could she get her husband, children, and boss to do what she wanted them to do? "When I was in college," she said, "I felt as though I was part of a Divine plan. I looked to my Higher Power to guide my actions. But when I got married, I forgot all about Divine will and instead let my life be ruled by some antiquated idea of what a mother was supposed to do." My friend realized that she was unconsciously following in her own mother's footsteps. Her mother spends hours each week entertaining people whom she claims she doesn't even like and doing tasks for her church that she feels duty-bound to carry out even though they bring her no joy whatsoever.

As you can clearly see, fifth-chakra (and thyroid) health is multifaceted. In order for this complex, entangled state of affairs to be resolved, many women would do well to begin a program of thyroid support while also taking an unblinking look at what parts of their lives and interpersonal relationships require change and upgrading (see Celeste's story below).

Program for Healing Thyroid Issues

STEP 1: Get your thyroid hormones tested. You'll want a test that gives your levels of TSH, antithyroid antibodies, T3, and T4. But remember that any blood test measures just one point in time, and even if all your levels are normal, you might still have suboptimal thyroid function. Trust how you feel more than a test result.

STEP 2: Add thyroid-nourishing supplements to your diet that also help your body quell EBV if it's present (and it probably is). These include the following:

- Curcumin (turmeric) (10 mg once or twice per day)
- L-lysine (500 mg to 2,000 mg once or twice a day)

- Vitamin C or Ester-C (2,000 to 10,000 mg per day; you will know you have saturated your tissues when your stools are loose, so when you hit that point, cut the amount slightly)
- Methylcobalamin, which is a methylated form of vitamin B_{12} (0.5 to 3 mg per day)
- Vitamin D, if your levels are below 40–80 ng/ml (take 5,000 to 10,000 IU a day until levels are optimal)
- Lemon balm extract (two to six dropperfuls per day)
- Cat's claw liquid extract (two to four dropperfuls per day)
- Zinc (7.5 mg of zinc in tablet form twice a day, or two to four dropperfuls of liquid zinc per day; I like the liquid zinc from vimergy.com)
- ReMag and ReMyte mineral solutions (½ to 1 teaspoon of each per day, although the dosage is quite individual, so start slow and build up; available from www.rnareset.com or Amazon)
- Pico silver solution (1 teaspoon per day; available from www .rnareset.com or Amazon)
- Chaga mushroom powder (1 tablespoon in 12 oz. of hot water as a tea; add a tablespoon of honey)

STEP 3: Take a good source of iodine, such as Atlantic dulse powder (1 tablespoon per day in smoothies or soup), kombu (place a piece of soaked kombu in the cooking water for oatmeal or brown rice or in any soup; remove the kombu after cooking), or Lugol's solution (1 to 7 drops per day in water, tea, or soup).

STEP 4: Follow an anti-inflammatory diet that includes foods such as celery, sweet potatoes, Brussels sprouts, spinach, kale, collards, carrots, broccoli, cabbage, cauliflower, tomatoes, bananas, mangos, dates, apples, and wild Maine blueberries. Celery juice in particular is very helpful—drink 16 oz. per day on an empty stomach, first thing in the morning. Also eliminate foods that feed viruses, such as eggs, dairy, soy, and gluten. Give this at least a month—it may be all you need to do to feel a lot better. For more on this, I highly recommend that you read Anthony William's book *Medical Medium Thyroid Healing* (Hay House, 2017). The work of Carolyn Dean, M.D., N.D., author of *The Magnesium Miracle* (Ballantine, 2003; updated in 2017), is also excellent.

STEP 5: Find a coach or good friend to assist you in finding your voice and your will. Some good ways to practice this include writing a letter to express something important to you (even if you never send it), toning (similar to chanting) or singing, and using affirmations (such as "My voice is powerful and readily received" or "I have a song to sing, and I sing it with joy and confidence"). Meditation and other stress reduction techniques such as the Emotional Freedom Technique (also called tapping) are also helpful because viruses can't live in the peaceful alkaline environment such practices help foster.

Particularly if you are in a close relationship with a narcissist, you need to know what you're dealing with and get the right kind of help. I highly recommend *The Empath's Survival Guide* (Sounds True, 2017) by Judith Orloff, M.D. Dr. Orloff also has a very active Facebook group for empaths. And then there is Melanie Tonia Evans's Narcissistic Abuse Recovery Program online and her large social media platform loaded with helpful information (www.melanietonia evans.com).

MENOPAUSE AND ADRENAL FUNCTION

The two thumb-size adrenal glands secrete three key hormones that help us withstand many of the stresses and burdens of life. However, if a woman has lived for a long time with the perception that her life is inescapably stressful, or if she is chronically ill, then chances are she has asked too much of her adrenal glands and has not given them adequate time to replenish themselves. Not surprisingly, EBV and other viruses thrive on the stress hormones produced by the adrenals, so many women with adrenal problems also have thyroid problems.

To understand what chronic exhaustion may do to the body and how it affects your menopausal experience, it's important to know what the adrenal glands do for you on a day-to-day basis, through the effects of three distinct but complementary hormones they secrete.

～ NOREPINEPHRINE (adrenaline) is the fight-or-flight hormone, produced when something is threatening you (or when you think that something is threatening you). It makes your heart pound, your blood rush to your heart and large muscle groups, your pupils widen, your brain sharpen, and your tolerance for pain increase, so you can be at your best in battle. In modern-day life your battles are likely to consist of daily challenges such as pushing your body to keep going when it's fatigued, dealing with a stressful job, and reacting with quick reflexes to avoid a traffic accident. Think of these adrenaline surges as withdrawals from a bank, to help you get through life's rough spots. If you have gotten into the habit of withdrawing adrenaline from your account too often, you'll eventually be overdrawn. Your adrenal glands will be overwhelmed, and you'll have too little adrenaline when you really need it.

~ CORTISOL increases your appetite and energy level while taming the allergic and inflammatory responses of your immune system. It stimulates the liberation and storage of energy in the body, helps the body resist the stressful effects of infections, trauma, and temperature extremes, and helps you maintain stable emotions. Synthetic versions of cortisol—prednisone and cortisone, for example—are prescribed often in human and veterinary medicine to help the patient perk up and feel better so he/she will eat, drink, and move around more and therefore be better able to fight off illness or heal from an injury. Ideally, cortisol is released into the system only on an occasional basis, rather than in response to chronic stress. Undesirable side effects can occur if cortisol levels become too high for too long. These include loss of bone density, muscle wasting, thinning of the skin, decreased ability to build protein, kidney damage, fluid retention, spiking blood sugar levels, weight gain, and increased vulnerability to bacteria, viruses, fungi, yeasts, allergies, parasites, and even cancer. If you've ever seen anyone on high-dose prednisone, you've seen how this drug can adversely affect the body.

~ DEHYDROEPIANDROSTERONE, also known as DHEA, is an androgen that is produced by both the adrenal glands and the ovaries. In both women and men, DHEA helps to neutralize cortisol's immune-suppressant effect, thereby improving resistance to disease. (Cortisol and DHEA are inversely proportional to each other. When one is up, the other goes down.) DHEA also helps to protect and increase bone density, guards cardiovascular health by keeping "bad" cholesterol (LDL) levels under control, provides a general sense of vitality and energy, helps keep the mind sharp, and aids in maintaining normal sleep patterns. Like norepinephrine and cortisol, DHEA also improves your ability to recover from episodes of stress and trauma, overwork, temperature extremes, and so forth. And if a woman is experiencing a decline in libido due to falling testosterone levels, often it is declining DHEA levels that are at the root of the testosterone deficiency, as DHEA is the main ingredient from which the body manufactures testosterone.

There is a price to pay for making too many demands on your adrenal glands. Excessive exposure of the body to adrenaline and cortisol can result in mood disorders, sleep disturbances, reduced resistance to disease, uncontrolled growth of EBV, and changes in vital circulation, all of which are common complaints in today's living-on-the-edge lifestyle. And because these side effects are not uncomfortable enough to be intolerable, the self-destructive lifestyle often continues. DHEA, which helps the body recover from this sort of chronic abuse, finds itself on duty full-time instead of only episodically. Gradually the adrenal glands become seriously exhausted, with the first and most profound effect being their waning ability to produce DHEA. As levels of this restorative hormone fall, cortisol and adrenaline levels begin to fluctuate as well, as the adrenal glands attempt to fill increasingly impossible orders for more support. One of the cardinal signs of adrenal exhaustion—relentless, debilitating fatigue—becomes a prominent complaint. Though this fatigue is often accompanied by depressed mood, irritability, insomnia, and loss of interest in life, this doesn't mean that the adrenal problem is necessarily the cause of the mood change, any more than similar problems are always caused by thyroid malfunction. That is why these emotional symptoms do not always go away with treatment—the underlying issues remain unresolved.

A woman in a state of adrenal exhaustion is likely to find herself at a distinct disadvantage when entering perimenopause, because in the simplest terms perimenopause is another form of stress. Furthermore, adrenal exhaustion suggests that there are long-standing life problems in need of resolution. These issues will loom all the larger when seen with the no-nonsense mental clarity of perimenopause, but not only will adrenal exhaustion make the transition needlessly unpleasant, it also can deprive a woman of the resources she needs to address those issues and to take full advantage of the creative promise of the second half of her life.

If a woman is feeling chronically tired or depressed, if she begins her day feeling inadequately rested, or if she finds that ordinary stresses are having an impact that is out of proportion to their importance, she may be suffering from adrenal gland dysfunction.

Adrenal Testing

Salivary or serum DHEA and cortisol levels can be easily tested through accredited laboratories. Conventional blood tests, taken at whatever time your doctor has scheduled your appointment, might indicate that your adrenals are "normal." However, a better diagnostic approach will test your levels at different times of the day, which is much more likely to reveal an out-of-whack pattern of cortisol or DHEA secretion. This is a case in which urine or salivary testing is far easier than having multiple blood tests in a day! If you want to be tested for adrenal function, see a healthcare practitioner who understands the complexities of adrenal testing. (Healthcare practitioners trained in functional medicine are a good choice. See the Institute for Functional Medicine's website, www.functionalmedicine.org, for referrals.) The DUTCH test from Precision Analytical, mentioned earlier, is an easy way to test cortisol levels in urine throughout a twenty-four-hour period; to order, see dutchtest.com.

ADRENAL STRESSORS

The following stressors can lead to fatigue and, ultimately, adrenal dysfunction—which may, in turn, make some stressors worse:

- Excessive, unremitting worry, anger, guilt, anxiety, or fear
- Depression
- Excessive exercise
- Chronic exposure to industrial or other toxins
- Chronic or severe allergies
- Overwork, both physical and mental (this applies only if you're doing work that doesn't fulfill you)
- Chronically late hours or insufficient sleep
- Unhealed trauma or injury
- Chronic illness
- Light-cycle disruption: shift work
- Surgery

How to Restore Your Adrenal Function

If, after testing, you find that you are producing inadequate levels of adrenal hormones, there are several available routes for increasing either DHEA, cortisol, or both. One is by taking the hormone directly. The other—which is ideal whenever possible—is to restore adrenal health and function so that these glands are eventually able to produce the hormones you need without outside supplements. That will require making changes in the lifestyle and relationship drains that caused the adrenal depletion in the first place. If you supplement your adrenal hormones in dosages that are too high, or if you take supplements for too long, the result can be permanent depression of adrenal function.

DHEA: DHEA is available as tablets, transdermal creams, or sublingual tinctures. Though DHEA is available over the counter in natural food stores, quality varies widely. It is always best to work with a healthcare provider who can help you monitor your dosage and your blood or salivary levels. Also, I recommend making sure you are taking pharmaceutical-grade DHEA. (See Resources.) Regardless of how you take your DHEA, blood or salivary levels should be retaken regularly until they return to normal. When levels return to the normal range, the dose should be gradually tapered until you're off the hormone completely.

DHEA can also be increased by focusing more on loving thoughts that bring you pleasure (such as thinking about loved ones, favorite pets, a delicious meal, or a sweet memory) and less on thoughts that are stressful. This learning to "think with your heart" is challenging at first, but because it short-circuits the harm done by the body's physiological reaction to stress, it's a valuable skill that is well worth learning. I recommend the HeartMath tools (www.heartmath.com), science-based technology that is proven to help reduce stress, anxiety, fatigue, depression, and more. Another choice is the Emotional Freedom Technique (also known as tapping), scientifically proven to reduce stress hormones, lower cortisol, and enhance well-being. (See www.thetappingsolution.com.)

It's also crucial to learn how to use your own power to change your life. And when I say that, I'm not suggesting that you "caused your problem." Using your own power to change anything simply means choosing how you are going to respond to a situation. Read empowering books such as the classic *You Can Heal Your Life* (Hay

House, 1987) and *Empowering Women* (Hay House, originally published in 1997, with a revised and updated edition published in 2019), both by Louise Hay, as well as *The Mind-Body Code* (Sounds True, 2014) by Mario Martinez, Psy.D., all the books written by Jerry Hicks and Esther Hicks (www.abraham-hicks.com), and *Outrageous Openness: Letting the Divine Take the Lead* (Atria, 2014) by Tosha Silver, one of my all-time favorite books. I also love everything written by Robert Fritchie, who runs the World Service Institute (www.worldserviceinstitute.org) and teaches about the healing power of Divine Love.

I recommend the work of Regena Thomashauer, also known as Mama Gena (mamagenas.com). She helps women all over the world find more pleasure and fun in their lives. If you have difficult people in your life (and we all do), you must learn how to stop the energy drain that happens unconsciously when you are around them. Read my book *Dodging Energy Vampires: An Empath's Guide to Evading Relationships That Drain You and Restoring Your Health and Power* (Hay House, 2018) or listen to the audiobook version by Audible (audible.com).

Focus on things that bring you pleasure and make you laugh, and take on fewer activities that feel like obligations. Spend more time with people who make you feel good and less with people who are draining. Dwell more on what you like about yourself and less on what you see as your limitations. In short, have more fun! Make pleasure a priority instead of a luxury. This takes courage, and it's worth it.

CORTISOL: Some individuals require very small doses of hydrocortisone, which can be used safely and effectively if prescribed by a healthcare provider knowledgeable about how and when to use it.[16]

DIET: The food plan outlined in chapter 7 is designed to support and recharge your adrenals, among other benefits. Be sure to get enough protein; every meal or snack should contain at least some protein. Remember that caffeine whips your adrenals into a frenzy; avoid it altogether. Also avoid fasting or cleansing regimens.

NUTRITIONAL SUPPLEMENTS: Supplement your diet at the higher ranges of the nutrients listed in chapter 7, pages 302–303, for at least three months for best results. After that, you can reduce them depending upon how you feel. Be sure you're taking plenty of vitamin C (1,000 to 2,000 mg a day in divided doses), a B complex (25 to 50 mg a day), zinc (15 to 30 mg daily), and magnesium (300 to 800 mg per day in divided doses—in fumarate, citrate, glycinate, or malate form). My colleague Norm Shealy, M.D., Ph.D., has had much success with transdermal magnesium (which you can order from Shealy-Sorin Wellness Institute; for more information, call 417-467-2124 or visit https://realholisticdoc.com). Dr. Shealy's Youth Formula supplement is specifically designed for raising DHEA. The topical and oral magnesium supplements created by magnesium expert Carolyn Dean, M.D., N.D., have been successfully used by thousands of people with great results; see www.rnareset.com.

SLEEP: Sleep is the most effective approach to achieving high adrenaline levels. Sleep restores adrenal function better than almost anything else. When I'm stressed, I routinely sleep ten hours or more a night! Shoot for at least eight solid hours per night.

EXERCISE: Regular light to moderate exercise, but not so much that you feel depleted afterward.

SUNLIGHT: Exposure to sunlight not only is good for your adrenal glands, but it boosts vitamin D as well. But do this wisely. Sunbathe with as much of your skin exposed as possible, starting out in the early morning or later afternoon, not at midday, and never enough to burn your skin. Work up to ten to thirty minutes of exposure three to four times per week. (Timing will depend on your skin tone. Those with dark skin need more exposure time.) Use sunscreen if you're out longer than that. This prudent sunbathing will not increase your risk of skin cancer.

HERBAL SUPPORT: Because one of the components of Siberian ginseng is related to a precursor for DHEA and cortisol, taking this herb can be very helpful in restoring proper adrenal function. Try one 100 mg capsule two times a day. It can have a stimulating effect, though, so if it interferes with your sleep, take it before 3:00 P.M. Licorice root can also help your adrenals because it contains plant hormones that mimic the effects of cortisol. Take up to ¼ teaspoon of 5:1 solid licorice root extract three times a day. Licorice tea is another good alternative. I prefer Traditional Medicinals' Organic Licorice Root tea. It's fine to drink three to four cups per day if your blood pressure is stable.

Note that everything I've said about thyroid healing very often applies to adrenal problems as well. In fact, thyroid and adrenal issues often coexist in the same individual. So please read and heed each section.

FIGURE 8: MENOPAUSAL SYMPTOMS TIMELINE

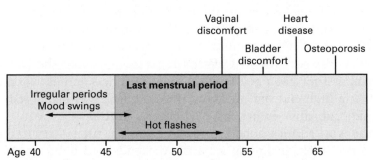

CELESTE: An Archetypal Story of EBV, Chronic Fatigue, Adrenal Exhaustion, and Thyroid Problems

Celeste was in her late twenties when her first marriage ended following a miscarriage and her husband's realization that he was gay. Heartbroken, she dealt with her grief by plunging into her work, earning a Ph.D. in nutrition and exercise, publishing academic papers, and embarking on a lot of successful speaking engagements. She told me that in her effort to achieve and rebuild her life, she "left her body" to some extent. Still, she was building a solid career and was successful and fulfilled in many ways.

About five years later, she met and married a tall, handsome, charismatic man named Charles who, much to her delight, was able to spend a lot of time with her. Compared to her first husband, who worked and traveled all the time, this relationship thrilled her. But it turned out that Charles was living off some interest from a family business loan and didn't have nearly the income and stability she thought he did. Two years later, their son was born. And within a year, Charles's family business started to fail and he had to get more involved in it. He began to travel two weeks out of every month. This coincided with Celeste's career really taking off. She was lecturing, publishing, and giving workshops all over the country. But with her husband gone half of each month, that had to be put on the back burner. And during the two weeks per month that Charles was actually home, Celeste also had to take care of Charles's young son from his first marriage.

When their son was two years old, they moved to Arkansas—back to her husband's hometown—so that he could "save the family business." That meant that Celeste's support system of family, reliable childcare, and referrals for her own business was left behind. Worse still, Charles's mother didn't like Celeste, and Charles was the apple of his mother's eye. The effect of losing her support system caused Celeste's immune system to plummet, and she was soon diagnosed with EBV and chronic fatigue syndrome. And within a few months of this diagnosis, Charles's family business declared bankruptcy.

They moved back to Celeste's hometown, where she was well known, and she got a good job running the fitness and nutrition program at a high-end spa. At about this time, she was diagnosed with thyroid problems—in her case, hypothyroidism.

She worked for about five years at the spa, often sixty to eighty hours per week, including a lot of weekends and holidays. Meanwhile, her husband developed back problems and had to have his gallbladder removed. To make ends meet, given the fact that Charles simply couldn't seem to bring in any money, Celeste started her own business in the nutritional supplement industry and became so successful she was eventually able to leave her job at the spa. But at this point, not only was she suffering from chronic fatigue, but she also had what she called "adrenal surges," in which she became so exhausted she could barely function. When Celeste went to a holistic medical center for a workup, got more rest, started a supplement program, and switched to good organic food, her chronic fatigue truly improved. But as soon as she returned to her regular life, her problems—EBV, chronic fatigue, hypothyroidism, and adrenal fatigue—returned as well. She became so miserable that she retained an attorney to file for divorce. But after discovering the work of Mama Gena's School of Womanly Arts and learning about the power of pleasure to heal relationships, she decided to give the marriage one more try. She was not aware that all of this just "fed" her husband more and more of her life energy while he continued to talk big but never really did anything to support her or the family. (In retrospect, Celeste realized that all she was doing was fueling him with "narcissistic supply.")

Celeste paid for her husband to go to real estate school and also helped him get his pilot's license. This resulted in him being gone from home nearly all the time "for work." Soon she found herself alone at home most of the time, being a single parent. At this point, she was diagnosed with ductal carcinoma in situ of the breast and had an abnormal thermogram. She began an intensive nutritional program to balance her hormone levels and started taking iodine. On the home front, she was exasperated. She wrote a letter to Charles (who was living with his mother because his current job in real estate was in Arkansas) and told him that she wanted a true partner who actually wanted to be with her and with their son. In a fit of rage, he quit his job and came home, saying, "There—now do you have what you want?" But he spent hours each day on the internet doing so-called work that never led to any income, and he was never truly present or helpful. She continued to pay the bills, support the family, and feel tired.

She also traveled abroad about twice a year to lead workshops in nutrition, yoga, dance, and empowerment for women—a task she was brilliant at. (Ironic, I know!) Her travel turned out to be the only way she could get Charles to assume any childcare or household responsibilities. Each time she traveled, she would return rejuvenated and optimistic, but at home her living situation was no better. She even tried to enroll Charles in helping her run her nutritional supplement business, but it didn't work. One day he blew up at her and said he had "given up everything" for her. At that point they decided to get divorced, but he wouldn't let her tell their son. Because she still hadn't found her own voice and her own will, she agreed. This led to another year of living with fatigue, thyroid problems, and misery. At about this time, she had yet another abnormal thermogram and mammogram, needed to increase her thyroid medication, and couldn't seem to lose weight no matter what she ate or how much she exercised. She realized that if she didn't change her living situation, she not only would continue to have health problems but also was likely to develop breast cancer. Charles finally moved out and they got a divorce.

After going through recovery for what she now understands was "narcissistic abuse," Celeste realized that her initial EBV infection, plus the stress of her marriage and her inability to have her say or get her needs met with a narcissist, had set the stage for all her health problems—problems that truly escalated during perimenopause. Her body had to speak louder and louder to get her attention, and it did so through a breakdown of her immune system that led to a rekindling of the EBV infection and subsequent thyroid, adrenal, and breast problems.

Celeste is now happy, healthy, and in better shape than ever. Her weight is where she wants it, she is sleeping well, her thermograms and mammograms are normal, and her relationship with her college-age son couldn't be better. She has also started a new and thriving business that involves empowering women at midlife and beyond to be at their best.

She still needs a small amount of Armour Thyroid daily, but otherwise she is doing well. She admits that it sickens her when she looks back at how long it took her to "wake up." But Celeste is typical of women who have what therapist Sandra L. Brown, author of *Women Who Love Psychopaths: Inside the Relationships of Inevitable Harm with Psychopaths, Sociopaths, and Narcissists* (Mask Publishing, 2009), calls "super traits." These women (and sometimes men) have personalities that are hardwired for loyalty, hard work, empathy, conscientiousness, optimism, and turning a blind eye to personal danger. These traits work beautifully in most all areas of life except relationships with narcissists. That is why such women are often highly successful in their workplaces but too often have disastrous personal lives. They are frequently targeted by narcissists, who use their empathy as a hook; for example, they might say something like "My ex-wife won't let me see the children and I am devastated." Celeste had been sure she could use her myriad skills and high degree of conscientiousness to "heal" her relationship with Charles, and it cost her many years of her life and took a huge toll on her health. But she, like so many others, eventually found her voice and the will to save herself.

It's easy to judge women like Celeste. But let us not forget how charismatic and charming those with character disorders can be. I have a good friend who is a psychologist with thirty-five years of experience. He told me, "I specialize in treating those who have been in relationships with people who have character disorders like narcissism and borderline personality disorder. And even I can be taken in by a charming, good-looking narcissist. That's how clever they can be."

WHAT TO EXPECT IN YOUR TRANSITION

Despite the fact that there are stacks of books describing the "normal" symptoms of perimenopause, many women escape most or all of them. Nonetheless, there are a number of symptoms that women in this culture report frequently, and you may want to review the list on the following pages in order to be informed and prepared. It may also decrease your anxiety about a particular symptom to know that it is related to a normal transition.

Bear in mind the following caveat: it is possible for your expectation of your menopausal experience to become your reality simply because it's what you believe will happen. Remember that in some cultures women rarely report any symptoms from perimenopause, and it is not necessarily written into your biological script that you will have any discomfort, either.

Remember also that your mother's menopause experience probably created a powerful unconscious blueprint for you. One of my readers told me that her mother always said that her life improved dramatically after menopause and that it was the best thing that ever happened to her. So when she herself went through it, she felt exactly the same way as her mother. If your mother's experience was negative, on the other hand, you need not assume that you will follow in her footsteps. Focus instead on the ways in which you are different from your mother, and choose a new and improved script for yourself. (See my book *Mother-Daughter Wisdom* [Bantam Books, 2005] for information on how to update the beliefs and behaviors you learned from your mother.)

The quotations that describe the symptoms below come from patients or from my online and social media community. I have indicated the chapters in which symptoms and solutions are discussed in more detail.

Hot Flashes

"I've had to give up wearing sweaters because I can suddenly get so hot that I feel the need to open all the windows (even in the winter) and peel off as many layers as I can."

Hot flashes are the most common perimenopausal symptom in our culture, occurring in about 70 to 85 percent of all perimenopausal women.[17] They can be very mild or so severe that they result in sleep deprivation and subsequent depression. They begin as a sudden, transient sensation of warmth that can then become intense heat over the face, scalp, and chest area; it may be accompanied by redness and perspiration. They are also sometimes accompanied by an increased heart rate, tingling in the hands, a crawling sensation under the skin, and/or nausea. They usually last from one to five minutes each, and in some cases the hot flash is followed by a feeling of being chilled. In the majority of women, hot flashes often start just before or during the menstrual periods during perimenopause. Triggered by falling estrogen and rising FSH, they tend to become more frequent as we approach our final period. That is the time when estrogen levels are lowest and FSH levels are highest. Hot flashes usually go away a year or two after actual menopause, although in some cases they may continue for many years, mostly because of a stressful lifestyle and adrenaline levels that are too high.

Also known as vasomotor flushing, the hot flash occurs when blood vessels in the skin of the head and neck open more widely than usual, allowing more blood to shift into the area, creating heat and redness. Besides hormonal changes, external factors can influence the intensity and duration of a woman's hot flashes. Anxiety and tension can magnify them, as can a diet high in simple sugars and refined carbohydrates such as those found in fruit juices, cakes, cookies, candy, white bread, wine and beer, and so on. Coffee—even decaf— also triggers them in some women. Excess weight and cigarette smoking have been identified as other risk factors.[18]

There are many approaches to cooling hot flashes. Estrogen therapy is about 95 percent effective, and until the Women's Health Initiative (WHI) study, it was considered the gold standard for hot flash relief. A 2 percent progesterone skin cream also works in many perimenopausal women; as little as ¼ teaspoon (providing 20 mg progesterone) rubbed into the skin once per day may provide relief.[19] (See chapter 5, "Hormone Therapy.") Certain antidepressants have been shown to reduce hot flashes, although the side effects include nausea, dry mouth, drowsiness, decreased appetite, and insomnia.[20] The drug clonidine, traditionally used for high blood pressure, reduces hot flashes up to 80 percent in transdermal form, but its side effects include low blood pressure, dry mouth, and sedation.[21] Because these meds are addictive and difficult to get off of, I don't recommend them. Fortunately, there are many other options. (See chapter 10, "Nurturing Your Brain.") Meditation and relaxation techniques work well. Examples include Herbert Benson, M.D.'s famous Relaxation Response and slow, deep, abdominal breathing that is started when each flash begins.[22] Studies show meditation can cool hot flashes in 90 percent of women, without any hormonal therapy at all.[23] This is because meditation lowers stress hormone levels. There are now a wide variety of apps available for meditation and stress reduction, including the Tapping Solution app and one called Calm.

Many women also find relief when they improve their diets. (See chapter 7, "The Menopause Food Plan.") Soy foods (a total of 45– 160 mg of soy isoflavones per day) provide relief, as do many herbs, such as black cohosh, dong quai, chasteberry, maca, or *Pueraria mirifica*. Acupuncture can also be very effective. (These approaches are detailed in chapter 6, "Foods and Supplements to Support the Change.")

SEEING HOT FLASHES AS A CRUCIBLE, NOT A CURSE

Here's an incredibly empowering perspective on hot flashes from my good friend and colleague Deborah Kern, Ph.D., a health scientist and mind-body researcher, who originally wrote this account in her blog. (To read more of Dr. Kern's inspiring wit and wisdom, visit her site at www.drdebkern .com.)

It's July and there are heat waves all over the country. I am no exception. I am a living heat wave. I am HOT! Since Sunday evening, I've been experiencing my first true waves of hot flashes—SIX the first night. . . . TWELVE the next day. This may sound crazy, but I've actually been awaiting this day with a sense of excited anticipation thanks to Joan Borysenko, Ph.D. While most women are afraid of hot flashes or complain about them, I've actually been looking forward to them. Why? Because in 1996 I read Dr. Borysenko's book *A Woman's Book of Life: The Biology, Psychology, and Spirituality of the Feminine Life Cycle* and I was captivated by a section about menopause and hot flashes. At the time I was in my late thirties and hadn't even given birth to my first son, but there was something so powerful in the way she described hot flashes that I committed it to memory and I've been waiting for my turn to experience them.

Here's what she says on pages 164–165 of her book: At the age of forty-seven, a spunky Frenchwoman by the name of Alexandra David-Neel left her privileged, protected life. Leaving her husband behind in Paris, she shaved her head, dressed in saffron and crimson robes, traveled halfway around the world to the forbidden mountains of Tibet, and sneaked into a monastery by impersonating a male lama. . . .

During the full moon one February she attended a ritual in which monks stripped naked in the freezing temperatures of a Himalayan cave, wrapped themselves in wet sheets and proceeded to dry them when their bodies liberated prodigious amounts of heat during a meditation practice called *tumo yoga*. The monk who dried the most sheets was considered the highest adept. *Tumo* means "fierce woman" in Tibetan. It refers to the life-force energy of every human being (regardless of gender) that circulates in thousands of small channels called *nadis,* similar to the acupuncture meridians. . . .

Tumo yoga was practiced primarily for spiritual reasons, however, rather than for physical healing. Through a series of meticulous visualizations and the repetition of sacred sounds, the monks raised the life-force energy through the lower energy centers up to the highest chakra at the crown of the head. In the process, they believe that they are burning away mistakes, erroneous beliefs, and ego attachments that keep them from fully recognizing the nature of their True Self.

What does tumo yoga have to do with my hot flashes? Well, as Dr. Borysenko points out in her book, menopausal women can use hot flashes in the same way the monks did: consciously thinking of their self-limiting beliefs, erroneous thoughts, stresses, and ego attachments and allowing them to be burned up in the inner fires of transformation. So six to twelve times a day (and night) I now have the chance to consciously burn off anything that might be blocking me from realizing my full potential. That thrills me! Am I still using my bio-identical hormones, following a healthy diet, exercising, meditating, and doing yoga in order to lessen the frequency, intensity, and severity of my hot flashes? You bet. But when they do come, I ride the heat wave with excited anticipation and I am grateful for all that is burning away.

When she sent this to me, Dr. Kern added, "I can truly feel old bonds being released by this fire." I suggest you try her strategy and see if it makes a powerful difference for you, too!

Night Sweats

"I sweat so much at night, I have to get up to change the sheets."
Night sweats are on a continuum with hot flashes. Traditional Chinese Medicine tells us, and many of my patients have confirmed, that 3:00 to 4:00 A.M. is the most common time for night sweats, which may wake you up drenched with perspiration. (This often happens postpartum as well. I like to think of it as the body's way of detoxing.)

Heart Palpitations

"It's like all of a sudden I'm aware of my heartbeat, whereas before my heart just did its job without me noticing it."
Like hot flashes, palpitations can range from mild to severe. They are rarely dangerous, though they can sometimes be very frightening. They are the result of imbalances between the sympathetic and parasympathetic nervous systems triggered by stress hormones and are often related to fear and anxiety. If they persist, see your doctor. (See chapter 14, "Living with Heart, Passion, and Joy.")

LESLIE: *Power Surges at Menopause*

Leslie is an art teacher at a local high school and doubles as an unofficial counselor for her students, who uniformly respect and love her for her obvious devotion. "I'm one of those art teachers you can spot a mile away," she wrote. "I look the part, I guess. I try to do more than just teach kids how to paint or sculpt—I mean, there's art all around us in this world, and much of the joy of life is in appreciating it. I try to demonstrate that in the way I live."

Leslie likes the image of hot flashes as "power surges," symbolizing a positive, transformative process. She did not find her hot flashes or any of her other symptoms to be troublesome, nor did she want to mask or muffle them with medication. "My doctor wasn't surprised when I told her I chose to forgo hormone replacement therapy. She knew I saw this as a way of honoring my body and the natural changes going on within me. At the same time, I did want to provide my body with support and help it adjust, so my symptoms wouldn't be severe." Leslie chose to provide that support through improved nutrition, herbs, and plant-based hormones (phytoestrogens). She takes black cohosh root, which softened her hot flashes within the first week and kept them mild enough that they were merely "interesting" rather than intrusive. She also drinks a glass of vanilla-flavored soy milk every morning and evening.

Migraine Headaches

"Ever since I turned forty, I've gotten a pounding headache the day or two before my period is due. This has never happened before."

Imbalanced hormone levels contribute to so-called menstrual migraine during perimenopause and menopause. This type of headache usually comes just before your period, when both estrogen and progesterone levels can fall dramatically. Hundreds of women have been able to completely recover from menstrual and menopausal migraines through the use of 2 percent progesterone cream. Apply ¼ teaspoon (providing 20 mg progesterone) on your skin daily for the two weeks prior to your period, or three weeks out of every month if you're no longer having periods. Or you can use progesterone capsules or vaginal gel, available by prescription in all conventional pharmacies. (For other headache remedies, see Resources.) Acupuncture and herbs (e.g., feverfew) also often help migraines.

Breast Swelling and Tenderness

"My breasts are sometimes so tender, it hurts to hug my children."

Many women have tender breasts just before their periods. This is often because of iodine deficiency. To remain healthy, the breasts require as much as 6 mg of iodine per day.[24] During perimenopause, you may notice that your breasts feel tender or swollen much more often. This is far more common when a woman is experiencing estrogen dominance. Relief can often be achieved by following a hormone-balancing diet (see chapter 7, "The Menopause Food Plan"), ensuring an adequate intake of B vitamins, making sure you get enough omega-3 fats such as EPA and DHA (start with 400 mg per day combined and work up to as high as 5,000 mg per day as needed), stopping caffeine, and/or using 2 percent progesterone cream (¼ teaspoon, providing 20 mg progesterone, twice per day). To add iodine to your diet safely, take several kelp tablets per day or add up to 1 tablespoon a day of Atlantic dulse powder to soup or a smoothie. Iodine supplements are available as well. (See "What Everyone Should Know

About Iodine" earlier in this chapter.) The addition of phytohormone-rich foods to the diet can also be very helpful. (See chapter 13, "Creating Breast Health.")

Heavy Menstrual Periods

"My periods have become so heavy that I soak through a couple of tampons and an overnight maxi pad in fifteen minutes. Sometimes I even soak through my clothing at work."

When estrogen levels are high or even normal but progesterone levels are too low from lack of ovulation, the monthly estrogen-driven buildup of the uterine lining (the endometrium) continues unopposed. When it finally breaks down, the result can be erratic, heavy bleeding that can go on for days at a time.

The problem can become so troublesome that some women resort to hysterectomy as a solution, but because heavy bleeding often resolves as a woman approaches menopause, hysterectomy is rarely necessary. The unopposed estrogen can often be treated with various types of progesterone or birth control pills. Since the problem is often worse in women who have too much body fat (fat produces estrogen), exercise and diet often help. Alternatives such as acupuncture and Traditional Chinese Medicine are also often helpful. In severe cases, the lining of the uterus can be cauterized via laser surgery in a procedure known as endometrial ablation. There are several different types. NovaSure is one that has worked well for many (see www.novasure.com). (See chapter 8, "Creating Pelvic Health and Power.")

Irregular or Erratic Periods

"I never know when I'm going to get a period. Sometimes I have a normal period. Then one week later I'll have some spotting. Then I'll go for three months before I have any bleeding again. I have to carry pads with me all the time, just in case."

When a woman is going through the hormonal changes of perimenopause, just about any kind of uterine bleeding is possible, ranging from periods that become very light and short to periods that space out to every three months or more. And some women have bleeding patterns that are so erratic, they don't seem like periods at all.

If you can live with erratic periods for a while, the problem will go away. It's not really abnormal. But if you also have other symptoms, such as mood swings or headaches, or simply want more regular periods, a very wide variety of treatments are available, ranging from conventional birth control pills to effective alternatives such as natural progesterone skin cream, the herb *Pueraria mirifica,* or the herb chasteberry (*Vitex agnus-castus*), which help regulate the hypothalamic-pituitary-ovarian axis to produce more progesterone. (See chapter 8, "Creating Pelvic Health and Power.")

Fibroids

"I was having irregular bleeding, and when I went in for my annual visit with my gynecologist, she told me that I had a growth in my uterus that was a fibroid. An ultrasound confirmed my doctor's diagnosis. My doctor tells me that we can just watch it."

About 40 percent of women develop benign fibroid growths in the uterus during perimenopause. Their growth is stimulated by estrogen, and they can become quite large. Fibroids shrink dramatically after menopause and, like heavy bleeding, do not usually require surgery or other treatment, especially if they don't produce symptoms. Some fibroids, however, can cause heavy bleeding, depending upon their position in the pelvis. Small ones can be removed through laparoscopic surgery or sometimes by surgical removal through the vagina. Uterine fibroid embolization (UFE, also referred to as uterine artery embolization) and magnetic-resonance-guided focused ultrasound (MRgFUS) are other nonsurgical treatments. Weight loss, acupuncture, herbs, dietary change, and natural progesterone are all effective alternatives in many cases. (See chapter 8, "Creating Pelvic Health and Power.") Many medical centers, such as the Cleveland Clinic and Johns Hopkins, have fibroid treatment centers that offer women a wide range of different options that do not require hysterectomy.

Loss of Sexual Desire

"There's nothing wrong with my marriage. I love my husband. But, quite frankly, I don't even get turned on by Matthew McConaughey anymore, let alone my husband."

There is nothing about a normal menopausal transition, per se, that lowers sex drive. But many women experience decreased libido as their attention turns inward toward themselves. Still, a healthy woman experiencing loss of sex drive should have her hormones checked. For reasons that aren't clear, some women experience a drop in their testosterone levels during perimenopause; this can result in lack of sexual desire. Adrenal exhaustion can be another factor. If these levels are low, supplementation with small amounts of testosterone or its precursor, DHEA, will sometimes restore libido to normal levels. Many women also find their libido returns when they take *Pueraria mirifica* in the right doses. For some women, libido problems are related to lack of estrogen or thinning of the vaginal tissue. (See chapter 9, "Sex and Menopause.") Women who've undergone removal of their ovaries surgically, or whose ovarian function has been compromised by illness, chemotherapy, or radiation, have lost a major source of their normal hormone production. A variety of safe alternatives, such as *Pueraria mirifica* or maca, can often help in situations such as these.

Vaginal Dryness and/or Painful Intercourse

"I just don't seem to be able to get lubricated during sex anymore. And when we do have intercourse, it hurts!"

The lining of the outer one-third of the urethra and the lining of the vagina are estrogen-sensitive. Symptoms may arise from a lack of estrogen, as well as from decreases in muscle tone and subsequent blood supply in the urogenital area.

For many women, the first sign of perimenopause is a decrease in normal vaginal discharge. This is a direct result of decreasing estrogen levels. Some may need to use a vaginal lubricant (e.g., K-Y Jelly) during intercourse because arousal and full lubrication take longer. Topical estrogen cream, vitamin E suppositories, systemic estrogen therapy, *Pueraria mirifica* vaginal gel, *Pueraria mirifica* capsules, or maca capsules can help. Some of my patients have been able to increase vaginal lubrication through creative visualization. (See chapter 9, "Sex and Menopause.")

Urinary Symptoms

"I keep getting symptoms that feel as though I have a urinary tract infection. I feel as though I have to urinate all the time, but my urine tests don't show any evidence of infection."

"I got my first-ever UTI at age forty-five—as it turned out, the first of many."

"Sometimes I lose urine when I cough or sneeze. I'm worried that if this continues, I'm going to end up using adult diapers!"

Recurrent urinary tract infections or urinary stress incontinence (the loss of urine with coughing, sneezing, laughing, etc.) may occur because of the thinning of the estrogen-dependent lining of the outer urethra. Urinary symptoms often resolve through the use of a small dab of estrogen cream applied locally. Pelvic floor rehabilitation can also increase blood flow to the area and help with stress incontinence. (See chapter 8, "Creating Pelvic Health and Power.")

Skin

"Almost overnight it feels as though my skin has become dry and crepey, especially around my eyes."

The collagen layer of our skin becomes thinner as our hormone levels fall. A wide variety of highly effective skin treatments are now available that help build collagen, resurface the skin, and prevent wrinkles. Systemic or topical hormones; phytoestrogens found in *Pueraria mirifica,* maca, and so on; and antioxidant supplements such as vitamin C, vitamin E, glutathione, and proanthocyanidins (from grape seeds or pine bark) help build collagen and rejuvenate the skin. Esthetic procedures such as intermittent pulse laser or microdermabrasion can help too. (See chapter 11, "From Rosebud to Rose Hip.")

Bone Loss

"My grandmother gets shorter every year, and more bent over. I don't want that to happen to me."

For many women, bone loss through the insidious process known as osteoporosis begins as early as age thirty—or even earlier. Because of chronic dieting, undereating, overexercising, lack of nutrients, or anorexia, many women do not reach the peak bone density they should when they are in their teens, twenties, and thirties. (Ideally, osteoporosis prevention should begin in childhood!) So when a woman turns forty and her hormonal levels begin to shift, her bone density may already be compromised. When estrogen, progesterone, and androgen levels start to shift, the collagen matrix that forms the foundation of healthy bone may start to weaken, especially when a woman's nutrition and exercise regimens are lacking. You can maintain the collagen matrix in your bones and also help rebuild healthy bone in a variety of ways, which include getting adequate phytohormones from foods such as soy, taking herbs, using hormone replacement, adding calcium and magnesium supplements, getting adequate vitamin D from sun exposure or supplements, and doing weight-bearing exercise. (See chapter 12, "Standing Tall for Life.")

Mood Swings

"I find myself crying during television commercials. Then I fly off the handle at my kids for no reason."

As I pointed out in chapter 2, many women experience an intensification of the kind of volatility in their moods that they once felt primarily before their periods, if at all. Part of the reason for this volatility, or for the increase in dark, negative moods, is hormonal. But it may also be a signal from your inner wisdom, trying to get your attention.

Insomnia

"I just don't seem to be able to get to sleep at night. When I do, I often wake up soaking wet and hot. So I throw off the blankets, and then get chilled!"

Many women wouldn't have insomnia if it weren't for their night sweats and hot flashes. For others, anxiety keeps them from sleeping soundly. And so does a refined-food, low-nutrient diet. If your sleep problems are related to hot flashes, they'll often resolve with hot-flash treatment. Many women find that simply taking *Pueraria mirifica* helps them sleep soundly again. If insomnia is due to anxiety, using a low dose of medical marijuana by mouth can help. Remember too that at midlife you may need to make some changes in your life, and the anxiety may be bringing them to your attention. You may also need to clean up your diet. Other sleep problems may be related to the fact that perimenopause, like adolescence, is a time of transition in sleep patterns. Some of us, like teenagers, will suddenly start requiring much greater amounts of sleep than before. Typically, this changes again after menopause, when we need less sleep than during our twenties and thirties. Some women find daytime naps help during the transition. (See the sleep section of "How to Restore Your Adrenal Function" in this chapter, and also see chapter 10, "Nurturing Your Brain.")

Fuzzy Thinking

"I keep losing my keys. I walk into a room and forget why I'm there. Sometimes my head feels like it's filled with cotton."

Many women report a feeling of forgetfulness and "cotton head" during perimenopause. It's not unusual to have trouble concentrating or to do things like put your cellphone in the refrigerator. The same thing often happens postpartum when a woman comes home with a new baby and suddenly feels incapable of balancing her checkbook. The difference between the postpartum period and perimenopause is that during perimenopause you're giving birth to yourself. It often feels as though the logical side of the brain goes to sleep for a while as a way to force us to become more intuitive and more in tune with our emotions and inner wisdom. Herbs such as ginkgo and St. John's wort can help keep your mind clear. So can following a diet that keeps blood sugar stable. (See chapter 7, "The Menopause Food Plan.") Some women find that soy isoflavones or hormones such as progesterone or estrogen are also helpful. The main thing to remember is that you're not getting Alzheimer's. You're just rewiring your brain for a whole new way of thinking. (See chapter 10, "Nurturing Your Brain.")

How Long Will My Symptoms Last?

Many women believe that the symptoms they are experiencing are what menopause—and life—will feel like from this day forward. The truth is that those symptoms, when present, are labor pains, as it were—part of our adaptation to the hormonal changes that take place as our biological focus switches from procreation to personal growth. In other words, the symptoms of the climacteric are temporary. How long they'll last depends on a number of factors, including the type of menopause a woman is experiencing (see page 129), what else is going on in her life at the time, and the ability of her body and soul to support her through this period of transition. In this culture the symptoms of perimenopause, in a natural transition, last anywhere from five to ten years, with a gradual crescendo in the beginning, a peak as the woman approaches the midpoint of the transition, and a gradual decrescendo toward the end as the body learns to live in harmony with its new hormonal support system.

Because all perimenopausal symptoms are interrelated, the treatment of one symptom may alleviate other symptoms as well. Since so many different treatments are effective, an individual woman will want to choose the ones that appeal to her most. Many women select several different treatments at the same time. An example of this would be taking bioidentical hormone replacement along with a soy product and a good multivitamin, and adding an exercise program. The bottom line is this: there's no need to suffer through perimenopause. As you read through the chapters that follow, choose the treatments that speak to you. Experiment. Your body is constantly changing. You can't really make a mistake.

5

Hormone Therapy:
An Individual Choice

The science of hormone therapy has been in continual evolution since estrogen therapy was first introduced in 1949 and the first birth control pills hit the market in the 1960s. The pill gave women a magic bullet that enabled them to go about their daily lives without being conscious of their natural hormonal and fertility rhythms. The downside is that these rhythms and the natural wisdom that created them have become pathologized, leading women to believe that synthetic, man-made hormones are safer and better than the "unpredictable" ones found naturally in our bodies. What became known as hormone replacement therapy, or HRT, was an extension of this thinking, in which the female body is deficient and needs to be fixed with substances not found in nature.

Today, however, new options exist that are much more respectful of the body's wisdom, as well as updated thinking about individualizing hormone levels instead of relying on one-size-fits-all recommendations. Taking hormones is now called HT (hormone therapy) instead of HRT. To understand how the current view of hormones and hormone therapy evolved, it helps to know where we're coming from.

A BRIEF HISTORY OF HORMONE THERAPY

When I was doing my family practice training in a small Vermont hospital, I remember going to the library and taking down a book that caught my eye, way up on the top shelf. It was *Feminine Forever* (M. Evans, 1966), by Robert Wilson, M.D. It described in graphic detail how the lack of estrogen at menopause led inevitably to the shriveling of a woman's body, leaving her old and decrepit. Moreover, he also suggested that the increasingly vocal and forthright self-expression of midlife women was a pathological sign of hormone deficiency.

His solution: estrogen pills to replace what her deficient body no longer produced. This was presented as a sort of magic potion that would leave her "feminine forever": youthful, resilient, moist, sexy, desirable, and compliant to the wishes of her husband and society. The way Wilson described estrogen's benefits, my then twenty-two-year-old self couldn't imagine a woman who would want to live without it at menopause—a life passage about which my medical training had taught me virtually nothing.

I was still unconscious about how embedded the devaluation of feminine bodies, minds, and spirits is within our culture, and how powerfully this devaluation influences the practice of medicine and the science that supports it. (At the time, anyone having her first baby at the age of thirty or older was referred to as an "elderly primigravida.") As was true of my peers, my own beliefs were clouded by my cultural legacy: just as male is superior to female, young is superior to old. Salvation would come through denying any differences between male and female, and endeavoring to stay forever young. Our better-living-through-chemistry society was poised to help us control our unruly female physiology through birth control pills during our reproductive years and estrogen during menopause. Not surprisingly, sales of Premarin—the first estrogen to be marketed—began to soar.

A Shadow Crosses over Premarin

When I was a third-year medical student, one of my mother's close friends confided to me that she had to stop taking her Premarin because she had started to have bleeding. She was later diagnosed with a condition known as adenomatous hyperplasia of the endometrium—indicating that her uterine lining was being overstimulated by the

Premarin. Although she never resumed taking Premarin, her bleeding didn't return, and she didn't suddenly shrivel up, either. She was climbing mountains and going on long hikes with her friends right up to the end of her life at age ninety.

My mother's friend was not alone. In the mid- to late 1970s, study after study appeared that proved beyond any doubt that taking estrogen resulted in an up to fourfold greater risk for developing uterine cancer. At about this same time, birth control pills were shown to increase the risk of stroke, pulmonary embolism, and heart attack—deadly complications in young women. Premarin sales plummeted. Women grew afraid of the pill. It would take several years before new studies of lower-dose pills, and major marketing efforts, quelled these fears—though never entirely.

Premarin Sales Revive

Then studies began to appear showing that estrogen could help prevent osteoporosis. I was intrigued. My then-husband was doing his training in orthopedic surgery, and he spent many nights repairing hip fractures in older women, many of whom never walked or lived independently again.

I researched the link between estrogen and bone health and did a presentation on it for the OB-GYN staff at the hospital. Many of my professors were dead set against Premarin for any indication—they had been burned too badly by the uterine cancer findings. And although I was convinced that estrogen replacement could help prevent osteoporosis, I was far more interested in alternatives such as nutritional supplementation and exercise. A colleague and I even discussed setting up a long-term study involving diet and exercise, but we were far too busy just trying to complete our residencies, and it would take another twenty years for those ideas to be proved and accepted by mainstream doctors.

Meanwhile, other studies showed that endometrial cancer could be prevented if a woman was given progesterone along with her dose of estrogen. Estrogen replacement slowly but surely made its way back onto the scene—this time in combination with Provera, a synthetic form of progesterone, which was given to all women on estrogen unless they had had hysterectomies. (In that case, doctors reasoned, there was no reason to give it.) Progesterone's role was thus reduced to that of a uterine vacuum cleaner—one that prevented excessive buildup of the uterine lining but had no inherent benefits of its own.

Premarin Becomes Synonymous with Hormone Therapy

Premarin is composed of estrogenic compounds derived from the urine of pregnant mares. Since its introduction in 1949, it has maintained a solid reputation as the queen of the hormone therapy world. In fact, when you say "hormone therapy," many people, including doctors, still think Premarin—end of discussion.

Its sales hit an all-time high during the 1980s and early '90s, when study after study (many supported by Wyeth-Ayerst, the maker of Premarin) began to support estrogen's role in keeping the cardiovascular system healthy. For example, it was shown to lower LDL cholesterol, which the famous Framingham study had identified as a risk for heart attack. Given that cardiovascular disease was also emerging as the number-one killer of women past menopause, doctors everywhere became convinced that all menopausal women needed estrogen to protect their hearts. Some even refused to care for women who wouldn't take it.

Other benefits were also touted. Premarin seemed to do everything: lift depression, thicken vaginal tissue, stop hot flashes, prevent heart disease, prevent osteoporosis, and even ward off Alzheimer's disease. Premarin was prescribed freely in a one-size-fits-all manner—the same dose for every woman, regardless of her size or her medical history. Provera was added for ten to twelve days of every month to protect the uterus. Later, Premarin and Provera were combined into one pill known as Prempro or Premphase. That was hormone therapy.

The End of the Premarin Empire?

But then a big fly found its way into the ointment. Multiple studies began to support an incontrovertible link between estrogen supplementation and breast cancer. This link makes biological sense, since estrogen is well known to stimulate the growth of estrogen-sensitive tissue, such as that in the breast and uterus. Still, the cardiovascular benefits seemed so strong that many women were persuaded to override their fear of breast cancer and continue to take Premarin or Prempro.

At the turn of the millennium, however, several large prospective studies challenged the heart-protection gospel. In the large HERS (Heart and Estrogen/Progestin Replacement Study) trial of women who already had heart disease, hormone therapy in the form of Premarin and Provera not only *did not decrease* their risk of subsequent heart attack, it actually *increased* that risk significantly in the first year of use, after which the risk leveled off.

Then, in July 2002, one branch of the huge Women's Health Initiative, a long-term government-funded study of hormone therapy, was stopped abruptly because the data showed that the risks of long-term Prempro use clearly outweighed the benefits. The study followed 16,000 initially healthy postmenopausal women randomly assigned to take either Prempro or a look-alike placebo. Those on the synthetic hormone combination were found to suffer more breast cancers, heart attacks, strokes, and blood clots than the women on placebo.[1] A second study from the National Cancer Institute, released on the same day, reported that women who used estrogen-only hormone therapy for longer than ten years doubled their risk for ovarian cancer.[2]

When this information was released, it created mass confusion for the millions of women and their doctors who had been convinced for over a decade that taking estrogen for life was the key to heart disease prevention, good skin, healthy bones, and a great sex life. Virtually overnight, there was a revolution in the way our culture views hormone therapy in general and Prempro in particular. Women stopped taking it in droves, and as a profession, we doctors realized that we needed to individualize our care.

Then, in early 2006, a reanalysis of the data from the Nurses' Health Study and the Women's Health Initiative study indicated that younger women who started taking hormones within ten years after menopause experienced an 11 to 30 percent decreased risk for heart attack—the kind of result that researchers had hoped to see when the WHI started. But those who started later (ten years or more after menopause—the majority of women in the WHI) experienced an increased risk for stroke, heart attack, and even Alzheimer's disease. Younger women on estrogen alone had a 44 percent decreased risk for heart disease as long as they started within ten years of menopause.[3] (At the time, I suspected that the difference between the risk of the younger HT users and that of the older ones had something to do with hormone therapy's ability to prevent the kind of vascular damage that tends to result from years of stress, high blood sugar, a nutrient-poor diet, and not enough exercise.) Yet another reanalysis of these studies published in 2010 added a new wrinkle: even the younger women who took estrogen-plus-progestin hormone replacement therapy slightly *increased* their risk of coronary heart disease within the first two years of starting their hormone therapy—although this increase was not statistically significant.[4] After six years of use, however, the increased risk disappeared, at which point, researchers found that hormone therapy might actually confer some protection. However, most women who use HT don't take it as long as six years anyway, so the potential protection claim may well be a moot point.

At the end of the day, here's what we're left with. After decades of trying to convince all women that menopause was a deficiency state that could be "cured" by hormone therapy, we finally realized the truth. There is no magic bullet, one-size-fits-all hormone prescription or drug regimen of any kind that is right and healthy for all or even most women to take indefinitely. And because each of us is an individual with differing needs, constitution, beliefs, and environment, there never will be—no matter how many studies are done. Quite frankly, I consider that good news.

On the other hand, there's no reason to throw out the baby with the bathwater. The science of hormone therapy is still evolving. The latest evidence-based position statement from the North American Menopause Society reports that, on the whole, the benefits of HT outweigh the risks for women who begin HT close to menopause (although the position paper also notes that those benefits decrease in older women and with time since menopause in previously untreated women).[5] And the newest data from the reanalysis of the WHI and Nurses' Health studies is encouraging. Hormone therapy has some very real benefits. Even in the Women's Health Initiative study of older women, the women who were using Prempro (which I consider the least desirable form of hormone therapy) were at decreased risk for bowel cancer and fractures compared to those who were on the placebo. And no one would disagree that hormone therapy offers many women one of the best ways to get relief from perimenopausal symptoms such as hot flashes. Thankfully, there are ways to get the benefits of hormone therapy while decreasing the risks and side effects.

BIOIDENTICAL HORMONES: NATURE'S IDEAL DESIGN

In contrast to Premarin, Provera, and Prempro, the hormones that I recommend are exactly the same as those found in the female body. Though they are synthesized in the lab from hormone precursors found in soybeans or yams, their molecular structure is designed to be an exact match of the hormones found in the human body. Hence we call them *bioidentical,* a term that is far more precise than *natural,* which can be used in confusing and ambiguous ways—for example, Premarin is said by some people to be a "natural" product because it is made from horse urine. As the late Joel Hargrove, M.D., a pioneer in the use of bioidentical hormones and the former medical director of the Menopause Center at Vanderbilt University Medical Center in Nashville, Tennessee, was known for saying, "Premarin is a natural hormone if your native food is hay."

Because bioidentical hormones are just like the hormones that our bodies were designed to recognize and utilize, their effects are more physiologic—consistent with our normal biochemistry—with less chance for unpredictable side effects at low replacement doses than with synthetic, non-bioidentical hormones.

Finally, large-scale clinical trials have begun to provide solid data on the effect of bioidentical hormones. The Early Versus Late Intervention Trial with Estradiol (ELITE) study, sponsored by the National Institute on Aging and conducted by researchers at the Keck School of Medicine at the University of Southern California, followed more than 600 postmenopausal women with no history of cardiovascular disease or diabetes to look at whether natural estrogen therapy would reduce the progression of early atherosclerosis if it is started soon after menopause. The results, reported in 2016, showed that women who took estradiol within six years of menopause had a slower progression of arterial plaque buildup than did women who began estradiol therapy ten years or more after menopause.[6] The ELITE researchers are now at work investigating the reasons why hormone therapy is more effective if taken earlier.

Similarly, the Kronos Early Estrogen Prevention Study (KEEPS), conducted by the Phoenix-based nonprofit Kronos Longevity Research Institute, was a multicenter prospective trial comparing the use of bioidentical hormone therapy with conjugated estrogen therapy (Premarin) in newly menopausal women. This randomized, double-blind, placebo-controlled study of more than 700 women reported that after four years, both groups showed similarly substantial reductions in hot flashes and night sweats,[7] and neither type of hormone therapy increased the buildup of arterial plaque.[8] A subgroup of KEEPS participants who then stopped hormone therapy were followed for an additional three years, at which point no rebound effect on atherosclerosis was found.[9] The National Institute on Aging is funding a continuation of the KEEPS study looking at whether cognition and brain structure change after hormone therapy has stopped. Results are expected in 2023.

To take advantage of the benefits of bioidentical hormone therapy, you first have to give up the notion that there is an easy, one-size-fits-all answer. There isn't. Some women need or want hormone therapy; some don't. Some will need to use it for only a year or two; some will want to stay on it longer. (For additional information and guidance about bioidentical hormones, read *The New Hormone Solution* [Post Hill Press, 2017] by Erika Schwartz, M.D., a pioneer in the bioidentical hormone field.)

When it comes to hormone therapy, the science we look to for answers is inconsistent, influenced by market forces, and confusing to researchers, doctors, and patients alike. The blessing is that this dilemma forces us to tune in more fully to our own inner wisdom, and to make our choices in partnership with our intuition *and* intellect. This approach is the essence of feminine wisdom.

THE PASSING OF A PIONEER

When Joel Hargrove, M.D., died in 2017 at the age of eighty, I lost one of the most beloved and influential mentors in my long career. In 1989, this pioneer led a group of researchers at Vanderbilt University in Nashville, Tennessee, doing the first-ever study comparing hormone therapy using natural progesterone and estradiol to the conventional therapy using equine-based estrogen plus progestins. The study followed ten women experiencing moderate to severe hot flashes and/or vaginal atrophy for one year. Dr. Hargrove and his colleagues reported that natural hormone therapy provided the same relief of menopausal symptoms but without the adverse effects on blood lipids associated with synthetic hormones.[10]

He was tireless in trying to get a major pharmaceutical company to manufacture the hormones that he knew worked, so that they would be more widely available. However, no pharmaceutical company wanted to spend money on something they couldn't patent. Only now, decades later, is this natural approach picking up speed, with delivery systems being patented, not the hormones themselves.

Dr. Hargrove intuitively knew that you can't get the ideal

biological result from something that does not naturally occur in the body. To him (and also to me), this was just common sense—the grasp of which is still very uncommon. Sadly, to this day, most physicians don't know the difference between a human hormone and a horse hormone. Decades ago, when he came to the hospital where I worked to lecture to the OB-GYNs on how to use bioidentical hormones, he gave me the confidence and courage to change my practice.

Dr. Hargrove worked with his college roommate, Joe Delk (one of the very first formulary pharmacists in the country), in writing individualized natural hormone prescriptions for women, teaching them how to titrate their own doses. Imagine that—individualized medicine because we're all different. Dr. Hargrove and I both grew up on farms, which I think explains a lot about our down-to-earth approach to medicine. He was a man far ahead of his time, a doctor who respected all women and knew how to help them—and one who had the courage of his convictions. His contribution to my life—and the lives of thousands of other women around the world—is beyond measure.

Moving Beyond Premarin

When Premarin was introduced, the technology to produce other types of estrogen was not yet available, so it became the gold standard. However, these equine estrogens aren't normally found in the human female body, and they are often associated with side effects such as headaches, bloating, and sore breasts. In addition, the metabolic breakdown products of Premarin in the human female are biologically stronger and more active than the original equine estrogens. A host of studies have shown that these breakdown products can produce DNA damage that is carcinogenic in tissue. Given this, it's no wonder that the incidence of breast cancer statistically increases when women are on this drug.[11] In contrast, the metabolic breakdown products of bioidentical estrogens are biologically weaker, so their effects on tissue do not last as long.

There's reason to believe that bioidentical estrogen at individualized low doses doesn't have the same carcinogenic effect on breast tissue as Premarin or Prempro. But until we have long-term studies of bioidentical estrogen to compare with the vast amount of data on Premarin, we won't have the scientific verification we need. Unfortunately, long-term studies are enormously expensive. The Women's Health Initiative study cost the American public well over $628 million.[12] It was also funded in part by Wyeth-Ayerst, the manufacturer of Premarin and Prempro, because the company hoped to be able to advertise its drugs as both preventives and treatments for heart disease, which is the leading cause of premature death among women.[13] Given the untoward results from the initial WHI study, what are the odds that a hormone manufacturer will take such a financial risk again? That remains to be seen. Nonetheless, many clinicians find that prescribing bioidentical hormone therapy for short-term relief of symptoms, such as vaginal dryness, hot flashes, and even mood swings, can work wonders for some women. The shifting news about Premarin and Prempro has actually opened the minds of many women and their doctors to these more physiologic and well-tolerated alternatives. Remember, this is all an ongoing process. So now, more than ever, you need to make the hormone choice in concert with your inner guidance.

HORMONE THERAPY: RESEARCH SUMMARY

Benefits of Estrogen

~ *Hot flashes:* Estrogen gives better hot flash relief than just about any other treatment. It can take up to four weeks to notice the effect.

~ *Skin:* Estrogen, either systemic or applied to the skin, can increase skin thickness and enhance the collagen layer in women whose estrogen is low. It can also help reduce wrinkling.

~ *Sexual function:* Estrogen can enhance sexual function by eliminating vaginal dryness and thinning, which in many women cause sexual intercourse to be painful. It works equally well either systemically or topically. Some studies suggest that estrogen enhances sexual desire. High-dose transdermal testosterone has been shown to increase desire in some women who've undergone surgical menopause.

~ *Urinary tract:* Locally applied estrogen may decrease the incidence of urinary tract infection. *Note:* Systemic estrogen has been shown to increase the risk of stress urinary incontinence.

~ *Cognition:* Estrogen and other steroid hormones have well-documented effects on nerve cells. Although estrogen does not improve already established dementia, research suggests that estrogen—particularly the estradiol patch—may give moderate protection against cognitive decline if the HT is begun soon after menopause.[14]

~ *Depression:* Estrogen may have an antidepressive effect in some women but shouldn't be used as primary treatment. Synthetic progestins may have a depressive effect in some women. Menopause itself is not associated with an increase in depression.

~ *Osteoporosis:* Estrogen has a well-documented beneficial effect on bone density that is equivalent to the bisphosphonates (e.g., Fosamax). It definitely reduces fracture risk and probably does so in a different way than the SERMs (see page 190) or bisphosphonates.

~ *Insulin resistance:* New studies show that estrogen may have the potential to lower insulin resistance, thus also lowering the chance of developing diabetes.[15]

~ *Heart and blood vessels:* Many studies have documented the positive effect of estrogen on the cardiovascular system. However, this has been a controversial subject since the WHI study released in 2002 showed that Prempro increased the risk of heart attack and stroke. This study followed mostly older women who started hormone therapy (in this case estrogen plus synthetic progesterone) ten years or more after menopause. The 2006 and 2010 reanalyses of the data on the WHI and Nurses' Health studies showed confusing data about the effect of estrogen on the risk of heart attack, but fortunately the more recent ELITE and KEEPS studies, mentioned earlier, show that hormone therapy initiated soon after menopause doesn't unduly increase arterial plaque buildup. Most authorities (and the latest evidence-based position statement from the North

American Menopause Society) don't recommend estrogen for the prevention of chronic diseases. And I wouldn't either. There are too many other factors involved.

Risks of Estrogen

~ *Breast cancer:* Several randomized clinical trials and observational studies have shown that estrogen increases the risk of breast cancer. The latest research on this is a meta-analysis of fifty-eight prospective studies that included more than 100,000 women; the study reported that women who had ever taken hormone therapy had a 26 percent greater risk for breast cancer than those who had never used it (roughly one additional case for every fifty users), and that the risk increased with how long they were on the hormones.[16] Even for those who stopped hormone therapy, the higher risk persisted for more than a decade. The researchers also noted that those women taking estrogen-only therapy (some of whom were on estradiol while others were on conjugated estrogen) had a lower risk than those taking combination hormones (estrogen plus synthetic progesterone), roughly one additional case for every 200 users. But the debate is far from over. Another recent study of long-term data from WHI showed that after sixteen years of follow-up, women who took conjugated estrogen-only hormone therapy had a 23 percent reduced risk for breast cancer (and a 44 percent reduction in deaths from breast cancer).[17] *Note:* Many well-designed studies do not show an increased risk of breast cancer with hormone therapy, including one of the largest studies to date comparing breast cancer risk with the use of natural bioidentical hormones and synthetic hormone therapy. The results of this study, which followed more than 80,000 postmenopausal women for more than eight years, showed that the natural hormones have significantly less associated risk of breast cancer.[18]

~ *Ovarian cancer:* Risk of ovarian cancer for women who use estrogen-only hormone therapy increases 63 percent compared with nonusers, according to findings from the

European Prospective Investigation into Cancer and Nutrition, presented at the 2010 conference of the American Association for Cancer Research.[19] Risk for ovarian cancer increased 29 percent for women on any form of HT compared to those not taking any hormones, although risk wasn't statistically significant for women taking a combination of estrogen and progestin.

~ *Pancreatitis and gallstones:* Women with high triglyceride levels are at increased risk for pancreatitis, which is sometimes fatal, when they take oral estrogen with or without progesterone. There is an increased risk of gallstones and problems requiring biliary tract surgery with the use of estrogen in all women.

~ *Blood clots and stroke:* Estrogen appears to double the risk of blood clots. It also increases the risk of pulmonary embolism. Embolism is most likely to occur in the first year of therapy and especially in those with a history of blood clots. Randomized trials also show an increased risk for stroke with unopposed estrogen. This risk is greater in smokers and older women.

Neutral Effects of Estrogen

~ *Weight changes:* Estrogen doesn't cause weight gain.

~ *Osteoarthritis:* Estrogen doesn't help or hurt those with osteoarthritis.

~ *Ovarian, endometrial, and bowel cancer:* Some studies show an increased risk of ovarian cancer when estrogen is used for ten years or more. Estrogen therapy without the addition of progesterone increases the risk of endometrial cancer, but adding progesterone eliminates this risk. Estrogen definitely decreases the risk of colorectal cancer, but experts agree that it shouldn't be prescribed solely for this purpose.

The Balanced Approach: Individualized
Bioidentical Hormone Therapy

A full range of bioidentical hormones—either singly or in combination—is available by prescription from formulary pharmacies (pharmacies that make up preparations to order). The dosages can be individually adjusted. Hormones can be prescribed based on a woman's test results and symptoms, so she is taking only what she needs to maintain the optimal levels of hormones in her body. This approach is standard with thyroid hormone, but it wasn't applied to sex hormones until recently. (See Resources for how to locate a formulary pharmacy in your area.) It is also possible to create a bioidentical hormone therapy regimen using hormone preparations available in all conventional pharmacies. You just have to know which brands are bioidentical and which are not. (See the chart on page 205.)

These individualized hormones can be taken orally, transdermally, or vaginally, whichever route works best for the patient. Though most women are accustomed to taking pills, the transdermal route is the more physiologically appropriate way to take hormones because they go directly into the bloodstream from the skin. You can also keep the dose much lower with this route because absorption is more direct than through the GI tract. (The body's own hormones are secreted directly into the bloodstream by the endocrine organs.) An important note: Don't allow pets (particularly smaller ones) to come into contact with any skin where you have applied topical hormones. Pets exposed to hormones in this way can experience breast or nipple enlargement (in male or female animals), vulvar enlargement, and hair loss. One of my good friends has two Pomeranian dogs she always carries around with her that lost all their hair from coming into contact with her transdermal estrogen. Once she realized what was going on, she stopped using her hormones and switched to *Pueraria mirifica*. Her dogs are now fine.

Oral preparations, on the other hand, have to be first absorbed from the gut and then transported to the liver, where they must undergo further metabolic breakdown before finally getting to the bloodstream. This process causes the liver to manufacture more clotting factors, which is one of the reasons that oral estrogen, especially at high doses, is associated with an increased risk of stroke, heart attack, and thrombophlebitis.

One popular form of hormone therapy is to have a prescription created especially for you using one or more of the bioidentical estrogens (estradiol, estrone, estriol) combined with bioidentical progesterone and an androgen in the form of DHEA or testosterone, if needed. These hormones are mixed into a lotion, cream, or other base and applied to the skin.

Research has clearly shown that these bioidentical transdermal hormone therapy regimens provide adequate blood levels of hormone, protect the uterine lining from overstimulation, prevent breakthrough bleeding, and give very effective relief for perimenopausal symptoms.[20] I prefer the transdermal method of hormone therapy because a woman can very easily adjust her dose as needed without danger of side effects. For example, if she is having PMS symptoms, such as water retention, headaches, and bloating, she's getting too much estrogen and needs to decrease her dose. The same is true if she develops vaginal bleeding. If she's getting hot flashes without PMS, she needs more estrogen and should increase her dose. The usual starting dose is 0.3 mg 17-beta estradiol and 100 mg bioidentical progesterone, applied as a cream to the inside of the wrists or elsewhere on the body. A woman can gradually increase the dosage to 0.6 mg estradiol and 200 mg progesterone daily.

Why So Many Hormones Are Synthetic

Though it should be intuitively and scientifically obvious that bioidentical hormones in individualized doses would give the best results, many scientists and physicians have turned a blind eye to this concept. The answer is simple: economics.

Bioidentical hormones cannot be patented, so there are no financial incentives for a pharmaceutical company to do the expensive research and development necessary to develop new products containing them. (Unique delivery systems *can* be patented, however, which is why patches such as Climara, Estraderm, and Vivelle-Dot, and the vaginal ring Estring, all of which contain bioidentical estradiol, can be profitable.)

Synthetic hormones, on the other hand, are made by altering the molecular structure of a hormone enough so that it can be patented. These maintain some of the activity of the natural hormone, but any change in the three-dimensional structure of a hormone, no matter how small, changes its biological effects on the cell in ways that are not completely understood. (*Note:* Premarin is bioidentical for a horse, not a human.)

Frankly, I trust the wisdom coming from Mother Nature's millions of years of experimentation much more than I trust fifty years of biochemical wizardry from Father Pharmaceutical. But not all women feel this way. Some feel far safer going with what their doctor prescribes. And since beliefs affect biology, what you believe can shape your experience. It's your decision, and my approach is not meant to undermine any individual's positive experience.

What About Birth Control Pills?

Birth control pills are widely prescribed as a convenient way to put the perimenopausal body and its symptoms on autopilot until it's time to move to conventional hormone therapy. There's a currently popular trend to convince women that our menstrual periods themselves are dangerous and that going on the pill as early as our teenage years, and staying on it except to have children, will prevent long-term health problems. Please note, however, that all birth control pills consist of synthetics that mask our natural hormonal rhythms and the messages about our health that they convey. Birth control pills are also associated with a wide variety of side effects, including blood clots, headaches, and PMS. Although they are appropriate in some cases, I'd rather keep my hormones tuned in to the cycle of the moon and the planets—as opposed to the energy of a pharmaceutical company. You may not be prepared to use other birth control methods right now, or you may be using the pill to quell symptoms such as heavy or irregular periods, but just be aware that other options are available. Some women love how they feel on the pill. Others hate it. Make your choice based on how you feel!

A HORMONE PRIMER: ESSENTIAL INFORMATION EVERY WOMAN SHOULD KNOW

It's important to keep in mind that hormone therapy involves more than just estrogen. It also includes the other hormones produced by the ovaries: progesterone and androgens such as testosterone. Some women might be perfectly comfortable with no supplemental hormones; some might need progesterone only; some might need all three. Understanding their original roles in a woman's body, and the kinds of responses some women see when levels drop, can help you make your own very personal HT decision.

Estrogen

For generations, estrogen has been the first (and often the only) hormone to be prescribed for women suffering from symptoms such as hot flashes, vaginal dryness, and mood swings. However, as I noted in chapter 4, estrogen levels don't fall until late in the menopausal transition, and the majority of perimenopausal symptoms in women with intact ovaries are related more to a lack of progesterone than to a lack of estrogen.

"Estrogen" actually encompasses three distinct estrogenic compounds produced naturally in the body: estradiol, estrone, and estriol. Estriol reaches its highest level during pregnancy; it has weaker biological effects on breast and uterine tissue than do estrone and estradiol. (Women with naturally higher estriol levels appear to have lower breast cancer rates than others, which has led some practitioners to prescribe estriol to decrease the risk of breast cancer.[21] Much more research is needed to establish the effectiveness of this approach.)

There is one area in which supplemental estriol is known to be particularly effective: urogenital symptoms. Applied locally in the vagina, it relieves urinary frequency, vaginal dryness, and other conditions associated with the thinning of these tissues.[22]

FIGURE 9: KINDS OF ESTROGEN

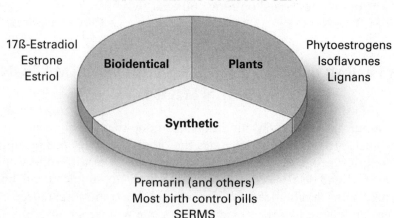

17ß-Estradiol
Estrone
Estriol

Bioidentical

Plants

Phytoestrogens
Isoflavones
Lignans

Synthetic

Premarin (and others)
Most birth control pills
SERMS

As I mentioned in chapter 4, there is reason to believe that estrogen's role during the childbearing years is quite different from its role after menopause. Before menopause, the primary role of estradiol is to stimulate growth in the breasts, ovaries, and uterus and to participate in the growth and maturation of egg-bearing follicles. It also is a major influence in stimulating maternal behavior. In other words, it promotes childbirth and childcare. After menopause, estrone becomes the predominant estrogen. No one knows exactly why this happens, but obviously it has nothing to do with procreation. It is likely that estrogen's ability to protect heart and brain function, as well as bone strength, is part of its purpose in this phase of life.

Recall as well that the ovaries continue to produce small amounts of estradiol, as do the secondary hormone production sites. As a result, it is biologically possible for a woman to produce enough of her own estrogen to support optimal health throughout the second half of her life. This is rarely taken into account, perhaps because stress, unmet spiritual needs, and cultural expectations conspire to impair a woman's natural ability to produce adequate levels of the estrogens.

The most obvious and immediate benefit of estrogen therapy is relief from the symptoms of estrogen deficiency. (See box below.) A longer-term benefit is estrogen's ability to help prevent excessive bone mineral loss leading to osteoporosis. Estrogen also helps maintain the thickness of the collagen layer in skin. Some early studies suggested that it may also help preserve mental function or at least delay the rate of so-called normal, age-related brain changes as well as dementia of the Alzheimer's type, but the initial results of the KEEPS study (mentioned earlier) concluded that hormone therapy did not improve memory or prevent age-related memory decline, although studies are ongoing. A recent observational study from Finland that included data from almost 85,000 women concluded that using hormone therapy for more than ten years might be associated with a small increase in risk for Alzheimer's disease.[23] It's safe to say that at this time there's not enough evidence to support prescribing estrogen for cognitive changes alone.

Estrogen is available in pills, skin patches, and vaginal creams. In low doses, even synthetic estrogen in vaginal creams has negligible systemwide absorption and is generally safe for women who need the local effect of estrogen but don't want any more exposure than necessary.

SYMPTOMS OF ESTROGEN DEFICIENCY

~ Hot flashes
~ Night sweats
~ Vaginal dryness
~ Mood swings (mostly irritability and depression)
~ Mental fuzziness
~ Headaches, migraines
~ Vaginal and/or bladder infections
~ Incontinence; recurrent urinary tract infections
~ Vaginal wall thinning
~ Decreased sexual response

SYMPTOMS OF ESTROGEN EXCESS

~ Bilateral, pounding headache
~ Recurrent vaginal yeast infections
~ Breast swelling and tenderness
~ Depression
~ Nausea, vomiting
~ Bloating
~ Leg cramps
~ Yellow-tinged skin
~ Excessive vaginal bleeding

A Note About "Designer Estrogens": SERMs

The selective estrogen receptor modulators (SERMs) are synthetic drugs such as tamoxifen and raloxifene. They get their name from their ability to bind with estrogen receptors and selectively modulate the effects of estrogen in different body tissues. Tamoxifen (trade name Nolvadex) blocks the estrogen receptors on breast cells while maintaining some positive estrogenic effects on bone, uterine tissue, and the cardiovascular system. Raloxifene (trade name Evista) also promotes bone density while decreasing the stimulation of breast tissue by estrogen. This selective activity is possible because there are two different estrogen receptors, ER-alpha and ER-beta, each of which predominates in certain tissue. The same estrogen can produce different effects according to the receptor to which it binds.[24]

Tamoxifen, the most widely used SERM, was first approved by the FDA for the treatment of patients with estrogen-receptor-positive (ER-positive) breast cancer in 1978. It is now prescribed for about half of all women diagnosed with breast cancer in the United States. It has been shown to reduce the risk of developing breast cancer in the remaining breast, as well as breast cancer recurrences and deaths. Tamoxifen is also approved for breast cancer prevention in women who are at high risk or perceived high risk for the disease. It helps prevent bone loss and also has a beneficial effect on LDL cholesterol but does not decrease the risk of heart disease.

Since the 2002 WHI study results underscored the risks of estrogen, especially in older women, raloxifene is being prescribed more than ever to protect women against osteoporosis. However, it doesn't protect bones as well as estrogen does. With or without estrogen, most women can get all the bone protection they need by doing weight-bearing exercise, getting enough vitamin D and minerals, and following the guidelines I've outlined for maintaining healthy bones in chapter 12. Why put yourself at risk with a relatively untested drug?

I'm very concerned about SERMs. They are not found anywhere in nature and have not been around long enough for us to truly assess their benefits and risks. Touted for their ability to stimulate the "good" effects of estrogen without the "bad" ones, these drugs are riding the current wave of panic about breast cancer and are being requested by women who really don't need them, or for whom there are far safer alternatives. If a young woman who fears breast cancer begins taking a SERM drug, she likely will be taking it for many years. This long-term blockage of some estrogen sites with stimulation of others is a double-edged sword. What if we find that these drugs actually increase the risk of Alzheimer's disease by blocking the estrogen receptors in the brain?

Troubling side effects of tamoxifen have already been documented, including an increased risk of certain visual disturbances, fatal pulmonary embolism, and endometrial cancer. Though studies indicate that raloxifene, unlike tamoxifen, can protect against endometrial cancer, both tamoxifen and raloxifene have been implicated in increasing the risk for colon cancer.[25] They also increase hot flashes in many women, the very symptom for which most perimenopausal women seek treatment in the first place.[26]

Even more disturbing is the finding that after five years of use, the antiestrogenic effects of tamoxifen on breast cells appear to reverse. A 2009 study showed that women who take tamoxifen for at least five years following a lumpectomy or mastectomy more than quadruple their risk of developing ER-negative breast cancer, a rare but more aggressive and difficult-to-treat cancer, in their healthy breast.[27] Although using tamoxifen for less than five years wasn't linked to the more aggressive cancer, it doesn't really matter all that much because women don't get the full benefit of the drug until they've taken it for five years. So while the majority of breast cancer patients will lower the risk of their cancer recurring by taking tamoxifen, 24 percent of them will actually *increase* their risk of getting an even more deadly form of breast cancer. I'm simply not comfortable with those odds, especially considering that tamoxifen also raises the risk of blood clots, stroke, and uterine cancer. Though this study involved women with cancer, not ductal carcinoma in situ (DCIS), women with DCIS are routinely put on tamoxifen. Given that most DCIS isn't likely to progress to invasive cancer in the first place, is tamoxifen really worth the risk?

The bottom line is this: unless you have no other alternative, I recommend that you avoid SERMs or limit their use to five years or less. Better yet, stick with bioidentical hormones or the alternatives I outline in chapter 6.

Progesterone

A decline in progesterone is the first hormonal change to cause symptoms in a woman approaching menopause—sometimes years before she suspects she may be nearing the change. Because the body is designed for progesterone and estrogen to be present in a dynamic counterbalance with each other, the result is estrogen dominance, with symptoms of both progesterone deficiency and relative estrogen excess.

Progesterone comes primarily from the ovaries both before and after menopause, but it is also produced in both the brain and the peripheral nerves.[28] Its main job during the childbearing years is to prepare and maintain the uterus for its most important function: pregnancy. It also is a uterine muscle relaxant, preventing premature contractions. Progesterone levels rise in anticipation of pregnancy and stimulate the uterine lining to thicken with rich, well-vascularized tissue to support an embryo, then fall precipitously if pregnancy does not occur. This abrupt drop-off in progesterone is what signals the shedding of the "nest" (that thickened uterine lining) in the form of menstrual bleeding.

Progesterone also affects brain function. It produces a sense of calmness, and its sedating, antianxiety effect helps promote rejuvenating sleep.

Progesterone comes from a temporary yellowish gland in the ovary called the corpus luteum, formed quickly in the small cystlike structure left behind when a follicle ovulates. The corpus luteum produces increasing amounts of progesterone until the body sends the signal "We're not pregnant," at which point the corpus luteum is reabsorbed. As a woman reaches her mid-thirties to early forties, the follicle is more likely (at least in this culture) to fail to ovulate, which means the corpus luteum does not form.[29] Over time, this contributes to an increasing deficiency of progesterone.

Note: Our bodies are designed to accommodate very high levels of progesterone during pregnancy. For that reason, symptoms from excessive progesterone are rare. However, depression is a common side effect of synthetic progestins such as Provera. And a few women are so sensitive to progesterone that they become depressed even on very small doses of natural, bioidentical progesterone. Women who have this side effect should try using chasteberry (*Vitex agnus-castus*) to increase their body's progesterone naturally.

SYMPTOMS OF PROGESTERONE DEFICIENCY

- ~ Premenstrual migraine
- ~ PMS-like symptoms
- ~ Irregular or excessively heavy periods
- ~ Anxiety and nervousness

SYMPTOMS OF EXCESS PROGESTERONE

- ~ Sleepiness
- ~ Drowsiness
- ~ Depression

Bioidentical Progesterone

Bioidentical progesterone supplementation can help alleviate the symptoms of both progesterone deficiency and estrogen excess, restoring the body's balance. This provides long-term as well as short-term benefits. As I've noted, a growing body of evidence points to estrogen dominance as a major factor in promoting breast or uterine cancer in susceptible women. Studies show that when estrogen therapy is taken in concert with an appropriate dose of progesterone, the incidence of uterine cancer does not increase. This is true whether the progesterone is synthetic or bioidentical. It is also clear that Prempro (Premarin plus Provera) at the dosages used in the WHI study increases the risk of breast cancer. An analysis of the WHI data published in 2011 shows the risk of breast cancer is greater for women using a combination estrogen-progestin than for those taking only estrogen.[30] The 2019 meta-analysis of fifty-eight prospective studies mentioned earlier also found breast cancer risk is greater for women taking combination hormone therapy than for those taking estrogen-only therapy, and that this higher risk lasted for more than a decade. The effect may not be the same with bioidentical progesterone, however.

One of the largest studies to compare bioidentical hormones with synthetic hormones showed that the bioidentical hormones (including progesterone) have significantly less associated risk of breast cancer. This 2008 study conducted in France followed more than 80,000 postmenopausal women for more than eight years.[31] A 2009 follow-up study by the same French researchers looked at when HT therapy was begun. The results showed no significant increase in risk for breast cancer among women using estrogen plus natural progesterone for short durations, whether HT use began three years or less after menopause, or whether HT use began three years following menopause.[32] (See chapter 13, "Creating Breast Health.")

Research also shows that natural progesterone is very helpful in relieving midlife chest pain from coronary artery spasm at very low doses (¼ teaspoon of 2 percent progesterone cream, providing 20 mg of progesterone) applied to the skin.[33]

Another advantage of progesterone supplementation relates to this hormone's relatively unique ability to be converted into other hormones as needed. If progesterone levels are adequate, for example, but testosterone levels are on the low side, supplemental progesterone can actually transform itself into testosterone. It also increases the levels of DHEA. (See "How to Restore Your Adrenal Function," page 152.) Under the right circumstances, supplemental progesterone can even be metabolized into estrogen. This is one reason that the use of natural progesterone cream in early perimenopause, when there's a great deal of variation in the levels of all three hormones, allows so many women to enjoy symptomatic relief.

Progesterone cream is available over the counter in a 2 percent strength, and I've been recommending it for years. You can rub the cream anywhere on your body. One of the best places is right into your hands, because they are very well vascularized. But many women love the way progesterone cream works as a face or body cream. I recommend Pro-Gest cream by Emerita—now made paraben-free and sold in both single-dose, 20 mg foil packets as well as in a tube (in fragrance-free, fragrance-free with added vitamin D, or lavender scent), available at Emerson Ecologics (www.emersonecologics.com) and Amazon—and PhytoGest cream by Kevala (available at kevala health.net). Research shows that even small amounts of topical progesterone are indeed absorbed by the body and increase salivary levels of the hormone.[34]

FIGURE 10: KINDS OF PROGESTERONE

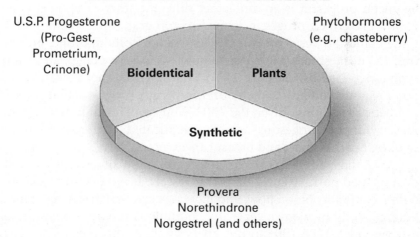

Natural progesterone is also available as a 4 to 8 percent gel (e.g., Crinone or Prochieve) or in an oral, micronized form (Prometrium). (Both require a prescription.) Though the manufacturer doesn't endorse this use, Prometrium capsules can be opened and the contents applied to the skin. I've found that this works very well for individuals who do not tolerate oral progesterone well but who require a higher dosage than is available with an over-the-counter cream.

THE YAM CREAM CAVEAT

Because bioidentical progesterone is often produced from wild Mexican yams, some women try to save money by buying one of a number of wild Mexican yam creams. The problem is, yam contains only a progesterone precursor, which remains inactive when it is absorbed through the skin. The conversion of wild yam into bioidentical progesterone can only occur in a laboratory setting. Yam creams may offer some beneficial phytoestrogens, but they certainly don't provide the documented benefits of laboratory-grade USP progesterone.

The Problem with Synthetics

Synthetic progestin is an altogether different story. The most commonly prescribed progestin is medroxyprogesterone acetate (MPA; trade names Provera, Amen). Others include norethindrone, norgestrel, and norgestimate. Progestin actually causes or exaggerates many symptoms. (See list on page 197.) That's yet another reason why I don't recommend any of the hormone therapy programs that employ synthetic progestins. Given the 2002 Women's Health Initiative findings, synthetic progestins are also implicated as a risk factor in strokes, heart disease, and breast cancer.

MPA has been shown to attenuate some of estrogen's well-documented positive effect on blood vessels. It increases vascular resistance, inhibits blood flow, and increases cerebral artery resistance. A large study of women receiving continuous therapy consisting of estrogen plus MPA (Prempro is an example of this type of therapy) showed a marked increase in myocardial infarction, death from coronary artery disease, and venous thrombosis (blood clots in the veins) during the first two years of therapy.[35]

The newer analysis of the WHI data released in 2010 confirmed that this risk is present even for women who began synthetic HT within ten years of menopause—although risk drops after six years of use (which is longer than most women take HT anyway).[36] An earlier reanalysis of the WHI and Nurses' Health studies data from 2006 is also interesting because it supports an adverse effect from synthetic progestin. Younger women taking Prempro had a 30 percent decreased risk of heart disease when they started HT within ten years of menopause. But those who were on estrogen only had a 44 percent decreased risk. I suspect that the difference in the two groups was due to the adverse effect of MPA.

Natural bioidentical progesterone contains no such risk and in fact has many benefits. In the famous PEPI (Postmenopausal Estrogen/Progestin Intervention) trial, oral natural progesterone in micronized form prevented the adverse effects on cholesterol that were seen in women on Provera.

SYMPTOMS FROM SYNTHETIC PROGESTIN

- Headache
- Depression
- Weight gain and bloating
- Moodiness
- Lack of sexual desire
- Potential narrowing of blood vessels, causing chest pain and lack of oxygen to the heart

ELLEN: Too Much Estrogen, Too Little Progesterone

Ellen, a potter and yoga instructor in a college town, noticed a subtle, fuzzy-minded feeling and morning dizziness during the spring of her forty-third year. One day, as she was placing a bottle of aspirin in her grocery cart, she also realized that though she'd never had headaches before, she'd gradually begun experiencing them regularly—attributing them to tension, a weather change, or PMS. On a visit to her doctor, he drew a blood sample and tested her FSH level, which was high, convincing him she was menopausal. He told Ellen that her symptoms—the mental fuzziness, dizziness, and headaches—were consistent with menopause and that they'd improve if she took supplemental hormones. He gave her a prescription for Premarin to take daily, with some Provera for the last twelve days of every month. Within days Ellen was miserable. What previously had felt like a tension headache now was a throbbing, splitting migraine; she felt depressed; she had restless legs that were keeping her awake; and most of her other symptoms persisted.

It's true that the symptoms Ellen experienced were consistent with the climacteric, but in light of her relative youth and the fact that she had not had these symptoms for more than a few months, it was probably early in the course of her perimenopause—which in many women is associated with low progesterone levels and a relative excess of estrogen. The blood test for FSH levels, upon which her

SAME DOLL, DIFFERENT DRESS

The latest wrinkle in the hormone therapy scene is prepackaged combinations. The synthetic hormones used in these preparations have been around for years; what is different is the packaging and the ways in which they are prescribed. A commonly used preparation, for instance, is Prempro (a combination of Premarin and Provera), the drug that was used in the WHI study. Others include Ortho-Prefest (a combination of bioidentical estradiol and the synthetic progestin norgestimate) and Femhrt (synthetic estradiol plus synthetic norethindrone). The advantage of these combinations is that they are convenient and women allegedly don't have any monthly bleeding on them. The problem is that many get spotting and intermittent bleeding for months before their bodies get used to the drug combos, causing many to stop taking them. The biggest drawback is that all of them contain synthetic progestin, which enhances a woman's chance of developing PMS-like side effects and also may increase her risk for heart disease and breast cancer. (To be fair, the 2006 reanalysis for the WHI and Nurses' Health studies data did, in fact, show a decreased risk of heart disease in younger women—even in those on Prempro, which contains a synthetic progestin. But why take any risk when other forms of progesterone are available?)

physician based his diagnosis of menopause, is an inaccurate way to assess the big picture. It's like looking at a single frame in a very long movie. In fact, the symptoms Ellen experienced after taking the prescribed estrogen were consistent with estrogen overdose.

Even without knowing this, Ellen did the intuitive thing: she stopped taking her estrogen. Within twenty-four hours she started feeling better, and she vowed to "tough it out" without going back to the doctor. But her original symptoms persisted, and eventually a friend referred her to another doctor, who ordered hormone tests for estrogen, progesterone, and testosterone. The results confirmed that Ellen was in an early stage of perimenopause, with her primary hormonal change being low progesterone. Eventually using a natural progesterone cream to gently supplement her body's own dwindling supply, Ellen felt much better, and she understood a lot more about the transitional process. "I'm a work in progress," she wrote. "My hormonal status is changing, and I know that what works for me now might need to be tweaked a little in six months."

Testosterone

Testosterone is produced in both the ovaries and adrenal glands. Its primary job is to provide vital assertive energy and sexual drive. Testosterone and other androgens can increase the ease with which a woman becomes sexually aroused, as well as the frequency with which she follows through by initiating sexual activity. Testosterone also increases sensitivity of the erogenous zones, frequency of orgasm, intensity of sexual fantasies, and incidence of orgasmic dreams.

Not all women's testosterone levels drop perimenopausally—in fact, androgen levels actually increase in some. But if a woman is suffering from adrenal depletion due to chronic stress (see chapter 4), a precipitous drop in testosterone may occur, with symptoms of declining libido and overall energy depletion. Surgical removal of the ovaries, uterus, or both, as well as chemotherapy, radiation, or autoimmune disease, can also contribute to a drop in testosterone levels severe enough to cause symptoms.

For reasons that have yet to be clarified, some women experience a gradual decline in testosterone from early adulthood to old age, while other women continue to produce plenty of testosterone throughout life. The adrenals surely play a role, but whether there are other factors remains to be seen. Before you decide to try testosterone supplementation, it is essential to have laboratory confirmation of a deficiency via saliva or blood testing for free (unbound) testosterone. As with other menopause-related symptoms, there is considerable overlap among the three hormones. In many women, for example, a decline in libido is due to an estrogen deficiency, while testosterone may be normal. There is no benefit from taking supplemental testosterone if there is no deficiency to begin with. And many women with low testosterone levels have a normal sex drive! (See chapter 9.)

This bears emphasis because testosterone supplementation is now being requested by many women who think it will jump-start a flagging sex life. If there is a deficiency, the benefits may include heightened sex drive and sexual function, higher levels of energy overall, better muscle tone, and improved mood and outlook. There also is evidence that restoring normal testosterone levels can help improve bone mineral density. Incorporated into a vaginal cream, testosterone can help restore normal vaginal wall thickness and lubrication. However, if there is no deficiency, supplementation will likely lead to overdose, which can produce symptoms most women find objectionable.

Bioidentical testosterone—or DHEA (dehydroepiandrosterone), an adrenal precursor for testosterone—is available from formulary pharmacies and can be used as a skin or vaginal cream by those women who require it. Some physicians are also inserting testosterone pellets under the skin. The problem with all of these androgens is that they tend to increase hair on the upper lip and chin and may also contribute to male-pattern baldness.

(Although DHEA is available over the counter, the quality varies considerably. I recommend pharmaceutical-grade DHEA, which is available from formulary pharmacies and Emerson Ecologics [visit www.emersonecologics.com]. I recommend 5 mg sublingual DHEA manufactured by Douglas Laboratories; the suggested dose is ½ to 1 tablet daily, or as directed.) Testosterone is also available in a patch as well as in gels.

A synthetic form, methyltestosterone, is available in pill form or mixed with estrogen and sold under the brand names Covaryx and EEMT; I don't recommend it.

SYMPTOMS OF TESTOSTERONE DEFICIENCY

- Decreased libido
- Impaired sexual function
- Decreased energy overall
- Decreased sense of well-being
- Thinning pubic hair

SYMPTOMS OF TESTOSTERONE OVERDOSE

- Mood disturbances
- Acne, particularly on the face and scalp
- Increased facial hair growth
- Deepened voice

HOW TO DECIDE WHETHER OR NOT TO TAKE HORMONES

Whether you should or should not take supplemental hormones at menopause depends on a number of factors, including your overall physical health, emotional and spiritual well-being, nutritional status, lifestyle, and so forth. All these factors can influence how well your secondary hormone production sites are able to keep up with your body's new needs. For some women, just learning that the symptoms of perimenopause are temporary is enough reassurance; they become willing to experience those symptoms without masking them with medicine. And once we relax and allow our fears and resistance to fade, the symptoms themselves may lessen. This is the "placebo effect" in action, and it is a significant factor in menopausal treatments as well. Knowing that we can ask for and receive help creates its own healing energy.

Taking Stock Before Making the Decision

Before deciding on hormone therapy, it is important to take an honest look at yourself and at your medical history—including that of your family members—so you can draw an accurate picture of your own goals and needs. Some women need hormones to feel their best. Others don't do well on them at all and much prefer nonprescription methods, such as herbs. Some women make enough hormones naturally in their own bodies to get through menopause without outside help. Others cannot make the biological conversions necessary to maintain the right hormonal balance. Still others have had their ovaries removed and need additional hormonal support, at least until they've reached the age when menopause would usually occur.

Despite the recent good news about HT and heart disease, I firmly believe that it is progesterone, not estrogen, that holds the biggest promise for preventing heart disease (or at the very least treating angina). I prefer a cautious, eyes-wide-open approach to long-term estrogen use to prevent chronic disease. Few would disagree, however, that hormone therapy can be very helpful for many women during the perimenopausal transition, when symptoms are at their worst. But for some women, the benefits of long-term hormone therapy may outweigh the risks—for example, when there is a strong family history of osteoporosis, or when a woman clearly feels much better on hormones than off them.

Given the nature of science, medicine, and the pharmaceutical industry, you can expect that the conventional wisdom on HT will continue to change. So stay tuned. If you have bothersome perimenopausal symptoms that aren't relieved by other methods, give hormone therapy a try, stay with it for a year or so, and then taper your dose. See how you feel. If you feel fine, then taper some more until you've weaned yourself off it. If, on the other hand, you clearly feel your best on hormone therapy, then stay with it and revisit your decision yearly.

The first step you need to take in making the HT decision is to identify your risk factors and decide how much weight you intend to give them.

When I say "how much weight you intend to give them," I mean that only you have the power to decide how much influence your cultural and family script will have on your reality. Perimenopausal discomfort is a reality for most American women, while women in some other cultures have a different experience. Studies show that while 70 to 85 percent of North American women are affected by hot flashes, only 18 percent of Chinese factory workers in Hong Kong experience them.[37] I can assure you that the basic biology of the ovaries in China is not different than in North America. This speaks to the strength of expectations and how an entire culture can come to dictate what each individual will experience. Notwithstanding, each of us has the power to acknowledge this influence and then change our response to it.

Statistics predict what will happen to groups in general, not to specific individuals. Studies have shown that a woman's faith in (or rejection of) her cultural and genetic/familial script can play a significant role in how her reality plays out. People who are known in their families as "black sheep" are the least likely to fall victim to diseases that run in the family, perhaps because it is their own personal attitude and style to reject rules and color outside the lines. Since most healthcare providers are trained to look at statistics when making decisions and predictions about our health, it is crucial that each of us emphasizes our innate ability to become "black sheep" when and if this stance can improve our health and outlook.

Although scientific studies may change how we think about something intellectually, our behavior and what we actually do with scientific information is shaped far more by our day-to-day relationships with friends and family than by any other factor. If, for example, you've watched your mother, sister, or best friend come alive again after going on some form of hormone therapy, you're apt to feel very positive about the benefits of this approach. If, on the other hand, you've watched a family member suffer from headaches, sore breasts, and weight gain from taking too high a dose of estrogen, you're not going to be very eager to try it yourself. And if you are surrounded by aunts, grandmothers, or other older female role models who are vibrantly healthy, live well into their nineties in good health, and have never taken HT of any kind, your inner blueprint for what is apt to happen after you go through menopause without medication will be quite positive.

My own personal legacy includes cardiovascular disease. My mother lost both her parents to heart disease, and my beloved father collapsed and died on the tennis court at age sixty-eight, a victim of a ruptured cerebral aneurysm, when my mother was only fifty-two and perimenopausal. She finished the climacteric as a widow, during an era when women were expected to fade physically and socially after menopause. Though my mother tends to avoid conventional wisdom in general and visits to the doctor in particular, her sister and her friends were told again and again that without supplemental estrogen, they would become little old ladies with fragile skeletons and weak hearts. But my mother greeted that prediction with a dismissive wave of her hand. She completed the entire Appalachian Trail and climbed the hundred highest peaks in New England in her seventies, and she trekked to a Mount Everest base camp at the age of eighty-four. She never took estrogen, but she did add some progesterone cream along the way as well as the herb *Pueraria mirifica*. At the age of ninety-four, she led all thirty-two members of her extended family on a reunion in the Adirondacks that included a daily hike.

Which of my family's medical legacies will I inherit? I firmly believe that through the physical and emotional choices I make—and the expectations and beliefs with which I live my life—I shape my own future. My daughters and granddaughters will do the same. Would I like to have the same level of health when I'm ninety-four that my mother now enjoys? Of course I would, but I believe it will happen because I have chosen it, not because I have inherited it.

What Are Your Goals?

Too many women see the HT decision as an either/or, yes/no decision. I'd like to reframe it as a process. As a first step, it is important to define the goals you hope to achieve with hormone therapy. Contrary to the message conveyed by pharmaceutical marketing efforts, HT will not give you a means of moving backward, of denying the wisdom that is part of growing older, or of keeping yourself young forever—though there is no question that lifestyle plays a huge role in remaining biologically youthful for as long as possible. Still, embracing the wisdom that comes from going through menopause is one of the true joys of life. And a personally tailored program—with or without supplemental hormones—can help reduce physical symptoms and health worries so that you can focus your energies on finding your creative passions, which in and of themselves can stoke the flames of your life force. Hormone therapy can help mask the heart palpitations and irritability often associated with perimenopause. And it can also promote healthy sleep (especially when natural progesterone is used). But hormones cannot resolve the underlying relationship problems (and ensuing high levels of stress hormones) that may be crying out for your attention.

Every day more and more studies are showing how effective modalities such as dietary change (in particular, a low-sugar diet), food supplements, exercise, and herbs can be in supporting a woman

Selected Hormone Options

Product	Route of Administration	Estrogen	Progesterone	Bioidentical or Synthetic (for humans)
ESTRING	Vaginal silicone ring	Estradiol	None	Bioidentical
VIVELLE-DOT	Skin patch	Estradiol	None	Bioidentical
DIVIGEL	Transdermal gel	Estradiol	None	Bioidentical
ESTROGEL	Transdermal gel	Estradiol	None	Bioidentical
AYGESTIN	Oral	None	Norethindrone acetate	Synthetic
PROVERA	Oral	None	Medroxyprogester-one acetate	Synthetic
AMEN ORAL	Oral	None	Medroxyprogester-one acetate	Synthetic
PROMETRIUM	Oral	None	Micronized progesterone	Bioidentical
CRINONE	Vaginal gel	None	Progesterone	Bioidentical
PROCHIEVE	Vaginal gel	None	Progesterone	Bioidentical
PREMPRO	Oral	Conjugated horse estrogens	Medroxyprogester-one acetate	Synthetic
FEMHRT	Oral	Ethinyl estradiol	Norethindrone acetate	Synthetic
ORTHO-PREFEST	Oral	17-ß-estradiol	Norgestimate	Bioidentical estrogen, synthetic progesterone
COMBI-PATCH	Skin patch	Estradiol	Norethindrone ac-etate	Bioidentical estrogen, synthetic progesterone
ANGELIQ	Oral	Estradiol	Drospirenone	Bioidentical estrogen, synthetic progesterone
ALORA	Skin patch	Estradiol	None	Bioidentical
CLIMARA	Skin patch	Estradiol	None	Bioidentical
CLIMARA PRO	Skin patch	Levonorgestrel	None	Bioidentical estrogen, synthetic progesterone
ESTRASORB	Cream	Estradiol	None	Bioidentical
EVAMIST	Spray	Estradiol	None	Bioidentical
FEMRING	Vaginal silicone ring	Estradiol acetate	None	Bioidentical
VAGIFEM	Vaginal tablets	Estradiol	None	Bioidentical
IMVEXXY	Vaginal inserts	Estradiol	None	Bioidentical

through her menopausal transition. Though some doctors still don't know about these approaches and may not mention them to you, they often work as well or better than hormone therapy. They can also be used in addition to hormone therapy, to reduce dosage levels, side effects, and potential risk. In other words, you don't necessarily have to choose between HT and alternatives. Think of your perimenopausal support as a smorgasbord. You get to choose what appeals to you at the moment and leave what doesn't.

Becoming an Active Partner in the Decision

For our mothers and grandmothers, the decision to take HT (or not) was very often a passive one, made by their doctors (or husband or best friend), with their own involvement limited to "being good patients." Or they decided by not deciding and simply let time go by. In those days there were very few HT preparations available, so the choices were only two: yes or no. And until recently, the potential benefits were too often clouded by side effects from the wrong type of medications or fear of long-term consequences. As of the late 1990s, less than 20 percent of American women used hormone therapy, and those who did often discontinued it within six months.[38] Now only 13 to 15 percent of women report ever having used hormone therapy.[39] As of 2008, the total number of women using hormones had dropped to less than 6 million, compared to nearly 18 million in 2001, the year before the initial data from the Women's Health Initiative was released.[40]

Today, the pendulum is swinging once again toward the benefits and away from the risks of hormone therapy. I recently was consulted for a media story about hormones by a journalist who had been told by her doctor that she had better get on estrogen soon because she was in the middle of that "ten-year window"—meaning that any benefits she might experience from hormone therapy would be attained only if she started HT in that ten years following her last period. She was very worried about getting Alzheimer's in later life and was hoping that taking estrogen early on might prevent it. I explained to her that nearly all studies on the benefits of hormones—or anything else, for that matter—describe their results in terms of an average of what happens in an entire population (what's called the mean). But let's not forget something known as the "ecological fallacy," an error that arises when we make inferences about individuals based on aggregate data about a group. It is not necessarily true that if something is true for the average of a group (the mean), it must also be true for the individual. The reverse also applies: if something is good for an individual, it doesn't mean it is also good for everyone in the group. We would do well to remember that in every population, outliers exist on either side of the mean—individuals whose biology, lifestyle, and beliefs fall outside the norm.

I suggest you try out saying "That needn't apply to me" on a regular basis. Here's how that works. You read a study that suggests that women over age fifty are more apt to get breast cancer, arthritis, or whatever. Instead of immediately starting to worry, you just say in your head, "That needn't apply to me." Start thinking like an outlier who defies the statistics about what is supposed to happen. In the case of that ten-year window with hormone therapy, remember that when it comes to health and disease, there are many, many other factors at play beyond simply your hormone levels. Ask your inner guidance if the information applies to you or not.

A great deal of confusion results, both for individuals and for doctors, if we rely only on the latest study to determine what an individual ought to do. Recall that the early reports on the Women's Health Initiative study seemed to indict all hormone therapy. In fact, the women in the original 2002 WHI study were all on the same dose of only *one type* of HT—namely, Prempro. But then came the 2006 analysis of the WHI data showing a decreased risk of heart disease in women who started taking it earlier. Still, there are a lot of unanswered questions, plus the irrefutable increased risk of breast cancer with some forms of hormone therapy.

One thing is clear: every woman is different. Some will do beautifully on some kinds of hormone therapies. Others will not. And coming up with a recommendation that is right for all women is simply not possible. Each of us should stop looking for that kind of prescription and instead tune in to our own individual needs.

At the same time, we also need to remember that medicine will always be an art, not an exact science. In the early 1990s, science seemed to indicate that the majority of postmenopausal women would benefit from hormone therapy. Some were even dismissed from their doctor's office if they questioned that belief. Then the pendulum swung all the way in the opposite direction. The truth for any given individual is almost always somewhere in the middle.

In addition to the question "Do I want or need hormone therapy, at least for right now?" we also have to ask: "What kind? What strength? What route of administration? In what combination? For what reason? For how long? At what risk?"

The number of options can be intimidating at first, but in the end you'll feel much better about your HT decision if you're armed with facts, know your options, and are willing to listen to your inner guidance as well as to your doctor's advice. And although I discourage using HT as a means of numbing yourself to what is happening in your body, mind, and spirit during the wake-up call of perimenopause, there is nothing to be gained from undue suffering. Given the range of formulations and dosages now available—as well as the many alternatives to HT—you can create an individual treatment program that supports you through the change, rather than helping you deny that it is happening.

EVIE: Brittle Diabetes, Brittle Hormones

Evie is an energetic, upbeat insurance saleswoman who steadfastly refuses to allow her diabetes—which she's had since the age of thirteen—to dominate her life. She checks her blood glucose levels regularly and gives herself two injections of insulin each day, but she's considered a "brittle" diabetic and still suffers at least one diabetic crisis each year.

Evie takes these episodes in stride, sometimes exasperating her friends and loved ones who wish she'd take her condition "more seriously," but she admits that she gets "prickly" when they dote on her. She has also begun to make the connection between the state of her diabetes and the state of her emotions. When she is upset with one of her children, her boss, or her husband, her insulin and dietary needs can change dramatically and quickly. It also came as no surprise to Evie's physician that because of her metabolic problems, her blood sugar levels went wild as she bumped and jolted through her menopausal transition. She wrote, "There's an amusement park nearby, with a really scary roller coaster. Let's just say I've got 'em beat. Estrogen, glucose, FSH—everything was bouncing all over the place."

Jerilynn Prior, M.D., a hormone researcher and professor of endocrinology and metabolism at the University of British Columbia and founder and scientific director of the Centre for Menstrual Cycle and Ovulation Research, calls this phase "estrogen's storm season" and has written a very helpful book with the same title (Centre for Menstrual Cycle and Ovulation Research, 2005). (For more information, see CeMCOR's website at www.cemcor.ubc.ca.)

Because Evie's levels were so erratic and sensitive, it was tough getting her regulated, but with trial and error Evie and her physician

managed to arrive at a hormone therapy program that gently alleviated her discomfort, stabilized her metabolism (and therefore her
glucose levels), and supported her body through the transition. "It
was a pretty tough trip for a while there, but I noticed a difference
within weeks of getting the right levels of hormones."

Clarifying Your Needs

In order to make the best choice for you, you need to clarify your
needs, then become an active partner in getting them met. This may
mean consulting more than one healthcare provider—an herbalist or
acupuncturist in addition to your OB-GYN, for instance. It may also
mean asking your physician to try an approach he or she is unfamiliar with—and sharing the responsibility for the results.

To begin, review the following eight health factors and determine
which, if any, apply to you. This will help you focus your thinking
about which replacement regimen to use, if any, and for how long.

FACTOR 1: YOU WANT RELIEF FROM DISCOMFORT, PARTICU-
LARLY HOT FLASHES THAT DISRUPT SLEEP. This is the most common reason why women choose hormone therapy, especially
estrogen. However, discomfort is also the most common reason for
women to stop taking HT—the formulation and/or the dosage prescribed may not be right for their particular metabolism, resulting in
persistent medication side effects and/or symptoms of overdose.

Many women have found relief from insomnia with meditation,
Pueraria mirifica, or maca. A few studies have shown that cognitive
behavioral therapy (a technique that involves modifying negative
thought patterns and behaviors so you can respond in more effective ways) may reduce hot flashes, depression, and sleep disorders
in menopausal women.[41] A new oral medication for hot flashes may
soon become available as well. Studies have shown that women
taking a neurokinin 3 receptor (NK3R) antagonist can reduce their
frequency of hot flashes by 72 percent by the third day of treatment.[42] At the current time the drug is still in trials, so stay tuned.
If relief from symptoms is your sole reason for seeking treatment,
treatment will probably be needed only until the perimenopausal
transition is complete, which can be confirmed either by a lack of
menstrual periods for at least a year or by the laboratory tests outlined in chapter 4. There might be a brief perimenopause-like adjustment when coming off hormone treatment, but if you are

weaned off the hormones over a period of several months, the symptoms generally are mild. Many women come off hormone therapy once they've become well established on regimens that include herbs, soy, exercise, or dietary supplements. This approach often smooths the adjustment.

If you want symptomatic relief but your personal preference is to stay away from supplemental hormones, there are many nonhormonal treatments available over the counter or from healthcare practitioners such as naturopaths and acupuncturists. (See chapter 6.)

FACTOR 2: YOU ARE SUFFERING FROM UROGENITAL SYMPTOMS. The health of the vaginal lining and urethral tissues is highly influenced by the hormonal milieu in our bodies. Women may seek relief from stress incontinence (they leak urine when coughing, sneezing, laughing, or lifting heavy objects), urge incontinence (they have difficulty making it to the bathroom without leaking), recurrent vaginal yeast infections, vaginal dryness and/or discomfort during intercourse, recurrent bladder infections, or urinary frequency (they need to urinate more than eight times during the day, or one or more times during the night).

Taking estrogen (by mouth or applied locally) and/or androgen hormones (by mouth or applied as a skin patch or as a cream formulated for vaginal application) helps maintain healthy vaginal and urethral tissue, even when relatively small doses are used. As little as 1 to 2 mg of natural testosterone in a cream base, applied to the vagina two to three times per week, for example, is often all that is necessary. And many times the phytoestrogens found in herbs like *Pueraria mirifica* can restore vaginal tissue to its premenopausal moistness and resilience. (See chapter 6.)

Some studies from the late 1990s found that systemic oral conventional hormone therapy actually increases the risk of urinary incontinence for reasons that aren't at all clear. What *is* clear is that urinary problems often clear up on their own with no treatment at all.

FACTOR 3: YOU CURRENTLY HAVE A HEALTHY HEART BUT ARE AT INCREASED RISK FOR CARDIOVASCULAR DISEASE. A woman's increased risk of heart disease is usually related to (1) a positive family history (heart disease or stroke in father younger than age fifty-five, or in mother or other first-degree female relative at age sixty-five or younger) and all the emotions that go with it, (2) lifestyle factors, such as a high-sugar diet, smoking, or lack of exercise, or (3) a predisposing factor such as low HDL cholesterol, high LDL cholesterol, or high triglycerides. Menopause is also a time when progesterone levels fall significantly, triggering the narrowing of coronary arteries in susceptible women. Preliminary research strongly suggests that low progesterone levels are far more likely to be associated with heart disease than estrogen deficiency is. Progesterone is, unfortunately, still largely underrated and misunderstood.[43]

Nevertheless, beginning in the late 1980s, doctors prescribed hormone therapy liberally to women to prevent heart disease because a large number of epidemiologic studies had shown a clear benefit. Estrogen decreases LDL (the bad cholesterol) and increases HDL (the good cholesterol).[44] It also has a positive effect on blood vessel walls that seems to involve nitric oxide, a chemical produced in the body that helps keep blood vessels dilated. (Viagra and other drugs for male impotence also exert their effect through nitric oxide pathways.)

But then in 2002 the Women's Health Initiative study branch that was testing Prempro against placebo in thousands of women was abruptly halted because the drug caused an increase in strokes and heart attacks, and the medical profession quickly backed away from its original position on HT and heart disease. The WHI was the first long-term placebo-controlled trial of hormone therapy, and it clearly showed that the cardiovascular risks of Prempro outweigh the benefits. While the 2006 reanalysis of the data from both the WHI and Nurses' Health studies showed that when women begin hormone therapy within ten years of menopause they decrease their risk of heart disease by at least 11 percent and as much as 30 percent, a 2010 reanalysis showed that the risk didn't drop until the women had taken HT for six years (longer than most usually take hormones) and that hormones actually *increased* this risk after only two years. As it turns out, most of the women in the original WHI study didn't start Prempro until they were in their sixties and well past the age of menopause.[45] No one knows exactly what to make of these data— but clearly estrogen can be heart healthy in some women.

The problem here is that Prempro isn't synonymous with all HT. It contains synthetic progestin, which is known to partially obliterate the beneficial effects of estrogen alone on blood vessels. In addition, all hormones in the WHI study were given orally. This increases the risk of blood clots because oral hormones must be processed in the liver, and increased clotting factors are the result—especially in older women. There are still solid data to suggest that low-dose, bioidentical estrogen, without synthetic progestin, given transdermally and at physiologic levels, could be beneficial for the cardiovascular systems of some women. Unfortunately, most of the conventionally available combination hormone therapies contain synthetic progestins, including Prempro, CombiPatch, Femhrt, and Activella.

I feel strongly that there is a far greater potential benefit for hormone therapy in women who use individualized regimens consisting of bioidentical hormones. Because of their deleterious effect on blood vessels, I believe that synthetic progestins (especially Provera or Amen) are more dangerous than taking no hormones at all. Tried-and-true methods to decrease heart disease risk also include avoiding smoking, doing regular vigorous exercise, taking supplements such as vitamin E, following a diet rich in fruits and vegetables, taking supplements, and keeping weight normal. (See chapter 14 for my heart health program.)

FACTOR 4: YOU HAVE ALREADY BEEN DIAGNOSED WITH HEART DISEASE. It is now clear that hormone therapy, at least in the form of Prempro (Premarin and Provera), increases the risk of stroke and heart attack in older women—the ones most likely to have full-blown heart disease.

Many scientists feel that this is due to a hormone-stimulated increase in chemicals called inflammation factors, such as C-reactive protein, which was found in the bloodstream in amounts that were 85 percent higher in women taking hormone therapy. However, this is once again a case where you need to read the fine print. As I've said, I believe that the increased risk from conventional HT boils down mainly to the adverse effects of medroxyprogesterone acetate (trade names Provera and Amen). It is also true that estrogens at high enough doses have long been associated with increased risk of blood clots that predispose to heart attack, especially in smokers.

Here's the bottom line: women with or without heart disease should avoid synthetic progestins and keep their estrogen doses as natural and as low as possible, and no one should take estrogen as a way to treat already-diagnosed heart disease. I would, however, consider transdermal natural progesterone.

FACTOR 5: YOU ARE AT INCREASED RISK FOR OSTEOPOROSIS OR ALREADY HAVE BEEN DIAGNOSED WITH BONE LOSS. A woman whose mother or grandmother has osteoporosis is at increased risk for this potentially disabling condition, though it is unknown whether this is because of a genetic inheritance or because we tend to "inherit" habits, lifestyle choices, and life expectations, which may predispose us to less-than-optimal bone strength. (See chapter 12 for additional risk factors, many of which are under our control.) Estrogen replacement definitely helps prevent bone loss associated with menopause, and continuous use of estrogen decreases the risk of fracture by 50 percent or more. The bone-preserving effects of estrogen are maintained only as long as a woman stays on it.

Androgens such as testosterone also play a role in preserving bone health. Those women with naturally high testosterone levels have a decreased risk for osteoporotic fractures. Low-dose testosterone supplementation has been found to help maintain bone mass.

A number of drugs—calcitonin; the bisphosphonates, such as alendronate (trade name Fosamax), ibandronate (Boniva), risedronate (Actonel), and zoledronic acid (Reclast); the SERMs, such as tamoxifen (Nolvadex) and raloxifene (Evista); parathyroid hormone analog (Forteo); and romosozumab (Evenity)—have also been shown to help prevent loss of bone and decrease fracture risk. These drugs have many adverse effects and their use must be approached with caution. (See chapter 12, "Standing Tall for Life," for a complete discussion of bone-building drugs.)

Regular weight-bearing exercise, vitamin D, vitamin K, and mineral supplementation are also very effective ways of maintaining bone density and decreasing fracture risk, both at perimenopause and beyond. (See chapter 12.)

FACTOR 6: YOU ARE AT INCREASED RISK FOR ALZHEIMER'S DISEASE. At this point in our limited understanding of this organic brain disorder, a positive family history is the strongest predisposing factor, although most individuals who get it don't have any genetic predisposition. Many authorities are now calling Alzheimer's "type 3 diabetes" because it is related to years of high blood sugar and high insulin levels—and the resulting inflammation in the blood vessels of the brain. There is less consensus regarding some studies' suggestion that high levels of aluminum intake (from using aluminum cookware or consuming food from aluminum cans) might also contribute to an individual's risk of developing Alzheimer's disease.

It is clear that all hormones can affect brain function—androgens and progesterone as well as estrogen—and that many women continue making enough of these throughout life to protect their brains. In fact, a 2000 British study of postmenopausal women not on hormone therapy found that those with the highest levels of endogenous estradiol were the least likely to have Alzheimer's disease.[46] But research has failed to prove that estrogen decreases the risk of dementia. Some studies even suggest that estrogen, plus or minus progestin, may actually increase a woman's risk. There are many additional things a woman can do now to protect her mental functions in later life. (See chapter 10, "Nurturing Your Brain.")

FACTOR 7: YOU ARE AT INCREASED RISK FOR BREAST, UTER-INE, OVARIAN, OR BOWEL CANCER. A positive personal or family history for one or more of these hormone-related cancers makes the hormone therapy decision particularly anxiety-provoking for many women. Here are the facts. Research suggests that the dose and for-mulation of hormone therapy are important factors in the cancer issue. All types of estrogen at high enough doses over a long enough period of time can potentially stimulate breast, uterine, and ovarian cancers because estrogen is a growth factor in these tissues. This in-cludes the estrogens produced in your own body. Premarin, because of its association with DNA damage and because it has a stronger biological effect than bioidentical estrogens, may be more carcino-genic than bioidentical estrogens, especially when they are used in low doses. In other words, the increased risk of breast and uterine cancer shown by past studies may have been related to estrogen over-dose or the wrong kind of estrogen, rather than estrogen per se. This issue is far from clear, however, because as mentioned earlier, recent analysis of long-term data from the Women's Health Initiative study showed that women taking conjugated estrogen-only hormone ther-apy had a 23 percent reduced risk for breast cancer. What is known is that the addition of synthetic progestin further complicates mat-ters. The WHI data clearly demonstrated that women taking the combination drug Prempro for five or more years had a higher risk for breast cancer than those on placebo. Not all studies show an in-creased risk for breast cancer with HT—some show that bioidentical hormones (including progesterone) have significantly less associated risk of breast cancer. And the estrogen-only branch of the WHI showed no increased risk. But these women had all had hysterecto-mies and were probably at a lower risk to begin with.

If estrogen is taken in a manner that more closely mimics the way it is produced in the body—in physiological doses calibrated to the body's needs, in bioidentical formulation, and partnered with bi-oidentical, not synthetic, progesterone—it begins to lose its sinister profile. (See chapter 13.)

For the woman who is in the highest-risk category for breast, uterine, or ovarian cancer but who desires support through the symp-tomatic phase of perimenopause, there are two options that are un-likely to adversely affect that risk. First, she can take bioidentical hormones at the lowest possible levels during the five years or fewer when her symptoms are the most troubling. This may involve fine-tuning her doses with the aid of hormone testing, so that she takes no more than the amounts necessary to achieve physiological balance and symptomatic relief. Second, she can opt for nonhormonal, herbal treatments. (See chapter 6.) Another support may be taking *Pueraria mirifica,* which studies show has an antiproliferative effect on breast cancer cells in vitro.[47]

With regard to colorectal cancer, the picture is clearer. Colorectal cancer is the third most common cancer after breast and lung (with the exception of skin cancer). In both prevalence and mortality it outranks endometrial, ovarian, and cervical cancers. A summary of ten studies with information on the timing of estrogen use indicates a 34 percent reduced risk of colorectal cancer in current users. The 2002 WHI study confirmed this data. This protection is nearly lost within a few years of stopping hormone therapy. Though no one knows why for sure, it appears that estrogen causes a decrease in bile acids, substances manufactured in the liver that are associated with the promotion of colorectal cancer.[48]

FACTOR 8: YOU REACHED MENOPAUSE PREMATURELY (PRIOR TO AGE FORTY) OR ARTIFICIALLY AND ABRUPTLY (DUE TO SURGERY, ILLNESS, CHEMOTHERAPY, OR RADIATION). Women with this history are more likely to need systemic hormone therapy, a program that provides physiologically appropriate hormone levels throughout the body, rather than more locally acting products, and rather than relying solely on herbal treatments and dietary approaches. This is because the physical and mental symptoms associated with a premature or abrupt cessation of natural hormone production are usually more severe than with a gradual perimenopausal decline. With premature menopause, the woman's body is left without endogenous hormone support for more years than if menopause had occurred later in life. I recommend using a combination of bioidentical hormones, with the dosage based on your symptoms and hormone levels.

SANDY: Surgical Menopause

Sandy had an "instant" menopause at age thirty-five, when her ovaries were removed because of severe endometriosis. This created the abrupt hormonal withdrawal characteristic of artificial menopause. Her symptoms were quite pronounced. Until her surgery, Sandy had believed that she would not take hormone therapy when she reached her natural menopause. Now, to say the least, her discomfort was intrusive. And the fact that she would be without her normal complement of hormones for approximately fifteen extra years meant that her bone density, heart health, and mental functioning might suffer in the future. As a result, Sandy felt she had no choice but to start HT. "Frankly," she wrote, "I was so miserable I couldn't give my full attention to the decision beyond that point." She and her doctor decided on a skin patch that delivered bioidentical estrogen (17-beta estradiol), along with natural progesterone oral capsules. With minimal tweaking, they arrived at the optimal dose for her, and her level of comfort vastly improved.

"At that point," Sandy wrote, "I could start applying myself to decisions that would affect my future. I really had not wanted to take HT after menopause, but I didn't want to increase my chance of osteoporosis, so it felt right to take HT under the circumstances. Then it hit me: I can have the best of both worlds! I decided I'll take these hormones until I'm fifty-five, when I'd probably have completed my menopausal transition naturally, and then I'll wean myself off the hormones and sail through my menopausal years au naturel. I feel much happier about this plan. I feel like the idea was a thank-you gift from my body for bending the 'rules' and providing it with hormones during these extra fifteen years of menopause."

When to Start HT

Over the years I've watched scores of women left to "tough it out" during their stormy perimenopausal years because their doctors didn't want to prescribe hormones until they were definitely past menopause. There's no need for this. You should feel free to start what you need when you need it—and that includes hormones, herbs, foods, lifestyle changes, or a combination of all these. Because menopause is really a retrospective diagnosis, you won't know you're there until you're there! And symptoms are generally at their peak during perimenopause, not later.

For the woman who wants help with perimenopausal symptoms and finds that a nonhormonal approach does not provide sufficient relief but who is afraid that supplemental estrogen might increase her risk for breast or uterine cancer, HT is not necessarily out of the question. (See chapters 8 and 13.) As I've said above, I'm not convinced that there is any significant risk from taking bioidentical estrogen at a low dose only during the five years or fewer that menopausal symptoms are likely to be the most intrusive. After that, she can wean herself off some or all of the hormones or replace them with other alternatives. And if you feel your best on hormones, any increased risk might well be worth the benefits!

PRINCIPLES OF HT

- ⁓ Establish your natural hormonal levels by getting a baseline test in your late thirties or early perimenopause.
- ⁓ Replace only those hormones that need replacing.
- ⁓ Use the lowest dose that does the job. Reevaluate your HT decision yearly and plan to use alternatives when possible.
- ⁓ Use bioidentical hormones that are an exact molecular match to those naturally occurring in your body.
- ⁓ Support your HT regimen with a healthy diet, the right nutritional supplements, and exercise.
- ⁓ Be realistic. The goal is not to turn back the clock. Rather, the goal is to optimize your comfort and overall health so you can live the second half of your life with maximal vitality and mental clarity.

WITH HORMONE THERAPY, TIMING MAY BE EVERYTHING

One of the hot topics for hormone researchers has to do with figuring out why hormone therapy might be beneficial for a woman who begins taking it early on (before about age sixty) but harmful to the same woman if she starts it later. Why those differences exist is part of what researchers are calling the "critical window" (or "timing hypothesis"), which involves both heart health and brain health, as well as relative risk for various cancers, osteoporosis, and mood disorders. This concept was even the focus of a January 2010 symposium called "Window of Opportunity of Estrogen Therapy for Neuroprotection," presented by the Stanford Center for Neuroscience in Women's Health and the Stanford Center for Longevity.

Here, in a nutshell, is why cutting-edge scientists now suspect age matters with HT. When estrogen is added to a healthy brain, its molecules act like tiny keys fitting into all sorts of locks that open the doors to a host of positive effects. It increases levels of HDL (the "good" cholesterol), protecting the heart. It regulates levels of the feel-good hormones serotonin and dopamine. And it assists brain cell growth and plasticity (the ability to adapt to various stimuli), which both strengthens and repairs brain tissue, protecting it from diseases such as Alzheimer's.

But when estrogen is added either to a brain that has already begun the natural aging process *or* to a brain in the early stages of Alzheimer's, some or all of the locks no longer open. Estrogen, then, either has no effect or, worse, it actually harms brain cells and hastens their death. So the timing hypothesis suggests that the degree to which HT helps or harms a woman depends on how healthy her brain is at the time she starts taking it.

Making that determination, however, isn't easy. So at the moment, women facing the HT decision are still left trying to balance unknowable factors (what they *do* know about what they *may* be at risk for in the future versus what they *don't* know about what is *already* happening inside their bodies).

Taking all the evidence into consideration, the latest hormone therapy position statement from the North American Menopause Society, released in 2017, calls for individualized decisions on when to take and when to stop hormones, making it clear that there is no longer a hard stop date for hormone therapy.[49] The statement notes that women under sixty (or within ten years of menopause) have the most favorable benefit-risk ratio, although those with persistent hot flashes or who are concerned about excessive bone loss may want to continue taking hormones even after age sixty, since both conditions worsen after hormones are stopped. The statement also recommends hormone therapy for those women who enter early menopause, at least until they reach age fifty-two (the average age of natural menopause). Finally, it adds that for women with a genetic predisposition for breast cancer, taking hormones does not appear to increase risk further (although more data is needed). As always, research continues.

RENÉE: Losing Control, Finding Compassion

Though many of us have fixed ideas about how we will negotiate menopause and what we will and won't do, we need to be willing to let go of all our preconceptions once we actually begin going through the experience. Renée's story is a beautiful example of this.

> I'd decided a long time ago that I wasn't going to color my hair when it went gray and I wasn't going to take supplemental hormones when I hit menopause. Menopause for me was going to be a beautiful thing. I had it all figured out.
>
> Then on my forty-seventh birthday my father died, without warning, of a massive heart attack. My mother, confused and scared and in need of support, moved in with us. Then my husband, David, lost his funding and suddenly was faced with the prospect of being unemployed by the end of the year. And I was practically blindsided one week later with my first hot flash, which was so powerful it actually steamed up my glasses. Emotionally, financially, hormonally, and in terms of my overall sense of security, it felt like the proverbial rug was being pulled out from under my feet. My hot flashes became increasingly bothersome, particularly when they happened in the middle of the night and interrupted my sleep. I was feeling short-tempered with my mom and with David, and the house felt claustrophobic—I guess I just couldn't handle all the unexpected stresses that came up at what felt like the worst possible time in my biology. When my gynecologist suggested that I needed a little hormonal support, I sighed with relief and accepted it, and I feel much better now. In fact, just making the decision to accept help made a big difference in the way I felt right away.
>
> The lesson I learned from all this applies to more than just menopause: you can't control everything. I've always been a big control freak, but now I understand that in some ways we're all just along for the ride, and we need to be compassionate with ourselves and willing to change direction once in a while, in order to adjust to and accommodate what life throws our way, no matter what stage of life we're in at the time.

A DUSTING OF HORMONES

Okay, let's say that you've decided that you may want to try hormone therapy. You are still having periods, but you're getting hot flashes before they start. You also have occasional night sweats. I'd recommend that at this point you get your hormone levels tested. The ideal time is about a week before your period is due, because you'll be able to see what your peak progesterone level is at that time, and it will also give you an idea of how much estrogen and testosterone is normally circulating in your system. These measurements will also give you a baseline to work toward once you start hormones.

The next thing you do, depending upon your hormone levels, is to start supplementing the hormone that is lowest. In most cases, this will be progesterone, and maybe estrogen. Increasingly we're finding that many perimenopausal women also have an androgen deficiency. As already mentioned, natural progesterone in the form of a 2 percent skin cream has been shown to give good blood levels and is available over the counter. This alone may be all you need. Try it for two weeks before your period, then take two weeks off after your period starts. You can also use it for three weeks on and one week off. Most women notice a reduction of their symptoms within a month of starting this cream. Continue with this as long as you're getting good results.

If your estrogen level is too low or you're having lots of hot flashes, you'll want to start with the lowest level of estrogen available. Estrogen is available by prescription only, so you'll need to work with a healthcare practitioner to get the right dose and blood levels for you. Many women like the convenience of the estrogen patch, which comes in many different strengths and can be left on the skin for several days. Others prefer to take a pill.

I particularly like the formulations that allow the individual to play around with her dose a bit to find what's best for her. For example, there is an estrogen gel called Divigel that comes in three dosage strengths—including the lowest approved dose of estradiol available, 0.25 mg—so you can take only as much as you need. Studies show the lowest dose significantly reduced the number of hot flashes after five weeks, and the highest dose significantly reduced symptoms after two weeks; further improvements were reported over eight to twelve weeks of treatment.[50] This clear, quick-drying gel is invisible and odorless when dry, and it leaves no sticky residue. In fact, it's similar in look and feel to hand sanitizer. (For more information, call 800-654-2299 or visit www.divigel.com.)

A relatively new delivery form for estrogen is a nonaerosol transdermal spray, used in a product called Evamist. Each pump of the spray delivers 1.53 mg of estradiol, so you can control your level—one, two, or three sprays a day. The spray dries in about two minutes and is invisible on the skin. (For more information, call 866-634-9120 or visit evamist.com.)

Another new option is Imvexxy vaginal inserts, which are small, soft, teardrop-shaped inserts containing estradiol; they are used to treat painful intercourse caused by vaginal dryness as well as vulvar and vaginal atrophy. The inserts come in two strengths (4 mcg and 10 mcg); in addition to delivering estrogen, they restore vaginal pH levels. For the first two weeks, use once a day (at the same time of day), and after that, use two times a week. Some women notice improvement in two weeks, with most experiencing relief after twelve. (For more information, visit imvexxy.com.)

If you're taking estrogen, you have to be sure that you have enough progesterone to prevent excessive buildup of your uterine lining. This can be accomplished in some women with 2 percent progesterone skin cream. Others may need a higher amount of progesterone, available only by prescription. I recommend Crinone vaginal gel, Prometrium capsules orally, one of the formulations I mentioned earlier, or another one from a formulary pharmacy.

The good news is this: many healthcare providers are now familiar with bioidentical natural hormones and work closely with pharmacists who specialize in compounding individualized prescriptions to fit a woman's unique needs. Look for a pharmacy that is accredited by the Pharmacy Compounding Accreditation Board (see www.pcab.org). At the very least, be sure that the pharmacy you use sends samples of its products to an outside testing lab to check their strength and purity. Some health plans cover prescriptions for formulary pharmacies and others don't. If your plan doesn't, I'd recommend that you advocate coverage if your plan covers conventional hormone therapy. Your doctor may be able to assist you.

It's always best to call ahead and make sure that your doctor is open to discussing an individualized natural hormone approach before spending the time and money on an appointment. If your doctor doesn't know about this approach, either educate him or her or find someone who already knows about it. Many nurse practitioners are familiar with individualized hormone therapy and will work with you to find the right solution.

CLEARING UP THE CONFUSION ABOUT COMPOUNDING PHARMACIES

Compounding (or formulary) pharmacies specialize in creating hormone prescriptions that are tailored to a patient's individual needs. These formulas are prescribed for patients by their physicians and compounded by state-licensed pharmacists using FDA-approved bioidentical hormones—the same hormones that drug companies use—procured by suppliers that are registered and inspected by the FDA. (Foreign suppliers also must be FDA-registered.) It is not true, as the American College of Obstetricians and Gynecologists and the North American Menopause Society would have people believe, that compounding pharmacies are not regulated. *All* pharmacies, including compounding pharmacies, are required to meet standards set by their respective state pharmacy boards (there is no such thing as an "FDA-approved pharmacy"). In addition, the Pharmacy Compounding Accreditation Board (PCAB) has developed national standards to accredit pharmacies that perform a significant amount of compounding. (See www.pcab.org for more information.)

HOW LONG SHOULD YOU STAY ON HORMONES?

The length of time you continue to take hormones depends entirely on why you are taking hormones and what other things you are doing to achieve the same benefit. For example, if you originally started estrogen to maintain bone health but have since incorporated regular weight training into your lifestyle, you can probably taper off the estrogen and still maintain your bone density. If, on the other hand, you are a confirmed couch potato, have been on steroids, or smoke and you know you are at risk for osteoporosis, then you'll want to do everything you can to maintain your bone density. Follow a low-acid diet and make sure your vitamin D levels are optimal. (I am very concerned about the long-term effects of bisphosphonate drugs, such as Fosamax. See chapter 12 for a discussion of this.)

With bioidentical hormones at low levels, the benefits of HT may far outweigh any risks—especially if you feel good on them, have risk factors that HT is known to ameliorate, or have a health history that doesn't include a lot of healthy ninety-year-old relatives! The vast majority of women start taking hormones, herbs, or both for immediate relief of menopausal symptoms such as hot flashes or vaginal dryness and will need them for only a few years. Others are far more concerned about osteoporosis or sexual function. Taking hormones for short-term symptom relief is very different from taking hormones for long-term disease prevention. The majority of women experience most of their menopausal symptoms during a five-to-ten-year period, after which the symptoms abate naturally. But many women, including me, have decided to continue on some form of herbal or hormonal therapy for life.

An increasing number of women have now been on bioidentical hormones for well over ten years, and they feel great when taking them and not so good when they stop. Here's an example from a sixty-two-year-old woman who just consulted me on this issue: "I've been on oral capsules of estrogen plus 100 mg of progesterone daily ever since I did some research after the WHI study stopped. I had already had my uterus removed as well as most of my ovaries when I was in my late thirties because of endometriosis, but I did not take hormones until I went through menopause and suffered from heart palpitations, fuzzy thinking, and awful hot flashes. Once I got on hormones, I felt reborn. When I'm not on them, I feel spacey and get urinary incontinence. I exercise and do yoga regularly, don't drink alcohol, and am happy with my life. Is it unusual to be taking hormones for this length of time?"

Given that this woman, and thousands like her, do not have normal ovarian function and feel great on small amounts of bioidentical hormones, I recommend staying on them. Yes, there is a potential risk. But why ruin one's quality of life right now to prevent a very unlikely event in the future? As with everything, this decision must be individualized.

If You've Been Taking HT and Want to Stop All Hormones

Don't stop cold turkey. Wean yourself gradually and slowly, giving your body time to adjust. Here's a sample weaning schedule:

Week one: Skip Sunday's pill

Week two: Skip Sunday and Tuesday

Week three: Skip Sunday, Tuesday, and Thursday

Week four: Skip Sunday, Tuesday, Thursday, and Saturday

Week five: Skip Sunday, Tuesday, Thursday, Friday, and Saturday

Week six: Off hormones altogether

During and after this tapering-off period, support your body by making sure you're getting enough plant hormones. You might want to start on something like *Pueraria mirifica* or maca at the same time as you start tapering your hormones. Then by the time you've tapered off your hormones, the herbs will have established a good level. Eat a wide variety of fruits and vegetables as well, plus ground flaxseed. (See chapter 6.) You'll also need a good multivitamin/mineral to help your adrenals and ovaries keep your hormones balanced.

Not Carved in Stone

After the initial Women's Health Initiative study results were announced back in 2002, many women went into a panic and stopped their HT cold turkey. A lot of them also worried that they'd done irreparable damage to themselves by being on HT. Of course none of that is true, and the current generation has mostly forgotten this history. To put matters into perspective, the vast majority of women in the WHI study—and other studies—did not experience any adverse outcomes from being on Prempro, and their risk of death was no greater than that for women taking placebo. The data indicate that if 10,000 women take Prempro for a year, eight more will develop invasive breast cancer than would develop it if they didn't take Prempro. An additional seven will have a heart attack, eight will have a stroke, and eighteen will have blood clots. But they will also suffer six fewer colorectal cancers and five fewer hip fractures.[51] And given that there are far better options than Prempro, we could assume that the risks with those other options are even smaller, with the same benefits. Every woman should know that she can decrease her risk of side effects from HT by switching from synthetics such as Prempro to low-dose bioidentical hormone therapy. Or, if she chooses, she can wean herself gradually off HT to avoid rebound symptoms and/or start an herbal regimen.

Because every woman's body is a work in progress, your hormonal status—and your need for a particular type of support program—may well change. If you elect to take supplemental hormones, it is wise to have your hormone levels checked every six months during the first year of hormone use. Compare the results to how you're feeling. This can help indicate if, and where, your prescription needs fine-tuning. After you have reached a comfortable level, you only need to test every year or so.

If you've been taking Prempro or another type of synthetic HT, feel good on it, but want to decrease any possibility of adverse side effects: I suggest that you switch to bioidentical hormones at the lowest possible dose. Your doctor or healthcare practitioner can give you a prescription for bioidentical hormones, which include oral Estrace and some of the patches (Estraderm, Vivelle-Dot, and Climara). If you have a uterus, you'll also need progesterone. Prometrium is available in all pharmacies. The usual dose is 100 mg a day, at least twelve days of the month. If you don't want to get a period, you may need to take it daily. These brands of bioidentical hormones are covered by most health plans that have prescription coverage.

Alternatively, you can have a formulary pharmacy make up a combination of estrogen and progesterone, and/or testosterone (if necessary), such as the formulations I've mentioned above.

Remember that formulations that work well for one woman do not necessarily provide optimal results for another. You may want to try a different formulation, a different delivery system, or a different dosage, or switch from hormone supplementation to nonhormonal herbal support or vice versa. Be calm and at peace about this decision process—you can always change your mind if what you've chosen falls short of your expectations.

6

Foods and Supplements to Support the Change

For thousands of years, long before our culture placed its trust in pharmaceuticals, women relied upon their intuition and Mother Nature to keep themselves and their families healthy. Guided by their inner wisdom, our ancestors plucked healing plants from nature's colorful pharmacy—fragrant chamomile for calming teas, fresh ginger to prevent nausea and calm the stomach, and foxglove to regulate the heartbeat.

It is remarkable that our herbalist ancestors, though separated by thousands of miles, often drew upon the same herbs to treat the same conditions. American Indian women and their Chinese counterparts, for example, both used angelica (dong quai) to treat menopausal symptoms.

Today this ancient, intuitive wisdom is being augmented by objective scientific studies confirming what wise women have always known: plants contain a wide range of ingredients, such as essential fatty acids, phytoestrogens, and antioxidants, that can heal and help keep us healthy at all stages of our lives, including perimenopause.

To use herbs and foods optimally requires an adjustment in thinking. Plant medicine and food do not work in the body the way drugs, or even bioidentical hormones, do. Modern pharmaceuticals and hormones usually consist of one purified active ingredient (often derived from a plant source and then altered biochemically so that it can be patented) that is carefully standardized and measured for its biological effect.

Whole herbs and foods, on the other hand, contain many different active ingredients that act synergistically in the body. And just like the flavor and nutrient density of food, the quality and exact chemical composition of an herb depend upon where it is grown and how. There is good reason to believe that to get the full range of benefits, you need to consume the whole plant—or a product made from part of the whole plant, such as leaves or roots—rather than a single ingredient. This is why some studies show that whole soy foods, for example, give better results than capsules or pills containing isolated soy isoflavones.

In allopathic Western medicine, we try to target a symptom or illness with a single drug—to take one example, we give birth control pills to stop heavy bleeding or to regulate irregular periods. Birth control pills control symptoms, but, as we've already discussed when it comes to thyroid function and thyroxine, they do nothing to treat the underlying imbalance. It is the same with antibiotics. They are designed to target a specific bacterial infection.

Herbs and foods, on the other hand, with their exquisite combinations of interactive ingredients, work to balance the body at a number of different levels simultaneously. Accordingly, there are many different herbs or foods that one might use to regulate the menstrual cycle or as overall perimenopausal tonics, including ground flaxseed, dong quai, *Pueraria mirifica,* chasteberry, and maca. All contain substances that help balance the endocrine system in slightly different but synergistic ways.[1]

Herbs also work best when considered as part of an overall plan that includes the right diet for a given individual, exercise, and improved relationships. In other words, we need to approach herbs and foods with a holistic mindset that asks, "What foods or herbs will best help me balance my body so that it can heal itself?" rather than the more dualistic "What pill do I need to take to remove this symptom?"

WHO SHOULD CONSIDER HERBS?

~ You know the power of natural medicine to heal and balance your body, and you want to avoid prescription medication if possible.

~ You believe that herbs are simply more natural and beneficial than prescribed hormones.

~ You'd like to avoid hormone therapy because of fear of breast cancer or another health concern.

~ You're on HT of some sort but would like the added benefits of herbs.

~ You cannot tolerate HT.

BASIC PRINCIPLES OF HERBAL THERAPY AT MENOPAUSE

In order to use menopausal herbs well and wisely, you need to understand the following basic principles.

~ All plant foods contain what are known as phytonutrients. (*Phyto* means "plant.") These are unique substances produced during the natural course of growth and are specific to a particular plant's genes and environment. In addition to providing taste and nutritional value, phytonutrients can play therapeutic roles by modifying physiological processes in our bodies. This is the basis for botanical medicine. An example of this is the phytochemical indole-3-carbinol, found in cruciferous vegetables such as broccoli. This substance appears to convert the most potent estrogens in the body into weaker, less carcinogenic forms. High consumption of cruciferous vegetables is associated with a decreased risk for breast cancer, breast tenderness, and bloating, all of which are related to estrogen levels that are too high.

~ The line between using herbs as foods and using them as drugs can be blurry. For example, ephedra (ma huang) was once used as an effective treatment for asthma and sinusitis, but it was never intended to be used as a daily supplement. But then it became popular with people using it addictively to lose weight who then suffered severe side effects from overdosing, and in 2004 it was taken off the market. In general, the greater your intake of an herb, the greater the potential for druglike effects. For safety, keep doses moderately low, and follow the directions on the package or an herbalist's recommendation. It is also best to let your healthcare provider know what herbs you take regularly, because some herbs interact with some drugs in a way that either decreases the drug's potency or changes its effect. This is because both use the same metabolic pathways in the liver.

~ Recent advances in the standardization of herbal supplements have led to more consistent quality and potency. The most effective products are those that combine the whole plant (or plant part, such as the root) with a standardized percentage of the primary active ingredient.

~ The common menopausal herbs mentioned in this chapter have been used safely and effectively for thousands of years and rarely have side effects. However, a few people may react to some of them, some of the time—just as with any food or drug. There are also many herbs with known toxicity that shouldn't be used except under the care of an experienced herbalist. Examples include belladonna, blue cohosh, lobelia, and poke root.

~ Phytoestrogens, the natural hormones found in plants, are not the same as the hormones found in the female body, although they may have somewhat similar beneficial effects.

Phytoestrogens are found in more than 300 plants, including some that we routinely eat in the United States, such as apples, carrots, oats, plums, olives, potatoes, tea, coffee, and sunflower seeds. Soy and flaxseed are particularly rich in these substances.[2] The herb *Pueraria mirifica* has the most potent phytoestrogen yet discovered, known as miroestrol.[3] Phytoestrogens can be divided into two main families: the *isoflavones,* which include substances such as genistein, daidzein, equol, and coumestrol, and the *lignans,* which include matairesinol, enterolactone, and enterodiol.

The estrogenic activity of phytoestrogens is lower than that of human estrogens—in the range of a hundredth to a thousandth that of estradiol. They also have antioxidant and antiproliferative activity that is still being elucidated. This means that they have the ability to prevent free-radical damage to cells, the number-one cause of premature aging of tissue, and they also help prevent abnormal cell growth.

Like other estrogens, phytoestrogens bind to estrogen receptors throughout our systems. (Research has shown that estrogen receptors are found on the surface of nearly every cell of our bodies, not just those of the vagina, uterus, and breast tissue.) When they bind, they exert a balancing, or "adaptogenic," effect.[4] This means that if your estrogen levels are low, the herbs will have an estrogenic effect, but if your estrogen levels are too high, they will block the stronger estrogens. That's why the same herb—dong quai, for example—can be used both for conditions in which there is too much estrogen (such as PMS) and for those in which there is too little (hot flashes).

Phytoestrogens do not stimulate the growth of estrogen-sensitive tissue such as in the breast and uterus; in fact, they have been shown to inhibit breast tumors in some animal studies. Mammalian hormones (standard prescription estrogen) bind to the alpha estrogen receptor in cells and promote cell growth. This is why excess estrogen is associated with cancer. Plant hormones, on the other hand, bind to the beta estrogen receptor and act, in part, like naturally occurring SERMs (selective estrogen receptor modulators). As a result, they've been shown to be protective against estrogen-driven cell growth.[5]

~ Menopausal herbs have never been implicated in promoting cancer in humans, either, and indeed, some herbs are noted for their anticancer properties.[6] For this reason, menopausal herbs are an excellent choice for those who are concerned about cancer.

~ Many plant extracts exert a tonic effect on the female pelvic organs, and other organs as well. What this means is that they stimulate blood flow and sometimes even increase the weight of these organs.[7] Herbs such as black cohosh and chasteberry have also been shown to reduce menopausal symptoms by acting on the pituitary gland.

~ In general, herbs exert their influence in a much slower, more gradual way than drugs or even the bioidentical hormones mentioned in chapter 5. That said, many women report almost immediate positive effects with the right kind of *Pueraria mirifica*. Still, it's best to be prepared to wait three or four weeks before noticing an effect from an herbal supplement.

~ Finally, menopausal herbs are often given in combination, since experienced herbalists have found that their actions are synergistic and produce better results when used this way. Chinese herbal formulations set the standard for this synergy.

Key Menopausal Herbs

The following are some of the best-studied herbs used for menopausal symptoms. They can be used singly or in combination. Please note that this list is far from comprehensive. Many others, such as peony, hops, motherwort, and false unicorn root, are also effective.

PUERARIA MIRIFICA (PM): Also known as Thai kudzu, PM is hands down one of the most powerful supplements a woman can take for menopausal symptoms. It has been used for 700 years by both men and women for its hormone-like effects. This herb has been shown to be extremely safe and effective at relieving no fewer than twenty different conditions associated with menopause and perimenopause, including vaginal dryness, hot flashes, night sweats, depression, insomnia, and irritability. In its phase I studies, every one of the menopausal symptoms evaluated was reduced from moderately severe to mild, with the most significant drop occurring in the first thirty days of use. Women typically start to feel relief in the first week of taking PM.

Of the thirteen different species in the genus *Pueraria* that are native to Asia, only one, *Pueraria mirifica,* contains the potent plant sterol known as miroestrol, which has estrogen-like effects on bone and vaginal tissue while also protecting the breasts and endometrium from the adverse effects of excess estrogen.[8] It works by interacting with estrogen receptors to balance the effects of the estrogen already in the body, not by changing the amounts of natural estrogen a woman's body produces. In one study comparing PM with conjugated equine estrogens (Premarin), PM had an estrogenic effect that was similar to Premarin but without the side effects.[9] In another study, conducted in Thailand by Chatsri Deachapunya, Ph.D., PM was shown to have no effect on endometrial epithelial cells (including both normal cells and cancerous cells), underscoring its safety.[10] Research further shows that PM can halt the growth of breast cancer cells in vitro (in the lab).[11]

Choose a brand of PM that contains standardized miroestrol (approximately 20 mg of miroestrol per 100 g). Research suggests the maximum safe amount of miroestrol is 10 mg per day per kg of body weight, so check the level in the supplement you purchase to make sure the amount is safe. I have been so impressed by *Pueraria mirifica* that I started my own company, AmataLife (www.amatalife.com), to bring attention to the benefits of this herb and also to make sure that the *Pueraria mirifica* used was the most effective and highest quality available. I also formulated a *Pueraria mirifica* vaginal gel that is highly effective. (See Resources.)

DONG QUAI (*Angelica sinensis*): Dong quai (also known as angelica, dang gui, and tang kuei) has excellent phytoestrogen activity and has been called female ginseng because of its ability to enhance energy and a sense of well-being. It is used for amenorrhea, irregular periods, and excessive uterine bleeding. My acupuncturist, who is from Taiwan, tells me that dong quai is one of the most widely used herbs in China and that many women take it throughout their reproductive and perimenopausal years.

Dong quai also has analgesic and antiallergy effects, is antibacterial, is a smooth-muscle relaxant, and can stabilize blood vessels.[12]

Dong quai is widely available over the counter. It is the foundation of almost all menopausal formulations and can be taken indefinitely. In Asia, women simmer the raw dried herb with chicken to make a soup or stew. Angelica root can be found in many herb shops or health food stores. It is also processed into capsules, tablets, and tinctures. (It is best to avoid alcohol-based tinctures.) The recommended dosages for most over-the-counter dong quai preparations are probably too low to be helpful (the usual dose is 4.5 g per day). Increasing the dosage on your own is unlikely to cause any problems, but it's always best to be under the supervision of a certified herbalist or practitioner of Traditional Chinese Medicine.

Note: Do not take dong quai if there's a chance you're pregnant.

CHASTEBERRY (*Vitex agnus-castus*): Chasteberry comes from the chaste tree, which is native to the Mediterranean. It is widely available at natural food stores, often under the name vitex. It has been shown to have a profound effect on pituitary function, increasing the secretion of LH (luteinizing hormone) and decreasing the production of FSH (follicle-stimulating hormone), which in turn shifts the production of hormones toward more progesterone and less estrogen.[13] This is thought to be the main reason why it helps balance the irregular periods that result from the hormonal swings of perimenopause. It also acts somewhat like the neurotransmitter dopamine. Chasteberry is particularly beneficial for women who are having PMS-like symptoms or are experiencing scanty, irregular periods. It has been shown to suppress appetite, relieve depression, and improve sleep. It can take several months to work.

The usual dose is 1 teaspoon of crushed fruit per cup of water one to four times per day, or 20–75 drops of the 1:3 liquid extract one to four times per day (or as directed on the bottle).

Note: Chasteberry can cause rashes in susceptible individuals. Don't take it with neuroleptic medicines such as haloperidol (Haldol) or thioridazine (Mellaril), or when pregnant or nursing.

BLACK COHOSH (*Cimicifuga racemosa*): Black cohosh has been used in this country for hundreds of years. Native Americans called it cramp bark. It is also a popular Chinese herb and is often used in formulations for perimenopausal symptoms. It binds to estrogen receptors, where it selectively represses the elevation of LH that occurs at menopause.[14] It decreases hot flashes, night sweats, irritability, and mood swings (although recent studies show black cohosh improves hot flashes in only about a third of those women taking it—far less than placebo).[15] It is also helpful for PMS symptoms. Although this herb was originally considered a phytoestrogen, studies show that it actually works by affecting the neurotransmitters dopamine and serotonin.

A standardized extract of black cohosh sold under the trade name Remifemin is one of the most widely used herbs in Europe, where it is a well-documented alternative to HT. Many women take Remifemin alone for relief of menopausal symptoms. Clinical studies show that it relieves depression, vaginal dryness, and menstrual cramps. While Denmark recently banned this herb because of concerns that it might cause serious liver damage, such cases of liver toxicity are rare and the evidence isn't definitive. (The culprit may actually be a related but different herb that was misidentified on product labels as black cohosh.)

The usual starting dose for Remifemin is 1–2 tablets (20 mg per tablet) twice per day. Or take black cohosh in any of the following forms, three times per day: powdered root or as a tea, 1–2 g; solid, dry 4:1 powdered extract, 250–500 mg; fluid extract, 1:1 tincture, 4 mg (1 teaspoon, or about 5 ml).

A newer form of black cohosh known as BNO 1055, used in the preparations Menopret (formerly Klimadynon) and MenoFem, was shown to suppress hot flashes in breast cancer survivors as well as conjugated estrogens did (completely eliminating the hot flashes in 47 percent of the women in the study).[16]

Note: Black cohosh can interact with medicines for high blood pressure and may result in excessively low blood pressure in some women.

MACA (*Lepidium peruvianum* Chacon): This herb is adaptogenic, which means that it helps modulate the body's response to stress of all kinds. Peruvian maca (a dietary staple in that country) traditionally has been used to benefit the endocrine and reproductive systems of both men and women, and research shows that it increases the production of sex hormones, enhances sex drive, increases energy, and also results in mental improvement in many. Its properties make it particularly useful for perimenopausal and menopausal women.[17] My colleague Anna Cabeca, D.O., has a company that provides high-quality maca and other products for menopausal women (see www.drannacabeca.com). Other maca products include Femmenessence MacaPause, a formulation of maca that has guaranteed potency and excellent bioavailability, made by Natural Health International (symphonynaturalhealth.com). The standard dose is two 500 mg capsules twice daily (morning and evening), although if you haven't noticed improvement in four to seven weeks, ask your health practitioner about taking slightly more or less until you find the optimal balance for you.

LICORICE ROOT (*Glycyrrhiza glabra*): Licorice is a perennial, temperate-zone herb that grows three to seven feet high. The parts used are the dried runners and roots. Licorice root is one of the most extensively used and scientifically investigated herbal medicines. The active constituents of licorice include both isoflavones and lignans. Licorice has many pharmacological actions, including estrogenic, anti-inflammatory, antiallergy, antibacterial, and anticancer effects. It helps regulate estrogen/progesterone ratios. It also helps replenish adrenal function, so it is very good for fatigue.

The usual dose is ¼ teaspoon of solid extract once or twice per day.

Note: Blood pressure should be monitored to be sure that it stays stable. The cortisol-like activity of this herb may cause a problem in those who are prone to hypertension. In those with low blood pressure, this herb can help correct and balance the problem.

Any of the key menopausal herbs above, either alone or in combination, often help to relieve a wide variety of symptoms, including vaginal dryness, sleep problems, hot flashes, and mood swings. My advice is to try one or more for at least a month. If you are still troubled by your symptoms, add another of the key herbs, or choose from the more specific remedies listed in other chapters.

Essential oils have been used for hundreds of years for their healing properties—and the menopausal transition is no exception. A deep dive into this approach is beyond my experience, but Mariza Snyder, D.C., has put together some very effective protocols in her book *The Essential Oils Menopause Solution: Alleviate Your Symptoms and Reclaim Your Energy, Sleep, Sex Drive, and Metabolism* (Rodale, 2021).

FOODS THAT HELP PERIMENOPAUSE

Many common foods contain vitamins, minerals, and phytoestrogens that are healthful for the perimenopausal transition, including freshly ground flaxseed, cruciferous vegetables (such as cabbage, broccoli, Brussels sprouts, and kale), and all of the colorful fruits and vegetables that are loaded with bioflavonoids. But before I get into what foods to eat, please understand that there is no one "magic bullet" food that can ever outweigh the benefits of a diet that keeps blood sugar and insulin at normal levels. High insulin and high blood sugar combined with an excess of the stress hormones cortisol and epinephrine wreak havoc with the body's other hormones, pure and simple. And over time, high insulin and blood sugar set the stage for almost all chronic degenerative diseases, including heart disease, cancer, and diabetes. So don't make the mistake of thinking that you can just add a couple of tablespoons of ground flax to your diet and all will be well. It doesn't work that way. I'll delve into this further in chapter 7, "The Menopause Food Plan." But as you read the next section, please keep that in mind.

A NOTE ABOUT PHYTOESTROGENS, ISOFLAVONES, AND CANCER RISK

There's a lot of confusion about the phytoestrogens (estrogens from plants) and isoflavones (a particular type of phytoestrogen) in foods such as soy and flax, with some saying they increase the risk of breast cancer. Many women have avoided these and other beneficial foods and herbs for fear that they may actually be harmful. But this is not the case. The literature shows that phytoestrogens and isoflavones do *not* increase your risk for breast cancer.

In 2009, the Council for Responsible Nutrition sponsored

a meeting in Milan attended by an international group of nearly twenty researchers from around the world to look at this very topic. Overall, the information presented in this conference strongly supported the idea that isoflavones are indeed safe for women with breast cancer as well as for women who are at high risk for developing breast cancer. Mark Messina, Ph.D., a well-respected soy isoflavone researcher, said this at the conclusion of the conference:

> According to the science presented at this meeting, isoflavones do not have an effect on breast cell proliferation or breast tissue density, which are two well-established biomarkers of breast cancer risk. In fact, epidemiologic data presented at the meeting showed that exposure to isoflavone-rich soy foods may improve the prognosis of breast cancer patients. Further, new findings strongly indicated that certain results from some animal studies that have raised concern about the impact of isoflavones on breast cancer are not applicable to humans.[18]

Margaret Ritchie, Ph.D., a world-renowned expert in phytoestrogens and associated breast cancer research at the University of St. Andrews in Scotland, explains that phytoestrogens simply cannot act the same way estradiol (the most biologically active form of estrogen) does in the body because of their chemistry and the shape of their molecules. Although research does exist indicating that rodents that are fed genistein (a single type of phytoestrogen) and then exposed to cancer-promoting chemicals did have a higher risk for cancer, Dr. Ritchie explains, "Since no person can eat only one phyto-oestrogen and rodents produce huge amounts of equol [a type of estrogen], these studies are of limited value. Additional studies carried out by the same researchers showed when animals were fed soy . . . with many other phyto-chemicals present, there was a reduction in tumour size and number."[19]

One phytoestrogen-containing herb in particular, *Pueraria mirifica*, is considered to be a selective estrogen receptor modulator (SERM) because the miroestrol and deoxymiroestrol it contains modify receptors in various tissues. Specifically, research shows that these compounds can actually help protect against the development of estrogen-dependent breast, uterine, and ovarian cancer because they inhibit estrogen receptors in the breast, uterus, and ovaries while also powerfully stimulating the receptors in other estrogen-sensitive tissues in the brain, bone, heart, lungs, kidneys, and other parts of the body.[20] In other words, *Pueraria mirifica* inhibits cancer cells rather than allowing them to proliferate because it binds to estrogen receptors in the cells, blocking estrogen from binding to them, so the cells don't receive the message to grow and multiply.

The Right Kind of Soy

In the previous editions of this book, I included a large section on soy and its benefits for menopausal women. Many studies exist that support a role for soy protein during and after menopause. And indeed, my own experience with various soy foods and supplements bears this out. However, over the last decade or so, the quality of many soy foods and supplements has deteriorated. Worse, poor-quality soy oil and soy protein have been added to far too many food items. As a result, when many people consume soy these days, they may experience allergy-like symptoms or gastrointestinal upset. In popular dietary approaches such as Whole30 (whole30.com), a popular detox and dietary reset program, soy is eliminated entirely. Indeed, it is estimated that about 20 percent of the American soy crop has undergone genetic modification to enhance drought resistance and other desirable traits. Such genetic engineering raises some disturbing ethical and health questions; in Europe, unease about this development has led to the banning of genetically modified organisms (GMOs). The same movement is now active in the United States. Until we know more about the possible health or environmental risks, make sure that any soy or soy food you consume is organic and non-GMO.

Traditional Asian cultures have used soy healthfully for centuries. In fact, in cultures like Japan, in which soy foods make up a large part of the diet, breast cancer is quite rare—as long as a woman is following a traditional non-Western diet. Traditional soy foods are often fermented, organically grown, and/or otherwise processed naturally. When that is the case, soy is a very healthful food that supports hormone balance. Think tamari soy sauce, organic tofu, natto, tempeh, miso, or fresh edamame.

Flaxseed: Super Source of Lignans, Fiber, and Omega-3 Fats

Flaxseed is a great source of anticancer and phytoestrogenic compounds known as lignans, with a concentration more than a hundred times greater than other lignan-containing foods, such as grains, fruits, and vegetables. Lignans are plant substances that get broken down by intestinal bacteria into two chemicals, enterodiol and enterolactone. These substances then circulate through the liver and are later excreted in the urine.[21] Flaxseed is also an excellent source of fiber and of omega-3 fats.

There are a number of reasons why we all should be interested in incorporating more lignans into our diet. The following are some of the most compelling.

Lignans

LIGNANS HAVE POTENT ANTICANCER EFFECTS. An impressive number of studies have shown that flaxseed lignans help in both prevention and treatment of breast and colon cancer because of their ability to modulate the production, availability, and action of the hormones produced in our bodies.[22]

LIGNANS ARE POTENT PHYTOESTROGENS. In women who consume flaxseed, studies have shown significant hormonal changes, including alterations in estradiol levels, similar to those seen with soy isoflavones. This makes flaxseed oil or ground flaxseed a great choice for women who can't use soy or who simply want another source of phytohormones.[23]

LIGNANS ARE GOOD ANTIOXIDANTS. Like soy and many herbs, lignans have antiviral, antibacterial, and antioxidant properties, which means they help prevent free-radical damage to tissues—the cellular-level injury associated with aging and disease.

LIGNANS HELP PROTECT THE CARDIOVASCULAR SYSTEM. Studies have also found that lignans in the form of flaxseed significantly lower LDL cholesterol (the "bad" cholesterol), raise HDL cholesterol (the "good" cholesterol), and reduce the incidence of atherosclerosis.[24]

Fiber

Flaxseed is an excellent source of fiber. In addition to its phytoestrogenic properties, flaxseed is rich in both soluble and insoluble fiber. Adding a daily serving of ground flaxseed to your diet may eliminate any problems you have with constipation. (Just be sure you take it with enough liquid.) While the fiber in wheat bran is quite hard and can irritate the bowel, the fiber in flaxseed is much softer. When combined with fluid, flax fiber forms a mucilage in the body that can significantly help reduce the risk for diabetes and cardiovascular disease. Fiber has been shown to reduce both total cholesterol and triglyceride levels in the bloodstream.

The total dietary fiber content in 45 g of flaxseed (about ¼ cup) is 11.7 g. This is nearly four times greater than the fiber contained in a ½ cup serving of oatmeal.

Note: Ground hemp seeds are also an excellent source of high-quality protein and fiber—⅓ cup contains 14 grams of fiber and 11 grams of protein. (For more information, see www.nutiva.com.)

Omega-3 Fats

Flaxseed is an excellent source of omega-3 fats. These fats are essential for the health of every cell in our bodies, including the cells in our brains and hearts. A deficiency of omega-3 fatty acids, which is quite common, can result in fatigue, dry skin, cracked nails, thin and breakable hair, constipation, immune system malfunction, aching joints, depression, arthritis, and hormone imbalances. Omega-3s are also linked to healthier weight and body composition. Research from Australia has linked higher blood levels of the omega-3 fatty acids EPA and DHA to lower rates of obesity. People with higher omega-3 blood levels had lower body mass indexes, narrower waists, and smaller hip circumferences. In addition, the cell membranes of the overweight and obese people in the study were nearly 14 percent lower in omega-3s than in those with healthy weights.[25] And a study conducted in Spain showed that for overweight and obese people participating in a weight-loss program, omega-3s boosted the feeling of fullness after a meal.[26]

Omega-3 fats are found not just in flaxseed but also in fatty fish (especially salmon, bluefish, mackerel, sardines, and anchovies), fish oil, organ meats, egg yolk, and marine algae. Flaxseed meal is an excellent source of omega-3 fats if it's freshly ground. (Flaxseed oil provides omega-3s, but it does not provide fiber. In addition, the oil must be kept refrigerated, or it will turn rancid.)

Fish, especially the cold-water fatty kinds, is a better source of DHA, the brain tissue building block that your body can't manufacture. That may be why studies show that individuals who consume fish exhibit a lower incidence of depression. Additional benefits of fish oil include lessening the frequency and severity of hot flashes (by 25 percent over twenty-four weeks, according to one Italian study)[27] and even increasing survival time in women undergoing chemotherapy for breast cancer.[28] A recent study following more than 25,000 people with no history of cardiovascular disease showed omega-3 supplementation reduced heart attacks by 40 percent in those who didn't eat fish at all or who ate less than 1.5 servings a week. The study also showed that omega-3 supplementation reduced heart attacks by a whopping 77 percent for African Americans.[29]

If you can't or don't want to consume fish regularly, I think DHA (200–2,500 mg per day) is one of the best supplements you can take. (See Resources.) If you take fish oil with EPA, be sure to take the lysophospholipid (LPC) form. Recent research shows it's the only type of omega-3 that can cross the blood-brain barrier and increase the levels of EPA in the brain.[30]

How to Take Flaxseed

Not all flaxseed is created equal. I recommend buying golden flax grown in the northern Great Plains regions of North America (Manitoba and the Dakotas), where the rich soil and climate produce flax that is high in omega-3 fats and flavor. (See Resources.) Although the brown flax found in most health food stores has all the nutritional benefits of golden flax, I personally prefer the taste of golden flax. For best results, use ¼ cup flaxseed three to seven days a week. Grind your daily serving in a coffee grinder and then stir the meal into soups and beverages, or sprinkle it on cereal or salad. You can add half your daily dose to a morning smoothie and consume the other half sprinkled on oatmeal, yogurt, or even fruit. This combination makes a wonderfully fiber-full, phytoestrogen-rich perimenopausal power breakfast. And it takes less than three minutes to prepare!

Bioflavonoids

Another rich food source for phytoestrogens is the bioflavonoids contained in many herbs and fruits. Bioflavonoids compete with excess estrogen for receptor sites and are therefore also helpful for balancing menopausal hormones and tonifying the pelvic organs. The white spongy inner peel of citrus fruits is a very rich source, so eat some of it along with your orange or grapefruit. (I usually just take the orange peel and eat the inner white part directly—the same as I would an artichoke leaf.) Other rich sources of bioflavonoids include cherries, cranberries, blueberries, bilberries, black currants, many whole grains, grape skins, and red clover. In supplement form, 1,000 mg of bioflavonoids with vitamin C daily has been shown to relieve hot flashes.[31]

TRADITIONAL CHINESE MEDICINE AND ACUPUNCTURE FOR MENOPAUSE

Over the years I've referred hundreds of women for acupuncture and Traditional Chinese Medicine (TCM), a system of medicine that is over 2,000 years old, for the relief of a wide variety of gynecological problems, including those related to menopause. I have personally used elements of Traditional Chinese Medicine, including various herbal formulas and acupuncture, to relieve menstrual cramps and hot flashes.

Traditional Chinese Medicine is by its very nature holistic, tailoring treatment to the individual's body, mind, spirit, and emotions. This system of medicine views our health as a balance between the two contrasting states of *yin* and *yang*. The following is a very simple explanation, courtesy of my own personal mother-daughter acupuncture team, of the most common pattern that occurs during menopause.[32]

According to Chinese medicine, the part of us that is referred to as *yin*—our vital fluids—begins to diminish as we grow older. This leads to an excess of *yang*—vital energy and heat—and/or stagnation of *chi* (life energy). Ideally, when our *yin, yang,* and *chi* are in balance, our bodies act something like a kettle containing liquid (*yin*) heated by fire (*yang*). The resulting steam (the enhanced *chi* flow) circulates throughout the body, warming and nourishing it.

How much and to what degree *yin* becomes depleted depends upon our lifestyle, diet, and genes. Depletion of *yin* causes the vital liquid in the kettle to burn off, so the fire burns without producing the steam necessary to moisten and nourish.

Excess heat leads to hot flashes, the most obvious symptom, as well as to dryness of the skin, eyes, and vagina. Excess heat can dislodge the *shen* (spirit) from the heart, causing restlessness and insomnia. If excess heat enters the blood, it can cause heavy menstrual periods. *Chi* stagnation can cause pain anywhere in the body, as well as moodiness and emotional instability. A combination of excess heat and *chi* stagnation can lead to restlessness and anxiety.

Diet

According to Chinese medicine, diet is the most effective way to relieve many symptoms, and my experience bears this out. All heat-producing foods and substances should be eliminated or greatly reduced. Caffeine, alcohol, refined sugar, food coloring, preservatives, and additives (including antibiotics and hormones fed to animals during the production of most meat, chicken, and eggs) will cause excess heat and *yin* depletion. Red meat should be consumed in small quantities, but being a complete vegetarian (vegan) is not recommended for most people either. Generally speaking, most people do best with at least 2–4 oz. of meat or fish every week or two, depending upon your size and lifestyle. It is also helpful to limit spicy, pungent foods, such as curries or chilies, and greasy, fried, or oily foods.

Foods should be lightly cooked, not raw or cold. You can dip your salad greens into boiling water for just a second or two, then add a little lemon juice to them. The body has to work much harder to digest raw food, which creates heat and *chi* stagnation. Cold food, contrary to popular belief, doesn't cool the body in a balanced way. Instead, cold and ice create blockages in the *chi* channel, which results in *chi* stagnation. The following foods are especially cooling and helpful: melons, bean sprouts, tofu, white ocean fish, celery, apples, asparagus, and grapes.

Smoking obviously makes everything worse. When you smoke you are quite literally breathing in fire and toxins that enter the brain and bloodstream directly. It is also well documented that smoking poisons the ovaries, decreasing our estrogen levels about two years sooner than would normally occur.

Practitioners of Traditional Chinese Medicine also discourage the regular use of ginger and Asian ginseng (*Panax ginseng*) and Siberian ginseng during perimenopause because both are considered heat-producing.

Chinese Herbs for Menopause

An incredible variety of Chinese herbs and herbal combinations are available to treat every condition known to humanity—and the symptoms of perimenopause are no exception. While many individual Chinese herbs have Western counterparts, the most effective Chinese herbal combinations are unique to this system of medicine. Many of these so-called patent formulations have been tested and refined for thousands of years.

A full discussion of Traditional Chinese Medicine and Chinese herbs is far beyond the scope of this book. The preparations mentioned below don't even begin to scratch the surface of what is available and safe for almost all people to take. Since most herbal prescriptions are based on an individual's unique constitution, it is best to work directly with a practitioner trained in this system.

Acupuncture

Acupuncture is an essential part of Traditional Chinese Medicine. Because it works to normalize the flow of life energy or *chi* in the body, it is particularly appropriate for perimenopause, a time when our energy is completely renewing itself. It is extremely effective for relieving hot flashes, insomnia, night sweats, anxiety, restlessness, emotional instability, moodiness, menstrual cramps, and excess bleeding.

Though most people resort to acupuncture only after conventional Western drugs and surgery have failed, and though it is often effective even in these difficult situations, acupuncture is best used as preventive healthcare or at the onset of symptoms. It can unblock stuck *chi* long before the problem manifests in actual illness. I consider it the first line of treatment, not the last, not something to be used only when all else has failed.

When I was in my thirties, I was able to eliminate my menstrual cramps with acupuncture treatment. They have never returned. I have also referred patients for acupuncture who have had illnesses ranging from migraine headaches to chronic urinary tract infections. Acupuncture can help regulate menstrual periods, control heavy menstrual bleeding, stop seizures, and even in some cases help shrink fibroids. Research has shown that acupuncture improves cortisol balance in the body, enhances immune function, and helps quell addictions to cigarettes and alcohol.

Acupuncture works by redirecting the flow of *chi* along energy pathways in the body known as meridians. Because the meridians have no known anatomical counterparts, allopathic medicine dismissed acupuncture's effectiveness for years, until the presence of meridians was definitively demonstrated in a French study. Researchers injected a radioactive tracer into both traditional acupuncture points and into random sham points. The tracer that was injected into the genuine acupuncture points could easily be tracked as it ran up the meridians.[33] The clinical evidence of acupuncture's effectiveness has also become too compelling to ignore.

START SOMEWHERE

Don't let all these choices overwhelm you or become another heavy list of "shoulds." The wisdom in nature is user-friendly, and you have a lot of it within you already. To tap into it, just pick the herb, the formula, or the foods that seem to jump out at you and say, "Try me." Because all of the herbs and foods I've mentioned contain phytohormones of some kind and have virtually no side effects, feel free to experiment.

7

The Menopause Food Plan: A Program to Balance Your Hormones and Prevent Middle-Age Spread

O ver the years, countless women in their late thirties or forties have come to me with one or more of the following complaints: "Where did this spare tire around my middle come from?" "Why can't I lose that last five to ten pounds I used to be able to shed within a few weeks?" "Why is it that although I weigh the same as I did in college, my body seems different?"

Some women find themselves gaining weight at midlife even if they are eating no more than before. Others simply change shape: their waistlines thicken, and fat accumulates on their abdomen, flanks, and shoulders. Most of us have to make changes in our diets and exercise regimens if we expect to negotiate menopause without ten, twenty, or more pounds of excess baggage, weight that, in addition to wreaking havoc with our appearance, is also a well-documented health risk.[1] This is especially concerning now because current estimates predict that about half the adult U.S. population will be obese by 2030.[2]

Midlife weight gain results from a series of metabolic changes from a variety of sources that actually begin decades before but then reach critical mass (no pun intended) during perimenopause. One such source is environmental toxins. Some researchers believe that our exposure to an increasing amount of synthetic organic and inorganic chemicals in use today (such as those used to fatten livestock) may have damaged our bodies' natural weight-control mechanisms.[3] Rapid changes in hormonal levels along with increased stress hormones also exacerbate midlife weight gain.

Thankfully, there are ways to negotiate the metabolic shifts and toxic load that often manifest at midlife. It is also possible to rebalance your hormones without any significant weight or fat gain. I know this path from the inside out, not only professionally but also personally.

MAKING PEACE (ONCE AGAIN) WITH MY WEIGHT

My weight has been an issue for me since I was twelve years old when, at 125 pounds, I was one of the heaviest girls in my eighth-grade class. This is when I went on my first diet. I am certainly not alone in this lifelong struggle. One of my friends—now in her mid-forties and naturally thin—told me that her father, a physician, told her that no woman should ever weigh more than 120 pounds. So she has been weighing herself several times a day for years, unconsciously validating herself in her father's eyes. Her story is in an important sense the story of a woman's body in patriarchy—always trying to measure up to some external standard that changes from decade to decade and that often has little to do with what is ideal and healthy for us.

In my teens and early twenties I was always trying to weigh ten to twenty pounds less than I should have, given my rather sturdy frame and large muscles. (No one understood at that time that weight could be a very misleading measure of health.) Throughout my teens, I struggled to weigh 115, a weight I achieved only for a month or so when I starved myself in college. The reason I chose 115 was that according to the fashion magazines of the time, that was supposedly the "ideal" weight for someone of my height: 5 feet 4 inches. Back then, no one made any distinction between lean body mass and fat! Now I clearly see that a goal of 115 pounds for my particular body was not only unrealistic, but also downright unhealthy! In my twenties, I ran regularly and was able to maintain my weight at around 125 with a great deal of effort, which included fighting constant cravings for sweets.

After my pregnancies I, like so many other women, was never

able to get my weight back to 125 no matter what I did. I had run headlong into another aspect of Mother Nature's wisdom, which has set up postpartum weight gain so that we new mothers will be likely to stay alive during lean times to nurse and care for our children.

In my thirties, after I had nursed my two daughters for a total of nearly four years, my weight stabilized between 137 and 140. During these years I added weight training to my fitness regimen, and I figured that my weight gain was as much muscle as fat. (Muscle weighs more than fat, but it also burns calories far more efficiently.)

Finally, in my early forties, I came to a place of peace with my weight and size, even though my skeleton will never be a size 4! Through careful attention to my diet—which has consisted mostly of whole foods, healthy fats, lots of vegetables, some fruits, and some animal protein, along with consistent exercise including weight training and classical Pilates, I managed to maintain my body fat percentage at a healthy 22 to 25 percent and my weight at about 140, plus or minus (mostly plus) a few pounds. Yes, I still wanted to lose five to ten pounds, but I wasn't willing to further change my lifestyle—or give up my regular, though modest, servings of chocolate—to lose them. I was certainly following my own recommendations and keeping my blood sugar stable!

My Fat Cells Take on a Life of Their Own

But then a month or so after turning fifty—about the time my periods became irregular—I began, inexplicably, to gain weight. Every day the scale showed another pound, even though I wasn't eating or exercising any differently. I was horrified. Yes, horrified. Lest you think that this is too strong a word, let me explain. I have the kind of body shape and metabolic rate that could very easily lead to obesity if I were not so disciplined about my diet and exercise routine. There was an upper limit on the scale beyond which I would not allow myself to go, and that number was 144. But now I stood by helplessly and—in the space of a few weeks—watched the scale climb to 149, one pound less than I had weighed at the end of my pregnancy with my first daughter!

I knew that a new plan of action was called for. But what should it be? I'd been so sure I'd finally won the battle of the bulge and found a comfortable way to eat that would work for me for life. Now what?

Ketosis and Me

I decided to try a more extreme form of carbohydrate restriction. Maybe I'd let too many carbs creep into my diet. I went out and bought a copy of *Dr. Atkins' New Diet Revolution*. The cover said two million copies had been sold; could that many people be completely wrong?[4] In any case, given the connection between carbohydrates, insulin, and weight gain (which I will discuss in more detail below), Atkins's research and clinical expertise made sense to me.[5]

I had also researched ketosis, the metabolic state that results when you cut down carbohydrates enough to begin burning body fat for fuel. The Atkins kind of ketosis from those days was achieved through a high-fat, high-protein diet. I knew that this metabolic state was safe for people with no kidney problems, at least for the limited amount of time recommended by Atkins and quite probably for much longer periods. More than that, it appeared to be associated with consistent and relatively fast weight loss.

I decided to follow the Atkins "induction" diet to the letter for at least fourteen days. I bought some urine testing strips at the drugstore to test for ketosis. (Ketone bodies, which result from the breakdown of body fat, are excreted in the urine and can be easily tested for at home.) According to Atkins, and now legions of others, the presence of ketones in the urine is a virtual guarantee that you're burning fat for energy. Then I cut my carbohydrate intake to less than 20 g per day, a level of restriction I'd never tried before.

According to Atkins, the vast majority of people reach a state of ketosis within forty-eight hours. That is how long it takes the liver's glycogen stores to be depleted so that the body begins to use its fat for energy. So I cut the carbs, waited forty-eight hours, and then began to test my urine two to three times every day. Nothing. The strips didn't turn purple. Though I actually felt good and had a lot of energy, I didn't go into ketosis.

After a full ten days of carbohydrate restriction, I managed to produce just a little bit of ketosis—the urine strips measured "trace." But even then I failed to lose weight or inches. In fact, I gained three pounds on the induction part of the Atkins diet. I had now plateaued to a new high. Talk about frustration! Here I was, exercising regularly, eating a very limited amount of carbohydrates, keeping the rest of my food portions normal, and following a diet that has helped millions lose weight. But it didn't work for me. Like many other perimenopausal women, I had hit a metabolic wall; our midlife bodies seem to hold on to fat for dear life! One of my good friends, an exercise physiologist who also has a Ph.D. in nutrition, had a similar experience. We each had followed diets as low as 500 calories per day for nearly a month and not only never lost a pound or an inch but even gained weight. According to every bit of science currently out there, this is not possible. But of course we now know that the old "calories in, calories out (via exercise)" idea is obsolete. All calories are not created equal. And weight loss or gain is about far more than what you eat and when.

Yet that was our experience, and the experience of so many women who are accused of "cheating" on their diets. Clearly the old "eat less and exercise more" adage that is still foisted upon so many— or even the more recent "eat fat to lose weight" advice—has some serious flaws when it comes to midlife women. And it is very demoralizing.

Finally, though, I was able to crack the code of midlife weight loss and weight maintenance, and you can too—though there is no "one size fits all" approach. Still, I can assist you in finally making peace with food and weight at midlife and beyond.

The following program is based on my own experience, reports from thousands of women in my social media community and e-newsletter subscribers, and leading-edge research on the effects of subconscious beliefs, excess blood sugar, stress, and accumulated toxins that get stored in body fat to protect internal organs. My program is designed to help you detoxify your body, change your subconscious programming, balance your hormones, maintain stable blood sugar, and safeguard your health on all levels—body, mind, and spirit. The side effect of all this is fat loss and improved health. In fact, my program is designed to give you a whole new body as you begin the second half of your life.

Let's start with upgrading your subconscious beliefs about weight.

HOW TO TRAIN YOUR MIND
TO RELEASE EXCESS WEIGHT

If you have ever tried to lose weight, you know that eating healthy food and moving your body are important components of any weight-loss plan. But did you know that reaching or maintaining a healthy body composition happens in both your body and your mind? In fact, if you have tried repeatedly to lose weight but have never succeeded, or if you lose weight but then gain it back—and then some (how many of us have lost and gained the same twenty pounds over and over again?)—it is most likely that your thoughts and beliefs are holding you back, not necessarily your diet (though I'll get into the diet part later).

The truth is that excess weight is often a reflection of your mental or emotional state. And the number-one reason people fail to lose weight is because they neglect to make changes in their subconscious mind to support their conscious goals. This aspect of weight loss was, in fact, the inspiration for the now-famous ACE (Adverse Childhood Experiences) study started at Kaiser Permanente in San Diego. Vincent Felitti, M.D., who originated the research that led to this study, was struck by the story of a young woman in the program who had gained 100 pounds following a rape. She said, "Overweight is overlooked. And that is what I need to be." Clearly she, like so many others, was holding on to a subconscious belief that her weight was a protection against a future adverse event. On some level, she felt that she needed the weight to feel safe. Her story is far too common.

I've spent more than forty-five years studying nutrition and its effects on women's bodies, minds, and spirits—both personally and professionally. Being born with a body that my parents termed "solid" (they used to say, "She's built like a Mack truck," I kid you not), I've had to work consciously for most of my life on accepting my size and weight. And having worked with thousands of other women with the same problem, I can assure you that I know what works and what doesn't.

How Your Beliefs Can Thwart Your Weight-Loss Efforts

Women receive negative messages about their bodies throughout their lives. Remember the colleague I mentioned earlier in this chapter whose father told her that no woman should weigh over 120 pounds? As you may recall, she has been naturally thin her entire life and yet still weighs herself several times a day, just making sure that she meets her father's requirement. It's no wonder that the diet business is booming. With more and more people turning to diets, exercise, and gimmicks to control their weight, it's a no-brainer that diets just don't work. Yet many women try to lose weight rapidly, often before attending a special event such as a wedding, school reunion, or vacation. But almost 90 percent of the time, they gain the weight back because the plan was not sustainable. Thus these women develop the limiting belief that they will never be able to lose weight or maintain their optimal weight. I too was in that mindset for most of my life—and I occasionally still step into it.

The reason this belief is limiting is that in order for you to release unwanted weight, your conscious and subconscious minds must agree. If your mind says, "I want to lose weight and I believe I can do so easily," and your subconscious mind agrees, you will lose weight. But if your subconscious mind holds the belief that you will never be able to achieve your optimal weight, then you will most likely struggle to lose weight despite your conscious desire.

The limiting beliefs that can keep you from achieving your weight and body size goals often stem from fear. For example, if you were sexually abused when you were younger, you may fear that if you lose weight, others will find you attractive and hurt you sexually. Or perhaps you are afraid that if you lose weight but then don't find a partner, you will be considered a failure. Some people hold on to weight out of the fear that more will be expected from them once they are thin. Others may fear that if they lose weight they will be rejected by their family or friends. There is also the common fear that if you aren't "the fat person," you won't know who you are.

How to Reshape Your Body with Your Thoughts

Assuming you don't have a metabolic issue or medical problem getting in the way of your weight-loss goals, the first step to losing weight is to become acutely aware of your story. This may be the story of your past, such as a relative always pinching your abdomen and calling you "chubs." Or it may be a more recent story that you began telling yourself. For example, you may repeatedly tell yourself that weight loss is hard because the long hours you spend at work keep you from being able to eat right and exercise.

Remember, your thoughts and beliefs create your reality. So before attempting to change your diet and exercise routine, it's a good idea to work on changing your thoughts and beliefs.

Here are thirteen practices to help you reprogram your subconscious to achieve permanent weight loss:

1. LISTEN TO YOUR SELF-TALK. Self-respect and self-acceptance are the cornerstones to achieving optimal weight. But most people can't lose weight because they engage in body-shaming talk and behavior. It's important to know how you've been talking to yourself

before you try to lose weight. If you have been telling your body for most of your life that you hate how it looks, or if you've been pinching your skin in the mirror in disgust because someone used to do this to you, your subconscious mind will believe the negative programming. By talking to your body in a positive, loving manner—the way you would speak to an innocent child—you can rewire your subconscious brain. Look in the mirror and identify what you love about your body. Touch the parts that you want to change and say, "Thank you for keeping me safe." One of my good friends did this while rubbing her belly. "I realized that my abdominal fat was quite likely full of stored toxins, and that my body was protecting my internal organs by storing those toxins in my body fat," she told me. Once she had thanked her belly and also gave up trying to control it, her belly fat went away rather quickly. It's important to assure your body that it is safe to lose weight. Do this every day. Over time your subconscious will align with your conscious desire to lose weight.

2. CHECK OUT YOUR METABOLIC STRESSORS. In her book *Fight Fat After Forty* (Viking, 2000), Pamela Peeke, M.D., a researcher with the National Institutes of Health, documents the connection between toxic stress and toxic weight gain—the kind of weight that accumulates in the abdomen and puts women at risk for premature death. Toxic stress can come from any daily challenge, but a number of circumstances make it especially common in women over forty: the resurfacing of childhood trauma, perfectionism, relationship changes such as divorce and caregiving, job stress, acute or chronic illness, dieting, and the effects of menopause.

This explanation clicked with me because my initial perimenopausal weight gain coincided with new stresses in my life. The scale started to climb just before Thanksgiving, when my older daughter arrived home for her first vacation from college and we officially launched our first holiday season as a "broken" family. My daughters were scheduled to split their holiday time between my house and their father's, a situation I had always been sure would never happen to us.

I was also caring full-time for a friend who was recovering from major spine surgery. I was preparing her meals, trying to anticipate her needs, watching her go through excruciating pain unrelieved by narcotics, and generally trying to provide a safe place where she could heal. For well over a month I was basically on call twenty-four hours per day, with only an occasional break. In retrospect, no wonder the pounds piled on.

CORTISOL STEAL SYNDROME

In functional medicine circles, it's now well documented that when cortisol levels are high from too much unabated stress, lack of sleep, and living in a constant state of "fight, flight, or freeze," your adrenals literally "steal" the building blocks of other hormones—such as DHEA, estrogen, and progesterone—to produce excess cortisol. When these resources get shunted into cortisol production, you don't have enough left over to produce the right hormonal balance. The only way to reverse this state of affairs (and the adrenal fatigue syndrome that results) is to put into practice the very things needed to metabolize excess stress hormones and stop the vicious cycle that keeps you tired and wired. That includes getting enough sleep, vitamins, meditation, and pleasure.

Get out your calendar, do some detective work, and see if you too have a stress pattern that could be leading to the cortisol steal syndrome and subsequent weight gain. Be particularly aware of what happens during the late-afternoon hours, when the main hormones that allow us to mount a response against stress—serotonin and cortisol—tend to fall, leaving us feeling more vulnerable to our underlying emotions. In particular, when serotonin, the "feel-good" neurotransmitter, is depleted, we are apt to eat anything in sight—particularly refined carbohydrates—to bring it back to a normal level.

The effect of stress on weight also works in the opposite direction. One of my perimenopausal physician colleagues recently went on a trip with one of her grown children, who is in medical school. They went to a stimulating medical meeting and then explored the Grand Canyon together. Though she paid no attention to her diet and ate whatever she wanted, she arrived home six pounds lighter! She told me, "I think that my cortisol levels returned to normal because for ten days I got to sleep through the night and not worry about being called in for an emergency. And besides that, my serotonin was up from all the exciting conversation and healthy sunshine I was getting!"

3. WRITE A NEW STORY. Instead of just saying you want to lose weight, write down exactly what you want to achieve and why.

Maybe you want to lose five pounds (or fifty pounds) so that you can keep up with your grandchildren, or because you want to look stunning for a wedding or a reunion. Or perhaps you want to make better food choices so that you have more energy. Be sure to write down how you feel now and how you will feel when you achieve your goals. For example, if being overweight keeps you from enjoying bike rides with your friends and this makes you feel left out, write down this specific situation and emotion. Then write down how you will feel when you lose extra pounds and can join in the fun. One of my colleagues was obese as a child, in part because of the stress of having a mentally ill mother and having to care for her younger siblings. She knew she would lose weight when she left home. And she did. It has been sheer joy for her to ride a horse and to ski at midlife and beyond, because she remembers how hard it used to be simply to get up off the floor.

As you start to uncover your emotions around reaching your weight goals, continue to write them down. Be sure to tell your new story to yourself every day. Let it seep into your subconscious and every cell in your body.

4. TRY TAPPING. Tapping, also known as the Emotional Freedom Technique (EFT), helps to align your subconscious mind with your goals on an energetic level by addressing the underlying emotions, patterns, beliefs, traumas, and more that lead to your weight gain. It involves tapping on specific acupressure points in sequence while you make certain statements. This reduces stress hormones and also helps to release the emotional memories and beliefs associated with the unwanted pounds so that you can break old habits and heal. Here's the basic technique:

STEP 1. Take three deep breaths, inhaling slowly through your nose for a count of five, holding your breath for a count of five, and then exhaling for a count of five. Repeat. Feel your body relax.

STEP 2. Start by stating your current limiting belief followed by a statement of how you love and accept yourself. For example, you can say, "Even though I have a hard time losing weight, I love and accept myself completely." As you say this setup statement, tap the outside of your hand (along the pinky edge) with the four fingers from your opposite hand. Say this setup statement three times while continuing to tap that one point.

STEP 3. Now begin the tapping sequence. Using your index and middle finger (on one or both hands), tap firmly between five and nine times on each of the following points as you voice your feelings as follows (feel free to change the statements to fit your situation):

eyebrow (EB)—"I can't lose weight."

outer side of the eye (SE)—"I'm so ashamed of how heavy I am."

under the eye (UE)—"I just want to hide from everyone."

under the nose (UN)—"I can't easily do the things I used to enjoy because of my weight."

chin (CH)—"The thought of wearing a bathing suit in public . . ."

beginning of the collar bone (CB)—". . . creates anxiety in my body."

under your arms (UA)—"I don't even want to buy clothes anymore because I look so bad."

top of the head (TH)—"I have all of this fear that I will always be overweight."

STEP 4. Continue tapping on the same points, saying the following:

EB—"Whether I ever lose weight or not, I'm still a good person."

SE—"I am beginning to appreciate my body just the way it is."

UE—"And maybe I can lose weight after all."

UN—"When I eat healthy and do exercise I enjoy . . ."

CH—". . . I honor my desire to take care of myself."

CB—"I choose what to eat and what to wear from a place of peace."

UA—"It's safe to let go of the anxiety I feel."

TH—"It's safe to love my body and appreciate all it does for me."

STEP 5. Take a deep breath and exhale with your hands over your heart.

STEP 6. With your hands over your heart, say the following: "What I think and feel matters. I matter. I choose to honor myself and my heart's desires."

Then reassess your level of discomfort and repeat the procedure above. If you only have partial relief after that, do more rounds of tapping, amending the opening statement to something like: "Even though I still have shame and fear about my weight, I deeply and completely love myself." Adjust your focus if necessary if you notice additional emotions you want to work on surrounding this topic. When you complete your tapping session, sit quietly and listen to whatever comes up. Answers or resolutions often begin to arise spontaneously from deep within you. In all likelihood, you will no longer feel stuck and powerless after tapping because the practice gets you out of your intellect and into your own heart and your own wisdom.

5. MEDITATE. Meditation is another tool that can help you become more aware of your thoughts and beliefs so that you can carve a path to successful weight loss. It also greatly reduces the stress hormones that keep excess weight on the body. You can use your meditation practice to uncover your motivations for wanting to lose weight, understand any emotional or subconscious blocks, and even use imagery of how losing weight may look and feel to positively rewire your brain and develop more compassion for yourself. If sitting in meditation is not your thing, try moving meditation such as yoga or qi gong. You may also like to listen to audio meditations, such as the free meditations from the Center for Mindful Eating (thecenter formindfuleating.org/free-meditations).

6. SET SUSTAINABLE GOALS. Your ultimate goal may be to lose eighty pounds. But if you set out to achieve that right away, you may be setting yourself up for failure. Instead, set smaller, sustainable goals. For example, start with goals you have control over, such as eating five servings of fruits and vegetables per day or drinking more water (and eating more foods high in water content). You can also set a goal to get eight hours of sleep per night. You may find that these sustainable goals alone help you lose weight. If you want to set an actual weight-loss goal, make sure it's no more than two pounds per month. I know this sounds low, but two pounds per month is sustainable. And in one year that amounts to twenty-four pounds!

7. EAT MINDFULLY. Studies show that mindfulness—concentrated awareness of your thoughts, actions, and motivations—plays an essential role in long-term weight loss when used with other weight-loss strategies.[6] Practice mindfulness as you go about preparing your meals and eating. Try to be mindful of feelings of hunger and fullness. Pay attention to tastes, textures, and the acts of chewing and

swallowing your food. Also, be mindful of how your body feels after you eat certain foods. This practice can help reduce bingeing and make you more aware of habits that don't support your weight-loss goals. When you start connecting what you eat with how you feel, you won't need to diet to lose weight. It will happen effortlessly. When you change your attitude about food as self-nourishment, your body composition and body image will also be transformed. That's because when you connect with your body and nourish it from a place of compassion and self-respect, the feelings associated with that self-respect create a metabolic milieu in your body that is conducive to optimal fat burning.

8. SAY AFFIRMATIONS. Affirmations help to reinforce the new story you are programming your subconscious to believe. They work well when they are believable. However, if you say "I will be eighty pounds lighter in one month," your subconscious won't believe it. Instead, try saying, "I am now that naturally slim person who lives inside of me!" Or "I now make healthy decisions that support my optimal weight." You can even make a ritual of saying your affirmations. For example, you can smudge your room or home to rid it of stagnant energy, light a candle, sit with your eyes closed, and say your affirmations three times in a row. Do this two to three times per day. You may want to say some version of your affirmations just before you fall asleep, when your subconscious mind is most receptive to suggestion. Remember, affirmations need to be in the present tense, as though they have already manifested. In the words of the Rev. Michael Bernard Beckwith of the Agape International Spiritual Center in Los Angeles, "Affirmations don't make something happen. They make something welcome."

I highly recommend the work of Jon Gabriel and the Gabriel Method for weight loss. Jon lost more than 200 pounds by using affirmations, visualization, and the power of the mind. He teaches people all over the world how to do the same thing. And he has a free ebook available online with a free subliminal meditation you can download and use nightly. It is one of the best I've ever heard (www .thegabrielmethod.com).

9. STOP WEIGHING YOURSELF. While weighing yourself is not inherently bad, many women put too much emphasis on the number on the scale and even allow their weight to determine their mood, thoughts, and actions. This behavior is self-destructive. Don't step on the scale until you are able to view the information from a place of

health and not use it to define your self-worth. The beauty of this practice is that once you stop weighing yourself, you'll learn when and what makes you feel good in your own body. Then the number on the scale doesn't matter. After decades of linking my self-worth with the number on the scale, I finally came to the conclusion that weighing myself wasn't worth the stress hormones that resulted. And as a result, I haven't weighed myself in several years. I go by how my clothes fit. And I make sure that I never go up a size. I have a pair of jeans that I use as my barometer. When they fit well, I feel good. When they become too tight, I make a few adjustments in my lifestyle, diet, or thoughts until the fit is right once again.

10. BREATHE. When you take time to breathe fully and deeply, you become more aware of your body. Breathing with intention can also help to lower your body's stress response. There are many breathing techniques. You can learn about them and how to do them on YouTube. Or simply breathe in deeply through your nose for a count of five, hold for a count of five, breathe out for a count of five, and hold for a final count of five. Repeat that sequence for several minutes. This is called "block breathing," and it instantly creates a parasympathetic "rest and restore" biochemistry in your body while digesting stress hormones.

11. TRY A DETOX OR CLEANSE PROGRAM. There are many forms of detox that are effective, from the Colorado Cleanse by my colleague John Douillard, D.C., to the 28-Day Cleanse created by Anthony William, the Medical Medium. These can all be very effective. I have often begun my day drinking 16 oz. of celery juice on an empty stomach first thing in the morning. Thirty minutes after that, I also drink the juice of three to five lemons. Both practices are very effective detox regimens. (More on this later.) Remember, however, that no detox or cleanse will work until you also do the necessary emotional detox. It is also true that doing a physical cleanse will assist with the emotional detox.

12. SAY GOODBYE TO ENERGY VAMPIRES. One of the most striking things I've observed in relationships between vampires (people with character disorders) and sensitive souls is the disparity in their tendencies to gain weight. Your life and your relationships reflect your ability to nourish yourself. If you are in an imbalanced relationship where you are constantly giving to and trying to please another person, your efforts to lose weight will be in vain because you are con-

stantly pouring your energy into the vampire (either a person or a situation) in order to make it better. There are some situations and people that can't be helped, and so it is your job to simply walk away. When you don't, or feel that you can't, an excess of the stress hormones cortisol and epinephrine is the result. And this makes it almost impossible to lose weight. Have you ever seen someone on prednisone? Notice how they often blow up like a balloon. Well, your body on excess cortisol does the same thing. As a result, you seek out sugar, carbs, and/or alcohol in order to take the edge off and feel a bit better. But this unabated stress too often results in excess weight no matter what you do—even when you stop eating the carbs—because it acts as an extra layer of "self-protection." It's cognitive dissonance in the body. And that, I realize in retrospect, is exactly what was happening with me, and also my colleague, back in the days when we were eating just about nothing and still couldn't lose a pound!

13. LIVE "AS IF." Your beliefs are your reality. That's why I love the advice of Mario Martinez, Psy.D. He suggests taking a picture of yourself today (or find a recent picture that represents how you look now). Then find a picture of yourself from a time when you liked how you looked and felt good about yourself. Once you have your two pictures, live for ten days "as if" you are still the self you felt good about. At the end of ten days of living "as if," take a new picture of yourself. You will look much more like your former self, whom you loved and respected.

WHAT SHOULD YOU EAT?

I want to give you some practical advice for how to get started on changing your hormones and your weight with the right food choices—keeping in mind that there is no one "right" answer that will work for everyone. There is, however, information that applies to everyone.

The Soil/Gut/Antibiotic Connection: Getting Down to Basics

Before we go any further, it's important to know about the profound connection between your gut microbiome and the foods you eat, the water you drink, the air you breathe, and the medications you take. Your microbiome is a diverse community of bacteria, fungi, and viruses that live on your skin, in your respiratory tract, in your reproductive system, and most especially throughout your digestive system—starting at your mouth and moving right down to the large intestine. The health of your microbiome—which in turn affects your cognition, your emotions, and the health of every system in your body—is determined by the health of the soil in which your food is grown and also by the health of the water you drink and the air you breathe. One gram of soil contains 40 million individual bacterial cells. And a milliliter of fresh water contains at least a million bacteria. All of these diverse life-forms are designed to live in harmony both in nature and in our bodies. In fact, the health of the soil directly and profoundly impacts the health of your digestive and immune systems.

Here's the rub. If you eat the same food over and over again or take antibiotics or other drugs repeatedly, your gut microbiome will not develop the diversity it requires for optimal health. One recent study from Ukraine showed that obese people had a higher level of some gut bacteria and a lower level of others compared to normal-weight and lean adults.[7] And if the foods you eat are mostly packaged and processed or filled with chemical preservatives and GMO grains, there will be many untoward effects on your health because our microbiomes haven't evolved to digest these foods. When you introduce a food that is new to your body, the right organisms may not be there to help digest it. Or the antibiotics you take may have wiped out a lot of your good gut bacteria, so you may experience some digestive upset (including gas, nausea, and diarrhea) until the right gut bacteria are replenished. A common example of this is eating a lot of beans when you haven't been eating them regularly. Excess gas often results. But if you consume legumes regularly, over time your gut bacteria will develop the ability to digest them far better. It's the same with other foods. It is also true that one's heritage partly determines what foods you can easily digest and which ones are more difficult. For example, people of Northern European heritage often have no trouble digesting dairy products because of evolutionary processes involving their genes and microbiomes that have developed over decades of regularly consuming cheese, yogurt, and milk.[8] But an individual of African descent would likely have far more difficultly digesting dairy.

We all know that a diverse diet is important to health. And it's the same for the soil. Yet our current agricultural practices of monocropping, which use chemical fertilizers, pesticides, and conventional livestock grazing, quite literally destroy the healthy microbiome of that soil. Using a plot of land to grow the same thing over and over again leads to degenerated soil even when no pesticides are used. And that is the state of much of the farmland in the United States. It is no different in your body. Many, many women approach midlife with highly compromised microbiomes from a lifetime of taking antibiotics, birth control pills, and other medications. This is not your fault, of course.

Losing Touch with Mother Earth: How We Got Here

When penicillin was discovered, we moved into the antibiotic era. Doctors began using antibiotics for everything from the common cold to acne. In fact, many patients have insisted on taking antibiotics even when they have not been indicated. Penicillin and all the other second-, third-, and fourth-generation antibiotics that have followed have been the "magic bullets" of the last fifty or so years. There is no question that they have saved many lives. But at what price?

When I was a girl, our family doctor used to drive up to our house in a big black car and give penicillin shots to whichever one of us was sick. But he didn't stop there. He often wanted to give everyone in the family a shot "just in case." We kids dubbed him "Shotsie," and when we saw the car coming up the driveway, we'd run and hide in the barn. My mother was given massive doses of an antibiotic called streptomycin for viral pneumonia during her pregnancy with my sister Bonnie, who later died at the age of six months. Bonnie wouldn't eat, and the doctors never knew why. I suspect that the antibiotics did something to her development.

My father often just let us hide in the barn and avoid the penicillin. I believe he intuitively knew that there was more to health than penicillin shots. He also wasn't afraid of dirt or germs. And neither am I. When I was little and a piece of food would fall on the ground, my father would say, "You can eat it. Let the earth pass through you. And then you will be immune to everything." He also had my mother make yogurt long before it was commercially available. He would take it down the street to give to his patients on antibiotics. In fact, we now know that children who are brought up with pets and who regularly get dirty are far healthier than those who are kept in more sterile environments by caretakers who are afraid of "germs."

We also have had to wake up to the reality that nature always finds a way. The constant killing of microorganisms with antibiotics as well as with antibacterial soaps and wipes has simply led to stronger and stronger bacteria that have now become "superbugs," increasingly resistant to even the most potent antibiotics. Hospitals are now full of antibiotic-resistant bacteria—a perfect example of "what we resist, persists."

I bring this up because so many people now have impaired microbiomes from fast food, nutrient-poor diets with food grown on depleted soils, and regular use of drugs and antibiotics. As a result, the health and diversity of our gut microbes is not what it should be. Digestive upset, depression, foggy thinking, autoimmune disease, fatigue, and even obesity are the result. The health of our bodies and the health of our soils are intimately connected. And right now, the vast majority of our soils (at least here in the United States) are vastly depleted of nutrients and the right bacteria because of monocrop farming, the overuse of nitrogen fertilizer, genetically modified seeds, and pesticides such as glyphosate, which kills pretty much all the good soil nutrients. Add to that the devastating effects of these things on our pollinators (bees), and you have a recipe for ill health.

The Solution

So—what to do? We must move from *anti*-biotic (anti-life) thinking to *pro*-biotic (pro-life) thinking in pretty much every area of our lives. And we must embrace the wisdom of Antoine Beauchamp, who was a chief rival of Louis Pasteur (the scientist who invented the process of pasteurization to kill bacteria in food). Beauchamp always argued that it was the environment, not the germ itself, that led to disease. Pasteur argued that it was the germ. It is said (but has never been proven) that on his deathbed, however, Pasteur finally admitted that Beauchamp was right. Specifically, it is the environment that a germ finds itself in that determines whether or not that germ becomes dangerous to life.

When I was an OB-GYN resident in Boston, I was involved in a study in which samples of peritoneal fluid were collected in a location behind the uterus known as the cul-de-sac of Douglas. We were trying to determine exactly what type of bacteria was involved in pelvic inflammatory disease. That fluid was then cultured to see what bacteria were growing in it. What was most astounding was that we often found some very "dangerous" bacteria, such as *Clostridioides difficile,* in perfectly healthy women. Obviously, these bacteria were held in check by a healthy microbiome. They were not causing any disease.

But when environmental stress of any kind messes with the balance of the microbiome, chronic inflammation and conditions such as asthma, chronic fatigue, colitis, constipation, gas, and diarrhea are often the result, in both children and adults. This is related to the fact that everywhere we look in the environment, we see degradation of our air, water, and soil—except in protected lands and those places where organic and regenerative agriculture are practiced. Here's the good news: nature always cooperates and restores balance in a relatively short amount of time, if given half a chance. We can do the same thing in our bodies.

Regenerative Agriculture/Cellular Regeneration

If you were to watch the 2018 documentary *The Biggest Little Farm,* you would see how a California couple took a defunct apricot farm from a wasteland of dead trees and dead soil to a thriving paradise within seven years. All the cells in our bodies are renewed within a seven-year period as well, though it doesn't take nearly that long to create an entirely new digestive system. How do we go about doing this?

Eliminate Certain Foods as an Experiment (But Not Necessarily Forever)

Every single one of us is exposed to multiple environmental toxins daily regardless of how pristine our environment or diet may be. There is no escaping this, given the impact of pesticides, plastics, and air and water pollution. Most municipal water contains chlorine and fluoride, both of which are known toxins. Most bottled water comes in plastic, and it has been clearly demonstrated that we all ingest a credit-card-size amount of plastic every week![9] In addition, the chemtrails in the air often contain ionized aluminum, which is a toxin. It's hard to believe that the United States routinely allows the use of eighty-five pesticides that have been banned in other countries, and that millions of pounds of toxic substances are used daily.[10] So I don't care who you are or where you are—you're exposed to toxins. Deadly glyphosate (the herbicide found in Roundup) can be found even in organically grown foods. I say all this not to scare you into giving up, but simply to let you know that some kind of regular detoxification program is necessary for optimal health for pretty much everyone.

The Whole30: A Good Place to Begin (But Not the Only Place)

Doing some kind of detox or cleanse program for starters—and then continuing it on a regular basis, such as at the change of seasons—is to your health like flossing is to your teeth and gums. It just makes sense in a world full of environmental toxins.

The best way to begin a detox program is to simply eliminate the foods that are problematic for the vast majority of people. Those foods include the following: grains of all kinds (including wheat, oats, barley, corn, amaranth, and quinoa), dairy (including goat's milk, cow's milk, sheep's milk, cheese, cream, and yogurt), added sugars (like sucrose, honey, and maple syrup), artificial sweeteners, and even natural sweeteners like stevia, monkfruit, and coconut sugar. Eliminate soy as well because so many people are now sensitive to it. Also, no tobacco products, MSG, carrageenan, or sulfites. Learn to read all labels.

You might not be sensitive to all of these foods, but doing the Whole30 for thirty days will detox your body in such a way that when you add back each of the "no-fly" foods, one at a time, you'll know which ones cause digestive upset, a runny nose, sneezing, gastrointestinal upset, or weight gain and which ones don't. You'll find that what works for someone else may not work for you. But your job here is to find what works for *you*—regardless of what any of the outside "experts" say.

When it comes to food allergies, the vast majority of culprits will be in the list of foods to avoid. Once you eliminate them for a period of time, your body will respond nicely. I urge you to go to the Whole30 website (whole30.com) for more information. Remember, it's only for thirty days.

So what *can* you eat? On the Whole30, you can eat any fruit or vegetable out there. Nuts and seeds are also fine, as well as any and all meats and eggs—but I urge you to eat only humanely raised grass-fed beef, pork, or free-range chicken. Healthy fats like grass-fed butter, olive oil, and avocado are also fine. You will be amazed by how easy it is to build meals around this healthy framework. It will also streamline your shopping—you just avoid the center of any grocery store and shop the perimeter, where the produce and meats are. And if you are a vegetarian, you just avoid the meat part. Another approach for detoxification is to eat just fruits and vegetables while avoiding all grains and legumes. It's easy to do this for thirty days.

Following this (or another) elimination diet does several things. It allows your body to "rest" from the stress of foods that may well be problematic but which you don't even realize are an issue. For many, many people this is certainly true of alcohol and grains. Also, because the foods that are allowed are nutrient dense and full of what are called "prebiotics"—the foods that good bacteria feed on in the gut—you will quickly be changing your microbiome for the better.

Here is what is likely to happen to you during the Whole30 program. You'll sleep better, you'll lose weight, you'll have far more energy, and your cravings may well decrease or be eliminated altogether. Your taste buds will change, too. You'll find that an apple tastes much sweeter than ever before. It's remarkable. You might also get a headache for a while, or maybe some skin rashes, and you may feel very tired initially. Expect this and don't let it stop you. This dietary approach is like clearing the weeds before planting a new garden.

There are, of course, other ways to do a detox or elimination diet. I just find this is one of the most well-thought-out and doable. Plus, there are Whole30 cookbooks and recipes all over the internet.

It's worth noting that recent research shows a diet high in both oily fish and fresh legumes is associated with a later onset of menopause, while a higher intake of refined pasta and rice was associated with an earlier onset.[11] Clearly your diet has an effect on your hormonal health.

Other Cleanses to Choose From

If the Whole30 doesn't appeal to you, then try the Colorado Cleanse, which was created by my colleague John Douillard, D.C. It is based on Ayurvedic principles and works very well to get rid of toxins and reboot the system. This cleanse is ideal to do at the change of seasons—in particular, spring and fall. It is all vegan except for the clarified butter (known as ghee) that is the backbone of the plan for an ancient Ayurvedic practice known as oleation, which draws toxins out of the gut, into the ghee, and then out of the body in the stool.

I have done the Colorado Cleanse several times and have found it very satisfying. It does allow grains and vegetables and a traditional food known as kitchari, a blend of basmati rice and mung beans. I also like the fact that it includes what are called "hot sips," small amounts of hot water throughout the day. This is very satisfying. Of course, this can be done anytime by anyone. To order the information and the necessary supplements, go to lifespa.com/cleansing /colorado-cleanse.

Then there is the Medical Medium's 28-Day Cleanse. This consists of a daily detox smoothie every morning, followed by fruits and veggies for the rest of the day. I have found this easy and also delicious, especially in the warm months. Anthony William also wrote a book called *Medical Medium Cleanse to Heal* (Hay House, 2020) that details the best foods to use for cleansing. These include Hawaiian spirulina, barley grass juice powder, cilantro, lemon balm, and a whole host of others.

DETOX SMOOTHIE RECIPE

The following recipe is based on the standard detox smoothie recommended by Anthony William, the Medical Medium.

Ingredients:

2–3 organic bananas

2 cups wild Maine blueberries (I use frozen ones that I buy in five-pound boxes and keep in the freezer)

1 orange

1 bunch fresh cilantro (just use a handful—about 1 cup)

1 teaspoon Hawaiian spirulina

1 teaspoon barley grass juice powder

1 tablespoon organic Atlantic dulse powder

1 heaping tablespoon CurrantC black currant concentrate (Available from www.currantc.com, this stuff is, in my view, the "secret sauce." It adds a tart flavor and beautiful color to this smoothie. Black currants also have one of the highest ORAC scores of any food. ORAC is an acronym for "oxygen radical absorbance capacity," and an ORAC score is a measure of the level of antioxidant and anti-inflammatory activity of a food or supplement.)

Directions:

Blend all the ingredients in a Vitamix or blender. This makes about one quart of smoothie, which is enough for one person to consume throughout the day. I like drinking this in two 16-oz. servings. I squeeze the juice of half a lemon on top of each serving and stir it in. If I have guests, I serve it in 8-oz. glasses as a morning libation.

Don't forget the lemon juice. You can also add many other things to this smoothie once it's in a glass. A few examples include liquid cat's claw herb, lemon balm, liquid B$_{12}$, zinc, or pico silver (I use the brand created by Carolyn Dean, M.D., N.D., available at rnareset.com). These individual herbs are all useful for various conditions, including Epstein-Barr virus problems.

CELERY JUICE: A MIRACLE FOOD

I first learned about the amazing health benefits of fresh celery juice from my friend Anthony William, the Medical Medium. It contains sodium cluster salts that are antiviral and which help heal the gut. I figured I'd give it a try, as have thousands around the world. Without going into all the benefits, let me share my experience.

I often drink 16 oz. of fresh celery juice every morning upon arising, on an empty stomach. Nothing else added. And I don't drink or eat anything for thirty minutes thereafter. I make it fresh each morning. The juice is hydrating, detoxifying, and cleansing—and it's delicious. It also stimulates normal bowel function far better than a cup of coffee.

If there were one dietary practice I would recommend to those who want to restore their health and digestive function, it would be to start the day with fresh celery juice.

For more information, read *Medical Medium Celery Juice* (Hay House, 2019) by Anthony William.

SIX STEPS TO MIDLIFE WEIGHT CONTROL

Step One: Understanding the Blood Sugar/Insulin Connection—The Real Key to Avoiding Chronic Disease

Like many women (and doctors), I used to operate under the delusion that the reason we tend to gain weight at midlife is because our metabolism slows down, our bodies become more efficient at storing energy in the form of fat, and falling estrogen levels result in increases in appetite.[12] As it turns out, these metabolic changes, though real enough, are not the result of menopause per se, but are instead the natural progression of metabolic processes that have been going on for years but have now reached critical mass.

Let's start with the first one: glycemic stress. Glycemic stress begins when blood sugar is too high and results in increased insulin levels.

When you eat too many refined carbohydrates (in the form of white bread, pretzels, cookies, candy, cakes, pastries, soda pop, mashed potatoes, or sugary foods—even the gluten-free ones) you get an immediate and substantial increase in blood sugar. This excess sugar in the blood is converted to triglycerides in the liver. At the same time, however, excess blood sugar causes inflammation in the lining of blood vessels throughout your body, starting in the skeletal muscles. This is known as "glycemic stress," a term coined by family physician Ray Strand, M.D., whose research has documented how glycemic stress, if left unchecked, eventually results in syndrome X, also known as metabolic syndrome. Syndrome X is characterized by central obesity (too much belly fat and fat around the upper back and shoulders—the classic apple-shaped figure), high blood pressure, high blood sugar, and abnormal cholesterol or triglyceride levels, leading to an increased risk for type 2 diabetes and heart disease.

Dr. Strand's observations have been backed up by further research, including the 2010 European Prospective Investigation into Cancer and Nutrition (EPICOR) study from Italy that followed 47,000 participants. The EPICOR researchers reported that women who ate the most high-glycemic-index carbohydrates had more than twice the risk of getting heart disease as those who ate the least (although the same association wasn't found in men).[13] In addition, another study published the same month and conducted by Emory University School of Medicine was the first to link eating food containing high amounts of added sugar with an increased risk for heart disease. This study, which looked at data from more than 6,000 adults who took part in the National Health and Nutrition Examination Survey (NHANES), showed that those who consume the most added sugar—the kind found in processed foods and drinks, not natural sugars found in fruits and fruit juices—were more likely to have higher levels of triglycerides and a higher ratio of triglycerides to HDL cholesterol (one of the most potent predictors of heart disease).[14]

Excess blood sugar over long periods of time eventually leads to insulin resistance. Let me explain. Insulin is produced in the pancreas and is responsible for ferrying glucose from the bloodstream into our cells, where it is used for fuel or stored as fat. Think of insulin as a storage hormone. Good health depends upon our body's ability to make and utilize just the right amount of insulin to keep our blood sugar at optimal levels and our metabolism working normally. Consumption of high-glycemic-index foods results in an immediate surge in blood sugar. This triggers the pancreas to secrete large amounts of insulin to take the sugar out of the blood and transport it into the cells. Every cell in the body has insulin receptors on the surface. These allow insulin to "open the door" so that glucose can enter the cell.[15] But over time, when blood sugar levels continue to be too high, the insulin receptors lose their ability to respond to this abnormal metabolic burden. The excess blood sugar is also stored as fat—a storage process that actually begins in the abdominal area, in and around the organs. Excess fat can be stored in the liver, around the bowels, in the walls of the abdomen, and in the omentum, a very metabolically active apron of fat that hangs over the abdominal organs. When performing surgery, surgeons often find that the abdominal area is packed with so much excess fat that the operation itself—whether it be a C-section, an ovarian removal, a hysterectomy, or something else—is far more difficult than it would be in a thinner person.

Over time the stored fat in and around the pancreas's islet cells (the cells that secrete insulin) actually puts mechanical pressure on the cells themselves, blocking them from being able to do their job. This in and of itself contributes to an all-too-common condition known as insulin resistance. But that's just one factor. As years go by, cells lose their sensitivity to the excess insulin that is being poured out to deal with the excess blood sugar. Eventually neither the body tissues nor the pancreatic islet cells can keep up with the blood sugar load. The metabolic state created by high blood sugar and high insulin affects virtually every cell in our bodies. In severe cases, an individual with this condition may be diagnosed with type 2 diabetes and require insulin injections. Even the brain is adversely affected by this condition, which is why Alzheimer's disease is now often called "type 3 diabetes."[16]

About 25 percent of the population appears to be genetically resistant to the adverse effects of overproduction of insulin and insulin resistance. These individuals usually manage to stay very slim no matter what they eat, though that doesn't mean that they are necessarily healthy. Fully 75 percent of the population is not so lucky, especially during perimenopause.

David Ludwig, M.D., Ph.D., an endocrinologist at Harvard Medical School and an authority on insulin and weight, says that the low-fat diets inspired by the old "calories in, calories out" model not only don't work but also have actually contributed to weight gain in many people.[17] It isn't overeating that causes weight gain, he says. It's the other way around—gaining weight causes us to overeat. He explains that the classic low-fat, high-carbohydrate diet raises insulin levels, which cause the body to store calories as fat instead of burning those calories as fuel. Because they don't then have access to those calories, our brains respond by making us hungry, to get us to eat more food, while at the same time slowing our metabolism to conserve energy. But our fat cells remain in storage mode, so those extra calories just pack on the pounds instead of providing energy. No wonder Dr. Ludwig describes insulin as "Miracle-Gro" for fat cells.

By cutting out processed carbohydrates in favor of eating the right balance of protein and fat from whole foods, his research shows, you can reprogram your fat cells to lose weight. His bestselling book, *Always Hungry?* (Hachette, 2016), outlines a plan that has been a game-changer for many. In it, he suggests first giving up processed carbohydrates, foods with added sugars, and all grain products for two weeks. During this time, half your calories should come from fat (which could include nuts, nut butters, full-fat dairy products, olive oil, fish, avocados, and dark chocolate), with 25 percent from protein and 25 percent from carbohydrates (non-starchy vegetables, fruits, and beans). This combination, he says, should eliminate cravings. Then, to retrain your fat cells, reintroduce whole-kernel grains, sweet potatoes (but not white potatoes), and a small amount of foods with added sugar. In this second phase, your diet should consist of 40 percent fat, 35 percent carbohydrate, and 25 percent protein until your weight reaches a lower set point. This could be a few weeks or several months, depending on how much weight you need to lose. Then you can reintroduce bread, white potatoes, and some processed carbs, aiming for a balance of 40 percent fat, 40 percent carbs, and 20 percent protein. See how your body handles the added foods—if you start to gain weight, stop eating whatever triggered the weight gain. Dr. Ludwig's plan works because it lowers insulin levels and burns fat for fuel—and it doesn't leave you hungry, which triggers overeating.

Most perimenopausal symptoms, such as heavy bleeding, cramps, fibroids, and PMS, will respond to a diet such as this that keeps your blood sugar and insulin levels stable—a diet that will also help prevent cellular inflammation. In general, insulin and blood sugar levels stay normal on a diet of unrefined whole foods that include carbohydrates with a low-to-moderate-glycemic index, such as fruits, vegetables, fish, chicken, pork, and legumes. The glycemic index is simply a measurement of the rate and degree to which a given carbohydrate-containing food raises blood sugar levels. High-glycemic-index carbohydrates—including alcohol, starchy and sugary foods such as cookies, candies, soda pop, alcohol, and white bread, and almost all refined, processed foods—are quickly metabolized into sugar, triggering a rush of insulin into the blood.

On the other hand, carbohydrates with a low glycemic index break down slowly, raising blood sugar to relatively low levels over a longer period of time. This allows them to be metabolized with only a small amount of insulin.

INSULIN RESISTANCE (SYNDROME X)

The medical conditions associated with insulin resistance are collectively known as syndrome X, a term first coined by Gerald Reaven, M.D., a world-renowned endocrinologist at the Stanford University School of Medicine.[18] They include:

~ Increased risk for type 2 diabetes[19]

~ Abnormal cholesterol levels[20]

~ Hypertension

~ Heart disease: coronary artery disease and peripheral vascular disease[21]

~ Obesity

~ Anovulation[22]

~ Overstimulation of ovarian testosterone[23]

~ Polycystic ovary syndrome

~ Excess hair on the face, hair loss on scalp (male-pattern baldness in women)

~ Adult acne

~ Increased risk for breast cancer and endometrial cancer[24]

Evolutionarily speaking, most of the high-glycemic-index carbohydrates are "new" foods that have been rapidly increasing in our
diets only over the last century. Up until then, for millennia, our food
supply and metabolism evolved side by side along with the active
lifestyles that also keep insulin levels normal. Traditional farming
methods ensured that we kept nutrient-rich soil alive with microorganisms. However, today's modern agriculture, with its pesticides
and herbicides, has contributed to nutrient-poor, dead soil—and as a
result, conventionally produced food (and almost all packaged fast
food) is woefully devoid of nutrients.

A diet high in refined carbohydrates makes all perimenopausal
problems worse because of its adverse effect on hormone balance.
It reinforces the tendency toward excess fat around the waist and
belly (central obesity), which in turn favors production of estrogen
and androgens. Central obesity and high insulin levels—which can
occur even in women of normal weight and BMI—are also associated with higher blood triglyceride levels and low HDL cholesterol.
(A low HDL level is one of the first signs of insulin abuse. I actually
had this in my early thirties but finally figured out the problem, and
all has been well since then.) This, of course, has a negative effect
on heart health, but it also interferes with the normal mechanism
by which the body deactivates free estradiol. A relative increase in
the amount of metabolically active estradiol in the bloodstream can
target estrogen-sensitive breast and endometrial tissue, resulting in
possible excessive growth of these tissues. This is one of the reasons why hyperinsulinemia (excess insulin in the blood) with insulin resistance is a significant risk factor for breast cancer as well
as polycystic ovary syndrome.[25] High insulin levels also increase
tissue sensitivity to a protein known as insulin-like growth factor
(IGF-1), which is known to stimulate the growth of breast and other
tissues.[26]

Skeletal muscles are designed to burn blood sugar effectively,
which is why maintaining adequate muscle mass and exercising regularly are important keys to maintaining stable blood sugar. But as
women grow older, they often stop exercising as much as they did in
their teens and twenties. Lifestyles become increasingly sedentary, so
by the time they hit perimenopause, many women have replaced their
muscle mass with fat, and years of insulin abuse have stored excess
energy as fat—particularly abdominal fat. (Fat weighs less than muscle but takes up more space. This is the reason why so many midlife
women notice that their clothes don't fit well anymore even though
they haven't gained any weight!) One of the earliest signs of insulin

resistance is increased belly fat—that spare tire around the middle. Body fat is loaded with insulin receptors, and the fatter you get, the more insulin it takes to get blood sugar into the cells. Type 2 diabetes will often disappear simply with fat loss alone.

Glycemic stress and insulin resistance are also associated with heartburn, insomnia, swelling, sugar cravings, fatigue, and excess daytime sleepiness—all of which are associated with tissue inflammation that is the result of the complex interaction between insulin, blood sugar, stress hormones, and essential fatty acids. People with excess body fat, from years of eating high-glycemic-index meals, actually produce high levels of inflammatory chemicals such as IL-6 (interleukin 6) from their body fat. They are prone to aches and pains, estrogen dominance, and PMS as a result. Ultimately, glycemic stress leads to insulin resistance and, later, diabetes and/or heart disease, if left unchecked.

Intermittent Fasting

Another dietary approach that works for many is intermittent fasting. The easiest way to do this is to make sure you have a twelve-hour window each day during which you eat nothing. You can drink water or have black coffee or tea, but the basic principle is that you want to fast long enough that your insulin levels become zero. It takes twelve hours with no food for this to happen. Intermittent fasting works especially well for those, like me, who are simply not hungry when they wake up in the morning. It's very easy to finish dinner at, say, 8:00 P.M. and then not eat anything until the next day at 8:00 A.M. or later. Over time, your body gets used to the rhythm of no food in the morning. But you can begin the day with a fasting tea or black coffee. Some people add MCT oil or grass-fed butter to the coffee. For many, this morning brew with healthy fat sustains them nicely until lunch. Please note that this doesn't work for everyone, but it's worth a try.

Step Two: Measure for Health—Waist/Hip Ratio, Body Mass Index, and Body Fat Percentage

Years of eating too many refined carbohydrates and exercising too little finally catch up with us at midlife. Slowly but surely, our lifestyles predispose us to central obesity (excess belly fat), which *is* a problem. Abdominal fat cells are more metabolically active—and potentially more dangerous—than the fat cells on your hips and thighs.

MORE REASON TO AVOID PROCESSED FOODS

The added sugars in processed foods aren't the only reason they're unhealthy for you. The preservatives and pesticide residues (such as glyphosate, the active herbicide in Roundup) that these foods often contain are also far from harmless. For example, not only does research show that glyphosate disrupts the endocrine system and harms our gut bacteria,[27] but the International Agency for Research on Cancer (which is part of the World Health Organization) also determined the chemical to be a probable human carcinogen (particularly associated with non-Hodgkin's lymphoma).

Research from the Harvard School of Public Health shows that processed meats can contribute to both diabetes and heart disease.[28] According to a 2010 meta-analysis that examined data from twenty different studies looking at 1 million adults from ten countries around the world, daily consumption of 50 grams of processed meat (the equivalent of either one typical U.S. hot dog or two slices of deli meat) was associated with a 42 percent higher risk of coronary heart disease and a 19 percent increased risk of diabetes. Processed meats were defined as those that had been preserved by smoking, curing, or salting (which also includes sausage and bacon).

However, eating *twice* as much *unprocessed* red meat a day didn't raise the risk of either heart disease or diabetes. It's time we all become aware of the dangerous effects of added ingredients in processed foods and eat accordingly whenever possible. The researchers found that while the red meats and processed meats had similar amounts of saturated fat and cholesterol, the processed meats had four times the amount of sodium as unprocessed meat—and they also contain nitrate preservatives. *Note:* Sodium—in the form of sodium chloride, regular salt—is not so healthful. But sodium as part of a complex group of minerals found in Himalayan salt and Celtic sea salt is a whole other story. This type of salt is quite healthful.

Abdominal fat increases blood triglyceride levels and is a sign of insulin resistance.

And belly fat cells also pump out too much estrogen and too many androgens. The classic apple-shaped figure is associated with an increased risk for heart disease, breast cancer, uterine cancer, diabetes, kidney stones, hypertension, arthritis, incontinence, polycystic ovary syndrome, urinary stress incontinence, gallstones, stroke, and sleep apnea.[29]

Your waist/hip ratio is a quick way to gauge your risk. Measure around the fullest part of your buttocks. Then measure your waist at the narrowest part of your torso. Divide your waist measurement by your hip measurement. A healthy ratio is less than 0.8. The ideal is 0.74. A ratio greater than 0.85 is associated with all the health risks listed above.[30] You can also use your waist measurement in inches because it directly measures belly fat. If your waist measurement is more than 34.5 inches, there's a strong likelihood that you already have insulin resistance and metabolic syndrome.

Body mass index (BMI) is another way to measure your health risk. To determine your BMI, simply find your weight and your height on the table on the following page. A BMI of 24 or below is ideal. For people who don't smoke and aren't chronically ill, a BMI of 30 or higher (considered obese) is associated with a two to three times greater risk of dying prematurely compared to a person with a BMI of 24 or less. For those with a BMI between 25 and 29 (considered overweight, but not obese), the risk of premature death is still 20 to 40 percent higher than for those at normal weight.[31]

Percentage of body fat is the final number you'll need. This can be measured by your doctor, at a health club, or at your YMCA. Though it's possible to purchase over-the-counter devices that measure body fat, I have not found them to be very accurate. It is possible to have a healthy body fat percentage (between 20 and 28 percent for women) and have a BMI that is higher than 24. This is especially true in athletes who have a great deal of muscle mass.

If your waist/hip ratio, BMI, and body fat percentage are all in the healthy range, then you simply have to fine-tune what you are already doing to maintain your weight and balance your hormones. If not, then do whatever you can to lower your risk. A 1999 study from Harvard Medical School found that women who gain approximately twenty pounds in adulthood experience a decline in physical function and vitality even greater than that associated with smoking. (And speaking of smoking, a 2010 study shows that obesity has now

FIGURE 11: BODY MASS INDEX CHART

Height (Feet and Inches)

Weight (Pounds)	5'0"	5'1"	5'2"	5'3"	5'4"	5'5"	5'6"	5'7"	5'8"	5'9"	5'10"	5'11"	6'0"	6'1"	6'2"	6'3"	6'4"
100	20	19	18	18	17	17	16	16	15	15	14	14	14	13	13	12	12
105	21	20	19	19	18	17	17	16	16	16	15	15	14	14	13	13	13
110	21	21	20	19	19	18	18	17	17	16	16	15	15	15	14	14	13
115	22	22	21	20	20	19	19	18	17	17	17	16	16	15	15	14	14
120	23	23	22	21	21	20	19	19	18	18	17	17	16	16	15	15	15
125	24	24	23	22	21	21	20	20	19	18	18	17	17	16	16	16	15
130	25	25	24	23	22	22	21	20	20	19	19	18	18	17	17	16	16
135	26	26	25	24	23	22	22	21	21	20	19	19	18	18	17	17	16
140	27	26	26	25	24	23	23	22	21	21	20	20	19	18	18	17	17
145	28	27	27	26	25	24	23	23	22	21	21	20	20	19	19	18	18
150	29	28	27	27	26	25	24	23	23	22	22	21	20	20	19	19	18
155	30	29	28	27	27	26	25	24	24	23	22	22	21	20	20	19	19
160	31	30	29	28	27	27	26	25	24	24	23	22	22	21	21	20	19
165	32	31	30	29	28	27	27	26	25	24	24	23	22	22	21	21	20
170	33	32	31	30	29	28	27	27	26	25	24	24	23	22	22	21	21
175	34	33	32	31	30	29	28	27	27	26	25	24	24	23	22	22	21
180	35	34	33	32	31	30	29	28	27	27	26	25	24	24	23	22	22
185	36	35	34	33	32	31	30	29	28	27	27	26	25	24	24	23	23
190	37	36	35	34	33	32	31	30	29	28	27	26	26	25	24	24	23
195	38	37	36	35	33	32	31	31	30	29	28	27	26	26	25	24	24
200	39	38	37	35	34	33	32	31	30	30	29	28	27	26	26	25	24
205	40	39	37	36	35	34	33	32	31	30	29	29	28	27	26	26	25
210	41	40	38	37	36	35	34	33	32	31	30	29	28	28	27	26	26
215	42	41	39	38	37	36	35	34	33	32	31	30	29	28	28	27	26
220	43	42	40	39	38	37	36	34	33	32	32	31	30	29	28	27	27
225	44	43	41	40	39	37	36	35	34	33	32	31	31	30	29	28	27
230	45	43	42	41	39	38	37	36	35	34	33	32	31	30	30	29	28
235	46	44	43	42	40	39	38	37	36	35	34	33	32	31	30	29	29
240	47	45	44	43	41	40	39	38	36	35	34	33	33	32	31	30	29
245	48	46	45	43	42	41	40	38	37	36	35	34	33	32	31	31	30
250	49	47	46	44	43	42	40	39	38	37	36	35	34	33	32	31	30

☐ Underweight ▨ Weight Appropriate ☐ Overweight ▮ Obese

become a greater health threat than smoking. The prevalence of smoking over the last fifteen years has declined by 18.5 percent, while the proportion of obese people has risen 85 percent.[32] And according to the Centers for Disease Control and Prevention, as of 2017–2018 an unheard-of 42.4 percent of Americans over the age of twenty are considered obese, with the percentage increasing steadily since 1997.) Weight gain in the Harvard study was also associated with an increase in bodily pain, regardless of a woman's baseline weight. The reason for this is that excess fat produces inflammatory compounds, such as cytokines and interleukin 6, that cause tissue damage and pain. Happily, this is all reversible. Once the overweight women lost weight, all characteristics of health and vitality improved.[33] This is very good news. You don't have to reach your ideal weight; even a modest five- or ten-pound fat loss—or achieving a BMI that is one number lower than your current number—can dramatically improve your health, lower your blood pressure, and balance your hormone levels.

THE OBESITY-CANCER LINK

As GYN oncology nurse practitioner Mary Welch sat in the audience of a medical lecture on obesity and cancer, she was stunned not only by one of the statistics she had just heard but also by what it meant for her personally: that her risk for endometrial cancer in particular was quadrupled because her BMI was 36. Indeed, more than 50 percent of endometrial cancers diagnosed today are attributable to obesity, which is recognized as an independent risk factor for this disease.[34] Obese and overweight women are anywhere from two to four times as likely to develop endometrial cancer, and for extremely obese women, the risk can be as much as seven times higher.[35] Thinking about this, Welch further realized that most of the newly diagnosed endometrial cancer patients in her practice had a BMI above 30 as well.

She became committed to changing her diet and lifestyle habits, eventually dropping eighty pounds and reversing chronic kidney disease—and then she decided to help others do the same. She's now on a mission to raise awareness that change is possible and to empower women to take control of their health and reverse or at least lower their risk for developing cancer and other life-threatening diseases. She offers a three-step program called Winning at Wellness that is designed to explore the root causes of excess weight, release old patterns so you can develop a new mindset with new habits that set you up for success, and empower you with new skills for achieving and then maintaining your health goals. For more on the program, join her Winning at Weight Loss community on Facebook (@releaseweightnow).

Step Three: Exercise

If you don't already exercise, there is no time like the present to start. Your muscles are loaded with insulin receptors. The more muscle mass you have and the more heat you generate from your muscles on a regular basis, the more efficiently you'll burn carbohydrates and body fat. You'll also be protecting your bones and your heart and boosting your health-related quality of life in a number of ways. (One study even showed that moderate physical activity improved these health-related quality-of-life factors in midlife women significantly more than hormone therapy did.)[36]

The government's Physical Activity Guidelines for Americans recommend two and a half hours a week of moderate exercise (such as brisk walking, water aerobics, ballroom dancing, or gardening) or one and a quarter hours a week of vigorous exercise (such as racewalking, jogging, swimming laps, jumping rope, or hiking uphill with a heavy backpack). The recommendations further suggest an additional two days a week of muscle-strengthening activities, such as weight training, push-ups, sit-ups, or heavy gardening.[37]

If you already exercise, change your routine. Perhaps you've found yourself, like me, stuck at a metabolic roadblock, even though you've already changed your diet and are exercising regularly. When this happens, it is usually because your body has adjusted to your current level of activity—just as it's possible to maintain your weight on as little as 1,000 calories per day, because the body's metabolic rate simply decreases to accommodate its perception of starvation.

In order to get your stubborn fat cells to release their load, you have to confuse them a little. Try a different exercise routine that recruits other muscles. If you've been walking, try a stair-stepper, an elliptical trainer, weight training, or a cross-country ski machine. The idea is to get your body out of its metabolic rut. I am also a big fan of circuit training; all that means is that you mix things up between aerobic and anaerobic exercise. Here's a sample routine:

Dance for a couple of tunes.
Get down on the floor and hold a plank for 30 seconds to 1 minute.
Get up and do some jumping jacks for 30 seconds.
Dance to two more songs.
Jog in place for 30 seconds.
Take a cool-down walk.

You get the idea. There are *many* ways to do circuit training and many apps available to take you through basic routines. The same is true with yoga.

I personally had to increase the intensity and length of my weight-training sessions while cutting back on my walking—something that had become so easy I barely even broke a sweat. The weight workouts were much harder. Over time this switch worked. Currently, my workouts involve an hour of Pilates twice per week, walking for twenty to thirty minutes a couple of times per week, and doing a Peak 8 workout on an elliptical trainer. Peak 8 just means doing thirty seconds of maximal exercise effort (such as using an elliptical trainer or bike) followed by a ninety-second recovery period, repeated for eight cycles. Peak 8 workouts are very quick and effective for cardiovascular fitness, giving you the same benefit in a twice-per-week schedule as daily workouts. You can do this with walking, a stationary bike, an elliptical trainer, a treadmill, or even a rebounder!

Your Built Environment

Let your daily environment promote fitness. I live in a house that was built from plans published in a magazine called *Popular Mechanics* back in the 1950s. It was constructed on three levels, with little staircases everywhere. That means I'm using stairs constantly throughout my day, which is a very good thing for fitness. It's simply built into the day. I had a friend visit who lives in a house in which everything is all on one level—a very popular trend these days, and completely understandable if you are in a wheelchair or have trouble with mobility, although my friend doesn't have these problems. Yet when she came to my house for a visit and had to negotiate all the stairs, it took her several days to regain her confidence. Living on one level had caused her to lose some of her innate coordination and ability to climb and go down stairs.

Biomechanics expert Katy Bowman, founder of the Nutritious Movement approach (www.nutritiousmovement.com), doesn't have any chairs in her living room. Instead, she and her family sit on cushions or a rug, which requires getting up and down regularly. She also doesn't use strollers—her children walk wherever they go. Katy regularly challenges her followers to incorporate more movement into their days, just as they would take vitamins and minerals to supplement their diets.

I include weights once or twice per week, although Pilates often takes care of the weight-bearing part of exercise and keeps my muscle strength at a good level. (This is a highly individual decision. I build and maintain muscle very easily without weights. But this is not true for many women.)

If your weight still doesn't budge, don't get discouraged. In a 2010 study following more than 34,000 healthy women for fifteen years, daily physical activity was associated with preventing weight gain only among women with a healthy BMI—not for women with a high BMI.[38] (For normal-weight women, one hour of moderate-intensity physical activity per day was enough to help them stay at their normal weight.)

But please remember that regular movement has plenty of other health benefits, including turning back the clock. Brisk exercise like running and racket sports has been shown to increase telomere length in cells, which is associated with longevity.[39] A British study of long-time cyclists between the ages of fifty-five and seventy-nine showed that the cardiovascular system and muscles of those in the cycling group were no different from those of other adults in their thirties.[40] A 2009 study found that one year of regular moderate-intensity exercise lowered levels of chronic, low-grade cellular inflammation, which is linked to a number of health problems, including heart disease and some cancers—but this effect was seen only in obese midlife women, not those of normal weight.[41] Also, when you do lose weight by following the other suggestions in this chapter, an already-established exercise routine will help you keep the pounds off for good.

SHALL WE DANCE? THE TRIUMPH OF ARGENTINE TANGO

It should come as no surprise that dance is wonderful exercise, and certainly more fun than doing crunches or jogging on a treadmill. But recent research indicates that the Argentine tango may be the dancing queen, trumping other forms of exercise and even other types of dance, for improving health.

Two studies done by researchers at Washington University School of Medicine in St. Louis looked at teaching people with Parkinson's disease how to tango. The first study divided patients into two groups—one taking Argentine tango lessons, and the other taking more conventional strength and exercise classes. Both groups attended one-hour sessions twice per week for a total of twenty sessions. The tango group focused on stretching, balance, footwork, and timing—and, of course, dancing the tango (both with and without a partner). The exercise classes focused on core strengthening and stretching in both seated and standing positions.

While both groups benefited, only the tango group showed improvement in all measures of balance, fall prevention, and gait.[42] They were also more confident about balance by the end of the study than was the other group. Even more telling, almost half the people in the tango group attended extra sessions after the study concluded, and demand was so great that free weekly tango classes for Parkinson's patients and their partners started up as a result. (Even some patients who had been in the conventional exercise group joined!)

The researchers have completed a second study comparing the effects of tango, waltz/fox-trot, and tai chi on health-related quality of life for Parkinson's patients. Each group got twenty lessons over a thirteen-week period. The results: those in the tango group significantly improved mobility and social support, while those in the other dance groups (plus a control group) reported no such gains.[43]

Many factors were credited for the tango group's success, including the dynamic balance, turning, moving backward, and initiation of movement at a variety of speeds that are required in tango. In addition, because tango is danced with a partner, researchers believe it can help people learn to work together to overcome problems. Social support certainly contributes in a major way to emotional well-being.

Thanks to the promise of these studies, the same researchers then followed tango-dancing Parkinson's patients for a year, holding the dance classes in a community center rather than in the hospital so that participants felt more like dancers than study subjects. Their results were similar.[44]

Parkinson's patients are particularly interesting because they lose functional mobility faster than healthy people. So if the tango can help this group make significant gains in mobility, just think how it can help the rest of us improve ours!

Other studies have been promising as well. The Albert Einstein College of Medicine in New York City conducted a twenty-one-year study of people seventy-five years of age and up that compared the effects of several different types of physical and recreational activities on cognitive health. Those activities included reading, writing, doing crossword puzzles, playing cards, playing musical instruments, playing tennis, golfing, swimming, biking, walking, dancing, and doing housework. The activity that offered the most protection against dementia (and the only physical activity to offer any such protection) was dancing. Frequent dancing reduced risk of dementia by an amazing 76 percent.[45]

Step Four: Get Your Thyroid Checked

As we already mentioned in chapter 4, thyroid problems are very common in midlife women. At least 25 percent of women (and probably more) develop or have preexisting thyroid problems by the time they reach perimenopause. Excess levels of estrogen relative to progesterone can lower thyroid function, and so can excessive stress hormone levels. This and Epstein-Barr virus activation are very common during perimenopause. Low thyroid function is associated with a decreased metabolic rate. If you have any symptoms of thyroid problems (fatigue, weight gain, cold hands and feet, thinning hair, or constipation), get your thyroid checked. See chapter 4 for a more detailed discussion.

Step Five: Quell Cellular Inflammation

The number-one reason for cellular inflammation—and all the diseases and symptoms associated with it—is a refined-food, high-glycemic-index diet, which has the following characteristics.

~ Too many refined carbohydrates, resulting in the overproduction of insulin. Too much insulin favors the production of pro-inflammatory substances such as prostaglandin F2-alpha and the cytokines.

~ Deficiencies in the polyunsaturated fats known as omega-3 fats. Omega-3 fats are necessary for the function of nearly every cell in the body, particularly those of the nervous system, brain, eyes, and immune system. Omega-3 fats also decrease cellular inflammation. Currently, levels of the especially important omega-3 fat DHA (docosahexaenoic acid) are 40 percent lower, on average, in American women than in European women.

~ Too many trans fats, usually from margarine and shortening, which increase cellular inflammation. (See page 298.)

~ Deficiencies in the micronutrients that are necessary for combating cellular inflammation. Too little vitamin C, vitamin B_6, and magnesium, for example, favor the overproduction of pro-inflammatory substances.

Unremitting stress is also a factor in cellular inflammation. It results in the overproduction of epinephrine and cortisol, stress hormones that promote cellular inflammation. Caffeine, which is often used to alleviate the effects of stress and fatigue, has the same effect. When you follow the hormone-balancing food plan below, supplement your diet with additional antioxidant nutrients (see page 301), and consciously decrease stress through meditation, relaxation, and regular exercise, you will be well on your way to quelling cellular inflammation.

BIOFILM: THAT STUBBORN, SLIMY MIX OF BACTERIA, VIRUSES, AND FUNGI THAT HIDES IN YOUR SYSTEM

Many women who suffer from mystery illnesses such as chronic fatigue, fibromyalgia, and chronic Lyme disease have what is called biofilm in their gut and other organs. Biofilm consists of microorganisms that hide in self-protective mucus-secreting colonies. If you leave food in your refrigerator overly long in a plastic or glass dish, you'll often notice that a kind of slimy substance collects around the spoiled food. This is biofilm. The same thing happens in those convenient single-serve coffee makers that have plastic tubing connecting the water to the coffee. Getting the biofilm out of the machine is nearly impossible.

When it comes to your physical body, there are a number of ways to cut through the biofilm. One of my favorites is to drink the juice of three to five lemons straight on an empty stomach first thing in the morning. The citrus cuts through biofilm very nicely, but it can take a while. And you also need to consume what are called "binders," substances that bind toxins in the body and help eliminate them. Some common binders include spirulina, chlorella, distilled water (up to a gallon of water a day if you can), cilantro, digestive enzymes, and zeolite.

If you start blasting your biofilm regularly, you may well feel a bit queasy at first. This is known as a Herxheimer reaction, and it happens when bacteria or yeast die off and toxins from them enter your system to be flushed out. This type of reaction is why you want to detox slowly, lest you get sick from toxins leaving too quickly.

Sinclair Kennally, co-founder and CEO of Vision Nation, runs an effective detox program backed by a great deal of research. She points out that biofilms have a kind of life of their own—much like the "pain body" concept of Eckhart Tolle (see page 96). Like the pain body, biofilms are semi-autonomous communities of organisms living within us. As with all life-forms, they are intent on their own survival. They feed on refined carbs, sugars, and other foods that aren't good for us. And they cause us to crave these foods. Sinclair teaches that when we crave an unhealthy food, it is our bio-film talking, not us. Because really, what would prompt any healthy mammal to eat unhealthy food if other choices were available? Of course, there are many factors that result in food cravings. Possibly the most common among them is the addition of highly addictive substances such as MSG to fast foods and junk foods. They are engineered so that "you can't eat just one."

As you are going through a detox and breaking down bio-film in your body, it's always best to drink a couple of glasses of distilled water and maybe take some detox supplements such as spirulina or chlorella tablets at the same time, to help bind the toxins and ferry them out of your body. By the end of that detox period, your cravings will have greatly decreased.

Another very effective way to detox from biofilm—and also the pathogens that live in it—is to follow the *MMS Health Recovery Guidebook*, written by Jim Humble with Cari Lloyd (self-published in 2016; see jimhumblebooks.co). Indeed, this is not approved by the FDA, but in my clinical experience, it is often very, very helpful.

THE HORMONE-BALANCING FOOD PLAN

Given the average lifestyle of today's perimenopausal women, it's not difficult to see why insulin and estrogen become unbalanced, putting us at increased risk for everything from heart disease and high blood pressure to arthritis and breast cancer. Fortunately, when you start with one of the detox food plans I suggest here, you won't have to wait long to feel better. In a matter of days, you'll probably notice that your sleep improves, you begin to lose excess fat, various troublesome symptoms begin to disappear, and your skin takes on a healthy glow. At the same time you'll be reducing your risk for the diseases of aging.

Focus on Portion Size, Not Calories

Instead of calorie counting, concentrate on eating the highest-quality food available, in smaller portions. Cup your two hands in front of you. That's how big your stomach capacity is. Limit your intake to no more than that at each meal or snack. And eat slowly. It takes twenty minutes for your stomach—and brain—to agree on the fact that you've had enough. It's always best to push yourself away from the table when you've had enough but could eat a little more, because in about ten to fifteen minutes your brain will register that you have indeed "had enough."

Overeating in general—regardless of the food—is associated with overproduction of insulin. In general, the food portions in U.S. restaurants are much bigger than in Europe, which is one of the reasons Americans are so overweight compared to Europeans. (That is changing, however, and obesity has become a global problem. The World Health Organization reports that worldwide, obesity has nearly tripled since 1975, with more than 650 million people now obese—13 percent of the world's adult population.) At one local restaurant, for example, the chicken dish I usually order comes with two halves of a chicken breast. I always eat just one and take the other home with me for another meal.

In order to keep my weight stable, I've had to cut down on my total food intake, eliminate grain products most of the time (see below), virtually eliminate desserts and decrease all sugars (see box on sugar, page 289), and increase my exercise time. Intermittent fasting has also helped a great deal. I often fast from dinner until lunch the next day. I don't count the 16 oz. of celery juice that I start my day with, and I sometimes have a cup of coffee as well. But I don't actually eat anything much until about 11:30 A.M., or sometimes even 2:00 P.M. That leaves me at least a twelve- to fourteen-hour window for low insulin levels.

Cut Down on Refined and High-Glycemic-Index Carbohydrates and Sugar, Including Alcohol

Remember, not all carbohydrates are created equal. One gram of carbohydrate from table sugar has a different metabolic effect than the same amount of carbohydrate from blueberries. This has been proven without a doubt by researchers such as endocrinologist David Ludwig, M.D., Ph.D., author of *Always Hungry?* (Hachette, 2016), who has spent a lifetime studying the effects of refined carbohydrates on metabolism, and pediatric endocrinologist Robert H. Lustig, M.D., author of *The Hacking of the American Mind* (Avery, 2017), whose

University of California video "Sugar: The Bitter Truth" went viral on YouTube. The bottom line is that a gram of fat has far different metabolic effects than a gram of refined sugar. Hint: the fat is generally healthier!

Keep your blood sugar stable and you'll experience:

~ More energy

~ Ability to sustain exercise

~ Clearing of brain fog

~ Ability to build muscle

~ Less hunger—ability to control portion sizes *and* cravings

~ Fewer PMS symptoms

~ Fewer hot flashes

~ Better-looking skin

~ Clear eyes without puffiness or dark circles

~ Deeper, more restful sleep

~ Stable moods and more optimism

Your success will be contingent on eating foods with a low glycemic index (GI). The glycemic index was created to measure how much the blood sugar rises after you eat a carbohydrate meal, using white bread as the benchmark. White bread has a glycemic index of 100, whereas the glycemic index of corn is 54, an apple is 38, and an avocado is 0. The rule of thumb is white and processed foods have a very high glycemic index, whereas whole foods and those high in protein typically have a low glycemic index. Research supports this way of eating. A 2010 study from the University of Denmark reported in the *New England Journal of Medicine* found that people who'd lost weight on a restricted-calorie diet were more successful keeping the weight off if they followed a higher-protein, lower-glycemic-index diet than if they were following diets that were either lower in protein or diets allowing higher-glycemic-index foods, or both.[46]

Eliminate as many refined carbohydrates from your diet as possible. That means cutting out foods made with refined white flour, such as muffins, rolls, bagels, biscuits, French bread, breadsticks, crackers, snack foods, and pretzels. A few exceptions do exist, however. Jennie Brand-Miller, Ph.D., of the University of Sydney, one of the world's leading authorities on the glycemic index, notes that pasta has a relatively low glycemic index because it is harder to digest than most other flour products. Al dente pasta has a lower glycemic index than overcooked pasta. Also, sourdough and pumpernickel breads are low-glycemic-index foods because of the acidity of the dough. (Similarly, if you add lemon juice, lime juice, or vinegar to a dish, you will lower its glycemic index.) You also need to eliminate soda pop, which is nothing but sugar water. The aspartame sweetener in conventional diet sodas is dangerous. (See chapter 10.) Soda sweetened with Truvia, made from the stevia plant, is a good alternative; one brand is Zevia. But don't use even this until you have done a detox and changed how your taste buds process sweetness.

Cutting down on sugar also means eliminating or cutting way back on alcohol in every and any form, including wine coolers, wine, beer, and hard liquor. Alcohol is nothing but sugar in a form that is so absorbable that its effects are felt within minutes in the brain. One of the first things women notice when they eliminate the empty calories found in alcohol is that they lose weight very quickly. Many also notice that their hot flashes go away as well. That's because alcohol significantly interferes with estrogen metabolism and causes an almost immediate hormonal imbalance, with too much estrogen in the blood relative to progesterone.

You also need to eliminate or cut way back on sweets: candy, cookies, cakes, and pastries. You may still want to have them on special occasions, but as your blood sugar stabilizes, you'll find that your craving for these foods will decrease dramatically and you won't like the way you feel after eating them. (Dark chocolate and full-fat ice cream, by the way, are low-glycemic-index foods—just don't gorge on them!)

According to Dr. Brand-Miller, you don't have to avoid *all* high-glycemic-index foods—just plan around them. For example, you could have a meal with a high-glycemic-index food as long as the other foods on your menu are low-glycemic-index. The net effect will be a low-glycemic-index meal. (For more information on the glycemic index, including a database of foods and their GI values, visit www.glycemicindex.com, a website maintained by the GI Group of the University of Sydney in Australia.)

Remember, your body will be able to burn stored fat and keep your insulin and blood sugar levels normal only when you don't eat or drink excessive amounts of the wrong kinds of carbohydrates. Otherwise excess blood sugar will be stored as fat, which will accumulate not just on your belly and hips but also in other places, including your arteries, heart, and brain.

THE SKINNY ON SUGAR

Sugar of all types (lactose, sucrose, fructose, glucose, etc.) is added to and hidden in all kinds of foods, even those that are moderate- or low-glycemic-index. But for most of human history, the average daily intake of sugar was no more 15 grams per day. Today, the average sugar intake is 47 teaspoons per day, which is about 200 grams!

Many women lose weight fast when they limit their intake of sugar to 15 grams a day or less. So read labels, and look specifically for the amount of sugar grams that are in each serving.

Once I started to read labels to determine sugar content, I was stunned. I found that foods such as yogurt, which we have been conditioned to think of as healthy, are actually loaded with sugar. But a handful of nuts or a hard-boiled egg is not. Once you begin to limit the total amount of sugar in your diet and focus on other healthy foods, you'll find that you sleep better and feel better. And heartburn will be a thing of the past for most. (That's because sugar raises insulin levels, which change the chemistry of gastric mucus, leading to heartburn.)

As you decrease sugar in your diet, you'll also notice that you can add back healthy fats without any adverse consequences. Cheese omelets, avocados, nut butters, and coconut oil have now become a regular part of my diet. And I've come to see that for many people, low-fat diets are part of the problem. They don't always work. Over the past thirty years or so, as we have replaced fat in the diet with hidden sugars, people have become fatter and fatter. (See the discussion of healthy fats on page 295.) So do yourself a favor: start decreasing sugars of all kinds—and go ahead and enjoy some healthy fat.

Even the government's dietary guidelines are getting on board with this idea. When the guidelines were updated in 2010, they emphasized for the first time ever the need to cut down on added sugars and solid fats (those that remain solid at room temperature, such as hydrogenated fats and saturated fats), which together make up 35 percent of the average

American diet without contributing any nutrients. The guidelines also suggested that Americans *avoid*—not just limit or allow moderate consumption of—sugar-sweetened beverages. It's about time! And the solid fat argument has some pretty big holes in it too.

Once you understand where the added sugar in your diet is coming from, you can experiment with eating more than the recommended 15 grams of sugar per day. Some people find that the sugar in fruits and vegetables doesn't cause any weight gain at all because those foods usually have a relatively low glycemic index. And more than that, those carbohydrates are digested very slowly. Other people have to be very careful, even with fruits. This is largely an individual issue.

Here's the bottom line: sugar is highly addictive. Though I had been following a low-glycemic-index diet for years, the information on grams of sugar has been a game-changer. To keep the pounds from creeping back, I had to decrease even what I'd previously thought of as "healthy" sugars. This has made a world of difference for me, and for many others as well.

IF YOU ARE A TRUE CARBOHYDRATE ADDICT

Women who grew up in alcoholic or chaotic family systems may have brain and body chemistry that is overly sensitive to the effects of food, and particularly to the neurochemical known as serotonin. Serotonin is released in the brain quite rapidly when you eat certain carbohydrate-rich foods, such as most breakfast cereals or cookies. True carbohydrate addicts cannot stop after eating a few cookies or potato chips. They don't seem to have a normal satiety mechanism in place, most likely because food is being used as a drug to soothe emotional pain. If this describes you, I recommend consulting one of the following books:

Potatoes Not Prozac (Simon & Schuster, 1999), by Kathleen DesMaisons

The Sugar Addict's Total Recovery Program (Ballantine, 2000), by Kathleen DesMaisons

Holy Hunger: A Memoir of Desire (Knopf, 1999), by Margaret Bullitt-Jonas

Bright Line Eating (Hay House, 2017), by Susan Peirce Thompson, Ph.D. (https://brightlineeating.com)

Consume Grain Products with Caution

Even if you have eliminated refined grains in all forms, you can still get into trouble with whole wheat, whole rye, whole oat, or millet flour. A fascinating line of research now suggests that the degenerative diseases that currently plague the human race didn't arrive on the scene until agriculture became widespread. Paleoarcheological studies show that many of the ancient Egyptians were fat and had dental caries—diseases associated with a grain-based diet and virtually absent in hunter-gatherers.

Many carbohydrate-sensitive individuals find that eating grain products triggers binge eating. (Not surprisingly, recent research indicates that a low-carbohydrate ketogenic diet may result in less binge eating and food addiction.)[47] I've certainly seen this happen with brown rice—a "health food" that I used to consume regularly but have had to virtually eliminate. I've also had to eliminate nearly all whole-grain bread products, even the unleavened ones. (One line of thinking suggests that yeast bread is difficult to digest because of the potential for yeast overgrowth in the intestines. Unleavened bread is better tolerated by many, but not everyone. Even a whole-wheat tortilla wrap sandwich at lunch can make me feel groggy and sleepy. Looking back, I can see that eating too much bread has been a problem with me for years. But at perimenopause, my body finally said, "Enough!"

In addition, about one in three people is intolerant of gluten, a protein found in grains (including oats, wheat, kamut, rye, and barley) used in many foods, such as wraps, breads, pasta, pizza, and rolls. About 1 percent of Americans have full-blown celiac disease, an autoimmune disorder of the small intestine characterized by an inability to digest gluten. But this isn't just a digestion problem. People with celiac disease or gluten sensitivity have a higher risk of death, mostly from heart disease and cancer. A study published in 2009 that followed 30,000 patients for about fifty years found a 39 percent increased risk of death in those with celiac disease, a 72 percent increased risk of death in those with gut inflammation related to gluten, and a 35 percent increased risk of death even in those who were sensitive to gluten but did not have a positive intestinal biopsy indicating celiac disease.[48]

Most people with gluten intolerance don't know they have it. You can find out if you have gluten sensitivity with a blood test that looks for specific anti-gluten antibodies, but an easier way is to eliminate all gluten from your diet for two to four weeks and then reintroduce it. That's what the Whole30 will do for you. (See earlier discussion in this chapter.) Be aware, however, that gluten hides in soups, salad dressings, sauces, and a host of other foods. For a complete list of gluten-containing foods, visit www.celiac.com. I also recommend the book *The No-Grain Diet* (Dutton, 2003) by Joseph Mercola, D.O.

Eat a Wide Variety of Fresh Fruits and Vegetables Daily

You want to shoot for at least five servings a day, but it's easy, at least in the summer, to get in more. Remember that a serving is small, as little as 4 oz. or ½ cup in many cases. The healthiest fruits and vegetables are the ones that are the most colorful. That's because the pigments in these foods, such as the carotenes or carotenoids, are very powerful antioxidants. Go for broccoli; red, yellow, and green peppers; dark green leafy vegetables such as collards, kale, and spinach; and tomatoes. Pigment-rich blueberries have been found to have the highest concentration of antioxidants compared to forty other fruits and vegetables.

Studies suggest that the carotenoid content of tissue may be the most significant factor in determining life span in primates, including humans.[49] Though beta-carotene (the vitamin A precursor found in carrots, other yellow-orange vegetables, and dark leafy greens) has received the most attention and is the carotenoid most commonly found in multivitamins, other carotenes that have little or no vitamin A–type activity exert much greater antioxidant protection. Alpha-carotene (usually found in the same foods as beta-carotene) is approximately 38 percent stronger as an antioxidant and ten times more effective in suppressing liver, skin, and lung cancer in animals.[50] Even more powerful is lycopene, the red pigment found in tomatoes. Some studies have shown a 50 percent reduction for all cancers among elderly Americans reporting a high tomato intake.[51] Food processing doesn't destroy lycopene, so tomato juice and canned tomato products also offer protection.

Every day the list of benefits from the natural antioxidants found in pigment-rich foods grows. They help balance hormones, protect the skin from sun damage, keep the skin and eyes radiant, maintain the lining of the blood vessels, and help prevent varicose veins. They also boost the immune system and help the body resist cancer and other degenerative diseases.

In addition to being good sources of cholesterol-lowering fiber, fruits and vegetables are also good sources of lignans, which are metabolized into phytohormones that help balance hormones and metabolize excess estrogen. Flaxseed is by far the richest source of lignans and is also very rich in essential omega-3 fats (see pages 597–599).

High-glycemic-index fruits and vegetables such as potatoes, corn, and bananas have a lot of nutrients in them, though their antioxidant content isn't as rich as that of the foods I've mentioned previously. You don't have to eliminate them completely. Just remember that the more processed they are, the higher their glycemic index. A baked potato is an entirely different food from a potato chip or french fry, and it is far healthier. And fresh corn on the cob in season is a better choice than canned creamed corn, which is often processed with added sugar in the form of corn syrup. Though fresh vegetables are always the best choice, research has shown that even canned and frozen varieties still contain many nutrients.

QUELL YOUR SUGAR CRAVINGS WITH SMART SUGARS

Most women find that their sugar cravings go away or are greatly reduced once they have stabilized their blood sugar. This can be done either with a low-glycemic-index diet or by keeping total sugar consumption to 15 grams per day or so. Cravings will generally cease in a couple of days. And believe me, this feels wonderful. Remember what I said about doing a cleanse or reset so that your taste buds get recalibrated.

You don't have to forgo sweetness for the rest of your life. There are now more safe non-nutritive sweeteners available than ever before.

My favorite is stevia, an extract from the leaves of the South American plant *Stevia rebaudiana*. It's easy to grow in your garden, and the leaves can be added to iced tea or lemonade. (See www.stevia.com for growing information.) A wide variety of extracts from stevia leaves are now available as well, in both liquid and powder form. These include Truvia, which is being added to commercially available foods such as soda pop. Some stevia preparations have a bitter aftertaste, but I have found that Truvia and NuStevia do not. Stevita is the brand name of a company that makes a variety of stevia-sweetened extracts that add delicious flavor to coffee and other foods. A number of animal studies have shown that stevia also improves the lipid profile in obese mice that consume it. It has yet to be determined if this benefit holds true for humans.[52]

Another safe sweetener is monkfruit, which comes in little packets. Other safe sweeteners include the sugar alcohols. Despite their name, they are neither sugars nor alcohols, but carbohydrates that are poorly absorbed. Hence, they're not converted into stored energy and they don't need to be counted as carbs in one's diet. They also don't cause cavities. Sugar alcohols include sorbitol, maltitol, xylitol, and erythritol. Sorbitol and maltitol can cause gastrointestinal upset, including gas and bloating, if you eat too much of them. Xylitol and erythritol don't have this effect.

Agave nectar has gotten a lot of publicity as a low-glycemic-index sweetener. Derived from a succulent grown in Mexico, agave nectar is highly refined and has more fructose in it than high-fructose corn syrup. Research suggests that it will trigger the same insulin response as sucrose or high-fructose corn syrup. I don't use it.

All the common artificial sweeteners are just plain bad for you. They include aspartame (NutraSweet—blue packet), saccharin (Sweet'N Low—pink packet), and sucralose (Splenda—yellow packet). Avoid them.

Eat Healthy Fats Each Day

For forty years, health experts have been pushing the idea that lowering dietary fat will lower your risk for cardiovascular disease—but the truth is that they've missed the mark by a mile. I'm not saying that eating gobs of lard is healthy. Far from it! But as Americans have jumped on the low-fat and nonfat chuck wagon over the past several decades, heart disease has not made a hasty retreat. Partly this is because food manufacturers replaced much of their saturated fats with trans fats, which we now know to be deadly. The other reason is that when Americans cut fat out of their diets, they tend to eat more carbs (and usually the wrong kind) to compensate. A 2010 meta-analysis from Harvard that looked at eight trials following a total of more than 13,000 participants showed that rather than simply lowering fats, shifting to eating *more* polyunsaturated fats in place of some saturated fats would reduce coronary heart disease risk by 19 percent.[53] It's ironic but true: the low-fat craze has actually made Americans fatter.

One caveat: My friend and colleague Anthony William teaches that excess fat contributes to all kinds of problems, including fatty liver. He advocates a plant-based, low-fat diet. He's not alone in this. So do many others, including doctors. I personally find that this kind of low-fat approach works well in the summer for those of us who live in colder climates, but not so much when it gets chillier; of course, some people manage very well with vegan soups and warm stews. There is no question that a low-fat, plant-based diet has helped many people heal. But remember that they are not including any refined foods; instead, they're advocating a whole-food diet of mostly fruits and vegetables, with no dairy, no grains, and no animal products. This can work for many but is not sustainable for some of us. So you'll have to experiment to see what works best for you.

That's a big reason why obesity is now at an all-time high—the experts have been telling us to eat the *wrong* foods all along. And it certainly didn't help that the food industry was able to successfully pressure the USDA into putting bread and grains at the base of the original food pyramid, suggesting Americans eat six to eleven servings a day! While the food pyramid has been replaced with much better guidelines, these guidelines still stress too many breads and grains for my liking.

In addition to encouraging weight gain and increasing risk for heart disease, cutting out fats has other health consequences. Back in the 1980s and early 1990s, when the low-fat craze reached its peak, I watched patient after patient come in complaining of sallow skin, brittle fingernails, difficulty fighting infections, inability to concentrate, and fatigue. None of these women were getting enough healthy fat in their diets, having been brainwashed into thinking that all fat was the enemy. Now we know differently. In fact, research published in the *Journal of the American Medical Association* in 2016 showed that those who consumed a high-fat diet had 16 percent lower rates of premature death than those consuming a low-fat diet.[54]

Essential fatty acids (EFAs) are indispensable for human development and health. Our bodies cannot synthesize EFAs, so we need to consume them in our foods. There are two essential types of EFAs: omega-6 fats and omega-3 fats. Omega-6 fats occur in relative abundance in the foods we eat. However, the current low-fat American diet is woefully deficient in omega-3 fats. In addition, because of agricultural practices, the fats in eggs and meat do not contain nearly the percentage of omega-3 fats that they used to. Farm animals raised on wild grasses instead of grain have a healthier, leaner body composition. Animals, like humans, get fat on diets composed mostly of grain, especially if they aren't allowed to roam.

WHAT SHOULD I DRINK? OPTIMAL HYDRATION IS KEY TO HEALTH

We all need to be optimally hydrated in order to feel our best. Most of us aren't. To accomplish this, we've been told to consume eight 8-oz. glasses of water per day. But this just doesn't work; in most of us, it just causes us to go to the bathroom all day. Why? Because to be really hydrated adequately, you need to get hydration into your cells. And that is accomplished by adding electrolytes to the water, making it a far more effective nutrient. Electrolytes actually "charge" water so that it carries electrical energy throughout the body. You do this by adding a tiny pinch of Celtic sea salt or Himalayan salt to your water. No more is necessary. I personally make what is called a "sole" (pronounced SOLE-lay). You do this by putting about ¼ inch of one of those salts in a jar with a plastic lid. Then add either distilled water or spring water, shake it up, and let the salt settle to the bottom. This creates a saturated salt solution. You just take out a teaspoon of this solution and add it to smoothies or plain water, and there you have your hydrating solution.

You can also "eat" your water. Gerald H. Pollack, Ph.D., has discovered a fourth stage of water (in addition to liquid water, ice, and steam), known as "gel" water. This is the water in plant parts—for example, lettuce, berries, and chia seeds—when they are swollen with liquid. This gel water is what keeps animals hydrated in the desert. When you eat your water in this way, it is very hydrating, and it stays in the right place in your tissues—in the cells—so you don't pee it all out quickly. Another great way to hydrate is to add a tablespoon of chia seeds to water. You can either drink them immediately or wait for the seeds to swell with gel water and then drink them. You can also make chia seed pudding. I personally like to add the seeds to some water and just drink it. Those seeds swell inside the body and help maintain optimal hydration. They are also excellent for optimal bowel function.

A different way to make regular water into more hydrating gel water is to add mint leaves, lemon, berries, or cucumber slices to it, since the plant material itself contains gel water.

I bought a water distiller recently and now use distilled water for cooking, making coffee, and drinking. But I make sure to add minerals to it regularly. My favorite minerals are the ReMag and ReMyte solutions from Carolyn Dean, M.D., N.D. Dr. Dean has spent a lifetime researching the role of magnesium and other minerals in cardiac function and nerve conduction. Her products have saved thousands of people from suffering with nighttime leg cramps, heart arrhythmias, and all kinds of other problems. (See www.rnareset.com.)

Coffee is a diuretic. If you drink coffee, just consume the same number of ounces in the form of hydrating water so that you don't get behind.

Too many women avoid water in the mistaken belief that they will put on weight if they drink too much. Then they end up dehydrated, and it shows in their skin. In fact, you need lots of water to help your body eliminate the breakdown products of fat if you are trying to lose weight.

Omega-3 deficiency often begins in utero, when our only source of these fats is our mothers, who are likely to be deficient in them already. Ideally, the omega-3 fats, particularly a fat known as DHA, are found abundantly in human breast milk, but DHA is absent in the baby formulas used in the United States and Canada. Research is rapidly accumulating that implicates DHA deficiency in the epidemic of attention deficit disorder in both children and adults. This essential fat is also one of the reasons why children who were breast-fed as infants have been found to have higher IQs than formula-fed babies.[55] Gratifying improvements in learning ability and mood stabilization have resulted when both children and adults have had their diets supplemented with omega-3 fats.

In addition to their role in nervous system and brain function, omega-3 fats also favor the production of substances known as series 1 and 3 eicosanoids, which help block the effects of cellular inflammation. It's not surprising, then, that supplementing the diet with omega-3 fats in either foods or pills has been shown to alleviate conditions associated with eicosanoid imbalance, including arthritis, PMS, eczema, breast tenderness, acne, diabetes, brittle fingernails, thinning and brittle hair, psoriasis, dry skin, and the sex hormone imbalance so common during perimenopause.

Good sources of omega-3 fats include pumpkin seeds, sunflower seeds, flaxseed or flaxseed oil, hempseed or hempseed oil, organ meats, cold-water fish or fish oil supplements, and docosahexaenoic acid (DHA) supplements. Nuts are also a good source, and they make a very satisfying low-carb snack—I take them to the movies in lieu of high-carb popcorn. Just make sure you enjoy them in moderation—no more than a handful once or twice per day. Raw chia seed is another excellent source and has a higher concentration of omega-3 fats than any other plant source (see Resources).

Trans Fats: The Bad Actors of the Fat World

The most dangerous fats by far are the trans fats—the partially hydrogenated fats and oils that aren't found anywhere in nature. They are present in shortening and margarine, which are made by blowing hydrogen into liquid vegetable oil at very high temperatures and pressures. Trans fats contribute directly to the overproduction of pro-inflammatory eicosanoids and have therefore been found to contribute to the development of cancer and heart disease.

Unfortunately, trans fats are added to just about every type of packaged baked good because they don't get rancid nearly as quickly as unprocessed fats. This prolongs the shelf life of the product. Since such products are also invariably high in refined carbs, it's best to simply eliminate them from your life. (If you have them once in a while, pray over them first.) The good news is that food manufacturers must now add information about trans fat content to labels.

Saturated Fat: An Overrated Threat

Saturated fat, as mentioned above, is not the culprit we've made it out to be as far as heart disease is concerned. The bottom line: if you're following a diet that keeps your insulin and blood sugar levels normal, then saturated fat isn't likely to become a problem. After all, the epidemic of heart disease didn't start in this country until margarine and shortening—which are trans fats, not saturated fats—were added to the diet back in the 1940s. Before that, lard and butter were widely used, and heart disease was rare. Some women, however, are sensitive to the arachidonic acid found in dairy foods, eggs, and beef, which contributes to cellular inflammation, and in turn to menstrual cramps and arthritis. The symptoms go away when they eliminate these foods. Other women have no problem. As with all things, I'd suggest that you enjoy saturated fat in moderation.

You don't have to count fat grams if you are keeping your carb intake relatively low. In the absence of excess insulin, it appears that fat in your diet is not stored as fat. But the minute that fat is combined with sugar or starch—as in a doughnut, for example—the pounds pack on.

Cooking and Salad Oils

Most salad and cooking oils contain omega-6 fats, and since an excess of omega-6 fats can lead to the overproduction of pro-inflammatory chemicals in cells, I suggest that you limit their use. Substitute flaxseed oil or olive oil whenever possible. (Olive oil is a monounsaturated omega-9 fat with metabolic effects that are neutral when it comes to eicosanoid balance.) You can also use a little clarified butter—also known as ghee—for cooking, since it won't burn at low temperatures like regular butter. My favorite salad dressing is made by mixing a little balsamic vinegar with some high-quality olive oil. For variety, try light sesame or nut oils.

EDUCATE YOURSELF

All of the following books contain meal plans and recipes that have helped thousands of women lose or maintain their weight. All of them will help balance hormones as well as insulin and will help decrease cellular inflammation. I recommend that you go to a library or your local bookstore and look through a few of them. Then choose the one that speaks to you.

Medical Medium Cleanse to Heal (Hay House, 2020) by Anthony William. Also check out Anthony's cleanse online at www.medicalmedium.com/blog/medical-medium -28-day-cleanse.

Colorado Cleanse 3.0 (LifeSpa, 2013) by John Douillard, D.C.

The Hormone Fix (Ballantine Books, 2019) by Anna Cabeca, D.O., which includes her Keto-Green diet plan

Always Hungry? (Hachette, 2016) by David Ludwig, M.D., Ph.D.

Always Delicious (Hachette, 2018) by David Ludwig, M.D., Ph.D., and Dawn Ludwig; a companion book to *Always Hungry?*

Medical Medium Celery Juice (Hay House, 2019) by Anthony William

Wheat Belly (Rodale, 2011) by William Davis, M.D.

Wheat Belly 30-Minute (or Less!) Cookbook (Rodale, 2013) by William Davis, M.D.

The Magnesium Miracle (Ballantine Books, 2003, most recently updated in 2017) by Carolyn Dean, M.D., N.D.

The PlantPlus Diet Solution (Hay House, 2014) by Joan Borysenko, Ph.D.

Recipes for Change: Gourmet Wholefood Cooking for Health and Vitality at Menopause (Dutton, 1996) by Lissa DeAngelis and Molly Siple

The No-Grain Diet (Dutton, 2003), by Joseph Mercola with Alison Rose Levy

The New Glucose Revolution: The Authoritative Guide to the Glycemic Index—the Dietary Solution for Lifelong Health (Marlowe & Company, 2006), by Jennie Brand-Miller, Thomas Wolever, Kaye Foster-Powell, and Stephen Colagiuri

The Plant Paradox (Harper Wave, 2017), by Steven R. Gundry, M.D. Dr. Gundry is a cardiovascular surgeon with years of experience helping people reverse cardiovascular disease. His work on diet is fascinating and has helped thousands restore their health.

Like me, you may find yourself vacillating between vegan, low-fat, and paleo, depending upon the season, with a cleanse added every six months or so. Keep trying new things, and remember—there is no magic bullet that works for everyone when it comes to diet. So don't be fooled.

Protect Yourself with Antioxidants

Every day, more and more research is showing the benefits of vitamins and minerals, especially those known as antioxidants. Antioxidants combat cellular damage from free radicals, which is one of the key underlying mechanisms leading to chronic conditions such as heart disease, cataracts, macular degeneration, and many cancers.

Free radicals are highly reactive unstable molecules that have lost one electron and are aggressively seeking a replacement—a process that, in your body, results in damage to everything from your DNA to the collagen layer of your skin. You can't escape free radicals completely, because they are a by-product of normal metabolism. They are formed in our bodies when, for instance, molecules of fat react with oxygen in a process similar to the one that turns fat rancid or makes iron rust. But free radicals are also formed by exposure to ozone, tobacco smoke, car exhaust, chemicals outgassed from new carpet, and other pollutants. Exposure to radiation, insecticides, and excessive amounts of sunlight can also lead to the formation of free radicals. Free-radical damage results in cellular inflammation and the release of too many of the "bad" eicosanoids that appear to be involved in virtually every disease process known.

The body was designed to fight off free-radical damage in the same way that your immune system is designed to fight viruses and bacteria. One mechanism that your body uses to fight free-radical damage is to repair the damage once it's been done. Another mechanism is to "scavenge" the free radicals before they cause harm: to supply the extra electron they need before they can grab it from vulnerable tissue. This is what antioxidants do.

Here's a great example from a 2010 study done in South Korea that looked at the effect of dietary supplements on high-risk human papillomavirus (HPV) infection and cervical cancer. The researchers found that women with HPV who also took the antioxidant vitamins C, E, and A (as well as calcium) decreased their risk of developing cervical dysplasia (precancerous lesions) by 79 percent.[56] That has certainly been my experience with hundreds of patients with cervical dysplasia who got better by adding good antioxidants to their diets.

Antioxidants are found abundantly in fresh fruits and vegetables, especially the brightly colored ones. One of the foods highest in antioxidants is black currants. I'm a huge fan of CurrantC black currant concentrate (available at www.currantc.com). I add it to all my smoothies. It's divine.

The amount of antioxidant in a given fruit, vegetable, grain, or protein source depends upon the soil in which it is grown or on which its food source is grown. Organically grown fruits and vegetables that are picked and eaten when ripe have the highest amounts of antioxidants and minerals in them.

Food is the best source for our antioxidants. They seem to work synergistically—that is, they're more powerful in balance with one another and with other nutrients as they occur naturally. However, if you don't manage to consume five servings of fruits and vegetables a day, supplements can still provide significant protection.

PERIMENOPAUSE SUPPLEMENT PROGRAM

Over the years I've seen hundreds of patients who have been helped by a good supplement program such as the one below.

Following this program means that you'll have to give up the idea of getting everything you need in one tablet. You'll probably end up taking ten or more capsules or tablets per day. Think of them as food, not medicine.

Antioxidants

Vitamin C	1,000–5,000 mg
Vitamin D_3	2,000–10,000 IU
Vitamin A (as beta-carotene)	25,000 IU
Vitamin E (as mixed tocopherols)	200–800 IU
Glutathione	2–10 mg
Alpha-lipoic acid	10–100 mg
Coenzyme Q_{10}	50–100 mg

Omega-3 Fats

DHA	200–2,500 mg
EPA	500–2,500 mg (total of 1,000–5,000 mg)

B Complex Vitamins

Thiamine (B_1)	8–100 mg
Riboflavin (B_2)	9–50 mg
Niacin (B_3)	20–100 mg
Pantothenic acid (B_5)	15–400 mg
Pyridoxine (B_6)	10–100 mg
Methylcobalamin (B_{12})	20–250 mcg
Methylated folic acid	1,000 mcg
Biotin	40–500 mcg
Inositol	10–500 mg
Choline	10–100 mg

Minerals

Calcium	500–1,200 mg (amount depends on calcium content of diet)
Magnesium	400–1,000 mg (I prefer ReMag because it's so absorbable; available at www.rnareset.com)
Potassium	200–500 mg
Zinc	6–50 mg (liquid zinc is very absorbable; I get mine from www.vimergy.com)
Manganese	1–15 mg
Boron	2–9 mg
Copper	1–2 mg
Iron	15–30 mg
Chromium	100–400 mcg
Iodine	3–12.5 mg
Selenium	50–200 mcg
Molybdenum	10–20 mcg
Vanadium	50–100 mcg
Trace minerals— usually from marine mineral complex	

OPTIMIZING MIDLIFE DIGESTION

Digestive problems, especially in the form of bloating and gas, are very common in women. Sometimes they begin at midlife and sometimes they develop only later, when you are in your sixties or seventies. I recently talked with one of my mentors from childhood, a woman who at the age of ninety still teaches yoga at a nursing home. Two of her biggest problems are constipation and heartburn, but otherwise she is doing well.

Being a Gut Reactor: Digestion and Your Third Emotional Center

One of the first things you need to do in order to heal your digestive problems at midlife is to shore up your third emotional center. The third emotional center is located in the solar plexus area, and the health of this area affects all our organs of digestion, including the stomach, liver, gallbladder, pancreas, small intestine, and upper large intestine. Women with substantial weight problems usually have unresolved issues in the third emotional center.

The health of the third emotional center depends on a balance between responsibility to ourselves and responsibility to others, and also on our sense of self-esteem. It is adversely affected whenever we feel overly responsible for the welfare of others or when we avoid taking responsibility altogether. Gloria, a former patient I followed for years, illustrates the conflicts in the third emotional center very well. Gloria is the oldest of four children. Her mother always told her that she was responsible for her siblings because she was the oldest and should "know better." Whenever any of her siblings was injured or got into trouble, she was blamed. As a result of having this responsibility placed on her at a relatively early age, Gloria developed a very acute "gut feeling" about when things were about to go wrong. This ability has served her well in her job as an executive assistant at a large hospital. Nevertheless, she still suffers from digestive upsets whenever there are conflicts at work—conflicts for which she always feels responsible. She once told me that she always seems to be caught in the middle between her boss and a co-worker, and this conflict quite literally goes into the middle of her body. It is not surprising that Gloria has problems with her weight and her blood sugar, and that she tends to overeat whenever she feels bad about herself for not doing enough at work. In fact, she does far more than most, but she still feels as though she hasn't done enough.

At midlife our job is to learn how to take care of ourselves instead of everybody else. If we don't grasp how to do this, we soon learn that no one will do this for us. But as we begin to go about mastering this important skill, we often find ourselves feeling guilty. Who will do everything around the house or the office if we don't? This feeling of guilt hits us right in our solar plexus, which is also the body center associated with self-esteem and personal power.

Self-esteem comes from feeling good about ourselves in the world. It is effectively created by developing skills in the outer world of work—one of the reasons why so many midlife women heal their lives and their digestion when they go back to college and get the degree they didn't finish after high school. Our third emotional center is also related to how good we feel about our relationships, our bodies, our homes, and our lives in general. Sometimes a lifetime of weight and self-esteem problems are solved at midlife as we finally learn the self-acceptance and self-celebration that are part of self-esteem.

WHAT TO DO ABOUT BLOATING

During perimenopause there is a shift toward fat-accumulating hormones (cortisol and insulin) and away from fat-mobilizing hormones (estrogen and growth hormone). If your body is under stress of any kind, this shift will worsen. In addition, your abdominal fat cells have more cortisol receptors on them at midlife, so fat is preferentially directed toward them. This often results in fluid retention and bloating.[57] Following the dietary guidelines I've outlined above will often take care of all digestive problems. Or try the following:

- DECREASE CONSUMPTION OF HIGH- TO MODERATE-GLYCEMIC-INDEX CARBOHYDRATES. Yet another symptom of cellular inflammation and too much insulin is excess stomach acid. A diet lower in carbohydrates and higher in fat and protein very often results in complete and fast relief of heartburn and indigestion.

- EAT THREE TO FIVE SMALL MEALS PER DAY. Consuming large quantities of food elevates insulin levels and makes bloating worse—even when the foods are healthy.

- INCLUDE SOME PROTEIN, HEALTHY FAT, AND LOW-GLYCEMIC-INDEX CARBOHYDRATES IN EVERY MEAL OR SNACK. However, fruit is best eaten alone. Consuming it with fat causes bloating and indigestion in many women.

- ELIMINATE ALL BREADS AND BAKED GOODS FOR AT LEAST A WEEK. See if this makes a difference. Many women are sensitive to gluten.

- DRINK PLENTY OF WHAT IS KNOWN AS STRUCTURED WATER OR GEL WATER. It helps the body rid itself of toxins. You can create it by adding fruit slices to water or a pinch of sea salt for electrolytes.

- TAKE PROBIOTICS. Every course of antibiotics you take disrupts normal gut flora. Over time, excess yeast can colonize the entire gut, causing allergies and indigestion. Taking a good probiotic regularly helps prevent problems. (Yogurt, by the way, generally doesn't contain enough bacteria to be helpful—unless you make the yogurt yourself.)

- LEAVE AT LEAST THREE HOURS BETWEEN YOUR LAST MEAL AND BEDTIME. Going to bed on a full stomach can cause acid reflux.

- STOP OR CUT WAY BACK ON ALCOHOL. Alcohol is a gastric irritant.

- USE ENTERIC-COATED PEPPERMINT. This supplement can be very soothing for digestion problems. Take 2–3 capsules between meals. If rectal burning occurs, reduce the dose.

- TAKE DIGESTIVE ENZYMES. Digestive enzymes are naturally occurring catalysts that help the body process sugars, starches, proteins, and fats. Taking the proper enzymes can dramatically improve bloating and gas as well as a host of other health problems stemming from faulty digestion. Look for a pH-balanced full-spectrum formula such as Wobenzym N (www.wobenzym-usa.com). For more information on this important topic, read *MicroMiracles* (Rodale, 2005) by Ellen Cutler, D.C., an authority on digestive enzymes, or visit Dr. Cutler's website at theramedixbioset.com.

MELBA: Stress and Antacids

Melba was forty-two and perimenopausal when she first came to see me. She had worked for ten years at the registry of motor vehicles. Every morning she had to face lines and lines of disgruntled drivers awaiting renewal of their licenses, getting new license plates, and the like. After several months of working in this job, Melba began to feel abdominal pain, bloating, and indigestion. After a routine check at her doctor's office, she was told to "reduce stress" and eat a high-carbohydrate, low-fat diet. Her problem became worse, but a co-worker introduced her to the world of antacids. Soon she would not travel without a few rolls of Tums in her purse. At first she noticed immediate relief upon taking antacids, but then after a while she began to take them earlier and earlier in the day, until she was popping antacids from nine until five, when she left her job. Over time, however, she noticed that she began to feel weak and tired, and she lost her appetite. In addition, her bowel movements became all messed up. When she first came to see me for a routine annual GYN checkup, I suspected that some of her problems were related to both her diet and her excessive use of antacids. Within a week of eliminating refined carbohydrates and grain products, and also learning some stress-reduction skills, Melba was able to cut way back on her antacid use. Some days she didn't need them at all.

Avoiding Antacid Addiction

Many women are addicted to antacids or the popular proton pump inhibitors such as Prilosec, Nexium, and Prevacid. Antacids have been known for many decades to be useful for indigestion, and even in the treatment of gastroesophageal reflux and ulcers. There are several types of antacids, but all of them work by blocking either the production or function of stomach acid. Conventional over-the-counter antacids such as Tums and Rolaids contain either aluminum hydroxide or magnesium hydroxide. Neither of them is without side effects. Aluminum hydroxide neutralizes stomach acid but tends to produce constipation. Prolonged and regular use may reduce the body's phosphate levels, with resultant fatigue and loss of appetite. In addition to this, the jury is still out about whether aluminum consumption contributes to Alzheimer's disease, so it's best to avoid it whenever possible. Magnesium hydroxide, on the other hand, produces loose stools or diarrhea in some individuals. Although some antacids combine both aluminum and magnesium, there may still be side effects.

Other antacids, such as Tums, have calcium carbonate as their main ingredient. (Tums has also been heavily marketed to women as a way to prevent osteoporosis.) Though these can help with indigestion, over time they cause acid rebound, a condition in which the excess calcium actually stimulates increased acid secretion. In addition, chronic excessive calcium carbonate intake is associated with a pattern of abnormal blood chemistry known as milk alkali syndrome, producing elevations of blood calcium, phosphate, bicarbonate, and other abnormalities. Over time, kidney stones and even progressive kidney disease may result.[58] The irony is that while many people believe that indigestion and heartburn are due to excessive stomach acid, which is why they are led to take antacids in the first place, chronic indigestion results, in part, not from excessive stomach acid, but from *deficient* stomach acid. It's no wonder that the most common side effect of the heavily promoted proton pump inhibitors is diarrhea and nausea—classic signs of digestive problems! And if stomach acid is chronically lacking, it can lead to nutritional deficiencies of vitamins such as B_{12}, which can set the stage for both chronic anemia and dementia over time.

If you have an imbalance of protein and carbohydrate in your diet, with refined carbohydrates predominating, this diet may be promoting a decrease in the production of gastric acid and overproduction of inflammatory substances, which may be (1) suppressing your immune system, (2) increasing inflammation in the stomach lining, and (3) increasing stomach discomfort and other pain. Since it is well documented that high blood sugar results in a decrease in gastric acid secretion, it's not surprising that refined carbohydrates are a setup for indigestion. Hundreds of individuals who switch to a low-glycemic-index diet have noted a complete disappearance of gastritis, reflux, and indigestion. I have personally experienced this myself since changing my diet. I used to have to take Tums or Di-Gel after dinner sometimes, and I never connected it with the bread I was eating until my problem disappeared along with the bread and rice (and cookies, I might add). This diet has been shown to improve the quality of the protective mucus in the stomach lining and also to normalize muscular control, preventing reflux and spasm.

If you find yourself popping antacids regularly, here's what I'd suggest.

⁓ GET OFF THE ANTACID MERRY-GO-ROUND. If you need to take one, use one without aluminum. And use it for as short a time as possible.

⁓ TAKE YOUR ANTIOXIDANTS. Low levels of vitamin C, vitamin E, and other antioxidant factors in gastric juice have been shown to encourage the growth of *Helicobacter pylori*, a bacterium whose overgrowth is associated with ulcers. Higher antioxidant intake may prevent these bacteria from growing and also improve the healing of the stomach and intestinal lining.

⁓ TRY DEGLYCYRRHIZINATED LICORICE (DGL). DGL may also help reduce *H. pylori* and stimulate the body's natural internal defenses. Unlike antacids, DGL does not reduce acid in the stomach. DGL improves both the quality and quantity of protective substances that line the intestinal tract, increases the life span of intestinal cells, and improves the blood supply to the intestinal lining.[59] DGL is available in most natural food stores.

⁓ TAKE THE RIGHT MINERAL SUPPLEMENT. Though the calcium in Tums is better than no calcium at all, you're much better off taking a calcium supplement that also contains magnesium and vitamin D, which help the body efficiently utilize calcium.

⁓ TRY SEACURE. Seacure is a polypeptide supplement made from pre-digested whitefish; it appears to nourish the bowel directly during the absorption process. It can be very easily absorbed by anyone who can take food by mouth, no matter how ill they are. Seacure has helped many of my patients recover from a broad range of digestive problems, including chronic indigestion, irritable bowel syndrome, and ulcerative colitis, as well as the side effects of chemotherapy. It also provides the many well-documented benefits of eating fish. The recommended dose is 3 capsules in the morning and 3 capsules in the evening.

⁓ TRY DIGESTIVE ENZYMES. (See "What to Do About Bloating" box on page 305.)

THE FINAL FRONTIER: ACCEPTING OUR BODIES

Ultimately, our digestive, food, and weight problems will not be healed completely until we have accepted our bodies unconditionally. Part of creating health at midlife is to regain the body acceptance and self-esteem that most of us lost when we entered adolescence. This is not inconsistent with wanting to make changes—and in fact may facilitate them. May the following story from one of my newsletter subscribers inspire all of us about what is possible when we cultivate enough compassion and self-acceptance and resolve to heal our third emotional center at last.

TRACEY: *Reconnecting with Body Acceptance at Menopause*

I disconnected from my body when I became pregnant at eighteen, an unmarried freshman in college who dropped out for my "shotgun wedding." I hated being pregnant—it was a daily reminder of my guilt and shame at having had sex before marriage, out there for the whole world to see and know. I never caressed my big belly, rubbed my aching feet or back, felt the wonder and magic that was going on inside me. I looked at myself totally nude only once and felt nothing but shame and disgust.

From that point onward, Tracey was anywhere from fifty to a hundred pounds overweight and at war with her body. In retrospect, she reasoned that the extra weight was a way to keep herself safe from sexual relationships, since the negative self-image it created kept intimacy at arm's length. Over the years, with maturity and years of self-discovery and therapy, Tracey slowly realized that she no longer needed such protection. Now, at the age of forty-seven and in the midst of perimenopause, her insights have clarified. She wrote:

I remembered something I said to my therapist many years ago. We were talking about what I liked about my body, and I honestly couldn't say there was anything I liked. I said, "Well, look at me—I look pregnant!" And it's true. In varying degrees of heaviness since my pregnancy, my body has always looked pregnant, patiently waiting for me to love it, which I never did when I was actually pregnant. Now I can mourn the loss of enjoying the real experience and move on. I love my essence. I'm very happy with who I am inside. I've come to understand that my physical body is the way my essence can have presence in this world. Therefore I can celebrate it now—I can reconnect my essence with my body. I can celebrate that my hands and senses allow me to express creativity and my body allows me to express my love.

No matter what your size, shape, percentage of body fat, or BMI, you and I, like Tracey, can start right this minute to express gratitude to our bodies for being home to our souls and allowing us to express our uniqueness on the earth at this time. The best way to do this is to stand in front of the mirror, look deeply into your eyes, and say, "I love you. You are beautiful." Over time, this will change every cell in your body!

8

Creating Pelvic Health and Power

The pelvis is the body center for our creative energy. The most obvious form this takes is making and birthing babies. What is less obvious is that our sexual energy, which is nothing more than life-force energy, is concentrated here. I like to think of the pelvic floor as an energetic trampoline from which our life force bounces to our heart and brain, then out into the world. Because perimenopause is a wake-up call that urges us to reevaluate how we're using our creative energy, it's not surprising that this is the most common time for women to develop problems with their pelvic organs, ranging from heavy bleeding to fibroids and urinary incontinence. It is also the most common time for women to undergo hysterectomies or other surgical procedures to treat these conditions. On the other hand, it can also be a time of complete renewal and rejuvenation of our creative and sexual energy once we understand the dynamics of this life stage.

Though numerous approaches help alleviate midlife pelvic symptoms, women can heal fully only when they acknowledge the message behind the symptoms. The emotional and energetic reason that so many women have midlife pelvic problems is associated with the rising need to undergo individuation at midlife and to transform the

312

relationship struggles that tend to make themselves known in the organs of the second emotional center: the genitals, lower bowel, lower back, and bladder. As the transforming *kundalini* energy rises through us, it often stops in our pelvic organs to create symptoms that will nudge us to address the money, sex, and power issues that are related to this area of our bodies. These blockages are known as *granthis*—psychic knots—in the ancient yoga traditions, and as the *kundalini* energy begins to rise at midlife, any *granthis* we happen to have will make themselves known, just as a blockage in a blood vessel will make itself known when blood pressure and blood flow increase! Whether or not we need surgery or other treatments, perimenopause is a crucial time to develop pelvic power by claiming and shoring up our boundaries, and by assuming more dominion over our creative energy.

WHAT IS YOURS, WHAT IS MINE, WHAT IS OURS? RECLAIMING OUR BOUNDARIES

The health of the second emotional center is tied into our creative drives: how well we balance going after what we personally want in the world versus spending time and energy on our relationships with family, friends, and colleagues. As I've pointed out, young women (or those who fall on the more *yin* end of the spectrum) are both biologically and culturally predisposed to funnel a great deal of creative energy into maintaining relationships. Men—or those who fall on the more *yang* end of the scale—are biologically and socially programmed to focus on the outer world. However, as the energy in our bodies shifts during perimenopause and our more *yang* nature arises, many women begin to turn their focus toward more worldly accomplishments. Men of the same age often turn inward and become more interested in relationships and nurturing.

Given both our cultural heritage and our shifting creative drives, it is not surprising that boundary conflicts often emerge as we begin, sometimes for the first time, to go after what we really want without being nearly as swayed by the needs and desires of others. This always requires us to claim or reclaim the healthy personal boundaries that allow us to access our power and autonomy. And given that we likely have spent thirty to forty years accommodating the needs of others first, this is often not so easy.

BETTY: *Unmet Creative Needs*

Betty was forty-two when she first came to see me for recurrent urinary tract infections. She seemed surprised when I asked her what was going on in her life and what gave her life meaning, but she clearly welcomed the chance to talk.

Betty had graduated from college over twenty years before and had made her living as a freelance writer before her marriage. She clearly had a keen mind and lots of ambition. When she was thirty-two Betty met a wonderful man named Ralph who was supportive of her writing. Ralph's dream was to run his own business, a family restaurant.

In the first year of their marriage, Betty became more flexible with her usual productive writing schedule. After all, Ralph needed help interviewing personnel for his restaurant. And could she help set up the accounting books?—it would take just a week or so, he said. But what started out as a week expanded into a month, and so on, until it became a nearly full-time job.

Despite Ralph's stated support for her writing, Betty's projects invariably took a backseat to the needs of his restaurant. As she started missing due dates, referrals began to dry up. More and more of her waking hours were spent on his business—which he was now calling "their" restaurant. Somehow, inexorably, "his" had turned into "theirs." And "hers" (Betty's writing career) had nearly disappeared.

It is imperative that in midlife, we assume responsibility not only for our current circumstances, but also for the often-outmoded beliefs that created them—beliefs that usually result from childhood programming. When I asked Betty about her family history, she told me that her father had been very demanding and invasive when she was growing up. He had a finger on every detail of their lives, and he kept after her about how she spent every minute: "You should be working on your homework now." "When are you going to do the dishes?" "Why aren't these clothes being put away as soon as you get home?"

Betty's body had registered this invasion of her second emotional center at an early age. She was only eight when she started to have bladder infections. They continued intermittently until she left for college, after which they cleared up for nearly twenty years. Five years into her marriage, they began again.

As she told her story, Betty realized that her bladder and its symptoms were part of her inner wisdom letting her know that her life was out of balance. She was, quite literally, pissed off! She had been overrun by her father as a child, and she had re-created a similar pattern with her husband. In addition to checking out her urinary system thoroughly, I suggested that it was time for Betty to begin shoring up her leaky boundaries. Simple. Not easy.

How Healthy Are Your Boundaries?

Every single one of us has experienced some violations of our personal identity—attempts to control how we think, dress, spend our money or our time, use our creativity, pursue a career. As children, we do not have the ability to form our own boundaries, and we need our parents to help us make healthy choices. But as we get older, we need more and more distance between our own choices and those of our parents. Individuation actually begins when we are two or three years old, which is why toddlers delight in saying no. In many cases, however, this process is incomplete, leaving us with less-than-ideal boundaries—which we may not even be aware of until the wake-up call of perimenopause.

Whatever our history, we must learn to live with healthy respect for our own boundaries—and for those of others. When we do, we'll have an easier time creating health in our second emotional center.

Become Aware of Ongoing Boundary Problems

What events seem to make your symptoms worse? What makes them better? When was the last time you felt really healthy? Betty noticed, for example, that her UTIs disappeared completely when she was in college and during the first few years of her writing career—times when she did not feel required to compromise her creativity to meet the needs of a loved one.

A boundary violation may be so unconscious or subtle that you do not notice it. For example, one of my patients couldn't buy shoes without checking with her husband first. When I questioned her about this, she said, "Well, he's paying for them, isn't he?" I pointed out that the shoes were for *her* feet, not his. Consider the following questions, and feel free to substitute for *partner* or *mate* another term, such as *friend, mother, father, employer, son, daughter,* and so on.

> Can you buy an article of clothing without asking your partner's opinion or permission? Do you feel guilty if you do so?
> Have you ever made a major purchase (such as a camera or appliance) without first running it by your mate? Does your mate make such decisions without consulting you?

Does your mate have the right to veto your decisions? Do you have an equal right to veto his/hers?

If you bring a purchase home and your mate doesn't like it, do you feel you must return it?

Do you feel compelled to dress in a way that is pleasing to your mate—even though you don't like the feel or style of what you're wearing?

Do you style your hair just for yourself or do you do it to please someone else?

At election time, do you and your mate decide together for whom you are both going to vote? How do you resolve any differences of opinion?

Do you find yourself eventually giving in to your mate's preferences for how to spend time and money?

Do you defer your career development needs for the sake of your mate's business or well-being?

If your mate makes more money than you, does that automatically mean that his/her career is taken more seriously and gets more support than yours?

Are you constantly on the receiving end of criticism or unsolicited advice from your mate or family about how you should live your life?

Sometimes awareness alone can help create healthier boundaries. However, if you think your boundary problems are affecting your physical health, it is almost always helpful to discuss your situation with a trusted friend or counselor. He or she can help you get clear on what healthy boundaries look and feel like in a relationship, and, most important, whether you are likely to be able to create them in your current relationship.

ALL EMOTIONS INDICATE A LEGITIMATE NEED

The late Marshall Rosenberg, Ph.D., the founder of the non-profit Center for Nonviolent Communication, taught that we all share the same basic human needs, and all human behavior is an attempt to get one or more of those needs met. Rosenberg believed that all people are compassionate by nature, and any verbal or physical violence a person employs as a conscious or unconscious strategy in getting those needs met is a learned behavior supported by the prevailing culture. (At this point, I disagree with him about the belief that all people are compassionate by nature. They aren't. But the majority are, so we'll go with that.) He identified three stages most of us work through as we progress in our personal development:

Emotional slavery. Seeing ourselves as responsible for what other people feel. For example, putting others' needs before our own because we don't want to disappoint or hurt anyone.

Being obnoxious. Feeling and expressing our anger at no longer wanting to carry the enormous responsibility we took on in the first step. In this phase, we defensively put our own needs ahead of the needs of others.

Emotional liberation. Taking responsibility for our intentions, for our actions, and for meeting our own needs, feeling free to be gracious and compassionate toward others while acting from a place of integrity and true well-being.

In the final stage, we cooperate with one another and feel a shared responsibility in true partnership. But to get there, we first need to learn to listen to our own needs, understanding that any emotional reaction we have is a valuable sign that alerts us to when our boundaries are being violated. It's easy to miss these signs, though, because of our early societal training to put others' needs ahead of our own. The process requires deep listening to ourselves as well as to others so that we can discover the depth of our own compassion, which of course begins with having compassion for ourselves. Dr. Rosenberg's process teaches people to clarify what they are observing and what emotions they are feeling, so they can learn to get their needs met without blaming, shaming, or judging themselves or others. For an extensive inventory of feelings—and a separate inventory of the needs our feelings point to—visit the website for the Center for Nonviolent Communication at www.cnvc.org, or read *Nonviolent Communication: A Language of Life* (PuddleDancer Press, 2003) by Marshall Rosenberg, Ph.D.

HORMONAL IMBALANCE: FUEL TO THE FIRE

The emotional imbalances that demand our attention at perimenopause are fueled by—and in turn contribute to—hormonal imbalance
at a cellular level. This hormonal imbalance is characterized by a
relative excess of estrogen, not enough progesterone, and, often, too
much insulin, all of which can also result in the overproduction of
androgenic hormones. Stress of all kinds, emotional, physical, or nutritional, is associated with an excess of the stress hormones cortisol
and epinephrine—and this leads to an imbalance in the evanescent
cellular hormones known as eicosanoids, such as prostaglandins and
cytokines, that govern every aspect of cellular metabolism and are
responsible for cellular inflammation. These same midlife metabolic
imbalances also contribute to physical conditions such as fibroids,
cramps, endometriosis, adenomyosis, and heavy bleeding. Some
women have all of these simultaneously.

Whether your problem is an asymptomatic fibroid or heavy
bleeding, the dietary and nutritional supplement approach to these
conditions is identical, because both estrogen dominance and eicosanoid imbalance are related to the same dietary factors. Follow the
guidelines in chapter 7 with regard to refined carbohydrates, protein,
types of dietary fat, and essential vitamins and minerals. In the sections that follow, I will discuss additional medical approaches to each
pelvic condition.

MENSTRUAL CRAMPS AND PELVIC PAIN

Starting in the teenage years, about 50 percent of all females suffer
from menstrual cramps (dysmenorrhea). During perimenopause, the
tendency toward cramping may worsen because of hormonal imbalance and the conditions associated with it, such as fibroids and adenomyosis. My own menstrual cramps started when I was about
fourteen and occurred on the first two days of each cycle until I had
my first child. They went away for a couple of years (which is very
common because of the changes that pregnancy makes in the uterus)
but came back in my mid-thirties. My cramps responded to acupuncture and dietary change, and by the age of forty I had recovered from
them completely. Looking back, I see how much they were associated
with excess stress hormones and feeling pretty much unsupported in
my medical and creative work.

Too Many "Bad" Eicosanoids

Cramps result when the uterine muscle and the endometrium produce too much of the eicosanoids called prostaglandin E2 and F2-
alpha. When these prostaglandins are released into your bloodstream
(usually within an hour or two after the onset of your period, but
sometimes even before) you begin to experience the effects of these
hormones: spasm in the uterine muscle, sweating, hot flashes, feeling
cold alternating with feeling hot, loose stools, and possibly feeling
faint. A gel made of prostaglandin E2 (one of the eicosanoids) is used
to induce labor, and it can produce exactly the same symptoms you
get when your period starts. However, in the case of cramps, the eicosanoid imbalance starts in your own body and is affected by the food
you eat and the amount of stress you're under, among other factors.

The Wisdom of Cramps

Are your cramps trying to get you to slow down, rest, and tune in to
yourself? Slowing down and resting can help balance eicosanoids.
How do you view your menstrual cycle? Is it merely a biological inconvenience for you—or do you see it as part of your wisdom?

The menstrual period is a natural time for rest and renewal. It's
nature's way of slowing you down so that you can replenish your
body for the next lunar cycle. In many ancient cultures, and even in
some contemporary societies such as parts of India, women were expected to take it easy during their periods. But in this society all of us
have been taught to try to be efficient, upbeat, and at 100 percent
energy all the time. No wonder our wiser bodily processes try to get
our attention! Women are lunar. Our bodies and our energies quite
naturally follow the phases of the moon. Though this has been considered a sign of female weakness, once you begin to listen to your
body, you will find that your cyclic energy shifts are a source of inspiration. If we have not been doing this regularly in our twenties and
thirties, our pain can become particularly acute during perimenopause, when the wake-up call to health becomes louder. As one of my
perimenopausal patients said, "If I just slow down, take a long bath,
and take care of myself, I rarely suffer during my cycle. But when I
try to bull my way through and ignore my needs, my body—and my
cramps—really try to get my attention."

As you learn to slow down during your premenstrual and men-

strual times, not only will your cramps diminish, you'll often find
that your intuition is at an all-time high. Insights may come to you
more easily. And you'll begin to look forward to this special time.

Keep the following in mind: Whenever the majority of a
population—in this case, the majority of women—suffers around a
perfectly normal function like menstruation, you can be sure that
there is a cultural blind spot in operation. Waking up and seeing the
blind spot—and how it might be related to your cramps—is part of
embracing your woman's wisdom.

In the past decade or so, women all over the world are aligning
their activities and work with their lunar menstrual cycles, learning
how to schedule rest during their premenstrual and early bleeding
time—just as the moon goes through waxing and waning times. One
of my good friends, who is self-employed, doesn't schedule any clients during her menstrual bleeding time. This allows her to tune in to
the energy of the earth and the moon and restore her energy. Since
she has started to do this, she finds that she is far more productive
than she was in the past, when she felt guilty for taking a day off and
always simply pushed through her fatigue and need for rest during
her period. My daughter Kate Northrup has created an entire online
business for mothers and entrepreneurs, teaching women how to
align their creative energies with their menstrual cycles (www.kate
northrup.com).

Treating Pelvic Pain and Cramping

Follow the Master Program for Creating Pelvic Health, later in this
chapter. If you need additional help, consider the following options:

⁓ NONSTEROIDAL ANTI-INFLAMMATORIES (NSAIDS). Nonsteroidal
anti-inflammatory drugs such as ibuprofen (Motrin, Advil),
naproxen sodium (Anaprox, Aleve), and ketoprofen (Orudis)
work by partially blocking your body's production of prostaglandin F2-alpha. (So do aspirin and acetaminophen [Tylenol], but
through a slightly different mechanism.) For best relief, NSAIDs
must be taken *before* you get uncomfortable. If you take them only
after the pain has begun, the prostaglandin will already be in your
bloodstream. The drug stops production of prostaglandin F2-
alpha, but it cannot stop the effect on your cells once the prostaglandin has been released.

~ BIRTH CONTROL PILLS. All pelvic conditions tend to quiet down when the natural hormonal cycles are put to sleep by the steady-state synthetic hormones in birth control pills. Take the lowest-dose pill available. Avoid birth control pills altogether if you are a smoker.

~ TRADITIONAL CHINESE MEDICINE. Acupuncture and Chinese herbs often work wonders for menstrual cramps. I highly recommend this approach.

HEAVY BLEEDING

Many women develop heavy and irregular bleeding in the years before menopause because estrogen dominance causes the lining of the uterus to overgrow. Stress of all kinds—whether emotional, dietary, or physical (including not getting enough sleep)—can make this worse. Instead of the normal monthly buildup and shedding of the uterine lining, too much endometrial tissue builds up and then breaks down in a disordered way that results in spotting or irregular heavy bleeding.

What do I mean by heavy bleeding? Many women experience a heavier flow on the first or second day of their periods, which slows them down a bit, but I consider this within the realm of normal. (You may still wish to try some of the gentler treatments listed.) However, if your bleeding prevents you from leaving the house or participating fully in your life for more than two days per month, if you routinely soak through a couple of tampons and a pad all in place at the same time and then through your clothes or your night-gown, or if you've been diagnosed with iron deficiency anemia, you need to take action.

The Wisdom of Bleeding:
Are You Leaking Life Energy?

I always ask women with heavy bleeding if they are leaking their life's blood into any dead-end job or relationship that doesn't fully meet their needs. Are you giving more than you are receiving in return? Is someone or something draining your energy by being a kind of Dracula? Take some time alone, sit right down on the earth, and pray for guidance and a boost of energy for yourself.

Physical Causes of Heavy Periods

In addition to hormonal imbalance, physical conditions may impede the normal uterine contractions that help stop menstrual blood flow each month.

Fibroid tumors are the most common physical reason for excessive bleeding. Whether or not a fibroid causes bleeding depends upon its location in the uterine wall. Bleeding is most often caused by submucosal fibroids, which are located right under the endometrium, the mucous membrane that lines the uterus.

Adenomyosis is another condition that can cause heavy bleeding. Adenomyosis results when the endometrial glands that line the uterus grow into the uterine muscle (the myometrium). When this happens, little lakes of blood form in the uterine wall that do not drain during menstruation. Over time, the uterus enlarges and becomes boggy, spongy, and engorged with blood, disrupting the normal uterine contraction patterns.

Since both fibroids and adenomyosis are associated with excess estrogen, minimal progesterone, too much prostaglandin F2-alpha, and frequently too much insulin, hormonal and physical factors are often present at the same time.

Treatment Choices for Heavy Bleeding

Follow the Master Program for Creating Pelvic Health, later in this chapter. If you still need assistance, and you've had a physical exam and a Pap test within the past year to rule out a more serious condition, consider the following options:

~ NSAIDS. Take a nonsteroidal anti-inflammatory drug, such as ibuprofen (Motrin, Advil), naproxen sodium (Anaprox, Aleve), or ketoprofen (Orudis), daily starting one to two days before your period, and continue it regularly through your heaviest days. Use the lowest dose that gives you results. The NSAIDs have definitely been shown to decrease menstrual blood loss because of their ability to interrupt excess prostaglandin F2-alpha.

~ LYSTEDA (TRANEXAMIC ACID). This nonhormonal therapy introduced by Ferring Pharmaceuticals in 2010 has been shown to reduce menstrual blood loss by nearly 40 percent over three and six cycles of use—and women see results as early as their first cycle after beginning the treatment.[1] Heavy menstrual bleeding is associated with an abnormally high rate of blood clot breakdown, and Lysteda works by inhibiting the breakdown of blood clots. The recommended dose is two 650 mg tablets taken three times a day for up to five days during the menstrual period each month. (For more information, visit www.lysteda.com.)

~ SYNTHETIC PROGESTERONE. When natural progesterone doesn't work, it is sometimes necessary to use a strong synthetic progestin such as medroxyprogesterone acetate (Provera). (This is the only circumstance in which I recommend the synthetic.) This is especially true if you have a fibroid that bleeds and you haven't been able to stem your problem with gentler approaches. Provera for heavy periods is prescribed at a dose of 10 mg once or twice per day for the two weeks before your period is due. Then you give your body a rest for two weeks and start over. Usually a three-month cycle of two weeks on and two weeks off will result in a significant decrease in excessive bleeding. Though Provera can have side effects, these are usually acceptable compared with losing your uterus.

~ BIRTH CONTROL PILLS. Many women who are having heavy, irregular periods due to fibroids, lack of ovulation, excess estrogen relative to progesterone, or a combination of these conditions often do well on birth control pills. Although they do not result in a true cure, they are a good option when the alternative is surgery.

~ D&C (DILATATION AND CURETTAGE). This standard surgical treatment for heavy bleeding involves scraping the uterine lining and removing excess tissue. It frequently decreases the problem, for reasons that aren't entirely clear. It is often used also to diagnose the specific condition causing the bleeding.

~ ENDOMETRIAL ABLATION. In this surgical procedure, the lining of the uterus is obliterated with a laser or with cautery. Because the procedure destroys the endometrial lining, it often results in complete cessation of periods or very light periods. It should never be used by anyone who wants to maintain her ability to have children.

Endometrial ablation (NovaSure) works very well initially for many types of intractable bleeding and is usually done as an outpatient surgery. Approximately 500,000 endometrial ablations are done each year. The most common complaint following the procedure is cyclic pelvic pain because the endometrial lining inside the uterus can grow back but the blood can't get out because of scarring. About 25 percent of women who've had endometrial ablation end up needing to have a hysterectomy later. As a result, many doctors are doing fewer of these procedures than in the past. When it works well, however, women are generally thrilled with it. If you do opt for this procedure, it should be done by someone highly skilled, with extensive previous experience. For a referral, consult a university medical center or teaching hospital. You can also call your local hospital and ask who does the surgery. Make sure the surgeon you choose is a board-certified OB-GYN.

I've referred a number of women for this procedure. For some it provides great relief. Here's an example: "Three months ago I underwent an endometrial ablation and tubal ligation. At age forty-four this sterilizes me two ways, for which I'm grateful, and has remedied the constant bleeding and clots for weeks on end. I now have no more periods! Yeah!" Though I don't like the connotation of the word *sterilize,* I certainly appreciate her relief! And she has continued to do well.

But as already mentioned, serious side effects and complications occur in about one in four women. It should be considered only if other treatments have not worked.

MARTHA: *Intractable Heavy Bleeding*

Martha wrote me the following about her midlife bleeding problem.

> I am forty-two years old. I weigh about 190 on God-given big bones, exercise regularly, and am generally healthy. My problem has been described as flooding. I have seen several doctors about this. They prescribed a double dose of birth control pills that I took for four months with no result. I have had a biopsy done, with negative results. My Paps are normal.
>
> My periods last twelve days and are very heavy with lots of clots. There is constant bleeding in between. I consulted a herbologist, who thought that because of my forty excess pounds, my fat cells could very well be overproducing estrogen. That is why the pill and the progesterone cream that I have used have not helped the constant bleeding.
>
> I have read Susun S. Weed's book *Menopausal Years: The Wise Woman Way.* In it she suggests using homeopathic remedies such as lachesis. I am also drinking raspberry leaf tea and using shepherd's purse. I am taking iron, as that has been low. Also *Lactobacillus acidophilus,* calcium, magnesium, and a good multiple vitamin.

The bleeding still has not stopped. I am becoming pretty tired of all of this, and as you can well imagine, my desire for sex is low with me having to constantly wear a pad. The bleeding has been going on for four months. Do you have any suggestions that may help?

I suggested to Martha that she seek help from an acupuncturist right away and also continue taking iron. I also recommended a Chinese patent medicine called Yunnan Bai Yao, which is superb for helping flooding problems. Many practitioners of Traditional Chinese Medicine carry it, and it's also available online from the Yunnan Baiyao Store (see www.yunnanbaiyaostore.com). This herbal combination generally works within a week or two. I suggested as well that she lose ten to twenty pounds, which could significantly reduce her excess bodily estrogen production.

It is possible that Martha has an undiagnosed submucosal fibroid. The diagnosis is made with ultrasound, MRI, or with a procedure known as hysterosalpingogram, in which dye is injected into the uterine cavity under X-ray visualization. If this is the case, she may need a surgical approach such as endometrial ablation or fibroid removal done via the vagina. I've also seen her type of problem respond well to a D&C done in the operating room.

The main point here is that there are many, many approaches to controlling heavy bleeding during perimenopause. In every case, it's helpful to have a diagnosis and treatment plan with alternatives to hysterectomy. Here is the bottom line: every perimenopausal woman who is experiencing heavy bleeding needs to know that there are many safe and effective treatment options. Hysterectomy, which amounts to killing the messenger, should be a last resort.

FIBROIDS

Benign fibroid tumors of the uterus are present in 70 percent of all women.[2] They occur in women of all races and backgrounds, but they are more common in women of African American or Caribbean descent. Fibroids arise from the smooth muscle and connective tissue of the uterine muscle itself. Though they can occur in women as young as their late teens or early twenties, they are most often diagnosed when a woman is in her thirties or forties.[3]

The majority of fibroids do not cause any real problems. In other words, they are just there. Sometimes, depending upon their location,

FIGURE 12: TYPES OF FIBROIDS

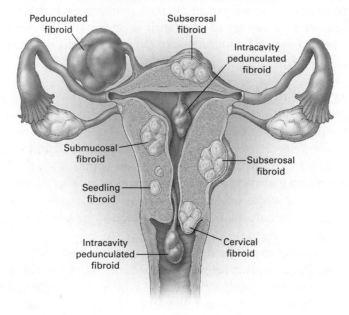

Pedunculated fibroid

Subserosal fibroid

Intracavity pedunculated fibroid

Submucosal fibroid

Subserosal fibroid

Seedling fibroid

Intracavity pedunculated fibroid

Cervical fibroid

you will be able to feel them. They feel like a smooth lump in your lower abdomen, just above your pubic bone. Because the female pelvis can accommodate growths the size of a newborn baby, it is obvious that small and even large fibroids don't necessarily lead to any problems. In other words, you may not even be aware that you have one unless you have a pelvic exam or pelvic ultrasound. Your periods may not be any different, and chances are you won't experience any pain or other symptoms. Fibroids may grow dramatically during perimenopause because of estrogen dominance (their growth is stimulated by estrogen), but they often shrink just as dramatically after menopause—nature's treatment.

The Wisdom of Your Fibroids

Though there are well-established dietary and hormonal reasons why so many women have fibroids, the baseline energetic patterns that result in fibroids are related to blockage and stagnation of the energy of the second emotional center. Women are at risk for fibroids (or other pelvic problems) when we direct our creative energy into dead-end relationships that we have outgrown. When my own fibroid appeared at age forty-two, for instance, I knew that it was related, in part, to my staying in a one-on-one direct patient care practice for several years longer than I really wanted to. I was afraid that I wouldn't be respected as a "real" doctor if I wasn't doing surgery regularly and maintaining a full office practice. Though I longed to channel my creativity into more writing and teaching, I also feared my colleagues would resent me if I worked only part-time. This is the classic second-emotional-center double bind. Our simultaneous ambition and need for love and approval create a logjam in the creative center of our bodies that, under the right circumstances, becomes a fibroid.

ELLEN: Birthing Her Creativity

Ellen, thirty-eight, was married with two children and worked as a research associate at a local university. She loved everything about her job, from the subject matter itself to the people she worked with daily. She was proud of the fact that her colleagues sought her out when they needed help with their own projects. But as the years progressed, Ellen found herself drawn to working more independently. Unfortunately, because she had become "indispensable," it was very difficult for her to set those other projects aside to birth her own individual creation. Her fibroid tumor was diagnosed at about this time.

Over the next several years, her fibroid continued to grow as she found herself torn between the needs of her own particular research and the needs of her colleagues, children, and husband. During an office visit in which she consulted me about possible surgery for the fibroid, I asked her to consider where she was "leaking" her energy. She said that a large part of her identity and sense of self-esteem came from being there for others. She told me that if she was to go off and work by herself, she was afraid that she wouldn't feel as useful—and that others would think she was selfish. As we talked about this, she realized that she had to make some long-overdue changes in her schedule and in her priorities. Then she told me that she wanted to give herself another six months before having any surgery.

The next time I saw her, her fibroid hadn't grown any further and was even a bit smaller. But more important, Ellen had told her colleagues what she was and was not willing to do for them—and had simultaneously made some big steps toward pursuing her own projects. In other words, she had started to birth her own creativity.

If you have or have had a fibroid, ask yourself the following questions: "What are the creations within me that I want to put out in the world before I'm no longer here? If anything at all were possible, what would my life look like? If I had six months to live, what relationships would I release from my life immediately? What relationships would I give more of my time and attention to? What relationships truly feed and nourish me? Which ones drain my energy?" Write your answers in a journal. Discuss them with supportive friends. Deep within you, you have all the answers you need. You just need to be open to hearing them.

ENERGY MEDICINE AND FIBROIDS

When we think of "energy" healing, we often don't think of it as affecting tissues and organs directly, but it does because at a quantum level everything is energy. It's just that the energy we call "matter" is vibrating at a much slower rate than things like thoughts and the signal from the heart that is picked up on an EKG. What that means is that when you impact the body's energy system, you are also affecting it physically—even at a distance.

This was illustrated beautifully by a case that my colleague Julie Ryan, a medical intuitive, recently shared with me. She had done an energy healing the day before on a woman with a fibroid that was causing some bleeding problems. The next day, Julie received this text message: "What a morning I have had! I was awake around 3 A.M. Got up and did some reading and went back to bed at 4:05 A.M. As I lay there, I started to feel blood pouring down. It seemed different, though, and I thought I should get up and change the pad but I continued to lie there. Then all of a sudden, I felt this rush like a lot of blood coming out and it seemed to have a solidness to it. Now I had to get up, and lo and behold, when I checked, I was staring at a lump of something solid that measured 4 cm by 4 cm. That must be the fibroid you cut away! I was mesmerized! Little fragments are still making their way out!"

Cutting the energetic "cords" that were anchoring the fibroid actually allowed the fibroid to be released physically. We are not trained to believe this, and therefore most people don't see it all that much. But I've seen this kind of thing repeatedly, simply because I'm open to the possibility. I believe that in the future, this kind of healing will become commonplace.

Treatment of Fibroids

Fibroids respond well to the suggestions outlined in the Master Program for Creating Pelvic Health, later in this chapter. After all, the first thing to consider is that a fibroid usually doesn't need to be treated at all. A watch-and-wait attitude is perfectly reasonable in many cases; you can live with fibroids for years with no adverse health consequences if they are not bothering you. What may well bother you, however, is simply knowing that you have them. Given our cultural inheritance about our pelvic organs, the perception that something *will* go wrong is often a bigger risk to a woman's well-being than the fibroid itself.

It would do most women a world of good to lighten up about their fibroids. At the time your fibroid is diagnosed, you usually will not know what has caused your second-emotional-center imbalances. Understanding comes retrospectively. Instead, commit to learning from the process, whatever course of treatment you decide upon.

An essential element of this learning experience is to release self-blame. It is never helpful to hold the idea that you have a particular illness or symptom because you are "doing something wrong." If you knew ahead of time what the condition was trying to bring to your attention, you wouldn't have had to manifest it. And in fact, all physical conditions have genetic, dietary, environmental, and emotional components simultaneously.

Of course, there are times when you may wish to seek treatment for a fibroid. Though most fibroids will shrink after menopause is complete, you may not want to live with a growth that makes you look pregnant until that time comes. If you find, as I did, that you are dressing to disguise your fibroid, and your menopause is six or more years away, then you may want to take action. And, of course, if your symptoms include pain, heavy bleeding, cramping, or backache, you'll definitely want relief. Thankfully, the treatment options are extensive.

Nonsurgical Treatments

~ BIRTH CONTROL PILLS. Birth control pills are a combination of synthetic estrogen and progestin that can smooth out the estrogen dominance that so often causes fibroids to grow or become symptomatic. Because they consist of synthetic hormones, I'd suggest that they be used only after more natural approaches such as dietary change or acupuncture and herbs have failed, or in situations in which a woman is unwilling or unable to try a more natural approach.

~ ELLAONE. Approved by the FDA in 2010 as a "morning-after" emergency contraception drug, ulipristal acetate (trade name ella-One) has also been shown to shrink fibroids and reduce heavy menstrual bleeding. Ulipristal acetate is part of a class of drugs called selective progesterone receptor modulators, which block the hormone progesterone. Blocking this hormone delays ovulation, preventing pregnancy. But because progesterone also feeds fibroids, they shrink in the hormone's absence. That means ellaOne (manufactured by HRA Pharma and available by prescription only) is effective in treating fibroids while still preserving a woman's fertility.

~ GNRH AGONISTS. GnRH agonists such as nafarelin (Synarel) or leuprolide (Lupron) act at the level of the pituitary gland and put the body into a state of artificial menopause. (Another GnRH agonist, elagolix [Orilissa], was approved in 2018 to treat pain with endometriosis and is now under development to treat uterine fibroids and heavy menstrual bleeding.) These drugs lower estrogen levels and shrink fibroids. Side effects include all the symptoms of late perimenopause, such as bone loss, hot flashes, and vaginal dryness, but these can sometimes be effectively countered with low-dose hormone therapy that doesn't cause fibroids to grow.

GnRH agonists can be quite effective as alternatives to surgery for some women. I do not recommend them if you have a family history of Alzheimer's disease, because the rapid withdrawal of estrogen from the brain may not be advisable in susceptible women.

Surgical Treatments

~ MYOMECTOMY. Fibroids can often be removed surgically. The size and location of a fibroid will determine the surgical route. Fibroids that are located just under the uterine lining deep within the uterus, for example, can sometimes be removed vaginally. Others can be removed via laparoscopy (sometimes known as belly-button surgery). Large ones, such as the one I had, usually require abdominal surgery.

If you decide to have your fibroid removed surgically, the procedure should be done by a pelvic surgeon who is trained in the repair and preservation of the pelvic organs and who philosophically is aligned with your desire to keep your uterus. When he was finished with my surgery, my pelvic surgeon told me, "Well, I'm happy to report that you now have completely healthy and normal pelvic organs. I didn't have to remove a thing except the fibroid!" That's exactly what I wanted to hear.

Having your fibroids removed can be a very empowering experience. As one of my e-newsletter subscribers wrote me:

> After having fibroids surgically removed, I also removed most negative issues from my life. It is wonderful! No headaches, no cramps, no backaches. I am still working on more dietary changes, but the ones I have already made have made me more positive, stronger, and carefree. I am also a praying person. So with this, and lifestyle changes, I am well on my way to healing and growing up at the age of forty!

~ HYSTERECTOMY. Hysterectomy should be the last resort for fibroid treatment, reserved for those women who, in addition to their fibroids, also have intractable bleeding or pain problems that simply have not responded to other measures. When this is the case, hysterectomy can be a real blessing, dramatically enhancing the quality of a woman's life.

Other Fibroid Treatments

~ FIBROID EMBOLIZATION. Uterine fibroid embolization (UFE), also referred to as uterine artery embolization, involves injecting a substance (usually polyvinyl alcohol particles) into the uterine artery. This causes clotting of the blood supply to the fibroid, which then shrinks over time. The procedure is done by interventional radiologists specifically trained in the technique. To reach the uterine arteries, a catheter is threaded into the femoral vein of the thigh. Most centers report good outcomes, with a worldwide success rate of about 85 to 90 percent. All types of fibroid symptoms, including heavy or irregular bleeding, uterine enlargement, and symptoms related to the size of the fibroid, such as urinary frequency, have responded.

The average patient who undergoes this procedure can expect

a 40 to 60 percent decrease in uterine size after about six months, but even those women who have no reduction in uterine size report improvement in symptoms such as heavy bleeding. The Society of Interventional Radiology reports that this procedure is vastly underused (especially in rural and smaller hospitals), even two decades after its introduction, despite the fact that the procedure has a low risk of complications and a shorter hospital stay compared with myomectomy or hysterectomy.[4] However, some serious complications, such as renal failure or an allergic reaction to the clotting agent, have been reported.[5] If this procedure appeals to you, seek out the advice of a specialist at a center where UFE is frequently done, call the Society of Interventional Radiology at 800-488-7284, or visit their website, www.scvir.org.

~ MAGNETIC-RESONANCE-GUIDED FOCUSED ULTRASOUND (MRgFUS). This technique uses magnetic resonance imaging to map out uterine fibroids and then follows that with high-intensity focused ultrasound to heat up and destroy fibroid tissue. Because the blood vessels in fibroids help the body to dissipate the excess heat generated during this procedure, it's particularly well suited for treating fibroids. The noninvasive, outpatient procedure leaves the uterus and ovaries intact. It involves lying on your abdomen in an MRI tube for up to three hours. Side effects may include blisters on the abdominal skin, cramping, nausea, and some pain (which is easily treated with over-the-counter pain medication).

About 70 percent of patients report that this treatment successfully reduces their fibroid symptoms, although 20 percent require additional surgery within a year. The FDA reports that though the MRgFUS treatment successfully reduces symptoms in most women, those symptoms—and the fibroids—may return. (Because of this, I recommend that *all* women suffering from fibroids also adopt lifestyle changes that alter hormone metabolism and reduce fibroid symptoms naturally.) Even so, I feel that MRgFUS is an exciting use of technology and has been a major step forward; in fact, if it had been available when I had my fibroid (which was very large), I would have strongly considered this treatment. *Note:* While women who wanted to get pregnant were initially told not to use MRgFUS, the FDA has approved labeling on this equipment stating that it is safe for women wishing to retain their fertility. For more information, call Insightec, the company that developed the technology, at 214-630-2000 or visit the company's website at www.uterine-fibroids.org; in addition, visit the Facebook page of the nonprofit organization Fibroid Relief (@fibroidrelief) for more information about focused ultrasound.

CAROL: *The Need to Let Go*

Carol was forty-six when she first came to see me for a second surgical opinion. Carol had multiple fibroids in her uterus that were causing her to bleed heavily each month, resulting in chronic anemia and fatigue. For the past four years she had tried desperately to keep her uterus, clinging to the hope that she'd be able to have a child of her own someday. Carol's condition had deteriorated to the point that keeping her uterus had become her career. In fact, she had even lost her job because of constant absenteeism due to doctors' appointments and episodes of heavy bleeding that required her to leave work. Though Carol had tried birth control pills, synthetic hormones, and multiple D&Cs to control the bleeding, nothing had helped. Her condition was too dangerous to suggest alternative treatments such as diet or acupuncture. I suggested that her health and overall well-being would best be served by a hysterectomy. (If I were to see her now, I would suggest uterine fibroid embolization or MRgFUS.)

Carol's uterine condition was preventing her from actually living her life. She was stuck in a holding pattern consisting of pouring her life's blood (literally) into unrealized hopes and dreams that had little or no chance of manifesting. Like all of us at midlife, Carol needed to let go of an unrealized dream from her past (having a biological child), allow herself to grieve fully, and then finally move on. Though this is never easy, sometimes it is the most healing choice.

AN EMPOWERED APPROACH TO SURGERY OR INVASIVE PROCEDURES

When you feel that you have been involved with the choice to have surgery, UFE, or MRgFUS and really know your options, then you've stepped out of the victim role and into the partnership model. This shift alone improves your chance for a good outcome. You can continue that partnership mode by reading *Prepare for Surgery, Heal Faster: A Guide of Mind-Body Techniques* (Angel River Press, 1996) by my colleague, psychotherapist Peggy Huddleston. Peggy has written the definitive manual for how to have a healthy and empowering surgical experience. Her healing statements and steps to prepare for surgery have been clinically proven to decrease blood loss, lessen pain (by 23 to 50 percent), and speed recovery. I personally used her approach when I had my own fibroid surgery. (See her website at www.healfaster.com, which also carries her MP3s and audio CDs designed to facilitate lasting healing; Peggy offers one-on-one consultations as well.)

I also recommend *Guided Meditations to Promote Successful Surgery* from my colleague Belleruth Naparstek (available on MP3 or audio CD as well as on the Health Journeys streaming app; see www .healthjourneys.com) as well as the Surgical Support Series developed by the Monroe Institute (available on MP3 or audio CD at www .hemi-sync.com). Both include meditations to prepare for surgery as well as music designed for you to listen to during the procedure itself.

Several major medical centers have divisions devoted to treating fibroids. A few that specialize in nonsurgical and minimally invasive options among their offerings include the Cleveland Clinic's Center for Menstrual Disorders, Fibroids and Hysteroscopic Services (http:// my.clevelandclinic.org/departments/obgyn-womens-health/depts /menstrual-disorders), the Johns Hopkins Fibroid Center (https:// www.hopkinsmedicine.org/gynecology_obstetrics/specialty_areas /gynecological_services/treatments_services/fibroid_treatment.html), and the Center for Fibroid Biology and Therapy at Duke University Medical Center (www.dukehealth.org/treatments/obstetrics-and -gynecology/fibroids).

Hysterectomy for the Wrong Reasons

Make sure that you get a second opinion if someone gives you one of the following reasons for having a hysterectomy for a fibroid.

1. *"You should have surgery before your fibroid gets any bigger. If you don't, your fibroid may grow and make the surgery much more difficult in the future."*
Unless a small tumor is causing intractable bleeding or fertility problems, it does not need to be removed. Not all fibroids are destined to grow, and even if they do, studies have shown that surgery to remove a uterus with large fibroids poses no increased risk to the patient. If necessary, the fibroid can be removed (see the section on myomectomy on page 330), leaving the uterus and the blood supply to the ovaries intact.

2. *"Your fibroid may become cancerous"* or *"We cannot be sure it is not cancerous unless it is removed."*

It is extremely rare for a fibroid to be cancerous (the incidence is less than one in a thousand). If a fibroid tumor does become cancerous, it is called a uterine sarcoma, and currently the prognosis for this condition is very poor, which means that diagnosing it via surgery will not greatly increase your chances for survival. In fact, the chances of dying from complications of hysterectomy, though small, are statistically a little greater than the chances of having a uterine sarcoma.

3. *"Your ovaries can't be seen on ultrasound."*

If you have had an ultrasound examination (or even an MRI) to confirm the diagnosis of a fibroid, one of your ovaries may not be visible because it's hidden behind the fibroid. Since doctors can be held liable for failing to diagnose an ovarian problem if it's present, they may suggest surgery to be absolutely certain that your ovary is okay.

However, if you have no reason to believe that your ovaries are diseased, you can ask to be simply followed by your doctor. Remember, inability to see an ovary on ultrasound doesn't mean that something is wrong with it—it just means that there are limits to technology! In this situation, some women will want to schedule laparoscopic surgery so that the pelvis can be examined from the inside with a light. (The uterus and ovaries can also be biopsied during this procedure.) Others will feel comfortable trusting that they are okay. Make whichever choice brings you the most peace of mind.

Should You Have a Hysterectomy?

Fibroids and heavy and irregular bleeding are the most common reasons why women have hysterectomies at midlife. Though hysterectomy is sometimes necessary, far too many women have it when they could have resolved their symptoms more easily and naturally using other means, including newer technologies such as uterine fibroid embolization. In addition, there is great value in keeping our pelvic organs intact when possible.

In an ideal world, every girl and woman would be taught the value of her pelvic organs from an early age; their benefits would be as well studied as those of the male organs, research on safe and effective natural alternatives to bleeding and pain would be common,

FIGURE 13: PELVIC ORGANS WITH SUPPORTING MUSCLES

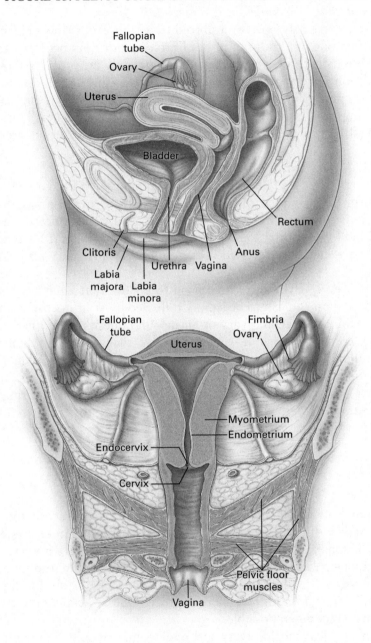

and hysterectomy with or without removal of the ovaries would be a very rare operation performed only when all other alternatives fail. This mindset is currently in place when it comes to male sexual organs. As a result, orchiectomy, the removal of the testes, is performed only as a last resort, though it is a very effective treatment for prostate cancer. And removal of the penis is just about unheard of, even in cases of penile cancer.

Unfortunately, the uterus and the ovaries have been the target of bad press for so long that many women have internalized a fear of their pelvic organs. I once overheard a woman talking to her friends at a party about her upcoming hysterectomy. Her fibroid was the size of a small orange, she told them, and she wasn't having symptoms. But, she explained, "I'm fifty, and at my age it's just a matter of time before something happens in that area. I might as well get it out now." Many physicians reinforce these fears. A patient who once came to me for a second opinion to avoid hysterectomy for a fibroid had been told by her gynecologist that her uterus (which had produced a healthy baby girl only seven months earlier) was "not her friend."

The Greek word *hystera* (womb) was used in ancient times to describe all manner of women's suffering, both psychological (hysteria) and physical, believed to be caused by the uterus. In the 1800s after the advent of anesthesia, hysterectomy became an enormously popular cure for women's ailments and was performed for just about anything that a woman's husband, father, or doctor thought was wrong with her: overeating, painful menstruation, psychological disorders, and most particularly masturbation, promiscuity, or any erotic tendency.

Surgical removal of the uterus remains one of the most commonly performed operations in the United States—both doctors and their patients have been taught that these organs are dangerous at worst or expendable at best, though this stance is now changing rapidly. Almost one in three women in this country has had a hysterectomy by the age of sixty. This is a staggeringly high number, especially considering that nine out of ten hysterectomies are performed for noncancerous conditions that are not life-threatening.[6] Not surprisingly, hysterectomy rates are very high among doctors' wives. And about 55 percent of women have their ovaries removed at the same time as their uterus, to prevent the possible development of ovarian cancer, despite the fact that the vast majority of us will never get ovarian cancer, but could definitely benefit from the hormones produced by our ovaries throughout our lives.

Good Reasons to Keep Your Uterus, Cervix, and Ovaries

~ Your uterus, cervix, and ovaries all work together to provide your body with hormonal support throughout your entire life. They also share much of the same blood supply. When the uterus is removed, the function of the ovaries is affected even if the ovaries are left in. Up to 50 percent of women who have had hysterectomies lose the function of their ovaries earlier than they normally would—and they go through menopause earlier, thus increasing their risk for heart disease and osteoporosis.[7]

~ Ovaries are the female equivalent of the male testes. As such, they are an important producer of androgens, the hormones that are involved in normal sex drive. Some studies have shown that up to 25 percent of women have decreased sex drive following removal of the ovaries. Removal of the ovaries literally castrates the female—and it is called that in medical literature.[8]

~ The uterus itself undergoes rhythmic contractions during orgasm, which contribute to the depth of sexual pleasure that many women experience during lovemaking. Some women who have had a hysterectomy complain that orgasm is not as satisfying anymore.

~ Hysterectomy with ovarian removal decreases pheromone secretion, which may decrease a woman's sexual attractiveness.[9] Fortunately, pheromone preparations are available to remedy this. (See chapter 9.)

~ Natural menopause, with ovaries and uterus intact, is a normal physiological event that takes place over a period of six to thirteen years. As your ovaries gradually shift function, the adrenal glands naturally take over some hormone production, as does the body fat. When a woman has her uterus, or uterus and ovaries, removed, her body goes through an instant menopause, which can be a shock to the hormonal system.

~ The cervix (the lower portion of the uterus that protrudes into the vagina) is part of the normal pelvic floor and helps to support the bladder. The nerves that go to the bladder are intimately connected to the cervix. When hysterectomy with removal of the cervix is performed, these nerves can be damaged, resulting in an increased risk for urinary incontinence.[10]

⁓ Only 10 percent of hysterectomies are done because of cancer. That means that up to 90 percent of the time, a woman's pelvic organs are removed for benign disease—disease that can often be treated effectively by nonsurgical approaches.

WHY KEEPING YOUR OVARIES COULD BE CRITICAL

Many doctors who do hysterectomies routinely remove the ovaries at the same time in order to prevent ovarian cancer in the future, even if the patient's ovaries are perfectly healthy. Currently, bilateral oophorectomy (removing both ovaries) is performed in 55 percent of all U.S. women who have hysterectomies, and in 78 percent of women between the ages of forty-five and sixty-four who have their uterus surgically removed. That makes for approximately 300,000 prophylactic oophorectomies performed every year.[11] If a woman has a strong genetic risk for ovarian cancer, this may be a sound decision. But the vast majority of women will never get ovarian cancer, and the routine removal of normal ovaries as prevention is a very high price to pay.

Indeed, statistics on bilateral oophorectomy (including a 2009 study following more than 29,000 women who had their ovaries removed before age forty-five, for twenty-four years) are simply too disturbing to ignore.[12] This and other studies show that women who have this procedure:

⁓ Double their risk of lung cancer—even if they don't smoke[13]

⁓ Increase their chances of coronary heart disease and stroke[14]

⁓ Increase their risk of dying from any form of cancer (although risk decreases for breast and, of course, ovarian cancer)[15]

⁓ Increase their risk of mortality for neurological or mental diseases fivefold[16]

⁓ Increase their risk for getting Parkinson's disease[17]

⁓ Increase their chances of cognitive impairment and dementia[18]

~ Increase their risk of hip fracture[19]

~ Report more depression and anxiety later in life[20]

Although taking hormone therapy after removing the ovaries can help prevent several of these outcomes, studies also show that long-term compliance is not sufficient to make up for the impact of hormone deficiency following the surgery.[21]

The bottom line: when in doubt, don't take it out.

Unearthing Your Hysterectomy Legacy

Over the years I've found that all the education and information in the world won't change a woman's life as long as she's operating from old, unconscious, and unexamined beliefs. Each of us carries a unique personal legacy passed down to us from family members. This is especially true when it comes to women's pelvic organs, a subject that has been shrouded in secrecy and misinformation for generations. Here are some questions to help you uncover your hysterectomy legacy.

Which of your family members, if any, have had hysterectomies? Why? Do you know what was going on in their lives at the time? Do you know what their diagnoses were and what symptoms they were having? Would it be possible to find out? Do you feel that you can't ask because this information is "too personal"? Does a belief in "better living through surgery" run in your family?

One of my patients believed that she would need a hysterectomy sometime during her forties because "all my sisters had them then." As a result, she became overly focused on her pelvic organs at midlife, noting every irregular or heavy period and every twinge. Ultimately, her mind-body connection—plus her unhealthy lifestyle—created enough symptoms so that she actually wanted a hysterectomy "for relief."

If, after going through these questions honestly, you still believe that hysterectomy is the best solution for you, then it well may be.

If You've Already Had a Hysterectomy

If you've had a hysterectomy and didn't know that you had any other choice, I know that it's upsetting to hear that the surgery may not have been in your best interest. One of my newsletter readers wrote:

> After reading your article on the benefits of keeping your ovaries and uterus, I wept. I was only forty-five when I had my hysterectomy for a fibroid that wasn't really bothering me at all. They took my ovaries, too. But that was twenty years ago. I didn't know that I had any other choice. And I also realized that I had never fully grieved for the loss of my pelvic organs. I have now completed that process, and I can let it go and move on.

The first step to healing after hysterectomy is to appreciate any benefits you've experienced from having the surgery. In a landmark study here in Maine, it was found that hysterectomy for noncancerous conditions of the uterus, such as bleeding and pain, was positively associated with improving the woman's quality of life in the vast majority of cases.[22] I want to stress that in this particular study, all of the women were given a choice: to have the surgery or to not have it and be followed. I referred many women to this study and even performed some of the hysterectomies that were included in the data. Many of the women who chose surgery were convinced that they'd be better off with a hysterectomy. Some had lived with pelvic discomfort or heavy bleeding for years that was cured by the surgery. Others actually had an improvement in their sex lives following the surgery. The moral is this: hysterectomy can be a healing surgery under the right circumstances.

Yes, your uterus and ovaries are important, but always remember that you are more than the sum of your organs. Your spiritual body, the field of electromagnetic energy that surrounds and nourishes your physical body, is always whole and intact. You cannot destroy this essential part of yourself, no matter what happens to your physical body.

Appreciate the fact that your body has the ability to rebalance your hormones and maintain its health if you follow a healthy diet, exercise regularly, and use bioidentical hormone therapies that match as nearly as possible what your body normally produces.

If you had a hysterectomy that you now regret, realize that you probably made the best decision you could have under the circumstances at the time. Give yourself credit for that. Our medical care system and its beliefs simply reflect those of the culture we're all a part of. And we can't help but be affected by these beliefs, at least to some degree. Maybe you would have avoided your hysterectomy if you had known more—but you didn't have that knowledge. Let any emotions you have around this issue come to the surface, even if they aren't pleasant ones. (One of my patients had a recurrent fantasy that she wanted to injure or even kill the surgeon who did her surgery. When she allowed herself to feel these unladylike revenge fantasies fully and express them out loud, she was able to release herself from the past and get on with her life, eventually forgiving herself and the surgeon.)

You can heal from anything—even events as life-changing as losing some body parts to surgery. And when you heal, your story can help someone else on her journey toward health. One of the most helpful things you can do to improve your health right now is to look back on the events leading up to your hysterectomy and see if you had any issues with boundaries or creative drive at the time. Making this link can be very empowering and will also give you greater appreciation for the wisdom of your body. Remember, too, that your second-emotional-center power and passion are still there. They don't get removed with your uterus.

The Mess Surrounding Transvaginal Mesh (the Pelvic Sling) for Pelvic Organ Prolapse

Pelvic organ prolapse (POP) is a disorder that occurs when the pelvic floor muscles weaken, become stretched, or are torn, allowing one or more of the pelvic organs (including the bladder, uterus, rectum, and bowel) to drop lower in the pelvis. This uncomfortable condition is extremely common—half of all women have some degree of prolapse—and it's the result of childbirth injury, genetics, aging, or chronic straining with constipation. POP is often associated with stress urinary incontinence (discussed later in this chapter).

In the 1970s, gynecologists began inserting mesh products through the abdomen to repair POP, inspired by two decades of good results reported by surgeons who had been using mesh to repair abdominal hernias as early as the 1950s. In 1996, the FDA approved the first pelvic mesh specifically designed for stress urinary incontinence; this product, known as the midurethral sling, was a thin strip of mesh (sometimes referred to as tape) placed under the urethra to support both the urethra and the neck of the bladder. In 2002, the FDA approved the first synthetic mesh used specifically for transvaginal repair of POP. This mesh (also known as "pelvic mesh," "pelvic sling," "transvaginal mesh patch implant," or "bladder mesh") is a netlike device (not unlike a hammock) typically made of a flexible plastic—specifically polypropylene—designed to support sagging pelvic organs. At the height of its use in 2006, synthetic mesh was used in one-third of all POP surgeries.[23] An estimated 10 million women worldwide have received mesh implants for POP. However, roughly 10 to 15 percent suffer complications.[24]

When the initial women who had this surgery first noticed feeling unwell, they reported persistent vaginal bleeding or discharge, pelvic or groin pain, and pain during sex. The adverse events (and, as it turns out, their treatment) were much worse than the condition the surgery was designed to repair. Doctors discovered that in many of their patients, the mesh had eroded and frayed, causing inflammation, infection, organ perforation, and autoimmune problems. Surgery to remove the mesh was required (which is complicated because the mesh is designed to bond with a patient's own tissue), with some women needing two or more surgeries. Tragically, some deaths were reported in women who had mesh implanted for POP.

In 2008, the FDA released a public health notification and additional patient information on serious complications in women who had surgical mesh placed transvaginally to treat stress urinary incontinence and POP.[25] It issued another safety communication in 2011 about the use of mesh specifically for POP.[26]

Women started filing lawsuits against various mesh manufacturers (including Johnson & Johnson's Ethicon, Boston Scientific, American Medical, and Bard) in 2012. The lawsuits eventually numbered well over 100,000 and claimed that mesh manufacturers intentionally misled the FDA, doctors, patients, and the public about the true safety and effectiveness of the product, and that they failed to properly test devices, research the product's risks, create safe and effective methods for removing problematic mesh, and adequately warn consumers of potential complications and injuries. The lawsuits also complained that manufacturers heavily marketed kits containing surgical tools and mesh for transvaginal prolapse surgeries to general OB-GYNs and urologists, describing the mesh as easy to implant, although the procedures were actually highly complex and suitable only for skilled and experienced surgeons.

Early on in these lawsuits, one plaintiff was awarded $80 million and another $120 million. The first manufacturer to voluntarily withdraw its mesh from the market did so in 2012, and not long after, several manufacturers began settling cases out of court. One of the largest transvaginal mesh settlements was $830 million for 20,000 cases. (The amount the injured women received after the lawyers' fees, however, was an average of less than $60,000 each, according to *The New York Times,* which is another story altogether.) To date, mesh manufacturers have paid a total of about $8 billion in settlements and jury verdicts.[27]

Some of the information made public during this time was truly horrifying. A December 2017 review published in the *British Medical Journal* revealed that sixty-one manufacturers sold mesh without conducting clinical trials and that the evidence they had submitted for safety and effectiveness was weak.[28] That same month, a BBC *Panorama* investigation claimed that Johnson & Johnson's Ethicon began selling its mesh implants after testing the product in only thirty-one women for five weeks, in addition to testing it in sheep.[29] The company withdrew its product in 2012, after six years on the market.

A May 2018 report broadcast on *60 Minutes* revealed that Boston Scientific used untested counterfeit plastic in its mesh products after its original supplier refused to continue selling the company its plastic (called Marlex) because the supplier determined it was not suitable for permanent implantation in the human body.[30] The *60 Minutes* report went on to say that Boston Scientific then began buying counterfeit Marlex from China. The show hired a plastics engineer as an independent consultant to analyze the tests Boston Scientific itself did on the plastic it bought from China (using test results *60 Minutes* found in court documents). The expert noted that the counterfeit product would likely last only a few months after implantation in the human body due to the fact that oxygen rapidly breaks up the polypropylene that the mesh is made from, even though it contains antioxidant additives. Boston Scientific denied its product was unsafe.

In April 2019, the FDA finally ordered the withdrawal of all mesh used for transvaginal POP repair from the market.[31] As of November of that year, more than 2,263 lawsuits involving the use of this mesh were still pending.[32] Notably, the FDA did *not* place restrictions on the use of mesh for POP surgery done through the abdomen (instead of through the vagina) or for surgery using mesh to correct stress urinary incontinence (instead of to correct POP). The midurethral sling used for incontinence is still in use, as is transabdominal mesh for treating POP. (Doctors also do transvaginal prolapse repair using the patient's own tissue, called "native tissue," a procedure associated with far fewer complications.)

Even though surgery using mesh to improve incontinence is less complicated than surgery done to repair POP, and while the piece of mesh used is smaller, 5 to 15 percent of women having this procedure still report complications.[33]

My friend and colleague Winnifred B. Cutler, Ph.D., first learned of this problem while attending the 2007 meeting of the American College of Obstetricians and Gynecologists—even before the FDA issued its initial warning. Dr. Cutler, president and founder of the Athena Institute for Women's Wellness in Chester Springs, Pennsylvania (www.athenainstitute.com), told me that during the meeting, one of the doctors gave a one-hour lecture castigating mesh implants that were doing serious harm to women. The doctor, Peggy A. Norton, M.D., a urogynecologist who specializes in POP at the University of Utah, told the assembled doctors that she'd conducted many three- to four-hour surgeries to remove mesh that had been implanted by other surgeons for women who began suffering months after their initial surgery. The mesh, she reported, had eroded, broken apart and embedded itself in various tissues, causing constriction, pain, and an inability to function normally.

"Dr. Norton described in great detail how she needed to open the body, search for the embedded tape, and use tweezers to delicately attempt to remove the pieces of mesh without tearing up the tissues in which it had embedded and constricted the normal movement of internal tissues and organs," Dr. Cutler wrote in the draft of an op-ed she shared with me. (Dr. Cutler also wrote about this experience in her book *Hormones and Your Health: A Smart Woman's Guide* [Wiley & Sons, 2009].) "Her hope was to relieve the pain and suffering in her patients," she continued. "More shocking to me was what happened next. She asked the approximately 120 attending surgeons for a show of hands if any of them had any problems with mesh implants; I counted about fifty men who raised their hands to answer 'yes,' although only one said he reported the problem to the FDA. Dr. Norton forcefully lamented both the lax approval criteria for new devices that were similar to existing marketed devices and the fact that surgeons' duty to report adverse experiences with medical devices like surgical mesh to the FDA was only voluntary." Despite this powerful presentation at the annual meeting of the premier professional membership organization for OB-GYNs, it would be twelve years before the eventual FDA ban of these products.

As for the FDA's order to take mesh used for transvaginal repair of POP off the market but not mesh used to treat stress incontinence, Dr. Cutler added, "As a biologist who is no surgeon, that defensive distinction eludes me! Is the surgically implanted mesh tape less harmful to women if the indication is incontinence?"

The bottom line is that if you have had transvaginal mesh implanted to treat POP, continue with all your regular checkups and follow-up care. If you are satisfied with your surgery and have not had any complications or adverse symptoms, you don't have to have the mesh removed or take any additional action. However, if you have experienced complications or symptoms, speak with your healthcare provider immediately.

Dr. Cutler concluded, "I strongly urge women to take charge of their health practices; to withhold informed consent until you are really informed about the recommended treatment; to view surgery as a last resort; and to never be embarrassed to get a second opinion." I strongly concur.

LICHEN SCLEROSUS: A BAROMETER FOR BOUNDARY ISSUES

Lichen sclerosus is a chronic inflammatory skin condition that affects both women and men at any age, although it's most commonly seen in women at perimenopause and beyond. It's also more common in those who have fair skin and red hair. It is characterized by white patches and thinned skin around the vagina and anus that can become itchy and irritated. This results in pain, bleeding, and sometimes scarring from scratching, as well as pain during intercourse and urination.

A homeopathic cream known as Emuaid (available in two strengths) can be very helpful in controlling this condition. In my practice I also often prescribed an ointment that was seven parts Valisone cream (a steroid) and three parts Eurax (an antihistamine). I would instruct the patient to rub this into the affected area twice per day for a week, then once a day for another week, and then once every three to four days thereafter.

Many women have found EFT to be helpful as well. I highly recommend Heilkunst practitioner Tammie Quick's self-published 2016 book, *How to Live Happily Ever After "Down Under": The How to Thrive with Lichen Sclerosis Guide,* which includes an EFT script specifically for use in treating the condition. (See www.quick-health.ca.)

To really get to the deeper healing needed, however, it's important to realize that the entire condition may be the result of either sexual abuse of some kind—even if it's not remembered—or some ancestral trauma stored in this area of the body. Given that one in three women will be raped over her lifetime, it is no surprise that the trauma of this might well show up in the genital area. Also, for those women living with a partner with whom they are not happy, the chronic irritation can show up in the genital area.

Over time, many women with the condition find they can use it as a barometer that lets them know how safe they feel and how well they are able to hold their boundaries within a relationship. When their boundaries have been violated, they will get a flare-up. When they are feeling safe, loved, and well cared for, the condition resolves.

MASTER PROGRAM FOR CREATING PELVIC HEALTH

The following program is effective for a host of pelvic health issues, including hormonal imbalance, menstrual cramps, pelvic pain, and pelvic floor disorders (including urinary health, discussed later in this chapter). Any dietary or alternative program such as this one that works to balance excess estrogen or enhance the flow of *chi* through the pelvis often works for treating fibroids and heavy bleeding, as well. However, let me repeat that before you start any treatment program for heavy bleeding, I recommend that you get a physical exam and a Pap test (previously known as a Pap smear) if you haven't already had one within the year. Though the vast majority of cases of heavy bleeding are benign and can be treated with the advice below, you want to be sure that you don't have some other condition that is contributing to your problem.

Diet, Nutritional Supplements, and Herbal Support

~ FOLLOW A HORMONE-BALANCING FOOD PLAN. (See chapter 7 for detailed instructions.)

~ ELIMINATE ALL DAIRY FOODS (CHEESE, ICE CREAM, CREAM, MILK, YOGURT) FOR ONE MONTH AND TOTALLY ELIMINATE RED MEAT if you suffer from menstrual pain. Though I do not have any statistics on this, I've seen many women get rid of their menstrual pain altogether (even in cases of severe endometriosis) by eliminating conventional dairy foods from their diets. Some are able to prevent cramps by avoiding dairy just for the two weeks before their periods. During perimenopause, when periods so often become irregular, you may need to stop dairy altogether for a few months to experience the benefits. (To make it easy, just follow the Whole30 program, as mentioned in chapter 7—that will cover it.)

One more thing: raw, unpasteurized dairy products do not appear to have the same adverse effects as conventionally processed dairy food. These products are considered a whole or complete food because they retain all of their natural enzymes, fatty acids, vitamins, and minerals (many of which are destroyed by the pasteurization process). Further, raw milk doesn't contain thickening agents such as carrageenan, which is often added to low-fat milk to improve the texture. Medical researcher Ted Beals, M.D., has shown that the risk of getting sick from unpasteurized milk is extremely low; in fact, you are 35,000 times more likely to get sick from other foods than from raw milk![34] (However, be aware that the risk is greater for the elderly, people with weakened immune systems, infants and young children, and pregnant women.) Although the U.S. Food and Drug Administration (FDA) requires all milk sold across state lines to be pasteurized, many states allow the sale of raw milk within the state in which it is produced. Look for it at farmers' markets, grocery stores specializing in healthy or natural foods, or online. To find where to purchase raw milk in your state, visit the Real Milk Finder website (www.realmilk.com/real-milk-finder), operated by the Weston A. Price Foundation. Always buy raw milk and dairy products made from it from a reputable distributor. Ask at your local farmers' market for recommendations and read customer reviews online.

Red meat, like dairy foods, is high in an eicosanoid precursor known as arachidonic acid, which results in symptoms such as cramps and arthritis in susceptible individuals. Eliminating it from your diet can cut down on the inflammatory eicosanoids associated with cramping and endometriosis pain.

⌐ TAKE ADDITIONAL SUPPLEMENTS. Follow the supplement program outlined on pages 302–303, with special attention to the following:

Omega-3 fatty acids: Omega-3 fats are precursors for series 1 and 3 eicosanoids. Take the recommended levels of fish oil (DHA and EPA) outlined on page 599, or commit to eating one serving of fatty fish (3–4 oz.) three or four times per week or taking either 4 tablespoons ground fresh whole organic flaxseed or 1 tablespoon fresh flaxseed oil daily.

Vitamin C: Take the recommended level of 1,000–5,000 mg per day, but increase to bowel tolerance (when tissues are saturated with ascorbic acid, loose stools result) when cramping occurs. This could be anywhere from 1,000 to 10,000 mg per day, or even more in some individuals.

B complex and vitamins A, C, and E: These vitamins are especially important for pelvic health because they help strengthen your blood vessel walls as well as help neutralize excess estrogen. Take the mid-to-high range of the B vitamins on pages 702–704.

Vitamin D: Higher vitamin D levels are linked to a lower risk for female pelvic floor disorders, according to the results from the National Health and Nutrition Examination Survey (NHANES).[35] Researchers reported that vitamin D levels were significantly lower in women with at least one pelvic floor disorder and for women of all ages who specifically reported having urinary incontinence. On the other hand, women age fifty and older whose vitamin D levels were 30 ng/ml or higher had a significantly reduced risk for incontinence. Optimal blood levels of vitamin D are 40–80 ng/ml. These levels are achieved by taking doses of 5,000 to 10,000 IU per day, plus or minus regular doses of sunlight, until optimal levels are reached. Once that happens, you can reduce the dosage to 2,000 to 5,000 IU per day, depending on sun exposure. It is well documented that the vast majority of the population has suboptimal levels of vitamin D. This vitamin is easy to measure, so you can determine what your status is. For crucial information on the importance of vitamin D, check out www.grassrootshealth.net.

Magnesium: 100 mg taken as frequently as every two hours during times of actual pain has been shown to help relax smooth muscle tissue and therefore decrease cramping. Do not exceed 1,000 mg per day, otherwise stools may become too loose. But don't only rely on magnesium when you're cramping. Most people have deficient levels of this mineral, which is especially concerning because vitamin D cannot be utilized properly without adequate magnesium. Yet unlike with vitamin D, there is no easy way to test magnesium levels, so knowing your status is more of an issue.[36] Magnesium requirements also vary a great deal from day to day, given that magnesium is a necessary cofactor for hundreds of metabolic reactions in the body.

To be sure that you are getting enough magnesium, I suggest you begin supplementing with this mineral slowly and build up. My favorite way to do this is with the ReMag and ReMyte liquid mineral supplements formulated by Carolyn Dean, M.D., N.D., a world-renowned magnesium researcher. (To order, see www.rnareset.com.) These supplements come with instructions to help you individualize your dose. You can also take magnesium in pill form in any number of ways, including magnesium threonate, which is quite well absorbed. The usual dose is 800 mg per day. But start slowly. You can't really overdose on magnesium because once tissue saturation is reached, you get loose stools.

Supplemental iron: In many women with heavy bleeding, the primary symptom is fatigue from iron deficiency anemia. Get your blood count checked, especially a serum ferritin level. If it's low, take iron. The recommended daily allowance is 15 mg per day. You may need to take three to four times this amount until iron levels are restored. (Iron supplementation itself has been shown to decrease menstrual flow in some women.) I recommend La Santé Iron Drops from Evolving Nutrition. (See Resources.) It is time-released, doesn't cause stomach upset or constipation, and is easily and readily absorbed. It has helped many women in my practice keep their blood counts normal—something they were previously unable to do with other iron supplements. It has even saved some women from needing surgery.

Pueraria mirifica: Many women find that when they take *Pueraria mirifica* either daily or cyclically (three weeks on, one week off), they can eliminate heavy bleeding. (See www.amatalife.com.)

⁓ REDUCE CAFFEINE INTAKE if you tend to have urinary problems. Caffeine is a bladder irritant. Eliminate it completely for two weeks and then reintroduce to see if symptoms recur. (Even decaffeinated coffee and tea still retain a small amount of caffeine.)

- DRINK PLENTY OF WATER AND CRANBERRY JUICE AND TAKE CRAN-
BERRY CAPSULES if you have frequent urinary infections. Drinking
copious amounts of water or unsweetened (or artificially sweetened) cranberry juice the minute you feel any bladder symptoms is
helpful. The reason is that the cranberry juice contains a substance
that prevents bacteria from sticking to the walls of the bladder,
making it easier for the body to eliminate the offending organism
so that microbiome balance is restored. You can also try cranberry
capsules, available at natural food stores; take as directed. Another
excellent supplement for preventing UTIs is femiNature, which
contains cranberry extract as well as inulin (a natural prebiotic for
rebalancing intestinal flora), D-mannose (a natural antibiotic and
pain reliever), phellodendron extract (a Chinese herb that helps
fight bacteria), and MSM (a mineral that fights pain). For more
information, see https://hmslaboratories.com.

- TAKE PROBIOTICS REGULARLY to help recolonize your gut with
"friendly" bacteria. The anus and urethra are so close anatomi-
cally that encouraging the growth of favorable bacteria in one area
of the body also helps the other. Two probiotic strains in particular,
Lactobacillus rhamnosus GR-1 and *Lactobacillus reuteri* RC-14
(formerly known as *Lactobacillus fermentum* RC-14), have been
shown in numerous studies to be helpful in both preventing and
treating genitourinary infections when taken as an oral dietary
supplement.[37] These strains are commercially available in Fem-
Dophilus from Jarrow Formulas (see www.jarrow.com), which is
perfect for women on birth control pills as well as women with
diabetes who get recurrent yeast or urinary tract infections.

Such approaches are always worth a try, as this letter from an
e-newsletter subscriber attests.

> I have been suffering for years with multiple uterine fibroid tu-
> mors, approximately twenty-five to thirty in number, in the wall
> of my uterus. For two weeks out of every month I had excruci-
> ating, unbearable pain. I was unable to sleep, would lie down
> curled up in a ball, and literally sweat in agony. I have had laser
> surgery through the laparoscope twice, and the surgeon was
> only able to remove three or four of the larger fibroids. Then I
> read your book and have been religiously following your advice
> to cut out dairy products and take B complex vitamins as well as
> 800 mg of magnesium. As a result, if I could, I would give you

my firstborn child in gratitude! My pain is gone! Though I was planning reconstructive surgery, I changed my mind when I realized that your suggestions were working. I feel like a completely new woman—reborn, revitalized, and empowered.

Acupuncture and Chinese Herbs

Acupuncture has been scientifically shown to alleviate menstrual cramps and pelvic pain.[38] I have seen its benefits hundreds of times in my practice, and I personally found it extremely helpful for severe cramping in my early forties. I also took individually prescribed Chinese herbs for about a year. If you cannot locate a trained practitioner of Traditional Chinese Medicine near you, it is safe to try Bupleurum (Xiao Yao Wan, also known as Hsiao Yao Wan). This patent medicine is widely available, and many of my patients have done very well with it. (See Resources.) Take four or five of the tiny tablets four times per day during the two weeks before your period is due, and continue through the first day of bleeding. It may take two to three months to see full results. Yunnan Bai Yao is a traditional Chinese medicine that can stop heavy bleeding within one to two weeks, sometimes sooner. Take 1 or 2 capsules four times daily. This treatment works very well for recurrent UTIs.

Topical Treatments

~ TRY HOMEOPATHIC REMEDIES, such as Menastil, which is available over the counter. The active ingredient is calendula oil—an essential oil extracted from marigold petals. The U.S. Food and Drug Administration and the Homeopathic Pharmacopoeia of the United States recognize this pure grade of essential oil for the temporary relief of menstrual pain. This all-natural product, which comes in a small roll-on applicator bottle, relaxes the uterine muscle and increases the flow of blood and oxygen, which in turn reduces pain. Claire Ellen Products manufactures and distributes Menastil; for information, call the company at 508-366-9378, or visit their website, www.bestpainrelief.com.

~ CONSIDER CASTOR OIL PACKS. Lying down with a castor oil pack on your lower abdomen for sixty minutes two to four times per week is often very helpful for both treatment and prevention of cramps and pelvic pain. Edgar Cayce, the renowned medical intuitive of the early to mid-1900s, recommended this immune-system-enhancing treatment for all kinds of conditions. (See Resources.) *Note:* Do not use these if they increase your pain or if you are bleeding heavily.

~ CONSIDER PROGESTERONE CREAM. Progesterone skin cream helps to counter estrogen dominance and can be used to decrease heavy bleeding, among other symptoms. It is available over the counter in a 2 percent strength (trade names Pro-Gest, PhytoGest). The usual dose is ¼ teaspoon (providing 20 mg progesterone) rubbed into your palms or the soft areas of your skin once or twice per day, three weeks on and one week off. If you are having regular periods, time the application so that your week off corresponds to the week of your period. If your periods are irregular, I suggest coordinating use of the progesterone cream with the phases of the moon, to which every human life is attuned. Plan to be off the progesterone during the dark of the moon—the time when women were most apt to have their periods before the advent of artificial lighting. Some women do best using the cream every day, with no week off.

For some women, 2 percent natural progesterone isn't strong enough to counteract their own estrogen. In this case, ask your doctor for a prescription for a stronger, natural progesterone cream, available from a formulary pharmacy, or for a prescription for a stronger vaginal gel, such as Crinone, which comes in 4 percent and 8 percent strengths. Micronized oral progesterone (brand name Prometrium) is another option if the creams are not effective. The dose is 100–200 mg once or twice per day for the two weeks before your period is due, although some women need to take it daily. Because oral preparations must be metabolized by the liver and the resulting breakdown products can cause excessive sleepiness or even depression in susceptible women, some women prefer the creams, which are absorbed into the bloodstream directly.

Strengthen Your Pelvic Floor

Getting in touch with your pelvic floor can be a most enjoyable experience. Remember that your pelvic floor is the seat of your life force and sexual energy. Since energy follows awareness, just placing your awareness in your pelvis can begin to change your experience of this area—you will probably notice a pleasant tingling sensation. After all, in addition to your pelvic organs and pelvic floor, the pelvis has a great deal of erectile erogenous tissue within it. (See chapter 9, "Sex and Menopause.") So when you do your pelvic strengthening exercises, make the experience as fun and juicy as possible!

Becoming aware of your pelvic floor and exercising it regularly—through either Kegels, Pilates, vaginal weights, the use of a jade egg, or Emsella treatments (discussed later in this section)—not only strengthens the pelvic floor but also increases blood flow to the vagina, bladder, and urethra, making the tissue more resilient. This will greatly improve both your sex life and your bladder control.

What Everyone Should Know About Kegel Exercises

Just doing Kegel exercises and expecting your entire pelvic floor to function optimally is not enough. Kegels can backfire. They work well in the short term for strengthening the pelvic floor, but a truth that has more recently come to light is that over time, doing Kegels can actually make your pelvic floor muscles *weaker*—unless you also develop strong gluteus muscles (the muscles in your butt). This is the central idea in the pelvic strengthening program developed by biomechanical scientist Katy Bowman, founder of Nutritious Movement (www.nutritiousmovement.com).

When I first read what she had to say about how Kegels have been overemphasized and why concentrating on your glutes is key for a strong pelvic floor for women *and* men, her explanation made an enormous amount of sense to me—even though it was the complete opposite of what most experts have been preaching for decades.

Bowman explains that Kegels keep the pelvic floor muscles short and tight, which actually makes them weak, not strong. Here's why: doing lots of Kegels certainly tightens your pelvic floor muscles initially, but over time it also pulls your sacrum (the large triangular bone at the base of the spine) forward, out of its natural alignment. (The first sign of this, she says, is not having a lumbar curve—that little curve in your lower back, also known as the J-spine.) This creates slack in your pelvic floor muscles, which run from your tailbone to your pubic bone. Continuing to do more Kegels—especially with a tucked pelvis—then tightens the slackened pelvic floor, but because your tailbone is still curling under, the tight pelvic floor muscles are now shorter. And shorter muscles are weaker because they have less range of motion.

To illustrate this, Bowman suggests thinking about curling your biceps with a weight. If you started in a curled position with your elbow bent but then lowered your arm only a little before bringing it back up, you wouldn't be getting much of a workout. To have proper form for such an exercise, you'd lower your arm the whole way, almost straightening your elbow, before bending your arm back up into the curled position. It's the same way with your pelvic floor muscles—for proper toning, they have to be able to stretch and relax the whole way instead of staying tight. Toning requires both strength *and* length.

On the other hand, maintaining strong gluteal muscles (the butt muscles you use when you squat) keeps the tailbone pulled back in its natural position. As Esther Gokhale, founder of the Gokhale Method (see gokhalemethod.com), says, "The behind is supposed to go behind." Keeping the behind behind you in turn keeps the pelvic floor muscles long and taut. In this position, the pelvic floor is much better able to hold up the pelvic organs and open and close what Bowman refers to as your "bathroom muscles" to keep you from leaking urine. In this position, the pubic bone will also be under you, holding up your pelvic organs. The most effective and natural way to strengthen your glutes, she says, is by doing two to three sets of squats daily, using proper form. I recommend ten squats three times per day. You can easily do these at your desk or even in the bathroom. Just hover above the seat for a moment, then stand up, and then squat down again. Repeat ten times. (As a bonus, squats are also good for your hips and knees.) *Note:* Just sitting down in a chair is a squat. You don't have to go all the way down to the floor—a position that young children are really good at, but which we manage to lose as we grow older and sit in chairs most of the time.

Because many people who live in third-world countries use squat toilets (which look something like drains in the floor, sometimes with places for your feet on either side of the hole) instead of the "throne"-style toilet Westerners sit down on, they naturally have stronger glute muscles, Bowman adds. Not surprisingly, women from these cultures have stronger pelvic floor muscles and often have an easier time giving birth because with their tailbone untucked and in proper alignment, their birthing space is bigger and they put less pressure on their pelvic floor, resulting in less tearing of muscles and tendons and less damage to ligaments.

As with most exercises, there's a right way and a wrong way to do squats, and even doing them the right way often requires working up over time to a proper full squat. Bowman's "Down There" for Women program in her Aligned and Well series presents a step-by-step guide to a safe and effective squat program, offering a progression that will gradually get you where you want to be. For a brief look at the squat exercises, including photographs of proper form, check out "You Don't Know Squat" from Bowman's website at www .nutritiousmovement.com/you-dont-know-squat.

I also highly recommend a stool to put your feet on when you sit on the toilet to get your body into the most squat-like position possible. This greatly enhances elimination. That's the whole point behind the very popular Squatty Potty; I suggest you watch the video that goes with this product so that you can clearly see why squatting while eliminating is so good for you. (See www.squattypotty.com.)

But remember, Bowman doesn't trash Kegels completely. She stresses that proper pelvic health and alignment requires maintaining balance. If you work only your glutes and don't ever do any Kegel squeezes, your pelvic floor muscles will be long but not strong, and you still won't get the support you need. Even so, Bowman insists that you don't need to do the hundreds of Kegels a day that the experts have been recommending. To keep your pelvic muscles balanced while you do Kegels (so you won't reverse the proper alignment you'll be trying to establish with the squat program), she suggests doing Kegels in a proper squat position (as detailed in her program), gently tensing and fully releasing the pelvic floor muscles ten times.

The release is a vital part of doing Kegels, she stresses, and she suggests you relax your pelvic floor muscles just shy of urinating for this stage. Otherwise, your pelvic floor muscles won't completely lengthen out and instead will stay short and tight, continuing to contribute to pelvic health problems.

Supporting healthy pelvic alignment also requires paying attention to the way you hold your body, especially your pelvis. Wearing high heels, for example, can contribute to pelvic floor dysfunction because high heels shorten both your hamstring and calf muscles and tilt your pelvis upward. Instead, you want the pelvis tilted slightly downward—think of your pelvic bowl the same way you would a bowl filled with water. A slight downward tilt allows the water to easily flow out of it. Wearing heels occasionally doesn't cause much harm, but working and walking all day in high heels is not good over time, despite what we see in the movies or on television.

If you're what Bowman calls a "tucker," someone who sucks in your gut and pulls in your backside, you're pulling your tailbone out of alignment and weakening your pelvic floor. So forget what your mother told you about not sticking your butt out! Women also tend to sit in this tucked position, Bowman notes. She suggests that when you'll be sitting for more than two hours at a time, sit on a rolled towel and tilt your hip bones forward just enough to establish a healthy lumbar curve in the small of your back. (This is also a good position for doing Kegels, she says.)

Many women are able to improve pelvic muscle tone, enhance sexual pleasure, and resolve or greatly improve their incontinence by strengthening the muscles of the pelvic floor and urethra. A strong pelvic floor can withstand increases in intra-abdominal pressure without giving out and also increases blood flow and innervation of the pelvic organs. That is exactly what Arnold Kegel, M.D., had in mind in 1948 when he told his patients to practice vaginal contractions in preparation for childbirth. Ideally, every pregnant woman should be doing Kegels regularly both before and after birth so that these muscles will be strong enough to withstand the rigors of labor and delivery. When Kegel exercises are done properly and consistently, they work very well. Kegel exercises actually condition the pubococcygeus (PC) muscle for sexual arousal. They also increase the flow of blood to the genitals, which enhances the ability to reach orgasm and also improves vaginal lubrication. Some studies report that up to 75 percent of women are able to overcome stress incontinence with Kegels alone.[39]

But again, doing Kegels effectively means both keeping your pelvis untucked and concentrating on developing strong glutes by doing squats three times a day. Unfortunately, the vast majority of women who are told to do Kegel exercises have not been instructed in how to do them properly and also give up too soon—which is why so many women think they don't work and why the reported results are so variable. Many women prefer using weighted vaginal cones or jade eggs as an alternative way to get the same benefits as Kegels (see below).

DEVELOP LIFETIME PELVIC POWER BY STRENGTHENING
YOUR PC MUSCLE (KEGEL EXERCISES)

1. Identify the PC muscle. Sit on the toilet with your legs
   spread apart. See if you can stop the stream of urine without moving your legs, your abdomen, or your buttocks
   muscles. The muscle used to stop the flow of urine is the PC
   muscle. This is the only muscle that should be contracting.
   Your PC muscle will not become stronger if you contract
   your abdominal, thigh, or buttocks muscles at the same
   time that you are doing a PC contraction. Check yourself
   by inserting two fingers in your vagina while contracting.
   You will feel the muscle tighten around your fingers.

2. Learn the exercises.

   Slow clenches. Squeeze your PC muscle and hold it
   clenched for a slow count of three. Work up to a slow
   count of ten after a couple of weeks or so. Though it's not
   necessary to hold your breath while counting, it may be
   helpful at first to establish your concentration. Release
   and exhale.

   Quick contractions or flutters. Now contract your PC
   muscle quickly, once per second.

   Push-outs. Clench your PC muscle and then push out as
   though you are bearing down to move your bowels. Hold
   for a count of three to ten. Note that your abdominals
   will contract when you do a push-out. Your anus will also
   contract.

3. Train your PC muscle gradually. Begin with ten slow
   clenches, ten flutters, and ten push-outs (one set) three to
   five times every day. After one week, add five slow clenches,
   five flutters, and five push-outs to the original ten. That's a
   total of fifteen reps for each set. Continue to do three to
   five sets a day. Next add five of these the following week,
   so a set equals twenty reps.

   Continue doing three to five sets per day to maintain optimal pelvic tone, urinary continence, and sexual function.
   In as little as a week's time you will definitely notice a dif-

ference in your ability to strengthen these muscles—if, that is, you are using the proper form by keeping your tailbone untucked and you're also strengthening your glutes. It may take three to four weeks to notice a change in urinary symptoms. You will probably notice a change in sexual responsiveness in a couple of weeks if you do both Kegels and glutes properly. *Note:* You can do Kegels anywhere and anytime: driving, watching TV, cooking, sitting in the bathtub—even riding the ski lift.

When you start training your PC muscle, you'll probably find that it doesn't want to stay contracted for the entire count of ten. It may also be difficult to do the flutters. That's because the muscle is weak. Don't worry about it. Take a rest during a set if needed. But be persistent. Like all muscles, the PC responds beautifully to resistance training. You'll be amazed by how fast you'll get results if you stick with it. Also, every time you do the exercises, you'll be giving yourself a powerful reminder that you have the strength and stamina to create and maintain healthy boundaries. (All this while also enhancing your sex life—what could be better?)

There's another way to do Kegels that doesn't require counting to ten or focusing on which muscles to contract. In this method, which is based on ancient Chinese techniques, you insert a weighted cone or a jade egg into your vagina and simply hold it in place for at least five minutes twice a day, gradually working up to fifteen minutes twice a day. You start with the heaviest cone or egg that you can easily hold in for one minute, gradually move on to the heavier ones, and finally shift to a maintenance program. (Cones range in weight from 15 to 100 g, and jade eggs come in a variety of sizes—see Resources.) Holding the cone or egg in the vagina automatically uses just the right muscles. I have been recommending these cones for years and my patients have had excellent results with them, provided there are no complicating factors such as infection, neurological damage, or use of diuretic medications or caffeine. About 70 percent of women can expect improvement or cure within four to six weeks of consistent use.[40] I also recommend the Kegelmaster (available on Amazon), which provides fifteen adjustable resistance levels, and the Perifit Kegel exerciser (www.perifit .co), which you use along with a smartphone app. There are also entire series of exercises available using jade eggs. These exercises are very effective in helping create vaginal dexterity and enhanced erotic potential (see www.kimanami.com or www.thedesiletsmethod.com).

BTL Emsella: The Kegel Throne

A relatively new treatment known as the BTL Emsella uses high-intensity focused electromagnetic energy to cause thousands of contractions of the pelvic floor muscles over a period of thirty minutes while you are seated in a special therapeutic chair. Think of it as an automatic Kegel exerciser. The treatment is painless and actually pleasant. You don't even need to take off your clothes. The recommended number of treatments is six—two per week for three weeks, although some women may need more. The cost is about $1,800 to $2,000 for the entire series, which is not covered by insurance.

I tried out an Emsella chair at Mindful Roots, a holistic women's health practice in my area, and I was extremely impressed. I intend to go back for all six treatments, just because I could tell how beneficial this was for my pelvic floor in general. To find a provider who offers Emsella, see https:// bodybybtl.com.

I highly recommend the Emsella chair treatments to anyone with urinary stress incontinence or simply those who want to enhance their pelvic floor strength and orgasmic experiences. I would certainly do this before undergoing incontinence surgery if at all possible, though I realize that the cost is prohibitive for many at this time. Still, I consider Emsella to be a boon to women (and men, who also can use it).

URINARY HEALTH

At midlife, the loss of hormonal support in the vagina and lower urinary tract is often accompanied by the loss of muscle tone in the pelvic floor. As a result, many women experience urinary problems, ranging from loss of urine when coughing or sneezing to recurrent urinary tract infections, and uterine prolapse (a condition with a hereditary component that is often exacerbated during midlife). The number of women suffering from these disorders is rising rapidly. Experts estimate that by 2050, one in three women will have some form of pelvic floor disorder. The number of women with urinary incontinence is projected to increase by 55 percent (from 18.3 million in 2010 to 28.4 million in 2050), while the number with pelvic organ prolapse is estimated to jump by 46 percent.[41]

Keeping Dry: Maintaining or Regaining Bladder Control

Urinary incontinence, the involuntary leakage of urine, is a major health problem that affects approximately thirteen million people in the United States. Though 10 to 30 percent of women age fifteen to sixty-four experience urinary incontinence at least some of the time, the condition tends to increase in frequency with age. It often makes itself known during perimenopause, when a great deal can be done to make sure it doesn't progress. By the time women reach age sixty-five and over, the overall rate of incontinence increases to about 15 to 35 percent.[42] In their book *The Bathroom Key: Put an End to Incontinence* (Demos Health, 2011), women's health physical therapist Kathryn Kassai and co-author Kim Perelli offer a comprehensive program to regain continence, pointing out that urinary incontinence is the number-one reason why women get put into nursing homes. I highly recommend their work. (See www.thebathroomkey.com.)

Many physical therapists are now trained in pelvic floor rehab, which reduces or eliminates urinary stress incontinence. Classical Pilates often takes care of it as well.

Though urinary incontinence does affect men, it affects women five times as often. Many women feel too embarrassed to bring it up with their doctors and therefore don't know about many of the new and effective treatments that are available. To compound the problem, many physicians aren't up on the latest treatments, either. In an editorial in the *Journal of the American Medical Association*, Neil M. Resnick, M.D., wrote, "Most physicians have received little education about incontinence, fail to screen for it, and view the likelihood of success as low."[43]

This doesn't mean that you should suffer in silence. Urinary incontinence is easily diagnosed and often treatable with excellent results. I've already covered the Emsella chair, Kegels, jade egg exercises, and physical therapy; these approaches will work for nearly everybody who has mild to moderate stress incontinence.

If you need more help, seek out someone who specializes in the evaluation of female urological problems. Determining exactly what type of incontinence you have will allow you and your provider to create an individualized plan of action. Many gynecologists are now trained in urogynecology and routinely do this evaluation in their offices.

Stress urinary incontinence (SUI) is the most common type of incontinence. It is diagnosed when a woman loses urine while performing any activity (such as laughing, standing up quickly, or exercising) that increases her intra-abdominal pressure and thus overrides the ability of her urethral sphincter to stay closed. This may result from problems with the sphincter muscle itself or from the fact that the angle of the urethral tube has changed, becoming too mobile to function properly—a condition known as urethral hypermobility. A number of factors that are increasingly common in perimenopause lead to the following situations.

- Weakened pelvic floor muscles. Unless you work out regularly and include your pelvic floor muscles, then these muscles, like your biceps, may be weaker than they should be.

- Thinning of the tissue of the outer urethral area, from estrogen deficiency.

- Nerve damage resulting from childbirth, major pelvic surgeries, a history of radiation, smoking, or excess intra-abdominal fat that pushes the urethra out of the proper position every time you urinate. Innervation of the urethral sphincter also tends to decrease with age, but age alone does not inevitably lead to loss of function. (Research has shown that nerve density in this area varies widely in perimenopausal women.)[44]

⁓ Underlying neurological disorders such as multiple sclerosis can result in other types of incontinence.

Whatever the exact cause of your problem, there are a lot of solutions besides spending the rest of your life wearing adult diapers!

Nonsurgical Incontinence Solutions

⁓ KEEP A RECORD. Keeping a record will help both you and your healthcare practitioner learn which substances and situations may be contributing to your incontinence. Record how often you experience the problem, any activity that precedes it, how much urine actually leaks, whether or not you experience a warning beforehand, if it wakes you up at night, and whether it follows the ingestion of certain foods, drinks, or medications. Sometimes you can alleviate your problem just by becoming aware of when it happens and making adjustments.

Many women also have an increased urinary output on the first day of their period, when they get rid of all that premenstrual fluid. On these days, stress incontinence will always seem worse because your bladder fills more quickly.

⁓ REDUCE OR ELIMINATE CAFFEINATED DRINKS. Many women have stress incontinence only when urine output is increased from drinking coffee or tea. Even decaf coffee is a diuretic—and so is cold weather (I never drink a cup of coffee in the morning if I'm going skiing, otherwise I'll have to stop at the lodge after every other run). Coffee is also a known bladder irritant. I've been able to help some women resolve their incontinence problem completely just by providing them with this information.

⁓ MEDICATION. Since there is a great deal of overlap between pure urinary stress incontinence and urge incontinence, many women are also offered medication to relax the bladder muscle regardless of what type of incontinence they have. (See section on urge incontinence, page 366.)

⁓ CONSIDER ESTROGEN CREAM. The outer third of the urethra is estrogen-sensitive, just as is the vaginal tissue. In post- or perimenopausal women with stress urinary incontinence, estrogen cream placed on the top surface of the outer third of the vagina has been shown to enhance nerve function and blood supply to the urethra, which in turn increases muscle size and strength. About 50 percent of women who have incontinence associated with estrogen depletion will be cured or greatly improved simply by re-estrogenizing their urethral area. This success rate increases for women who strengthen their pelvic floor simultaneously. Vaginal cream made with the phytohormone *Pueraria mirifica* also works very well. (See www.amatalife.com.)

~ STRENGTHEN YOUR PELVIC FLOOR. See the Master Program for Creating Pelvic Health, earlier in this chapter.

~ URETHRAL PROSTHESES. Urethral prosthetic devices are very useful for stress incontinence caused by urethral hypermobility, a condition in which the angle of the urethral tube has changed, becoming too mobile to function properly. These devices work by stabilizing the bladder base and reestablishing a normal angle between the bladder and urethra. (You may have noticed that it's more difficult to urinate with a tampon in. This is because the tampon elevates the bladder neck. A diaphragm can do the same thing.) Urethral prostheses are virtually risk-free and can be used on an as-needed basis, making them especially good for those women who have incontinence only during specific activities such as golf or aerobics. They can also be used temporarily while you're strengthening your pelvic floor muscles. Available products include the Incontinence Ring, Incontinence Dish, and Incontinence Dish with Support (all from Milex). Many users of these devices report a heightened sense of self-confidence and freedom.

~ MAINTAIN OPTIMAL VITAMIN D LEVELS. See the Master Program for Creating Pelvic Health, earlier in this chapter.

Surgical Techniques to Relieve Bladder Symptoms

If you've strengthened your PC muscle maximally and still have incontinence problems, then a surgical solution may help.

~ STANDARD SURGICAL REPOSITIONING PROCEDURES. There are a variety of tried-and-true surgical techniques for treating stress urinary incontinence that give long-term success rates of 80 to 95 percent in the hands of an experienced surgeon. In all of these procedures, sutures are placed in the tissue near the urethra to elevate the bladder neck so that it functions properly. The disadvantage of these approaches is that they require an abdominal incision and a fairly long recovery period.[45]

~ MINIMALLY INVASIVE REPOSITIONING PROCEDURES. A whole host of new surgical techniques have recently been developed to help permanently reposition the bladder neck so that urethral function is restored. They are done laparoscopically on an outpatient basis. Short-term results with the new techniques are also favorable, with a cure rate of about 82 percent. Long-term results are not yet available.[46] In addition, several surgical techniques are now available to suspend the uterus, including laparoscopic suspension—thus "curing" prolapse without removing the uterus. Results have been mixed so far.[47]

~ INJECTABLES. A variety of agents, including body fat or bovine collagen, can be injected around the urethra under local anesthesia. These injections increase the volume of urethral tissue, allowing it to close properly and prevent the passage of urine during times of increased intra-abdominal pressure such as coughing, laughing, or changing position. They are effective immediately and can be done as an office procedure. A skin test is necessary four weeks prior to the procedure to be certain that there will be no allergic reaction to the material. It usually takes two or three injections over time to get the desired result, and they may eventually have to be repeated. The improvement or cure rate ranges from 82 to 96 percent, depending upon the type of incontinence being treated.[48]

~ STEM CELL THERAPY. This is one of the most promising new procedures for stress urinary incontinence, with several preliminary studies showing good outcomes. However, the studies so far have reported only short-term results on small numbers of women, and more research needs to be done on which sources of stem cells are the most effective, as well as on which patients are most likely to benefit from this therapy.[49]

Here's how it works. Doctors take cells from the patient's body (for example, from the thigh muscle) during a needle biopsy procedure. The cells are then sent to a lab, where they are refined and grown into stem cells. Four to six weeks later, the doctor injects the stem cells into the bladder's sphincter. These cells then help to strengthen the muscles that control voiding. Both procedures—the biopsy and the injection—each take half an hour or less and are done on an outpatient basis. Serious side effects have not been reported so far, and some subjects have achieved complete bladder control—although improvement may take several months. Stay tuned for more news on this promising procedure.

Irritable Bladder: Urge Incontinence

Some incontinence is caused by involuntary contractions of the bladder muscle (the detrusor muscle). These involuntary contractions cause strong, sudden urges to urinate and the feeling that you might be about to wet yourself—which sometimes happens. Women with an overactive bladder often find themselves missing out on normal activities because they have to go to the bathroom so often and worry whether or not one will be available.

Urge incontinence is commonly treated with drugs such as tolterodine (Detrol), which inhibit detrusor contractions. Side effects include headache, dry mouth, dry eyes, constipation, and indigestion. Another drug, called oxybutynin, is also useful. It's available by prescription as Oxytrol (a transdermal patch) and Gelnique (a transdermal gel). Though this type of medication can be helpful, there are other options, including biofeedback training. Women's health physical therapist Kathryn Kassai, mentioned earlier in this chapter, suggests contracting your pelvic floor several times when you feel the urge to urinate, and then avoid going for ten minutes or so. Over time, you'll train your detrusor muscle to calm down so it doesn't send you the signal to urinate so much.

Sometimes bladder irritation is caused by the localized lack of estrogen in the bladder and urethral area associated with perimenopause and menopause. The problem resolves with local or systemic estrogen or phytoestrogen therapy. Caffeine is also a bladder irritant. As little as one cup of coffee per day can result in bladder symptoms in some women.

Sacral nerve stimulation (first offered with InterStim from Medtronic; see www.interstim.com) became available for women with urge incontinence in the late 1990s. This pacemaker-like device is surgically implanted just below the skin's surface on the lower back. It then delivers mild electrical impulses to the sacral nerves, which influence bladder function and improve control.

A newer technique, called percutaneous tibial nerve stimulation (PTNS), is a less invasive version of sacral nerve stimulation and was inspired by acupuncture. PTNS involves having a doctor insert a thin, needle-like electrode into the ankle to deliver a low-frequency current to the tibial nerve, which is connected to the sacral nerves, which in turn regulate bladder contractions. Each treatment lasts about a half hour and, like acupuncture, is basically painless. Patients return once a week for about three months and can have more treatments later if they are needed. Researchers report a 60 to 80 percent positive response rate.[50]

Injecting botulinum-A toxin (commonly known as Botox) into the bladder and the bladder's sensory pathways is a relatively new treatment for urge incontinence. It works by blocking the ability of some nerves to communicate with the bladder or sphincter muscles. This outpatient procedure takes about twenty minutes and can be performed under either local or general anesthesia. Patients begin to experience improvement in about a week. Research shows the treatment is 70 to 80 percent effective. However, repeat injections (probably three to nine months after the initial treatment) are necessary, as the Botox wears off. More worrisome is urinary retention, a complication seen in many women.[51] The Mayo Clinic is conducting trials that involve injecting a solution containing Botox and dimethyl sulfoxide (currently FDA-approved only for interstitial cystitis) into the bladder with good results and no side effects.[52]

Irritable bladder syndrome can also be associated with stressful psychological situations such as taking an exam, being evaluated at work, or worrying about some aspect of your life that isn't working. I'll bet you've had the experience of going to take a final exam, going into a job interview, or being in some other stressful situation and finding that you had to pee repeatedly before the event.

Many perimenopausal women find that they repeatedly have to get up at night to urinate when their sleep is interrupted by chronic worry or anxiety. In my experience, there is an exquisite connection between the worry-and-obsess area of the brain and the bladder. Happily, we each have the ability to interact consciously with this area and get it to cooperate with us.

Biofeedback-assisted behavioral training, for example, has been shown to reduce involuntary incontinence episodes by about 80 percent (drug therapy results in a 68 percent reduction).[53] In one controlled study, women were asked to keep a voiding diary in which they recorded the time of day of the urgency and what they were doing at that time, so that their voiding patterns and the circumstances surrounding them would become clear. They were then shown how to identify their pelvic muscles and contract and relax them voluntarily while keeping abdominal muscles relaxed (the same as with Kegels)—a procedure that took only one session. Next, the women were taught to respond to the sensation of urgency by pausing, sitting down if possible, relaxing their entire body, and then contracting their pelvic muscles repeatedly to diminish urgency, inhibit detrusor muscle sensation, and prevent urine loss. When the urgency subsided, they proceeded to the toilet at a normal pace. Women were encouraged to practice pelvic muscle contraction at home in various positions and also during activities when urge incontinence is most apt to occur. Finally, they were taught to practice interrupting or slowing their urine stream during voiding once per day.

I strongly recommend that women with incontinence problems (who have faithfully strengthened their pelvic floor and brought awareness to the area in the ways I've described above) consult a gynecologic urologist, a relatively new type of specialist. Doctors trained in this area are the best resources to discuss both medical and surgical options for women with bladder problems of any kind.

LIANA: *Addressing Long-standing Urinary Health Issues*

My friend Liana's story is a great example of how successful treatments for urinary incontinence can be when combined with a few additional techniques to create an entire mind-body approach. Liana's issues with urinary health stretch back to the second grade, when she had recurring urinary tract infections caused by her refusal to use the bathroom at school. (The school had taken the locks off the stall doors, and she was so afraid someone would walk in on her that she just held it until she got home.) She was even hospitalized once for a special test that involved being catheterized. "What I remember most about that was how badly it burned to urinate after having the catheter in me," she remembers.

Liana's problems worsened after she gave birth at age forty and ended up with a severely prolapsed bladder, which caused her to leak urine constantly. A surgical procedure she hoped would help actually ended up backfiring, leaving her with incontinence *and* chronic pelvic pain.

Not surprisingly, her sex life had pretty much fizzled out, but she certainly wasn't ready to give up. "After seven years of chronic pelvic pain," she told me, "I began studying sacred sexual practices in hopes that I might somehow find a way to feel sexually intact and whole again. But within a month, I began experiencing a searing hot pain deep inside my pelvis. It felt like someone was stabbing me with a red-hot sword. Sometimes the pain was so intense that I would be incapacitated for hours at a time, although my doctor couldn't find anything wrong. It was a mystery."

I recommended that she have her bladder repaired by a urogynecologist and also that she work with Doris Cohen, Ph.D., a clinical psychotherapist, medical intuitive, and healer who is the author of *Repetition: Past Lives, Life, and Rebirth* (Hay House, 2008). Here is Liana's account of what happened:

> Dr. Cohen's guides linked my current pelvic pain to a past life in which I was three years old when my mother died in childbirth. My name had been Amelia then. We were a pioneering family living far from anyone, and my father was so distraught by my mother's death that he lost his mind and began abusing me nightly with a hot fireplace poker. As soon as Dr. Cohen gave me this information my entire body began shaking. I knew it was true! The guides told me that Amelia's trauma was being repeated in my body in this lifetime. In order to heal my pelvis, Dr. Cohen said, I needed to go back to the lifetime when the wounding happened.
>
> She gave me an exercise to do for forty days to release this pattern of repetition. Each day I was to take four deep breaths and imagine a magical garden. In the garden is a body of calm water, trees, flowers, butterflies, angels—and Amelia, at whatever age she chose to be. I was to enter the garden as the adult Liana and reassure and comfort Amelia, telling her that the garden was a safe place filled with angels who would take care of her. Then I was to say goodbye to Amelia and come back into the present as my adult self. When I first started this exercise, Amelia showed up as a young woman. But each day that I went to the garden, Amelia became younger and younger until finally she was four years old.
>
> In the meantime, I found a urogynecologist who agreed to do my bladder repair surgery. During one of the presurgery tests, a nurse practitioner inserted a catheter in my urethra and electrodes in my vagina. Even though I wasn't either frightened or cold, my legs began to shake uncontrollably. I knew instantly that little Amelia had been activated, so I closed my eyes, breathed deeply, and went to meet her in the garden. I found her running around like a wild animal, trying to pull her hair out and screaming, "*Stop!* Make them *stop!*" She wouldn't let me get near her, so I called on the angels in the garden to help. Sud-

denly a natural hot springs appeared, and the angels coaxed
Amelia to get into the hot water. They began brushing her hair
to soothe her, and she finally began to relax. The moment she
began to calm down, my legs stopped shaking! I left Amelia with
the angels and came back to the present moment, completing the
testing with no discomfort.

I continued to do the Magic Garden exercise as I prepared
for the surgery, and I also used Belleruth Naparstek's guided
imagery [*Guided Meditations to Promote Successful Surgery;*
see www.healthjourneys.com]. The results were astounding! I
was awake and able to urinate without pain within a few hours.
My healing was swift and relatively pain free. And best of all,
one year later I am still 100 percent continent and have had zero
pelvic pain. None! I am sexually intact and am able to enjoy
physical intimacy with my husband with no pain!

Liana's story illustrates how multifaceted and mysterious the
healing process can be. Past-life influences on health are, in my view,
both real and important. The research of Brian L. Weiss, M.D., a
prominent psychiatrist and the author of *Many Lives, Many Masters*
(Simon & Schuster, 1988), bears this out. So does the work of many
others, including the famous Edgar Cayce.

For more information about urinary incontinence, contact either
the National Association for Continence at 800-252-3337, www
.nafc.org, or the Simon Foundation for Continence, 800-237-4666,
847-864-3913, www.simonfoundation.org.

Recurrent Urinary Tract Infections

Urinary urgency and frequency are often the result of recurrent urinary tract infections. Get a medical evaluation to be sure that you
don't have some anatomical problem that is contributing to your infections. Make sure that the outer third of your urethra is well estrogenized. Your doctor should be able to evaluate this during a pelvic
exam, because the urethra runs right under the top part of the vagina
and is easily felt and observed. If there is any evidence of thinning of
the outer urethra, get a prescription for estrogen cream or use *Pueraria mirifica* vaginal moisturizer (www.amatalife.com). Low-dose
Premarin vaginal cream used twice weekly has shown good results
with no endometrial problems.[54] Estrace is another brand of bioidentical estrogen cream that I would recommend over Premarin.

Also follow the food and supplement plan as well as the advice on acupuncture and Chinese herbs outlined earlier in this chapter in the Master Program for Creating Pelvic Health.

There you have it. I hope this information has given you hope and let you know how much can be done to improve all aspects of your urinary and pelvic health. Don't resign yourself to using adult diapers the rest of your life when so many other solutions are available. You are not alone—incontinence is more common than diabetes. It is also often easier to treat! But you have to take the first step. Ask for help.

9

Sex and Menopause:
Myths and Reality

It's no secret that many women experience a decrease in their sex drive during perimenopause. What's not so obvious is the wisdom behind this decrease—and why it is often a necessary step toward having the best sex of your life. (More about that later.) As previously discussed, perimenopause puts all your relationships, including the one you have with yourself, under a microscope. This transition forces us to reevaluate every aspect of our relationships and update them. And this includes our sexual relationships.

Libido at perimenopause can be likened to sap in a tree. In the fall and winter, that sap goes deep into the roots of the tree, where it lies waiting for the inevitable rise and new growth that begin in the spring. During the winter, there are no leaves on the tree and it may seem as though nothing much is happening. But deep inside, the tree is undergoing rest and renewal before another cycle of growth. In many women, libido turns inward to nourish the new growth that is under way on a soul level but which cannot yet be seen on the outside. Here's what that means: if a woman's sexual relationship needs to be updated, if she is not getting the tenderness and care she desires, or if she has unfinished business with her mate or a history of sexual abuse, then any or all of these issues may well arise during this time so that the deck is cleared for the next stage of life.

This change in sex drive often has absolutely nothing to do with hormone levels and everything to do with a woman's deepest unfulfilled desires, desires that are now rising into her consciousness—desires that she may have pushed down for decades. The heart in our chest is the high heart, and the uterus and genitals are the low heart. The high heart and the low heart are energetically connected. At midlife, the dictates of our high heart's desires become increasingly urgent, and our low heart and genitals will no longer willingly participate in sex that is not connected to our high heart and our deepest yearnings.

For many women, libido resurfaces after they have identified their unsatisfied needs and taken steps to get them met. (As discussed in chapter 2, I recommend visiting www.cnvc.org, the website of the late Marshall Rosenberg, Ph.D., founder of the Center for Nonviolent Communication; here you'll find both an inventory of human needs and an inventory of the emotions that signal when those needs aren't being met.) Listing our needs and desires and trusting that we have the power to get these met is the first step toward recharging the batteries of our libido. At midlife, our task is to broaden our concept of sexual energy and appreciate it as life force that may have nothing to do with sex per se. Our culture, through its books, movies, and media images, promotes love and sex as the major—if not exclusive—route to happiness. But this is only part of the truth. When we are fully open to the energy that created the universe in the first place—which is another way of saying when we are in love with our own lives—then we have the ability to tune in to and become part of the vitality of the world around us and in us. It's everywhere—in the beauty of nature, the pursuit of a cause we believe in, and the exercise of our creative powers. We find that we are capable of becoming passionate about life itself, whether or not we have a sexual partner.

In other words, if we think of sexual energy in the largest possible context—as life force, or as Source energy—then the relationship between the two becomes clear: the health and vitality of our sexuality is inexorably linked to the health and vitality of our lives.

THE ANATOMY OF DESIRE

By the time we reach midlife, the challenge for each of us is to be able to access life force or passion in other ways besides looking to another person for fulfillment and gratification. The call goes out for each of us to expand our personal repertoire for accessing Source energy in our lives.

Many women who are in the midst of negotiating this step for themselves find that in order to tap into their Source energy directly, they first have to withdraw from the outer world for a while as they do the inner work of reassessing their goals, boundaries, and relationships. With this more inward focus, the sex drive of many wanes for a period.

Though a menopause-related deficiency of hormones most often gets the blame for a drop in sex drive around this time, the most recent research on sexual function at midlife (which is increasingly being carried out by women) has found that menopausal status, per se, is not related to most aspects of sexual functioning. The truth is that midlife women are having sex more often and enjoying it more than ever before! An ongoing study on midlife presented at the 2007 meeting of the Gerontological Society of America reported that American women age fifty-five and older enjoy sex more and put more thought and effort into their sex lives than women a decade ago who were the same age.[1] The good news gets even better: the women in the study who were in their mid-sixties to mid-seventies reported the biggest increase. The researchers noted that women who've reached midlife and beyond feel younger, are more open about their sexual needs, and are more interested in health than women at the same age a decade ago. They also consider a healthy sex life to be part of having a healthy lifestyle. This trend holds up over time. A 2017 national survey of adults between age sixty-five and eighty conducted by the University of Michigan reported that women in their seventies often express more satisfaction with sex than women in their forties.[2] Of course, sexual satisfaction can continue well beyond the seventies. A 2012 study found that those women most likely to report satisfaction with their ability to achieve orgasms were either under fifty-five or over eighty![3]

These results echo those of a 2007 study published in the *New England Journal of Medicine* showing that midlife men and women have sex an average of two to three times a month—the same frequency that younger adults report. Even more encouraging was that more than 25 percent of the oldest group surveyed (seventy-five to eighty-five years old) were still having sex.

Not surprisingly, the survey further showed that those in poor health reported having sex the least, while those who said they were healthy reported having the most sex. The researchers concluded that a strong sex life has less to do with how old you are and more to do with how healthy you are.[4]

Though some women do indeed report a decrease in desire, less interest in sex, and changes in arousal, research on healthy nonsmoking menopausal women with partners shows that there's no change in sexual satisfaction, frequency of sexual intercourse, or difficulty reaching orgasm.[5]

Researchers have also demonstrated that a woman's perceptions of "being menopausal" may also affect her sexual functioning, especially if she has been led to believe that her sexy years are finished. For ages, women have been brainwashed into thinking that menopause is the end of their sexual attractiveness. When you have been led to believe that you are no longer desirable or attractive, this belief itself certainly can affect sex drive—not to mention one's body image and self-esteem. Older studies done on women seeking treatment for menopausal symptoms have reinforced this cultural bias. It is well documented, for example, that women who seek treatment for menopause tend to report more life stress, and they suffer from more clinical depression, anxiety, and psychological symptoms than women who don't seek care. Of course, these factors are all strongly related to sexual functioning.

The Truth About Sexual Functioning and Menopause

Sexual function is a complex, integrated phenomenon that reflects the health and balance not only of the ovaries and hormones but also of the cardiovascular system, the brain, the spinal cord, and the peripheral nerves. In addition, every factor that affects sexual function has underlying psychological, sociocultural, interpersonal, and biological influences of its own. Happily, current research on women and sex is finally taking into account how complex female sexual arousal really is. Consequently, the entire concept of so-called female sexual dysfunction is being updated. New research (much of it done by women) is shedding increasing light on how seamlessly psychological states affect biological responses. Finally research has begun to validate what women already know: a woman's experience of sexual arousal is more influenced by her thoughts and emotions than by feedback from her genitals. In other words, her emotions and thoughts must be in sync with the goal of sexual satisfaction for her body to perform sexually.[6] This is very good news! When you learn how to change your thoughts, you can change your sexual response.

⌐ The truth is that a woman's relationship satisfaction, attitudes toward sex and aging, vaginal dryness, and cultural background have a much greater impact on sexual functioning than does meno-pause, per se.[7]

~ What is commonly called female sexual "dysfunction" may well be a logical adaptation to such things as past negative experiences, pain with intercourse, fatigue, depression, and medication—or lack of emotional intimacy with a partner.[8] A 2008 Harvard study of 32,000 women age eighteen and up found that 43 percent reported having sexual problems, yet only 12 percent said they were upset by them.[9] What's particularly ironic about this study is that it was funded by Boehringer Ingelheim, the company that makes the female sexual dysfunction drug flibanserin. Interestingly, the FDA originally denied approval of this drug because of lack of evidence that it offered any benefit that was worth the considerable side effects.[10] In 2005, the FDA changed its position and approved the drug—in my opinion, probably because of pressure from the pharmaceutical industry. Though drug companies will continue to want to cash in on the discovery of a female Viagra, female sexuality is way too complex for a quick fix like that. Female sexual dysfunction is, at its core, a reaction to our cultural programming about sexuality—and there's no drug yet that can cure that!

~ There is nothing about the menopausal transition, per se, that results in decreased libido in healthy, happy midlife women. In fact, the number-one predictor of good libido at menopause is a new sexual partner—even in those women who previously had sexual problems in prior relationships.[11] In my view, it is not necessary to get a new partner during menopause if you are mostly happily coupled. What you must do instead is focus on yourself and your needs and *become* a new partner. This is true even if your partner is yourself.

~ Genital sexual responsiveness of premenopausal and postmeno-pausal women doesn't differ significantly.[12]

~ Male sexual function is an issue for many midlife women. More studies need to address the effect of a male partner's erectile dys-function on a woman's sex life. Many midlife men experience this problem and most are not comfortable talking about it or seeking treatment. A fiftysomething woman recently told me that ever since her husband's treatment for early prostate cancer, he hasn't touched her sexually. She said, "He won't even talk about it. I love this man and I'm not going to take this sitting down. There must be something that can be done!" Thankfully, there is. For example, I've known men who have regained full sexual functioning even after prostate removal, improved their health, and also learned how to open their hearts.

Other health challenges in men can also be an issue. A 2019 study based on surveys of more than 24,000 British women ages fifty to seventy-four found that often a woman's sex life wanes because of the health of her partner.[13] Twenty-three percent of the women who responded said their partner's physical problems were the main reason for their not having sex, with 21 percent saying their partners were the ones who lost interest.

FEMALE LIBIDO DRUGS: ARE THEY WORTH IT?

Addyi (flibanserin) was the first "female Viagra"–type drug to be approved. This drug came to market in 2015—after two failed attempts to convince the FDA that it should be approved. It must be taken daily, it works on the serotonin system in the brain, and if you have a glass of wine within two hours of your dose, you're likely to have a severe drop in blood pressure and also faint. So much for setting the mood. Other common side effects of this drug include the following:

~ Blurred vision

~ Confusion

~ Dizziness, fainting, or lightheadedness, especially when getting up suddenly from a lying or sitting position

~ Sleepiness or unusual drowsiness

~ Sweating

~ Unusual tiredness or weakness

Somehow this just doesn't seem worth it, given that sexual encounters are designed to be uplifting and health-enhancing! At least the FDA required a boxed warning to be included on the packaging, warning women not to take the drug with alcohol.

In June 2019, the FDA approved a second drug to enhance female sex drive. Vyleesi, generically known as bremelanotide, was created to "treat acquired, generalized hypoactive sexual desire disorder (HSDD) in premenopausal women." This is not the same as erectile dysfunction in men. Here's how the press release put it. "HSDD is characterized by low sexual desire that causes marked distress or interpersonal difficulty and is not due to a co-existing medical or psychiatric condition, problems within the relationship or the effects of a medication or other drug substance. Acquired HSDD develops in a patient who previously experienced no problems with sexual desire. Generalized HSDD refers to HSDD that occurs regardless of the type of sexual activity, situation or partner."[14]

Given the complexity of the mind/body/spirit connection, especially when it comes to sex, this drug really doesn't make much sense. The FDA admits that the mechanism by which it works is unknown. Taking this drug to enhance sex drive is like sitting down to start your car when you don't know where the starter is or how the car even works. Vyleesi is administered via a shot in your abdomen or thigh up to forty-five minutes before sex. Moreover, it causes nausea 40 percent of the time. So imagine this: you are already distressed by the fact that you have no desire for sex, and then to treat it you have to inject yourself with a needle—and there's nearly a 50/50 chance that the drug will make you sick to your stomach. (But of course, you can take yet another drug for that side effect.) Does that seem sexy to you? And when you look at the data, it's not very robust. About 35 percent of patients using Vyleesi said they were no less stressed about sex, while 31 percent of the placebo group reported the same result.[15] And in the clinical trial, only 25 percent of the patients said their desire improved significantly, while 17 percent of the placebo group had the same result. There is essentially no appreciable difference between these two groups.

The truth is that men go through midlife change as well. It's often called the "midlife crisis." In her book *The Liquid Light of Sex* (Bear & Company, 1991), astrologer and esoteric teacher Barbara Hand Clow points out that men generally source their erections from their second chakras during the first half of their lives. Recall that the second chakra is all about money, sex, and power. But at midlife and beyond, they need to source their erections from their hearts. There can be a time when they are moving from one center to the next and go through a period of impotence. If a man doesn't understand this, he may "act out" by having an affair or getting a hot new car—just to prove to himself that he's still "got it." A little patience goes a long way at this point if you've got a good man (not a narcissist). A new workout routine, a new puppy, and a better diet can also help.

For more information about prostate issues, I recommend *Invasion of the Prostate Snatchers: No More Unnecessary Biopsies, Radical Treatment or Loss of Sexual Potency* (Other Press, 2010) by Ralph H. Blum and Mark Scholz, M.D., as well as *The Male Biological Clock: The Startling News About Aging, Sexuality, and Fertility in Men* by Harry Fisch (Free Press, 2005).

HELP YOUR MAN AVOID THE SEXUAL SIDE EFFECTS OF PROSTATE CANCER TREATMENT

Aaron Katz, M.D., chairman of the Department of Urology at New York University's Winthrop Hospital, has been a leader in what is called "active surveillance" of men with slow-growing prostate cancers. Fifty percent of men who have total prostatectomies have urinary and erectile problems. Acknowledging the fact that far too many men are overtreated for slow-growing prostate cancers, Dr. Katz has pioneered nutritional and lifestyle protocols that actually result in men who are healthier than when they started—despite their slow-growing prostate cancers, 90 percent of which never grow outside the capsule surrounding the prostate gland. Dr. Katz and now many other urologists place those who want to avoid the sexual side effects of surgery and/or radiation on a program that includes aerobic exercise, dietary improvement, antioxidant-rich supplements, optimal levels of vitamin D, and active hexose correlated compounds (AHCCs), an immune-enhancing nutritional supplement derived from several species of mushrooms. This program has allowed many men to not only avoid the adverse sexual side effects of standard prostate cancer therapies, but also vastly improve their health. Check out *Dr. Katz's Guide to Prostate Health: From Conventional to Holistic Therapies* (Freedom Press, 2006).

~ A woman's overall mental and physical health are more important to sexual functioning than menopausal status.

~ Smoking has a much greater impact on a woman's sexual functioning than her menopausal status. Smokers have decreased blood flow to the genitals and other organs. Toxic substances in cigarettes also poison the ovaries, changing hormone levels.

~ Vaginal dryness is more common at midlife because of the effect of lower estrogen levels on the vagina. As a result, midlife women suffer from painful intercourse more often than younger women unless they are fully aroused or adequately lubricated prior to intercourse.

~ There are significant ethnic and cultural variations among menopausal women. Compared to white women, studies have shown that African American women have a higher frequency of sexual intercourse, Hispanic women report lower physical pleasure and arousal, and Chinese and Japanese women report more pain and less arousal.[16]

~ Sexual preference may change at midlife. Several of my patients reported to me that after menopause, they became sexually attracted to women, even though they had defined themselves as heterosexual their whole lives. Research now shows us that women's sexuality is much more fluid than we ever knew before, so this makes sense.[17]

~ Although orgasm certainly shouldn't be the "goal" of having sex, it's still well worth noting that orgasm is incredibly healthy in more ways than you might imagine. The hormone oxytocin (released by the pituitary gland during labor and breast-feeding as well as during skin-to-skin contact with others and during orgasm—in both men and women) encourages bonding and helps prevent blood pressure spikes in response to everyday stress.[18] It also reduces cravings for sweets and for drugs and alcohol in those who are addicted. Research shows that oxytocin can reduce cell death in damaged hearts as well as lower certain inflammatory factors known to slow healing.[19] This hormone is probably what's behind the findings that couples generally live longer than single people, support groups work for those battling addictions and chronic diseases, and pet owners heal more quickly from illnesses than do those who don't have pets. Healing touch, including touch from massage, also increases oxytocin. Orgasm is also associated with a huge burst of nitric oxide (see below).

Resolving problems in an existing relationship can have an effect on your sex life that's comparable to that of a new sex partner—when a woman makes a decision to have more fun and pleasure with the man or woman she loves, she experiences a boost in her life energy, which translates to an equivalent boost in sexual energy. Hanging on to old anger and resentment, on the other hand, quells libido rapidly.

THERESA: The Restorative Power of Passion

When Theresa became a widow at the age of fifty-seven, she thought her heart would never be the same again. When her husband of thirty years was diagnosed with cancer, she'd been right by his side every step of the way. But when Stan started what was to become a long, slow decline, Theresa felt as though her whole world was slowly slipping away. He'd been the love of her life, and she couldn't imagine being without him.

When Stan died, she took it very hard. She kept busy with friends and work, but she still felt the loss deeply. The summer Theresa turned sixty, she decided to follow a dream she'd not yet had a chance to fulfill—she went to Italy for two weeks. And she took her best friend, Margo, along for support.

Two days after they arrived, the two women found themselves wandering around an almost-deserted Sorrento. It was a Sunday and everything was closed. A forty-nine-year-old artist named Antonio who happened to be in the same café having coffee struck up a conversation with them. His warm eyes and heartfelt laugh instantly won Theresa and Margo over. Antonio was also a race car driver, and when he talked about racing, the women could tell that this was a man who was genuinely in love with life.

Antonio offered to drive the women around for the day to share the sites with them, and they eagerly agreed. In no time, they were all on their way to an ancient Greek temple, singing Frank Sinatra tunes at the top of their lungs. It was the most fun Theresa had had in a long time.

Antonio joined the women regularly throughout their trip. He innocently flirted with Theresa the whole time, and she allowed herself to flirt back. Margo, in the meantime, aided and abetted the relationship, finding excuses to leave Theresa and Antonio alone together for an hour here and there so they could get to know each other better.

After a few weeks, the women flew home to New York, and Theresa and Antonio continued to talk on the phone and text each other. Theresa went back to Sorrento to see Antonio the following fall and spent a month with him. He in turn flew to New York to visit her several times and even came to spend Christmas with her.

But here is the best part: when Theresa and Antonio are together, they often make love four times a day—and Theresa has even had orgasms when Antonio has merely touched her nipples! She's truly come alive again in a way she could never have imagined. In fact, she's more passionate and sensual now than she was at twenty. And she didn't need hormones to do it—she's never been on any hormone therapy of any kind. What brought her back to life was not only being in a new relationship, but also allowing herself to be a new woman.

An active and joyful sex life can have amazingly restorative effects on life force. And the good news is that you really don't need a partner. Start with yourself. For more on this, please read my book *Goddesses Never Age* (Hay House, 2015).

NITRIC OXIDE: THE MOLECULE OF LIFE FORCE AND PLEASURE

Back in 2005, I found a book on my shelf called *ESO: Extended Sexual Orgasm,* published in 1983. I went to Amazon to see if an updated version was available. It wasn't, but what *was* available was *The Illustrated Guide to Extended Massive Orgasm* (Hunter House, 2002), by Steve Bodansky, Ph.D., and Vera Bodansky, Ph.D. I figured that massive and extended was better than just plain old extended anyway. Amazon said that those people who'd ordered the Bodanskys' book had also ordered *Mama Gena's Owner's and Operator's Guide to Men* (Simon & Schuster, 2003) by Regena Thomashauer (a.k.a. Mama Gena). I couldn't figure out how they were related, but I bought both. The Bodanskys' book was an extraordinarily helpful tool for teaching individuals and couples to feel more pleasure, and it is beautifully illustrated. It is, in truth, a biofeedback manual for how to wake up your female erotic anatomy. Much to my surprise, I found that *Mama Gena's Owner's and Operator's Guide to Men* was based on the same principles in the Bodanskys' book. I later found out that Regena and the Bodanskys are friends and colleagues and have been collaborators for years. You can think of the Bodanskys' book as the medical text for the work, while Regena Thomashauer provides the laboratory for the work—how you take it out into the world and use it. I was so impressed with their work that I soon thereafter began teaching at the former Mama Gena's School of Womanly Arts in New York City, which closed in 2019 after two decades (although Regena plans to continue teaching in a new format in the future).

After attending a couple of sessions and doing some lectures, I observed that many of the women finishing Mama Gena's program seemed to be far happier than when they'd started. And I had a hunch that they were also getting healthier. I asked women who had experienced physical healings or improvements in health conditions to stand up and form a line. The line stretched to the back of the room as, one after another, women told me how they had healed from chronic pelvic pain, abnormal Pap tests, ovarian cysts, and even the symptoms of lupus. Thus I began to study pleasure as a health strategy.

About that time, I was introduced to the work of Ferid Murad, M.D., Ph.D., who won the Nobel Prize in Physiology or Medicine in 1998 for his work with nitric oxide. He and his colleague Edward Taub, M.D., had, in fact, written an entire book about the role of nitric oxide called *The Wellness Solution*. This raised the possibility of a link with pleasure, because the mechanism through which erection-enhancing drugs such as Viagra work is by increasing nitric oxide in the blood vessels of the penis, which increases blood flow.

From my observations at Mama Gena's and my own research, it soon became clear to me that the path of pleasure involved raising nitric oxide levels in both men and women. This fact was brought home to me very clearly during one of Regena's Men's Nights—an event in which men are invited to learn all about women in a very fun and festive setting. The husband of one of the participants, a man in his seventies, had had to use Viagra to get erections before his wife took Mama Gena's mastery course. But he no longer needed the drug because his wife had become so turned on by pleasure and by life that she was now turning *him* on without his having to take the drug.

Nitric oxide is a gas produced by the endothelial lining of

every blood vessel in the body as a result of healthful pleasures such as exercise, taking antioxidant vitamins, laughing, and having sex. In fact, orgasm can be thought of as a big burst of nitric oxide. Drs. Murad and Taub dubbed nitric oxide the molecule of the fountain of youth. Nitric oxide not only increases blood circulation, it's also an über-neurotransmitter that balances the levels of all other neurotransmitters, including serotonin, dopamine, and endorphin. Plus it also helps quell cellular inflammation, which is the root cause of most chronic degenerative diseases.

I was so fascinated by the connection between pleasure and nitric oxide that I wrote a small book called *The Secret Pleasures of Menopause* (Hay House, 2008) along with Drs. Murad and Taub. This little book tells the whole nitric oxide story, and along with its companion, *The Secret Pleasures of Menopause Playbook* (Hay House, 2009), it gives women all kinds of ideas for enhancing their levels of nitric oxide by deliberately pursuing pleasure in their lives.

Many foods and supplements also enhance nitric oxide production. One of my favorites is Cardio Miracle (see www .cardiomiracle.com). I also love the beet chews produced by HumanN, which increase nitric oxide (see www.humann.com).

Nothing illustrates the parallel circuitry between sexual energy and life energy better than the power of sexuality to heal when it is able to express itself freely. In *Reclaiming Goddess Sexuality: The Power of the Feminine Way* (Hay House, 1999), Linda Savage, Ph.D., writes about her experience of recovering from Crohn's disease, a chronic condition involving inflammation of the gastrointestinal tract that can result in weight loss, bloody stools, bloody diarrhea, and an increased risk of bowel cancer. Her weight had dropped to eighty pounds when she met a man with whom she began a very remarkable relationship. Within a few weeks all traces of her Crohn's were gone. She attributes her recovery entirely to the healing power of sexual energy, which is simply one of the many forms the life force takes.

This doesn't mean I'd recommend running right out and having sex in order to heal yourself of a disease. This doesn't work. Besides, sexual energy and its rejuvenating power don't even need to be connected with the act of having physical sex with someone. The only way sexual energy can act as a healing force is if you experience it in the context of an unconditionally loving relationship in which your body, your soul, and your psyche are all cherished by another—or by yourself. *Remember, you do not have to have a partner to experience the rejuvenating energy of your own sexuality. You simply have to realize that your body was created from sexual energy and is also rejuvenated by it.*

With all this in mind, it is also important to remember that as a woman traverses the perimenopausal transition and all the changes it invites, her libido may seem to go underground for a time, while she reprioritizes her life and the manner in which she uses her energy on a day-to-day basis. This is a perfectly normal diversion of life energy— an investment that can yield great dividends—but it is only temporary. There is no reason for a diminished sex drive to become a permanent feature in the life of a menopausal woman. As a matter of fact, the work of the late sex researcher Gina Ogden, Ph.D., found that it is women in their sixties and seventies who are having the best sex of their lives. My own personal experience and that of many of my friends absolutely bear this out.

MIDLIFE CHANGES IN SEXUAL FUNCTION

All of the following changes in sexual function have been as-sociated with perimenopause. Reading through the list, you can quickly appreciate that change itself—and not the nature of the change—is one common theme.

~ Increased sexual desire
~ Change in sexual orientation
~ Decreased sexual activity
~ Vaginal dryness and loss of vaginal elasticity
~ Pain or burning with intercourse
~ Decreased clitoral sensitivity
~ Increased clitoral sensitivity
~ Decreased responsiveness
~ Increased responsiveness
~ Fewer orgasms, decreased depth of orgasm
~ Increase in orgasms, sexual awakening

SEXUALITY AT MENOPAUSE:
OUR CULTURAL INHERITANCE

Like it or not, our sexuality has been, and continues to be, influenced by a male-dominated culture with an inherent double standard. In a bestselling book I read a while back on how to slow the aging process, it was reported that the quality of a man's sex life and its purported effect on his health were determined solely and meticulously by his annual number of orgasms—with a figure over 300 being considered the most healthful. (Though this is slightly off topic, I feel compelled to tell you that orgasm and ejaculation in men are two separate things. Master Mantak Chia, a world-renowned teacher of the Universal Healing Tao system of sexual health and energy, points out that a man's health [especially as he gets older] is greatly enhanced when he limits his ejaculations—but not his orgasms [www .mantakchia.com].)

Yet when it came to women, the author of this book never even bothered to tabulate or quantify how many orgasms a year could promote longevity. We women got points only for being "satisfied with quantity and happy with quality" of orgasms. Happily, the data on women are starting to catch up to the data on men!

Still, the double standard is also apparent in the fact that men can buy Viagra at any of hundreds of internet sites without seeing a doctor, while women still can't get birth control pills anywhere without a doctor's visit and a prescription. There are even television ads addressed to the one-third of men who allegedly suffer from erectile dysfunction, letting them know they can buy themselves a cure in the perfect form: take a pill and get a reliable erection without having to connect your heart with your penis in any way. It's no wonder the most notorious side effect of this medication is sudden cardiac arrest. The other black box warning associated with erectile dysfunction drugs is unilateral blindness—which happens because when blood flow is suddenly diverted to the penis, it leaves the tiny retinal vessels vulnerable and without enough pressure to keep them open and functional. As you might imagine, when I share this fact with people, I get a lot of comments like "I guess they were right about going blind if I . . ."

Along those same lines of phallocentric reasoning, I once read about an ongoing study testing Premarin vaginal cream as a kind of "female Viagra" for women whose husbands are already on Viagra.

The premise is that women's sex drive decreases at midlife because of vaginal thinning and dryness. Inserting Premarin cream in the vagina, the researchers posit, would result in a reestrogenization of the vagina, making the experience of sex more comfortable for the woman (who, we assume, is already having intercourse regularly with a Viagra-enhanced penis). This is like reducing the vagina and female sexuality to a runway that requires de-icing for the plane to be able to take off more comfortably. For most women, sexual desire is related to far more than the estrogenic state of the vagina (though estrogen cream has been found to help some women).[20] That said, however, there is no question that enhanced lubrication of the vagina can be associated with the return of optimal sexual functioning (see "Awakening the Goddess Within" box).

I am reminded that our word *vagina* is derived from the Latin word meaning "sheath for a sword." It would appear that we have not come very far in this respect since the ancient Romans. Too many women still see female sexuality predominantly in terms of how well our bodies meet and satisfy the needs and desires of males, rather than ourselves. Although this is changing, that attitude and the beliefs associated with it make their way into every aspect of our lives, including the medical research upon which women's health treatments are based.

In a study entitled "Vaginal Changes and Sexuality in Women with a History of Cervical Cancer," the authors note that women who had been treated for cervical cancer experienced changes in their vaginal anatomy and function that had negative effects on their sexual function, including decreased lubrication, decreased elasticity, and decreased genital swelling during arousal. The authors said that the women experiencing these changes reported them to be "distressing," and then went on to make the following observation:

> Although numerous studies have documented the distress associated with the loss of a breast, changes in the vagina have been neglected in this respect. A [literature] search performed in mid-1998 with the combined terms "cancer," "breast," and "distress" yielded 197 references. In contrast, a search in which the term "vagina" was substituted for "breast" yielded only 2 references. One might assume that vaginal changes would affect sexual function at least as much as the loss of a breast. An obvious reason for the predominant interest in the breast is that, in developed countries, breast cancer is more common than cancer of

the female genital organs. Nevertheless, the paucity of literature on the effect of vaginal changes is noteworthy, and it may not be irrelevant to speculate about nonscientific reasons. For men, female breasts have aesthetic as well as sexual value, which may influence research policies in academic medicine, where male investigators predominate.[21]

Identifying and Awakening Your Female Erogenous Anatomy

Women are, by design, orgasmatrons—capable of far more sexual pleasure at any age than we've been led to believe. We have as much erogenous erectile tissue as men do. It's just that it's mostly on the inside. And, unfortunately, the full extent of this anatomy and how to stimulate it is virtually unknown, even to most gynecologists! I am eternally grateful to registered nurse and midwife Sheri Winston, author of *Women's Anatomy of Arousal: Secret Maps to Buried Pleasure* (Mango Garden Press, 2009), for her work in waking women up to the fullness of their erotic potential. The first step toward awakening this potential is knowing where it is. (See Figure 14, on page 389.)

Let's start with the clitoris. This organ has 8,000 nerve endings whose sole function is pleasure. And it's connected to the so-called G-spot (Grafenberg spot, or what I often call the sacred spot, the term used in the tantric yoga tradition) by a rich network of nerves that run throughout the pelvis. I like to think of the clitoris as the north pole and the G-spot as the south pole. The G-spot is connected to the pineal gland—the seat of the soul—via an energetic pathway known as a *nadi*. No wonder sexuality and spirituality are so intimately connected.

When you stimulate the G-spot, you are actually stimulating your connection to your soul and spirit. You can stimulate both the sacred spot and the clitoris together. But know this: if a woman has had a history of sexual abuse, stimulation of the sacred spot may well be incredibly painful at first, or the spot may be numb. A woman can awaken this area and work through the pain with loving massage from a partner or from herself. Over time, the pain and numbness will leave, and she will feel exquisite pleasure. And since the sacred spot is also connected to the glands that result in the female ejaculate, a woman may experience female ejaculation

FIGURE 14: THE CLITORAL SYSTEM

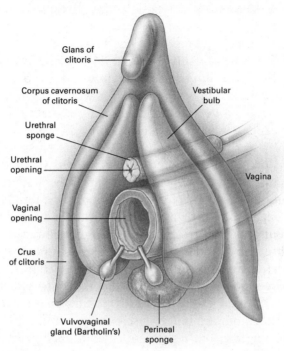

Glans of clitoris

Corpus cavernosum of clitoris

Vestibular bulb

Urethral sponge

Urethral opening

Vaginal opening

Vagina

Crus of clitoris

Vulvovaginal gland (Bartholin's)

Perineal sponge

as well. It is well worth the time and effort required to awaken this area, because once you do, you will begin to realize that you can trust this area of your body to guide you toward what is life-giving and away from those things that are not. In other words, your female erotic anatomy becomes a kind of GPS toward life force. In the former Mama Gena's School of Womanly Arts, Regena Thomashauer used to call this "being in your pussy." She expounds upon this in her book *Pussy: A Reclamation* (Hay House, 2016). I know that word is very difficult for many people to hear, let alone say. But I certainly appreciate where Regena is coming from—and her work has been liberating for women all over the world. The curriculum of her school taught women how to feel and inhabit this most essential part of their bodies and use it as a guidance system. And trust me, it works. Your female erotic anatomy will always guide you toward what is most life-affirming (eros) and away from what is deadening (thanatos).

AWAKENING THE GODDESS WITHIN

I recently had the pleasure of doing a Facebook Live session with Denise Linn, who has been a renowned spiritual teacher for decades, runs a mystery school for women, does past-life healings, and for years taught women's sexuality classes. I sent her some of my company's *Pueraria mirifica* vaginal moisturizer to try. After she and her clients had used it for several months, she told me that she wished she had had a product like this during the years that she was teaching women about their erotic anatomy. She told me that both she and her clients found that the product not only rejuvenated the vaginal area and restored moisture but also had a profound effect on libido. Better yet, after a couple months of regular use, her clients no longer needed to keep using it. The *Pueraria mirifica* and other ingredients in the moisturizer somehow "turned on" a woman's goddess nature and enhanced her libido and innate lusciousness—and once turned on, they remained on, regardless of continued product use. Denise said it has been an absolute game-changer. Hearing this kind of feedback has been very gratifying for me, knowing that my efforts in creating this product can assist so many women with remembering their goddess selves and their innate sensuality and sexuality.

Overcoming Cultural Barriers: The First Step Toward Waking a Sleeping Libido

Although progress is being made, change in our culture's attitude about women and sexuality is slow in coming, and many women have never felt as though they had permission to explore their own sexual energy on their own terms. In *Reclaiming Goddess Sexuality,* Dr. Savage writes:

[Women] want the beauty of the context of sexual encounters to be more important than the act. They want to be touched in slow, sensual ways. They want to be ravished with intense passion that demonstrates how much their partners need them, rather than just needing an orgasm to relax. All in all, women want to be adored as precious feminine beings.[22]

The fact that this need is incompletely met for so many women in our culture is what drives the multimillion-dollar romance novel industry, with books that have increasingly explicit and very erotic sexual content. Many women are absolutely addicted to these stories (which a friend of mine calls "cliterature"), because they invariably show women being adored for who they are, not just for their bodies. Novelist Isabel Allende writes that the G-spot is in the ears and that anyone who looks for it anywhere else won't find it. I so agree. Women fall in love through words and being talked to!

LORI: *What I Did for Love*

Over the years, Lori had become gradually aware that her sex life with her husband, Roy, was not meeting her needs. "There was never any cuddling, caressing, nothing to get me in the mood. And he wanted it at least once a day—the harder his day had gone at work, the more he needed it. For him it was a tension reliever. For me it had become mechanical and pretty much unsatisfying." With the help of a marriage counselor, Roy became aware of Lori's needs, and together they learned techniques that opened up a whole new world for them both. "The sex became great," Lori wrote. But Roy's needs for regular "pressure release" after work didn't go away, and to engage in that sort of sex seemed to Lori like a step backward. "To be honest, it made me mad," she reported. "I felt like screaming, 'Haven't you been listening?'" Their counselor, in subsequent sessions, led Lori to believe that to be in a fair partnership, she must be willing to meet Roy's needs, too.

Generally speaking, Lori's counselor was correct. All couples must learn how to negotiate each other's needs, and sex is no different from any other area of need. But there were parts of Lori and Roy's story that deeply concerned me when I first spoke to Lori, who came to see me about hormone replacement at the age of forty-five, when she started skipping periods.

I wanted to be sure Lori didn't believe that it was her "job" to relieve Roy's tension and stress by allowing her body to be used in this way every day. I validated her anger at this and told her that it was her barometer, letting her know that the problem it signaled was real and needed to be addressed. Second, I suggested that when an individual needs that much sex to medicate his (or her) stress, something is wrong in his (or her) life. I asked if their therapist had suggested that Roy examine his life, his job, and his stress levels. Lori said that she had raised this in therapy but had been told that this was an individual issue, not a couples issue. Since Roy had refused individual therapy, there was nothing further she could say on this subject during their sessions.

This is a perfect example of what can happen when couples therapy goes awry. Fully 96 percent of all couples therapy involving heterosexual relationships is initiated by the woman, who usually holds it over her husband's head as a last-ditch effort to save the marriage. He goes in, usually reluctantly, often feeling, "It's her problem, but I'll go along," and unable or unwilling to understand that his own issues are part of the couple's dynamic.

Candidly, many therapists have told me that if the man's issues were addressed directly, he'd be sufficiently uncomfortable that he'd probably terminate therapy altogether. So the therapist tries to keep him engaged with so-called couples issues. Too often, the woman's individual concerns also get subverted to the needs of the "couple." This kind of therapy can go on for years, relieving the relationship tension just enough so that the couple stays together, while the fundamental power dynamic of the relationship never changes because key individual behaviors never change. When this happens, there's no chance for the transformational power of true partnership. And far too often, the person who is blaming their partner and who doesn't want to go to therapy is actually a narcissist who is never going to change. This is a subject I've covered thoroughly in my book *Dodging Energy Vampires: An Empath's Guide to Evading Relationships That Drain You and Restoring Your Health and Power* (Hay House, 2018).

To create a true partnership, Roy needed to see that he was using Lori sexually as an opiate, to medicate himself for stress. There was no way Lori could have a sense of true communion or of being cherished by him as long as stress relief was the main energy driving his lovemaking. Though it would be perfectly reasonable for them to compromise with a "quickie" now and again, for Roy to make a daily pattern of using sex to self-medicate for stress sounded like sexual addiction and dysfunction to me. It was certainly undermining Lori's ability to feel good about their sexual relationship. Roy needed to take responsibility for his own stress reduction needs, and he needed a wider repertoire of behaviors to accomplish this. This might include exercise, meditation, or even self-pleasuring. Though wives have been expected to carry out their "wifely duty" in this way for centuries and have acquiesced for fear that their husbands might go elsewhere to "get their needs met," there is no place for these assumptions today if a couple is to reach the joyful communion that's possible at midlife. I might also add that self-pleasuring is a completely natural and normal way for people to get their individual sexual needs met, even for those people who are in a sexual relationship.

At the time of her next annual exam, Lori told me that over the past year Roy had begun to realize he needed to change his job if he didn't want to follow in the footsteps of his father, who had died at age sixty, only one year after retiring from a job he had hated. He had also found several ways of achieving stress reduction, including going to twice-weekly yoga classes and joining a basketball league at work. Thanks to these changes, Roy's blood pressure and cholesterol dropped to normal, and he began to feel better about himself, knowing that he had been able to assert this kind of control over his life and free himself of the pattern that had probably helped bring about his father's premature death. Once Lori saw that he had become more emotionally self-sufficient, she found him more sexually attractive—to the point that she was actually initiating sex.

What Viagra Tells Us About Our Sexuality

Viagra and the enormous publicity surrounding it speak volumes about the values of our culture. There is no question that Viagra and related drugs such as Cialis can be a boon to quality of life for many couples in which the male partner suffers from erectile dysfunction. (Note, however, that these drugs have been linked with an increase in a condition called ischemic optic neuropathy, which leads to vision loss. In October 2005, Public Citizen petitioned the FDA to immediately require a black box warning on the labels for each of the three erectile dysfunction drugs. If your partner relies on these drugs, take heart—there are all kinds of ways to treat erectile dysfunction with nutrition, herbs, and exercise.) There are also other ways to enjoy sexual fulfillment besides intercourse. Enhanced sexual performance through medical manipulation of the male's genitals only cannot heal a relationship that needs more love and attention or may need to end.

Our culture is quick to forget the holistic nature of sexual function and how profoundly it is enhanced when a couple is truly connected via their hearts and minds. It is well documented, for example, that the excitement and plateau phase of the sexual response can be prolonged if the connection between the man and woman is not only genital but also related to heart and mind. In fact, both men and women are capable of experiencing far more sexual pleasure and fulfillment than most currently enjoy. A first step toward experiencing this pleasure is knowing that it's possible and health-enhancing.[23] At midlife many couples find that they have the time and the desire to be fully present to each other in this way, and as a result they experience the best sex of their lives. This is in part because older, more experienced women tend not to be as inhibited as when they were younger. They know their bodies better. I've heard their stories repeatedly in my office. But for some, making love is just another task on the to-do list. Sex therapist Patricia Love, Ed.D., wrote:

> Sensuality—the ability to be comfortable in one's body, suspend time, and communicate through the skin—is what is missing in many marriages. . . . All too often husbands and wives go to bed feeling distracted and numb, reflexively groping for each other's genitals. The unspoken goal is to go from neutral to orgasm in fifteen minutes, like a car zooming from zero to sixty.[24]

This results in what sex therapists call "spectatoring," which is a mental disconnection during lovemaking, thinking more about work or household chores than about the partner beside you. For the man, this may translate to erectile difficulties; for the woman, difficulty reaching orgasm. The man who looks first to Viagra to "save" him may be discounting the importance of making a deeper connection with himself and his lover. A woman involved with a man who feels he needs Viagra for psychogenic impotence would be wise to ask herself about the quality of their connection. Those things that remain unspoken between them, the issues and feelings that are too uncomfortable to talk about, may be blocking full erection and orgasm, and may also be putting their health at risk in other areas.

GINNY: *Victor and Viagra*

Ginny and Victor had been married for thirty years and had a pretty happy relationship. Victor had always prided himself on his virility, and he and Ginny had enjoyed a vigorous sex life for years, making love about three times per week. When he turned fifty-five, however, Victor noticed that his erections were not as hard as they used to be, and it sometimes took him longer to achieve them. Occasionally he even found that he was unable to sustain an erection long enough to bring Ginny to orgasm. He and Ginny had gradually slowed down in their lovemaking to about once every two weeks. This didn't bother Ginny, particularly because she was very busy starting a new catering business—something she'd always dreamed of. Her business was taking off, and now that their youngest child had left home for college, her life was no longer focused solely on the needs of her husband and children. But Victor, who was planning to retire in a year or two, was not nearly as happy with his life. It seemed that just as he was starting to slow down, Ginny was taking off in the outside world.

Victor sought a consultation with his doctor, who prescribed Viagra. Victor was elated with the results. Ginny wasn't. The Viagra introduced a "mechanical" element to their sex life that had never been present before. She didn't like having to be sexually available just because Victor had taken his pill, and she began to spend more and more time away from home, partly because she was having so much fun at work, partly because she didn't want to have sex "on demand." When asked how she felt about Viagra, Ginny replied, "I think we were better off without it. I love Victor and it really didn't bother me when it took him a little longer to get hard. I usually knew how to help. Now I feel as though a vital emotional component of our lovemaking has been replaced by a pill." Ginny, like so many other women, also needs to own her ability to "be the party." What I mean by that is that she needs to learn how to consciously seek pleasure and joy in her life, regardless of what Victor is doing. I watched the results of this in the women who, along with me, took the Mama Gena's School of Womanly Arts Mastery Program in New York City. As we learned about the deliberate pursuit of pleasure (and its effect on our female erotic anatomy), we all became far less dependent upon the men in our lives and instead learned an incredibly valuable lesson: that when you finally see yourself as the source of your own pleasure and fulfillment, the men in your life (or those who identify with a more *yang* polarity) quite naturally gravitate toward you and enjoy fulfilling your needs. This doesn't happen as long as you're unhappy and complaining (no matter how justified those complaints might be).

Ginny and Victor's situation is not unusual. Victor's change in sexual function is, in part, related to his sense of decreasing power in the outer world, even though it is his own choice to retire from work.

Though Viagra is probably a relatively safe solution for him for a time, I would strongly recommend that he also find a new life's purpose into which to pour his energy. Otherwise he won't be able to keep up with his wife, in the bedroom or otherwise, without resorting to a drug for support. That doesn't mean there aren't valid indications for Viagra. Rather, it is to point out that sexual function is related to much more than the size and duration of an erection. There is also a great deal that men can do to improve their health, circulation, and erectile function. Exercise, an inflammation-reducing diet, and a good supplementation program are the first places to start.

MENOPAUSE IS A TIME TO REDEFINE AND UPDATE OUR RELATIONSHIPS

Before the first edition of this book, I would have written all of this while thinking it did not apply to me. Similarly, many of you may be thinking, "That's interesting, but my relationship with my significant other is good," and you may be right overall. For many of us, the relationships we have maintained over the years have served us well and have been mutually beneficial, even passionate. But it is very often necessary to renegotiate some of the terms of the old relationship as you enter the transformative years of midlife. No matter how good that relationship may have been, what worked for you in your "previous" life will, in all likelihood, need some updating in order to serve the person you are becoming.

One area in which the necessity for change may become apparent is in the waning of a woman's libido. Just as wild animals refuse to breed in captivity unless everything is in balance in their environment, a woman and her significant other may notice problems in their sexual intimacy if their relationship is in need of rebalancing. Menopause is also a time when what a woman wants from a relationship begins to change. And that change has to start with her relationship with herself.

As we have seen, it has usually been the woman who sacrifices career and personal growth for the sake of maintaining and nurturing the family, even if she works full-time outside the home. Not only the unwritten rules of society but also the hormones flowing through her veins encourage her to give high priority to family, nurturing, nesting, and protection of loved ones. At menopause the hormonal changes are only part of a woman's ongoing transformation, which begins at an energetic level and triggers changes not only in her biology but also in her perception, intuition, neural pathways, emotions, creative drive, and overall focus. While she spends the first half of her life giving birth to others (literally and figuratively), everything about her menopausal transition suggests that the second half of life is when she is meant to give birth to herself.

If, through the lens of your transforming self, you discover that you are not in love with your life, your libido may suffer as a result. The same thing may happen if you've given too much of yourself away in your relationship. In fact, a fading sex drive may be one of the first places a red flag will pop up, as a signal of a fading love of life—a waning life force. Only if both you and your significant other are willing to question what is no longer viable in your relationship and work together on the necessary remodeling can you open the door to rejuvenation of your life energy and the rekindling of your passion, sexual and otherwise. Healing will require a bilateral effort—both you and your partner must be willing to ask, and hear the answers to, some difficult questions in order to restore and renew your relationship.

Terminal Busyness Leads to Exhaustion and Waning Libido

Someone sent me the following anonymous posting from the internet. This one paragraph summarizes the plight of many midlife women—and the difference between their lives and those of their husbands.

Mom and Dad were watching TV when Mom said, "I'm tired, and it's getting late. I think I'll go to bed." She went to the kitchen to make sandwiches for the next day's lunches, rinsed out the popcorn bowls, took meat out of the freezer for supper the following evening, checked the cereal box levels, filled the sugar container, put spoons and bowls on the table, and started the coffeepot for brewing the next morning. She then put some wet clothes into the dryer, put a load of clothes into the wash, ironed a shirt, and secured a loose button. She picked up the newspapers strewn on the floor, picked up the game pieces left on the table, and put the telephone book back into the drawer. She watered the plants, emptied a wastebasket, and hung up a towel to dry. She yawned and stretched and headed for the bedroom. She stopped by the desk and wrote a note to the teacher, counted out some cash for the field trip, and pulled a textbook out from hiding under the chair. She signed a birthday card for a friend, addressed and stamped the envelope, and wrote a quick note for the grocery store. She put both near her purse. Mom then creamed her face, put on moisturizer, brushed and flossed her teeth, and trimmed her nails. Hubby called, "I thought you were going to bed."

"I'm on my way," she said. She put some water into the dog's dish and put the cat outside, then made sure the doors were locked. She looked in on each of the kids and turned out a bedside lamp, hung up a shirt, threw some dirty socks in the hamper, and had a brief conversation with the one still up doing homework. In her own room, she set the alarm, laid out clothing for the next day, and straightened up the shoe rack. She added three things to her list of things to do for tomorrow.

About that time, the hubby turned off the TV and announced to no one in particular, "I'm going to bed," and he did.

MARY: Overcare and Burnout Send Libido Underground

Mary was a registered nurse. As the eldest of five children from an Irish Catholic family, she had always been expected to take care of her parents and younger siblings. When her mother died suddenly, Mary's alcoholic father, a man in the early stages of dementia, came to live with Mary and her husband, Jeff, a police officer. Despite having four siblings, Mary had never questioned her role as the designated family caregiver. But the increased need for "alone time" so many women experience at menopause led Mary to feel not only a total loss of sexual desire, but also complete emotional burnout. She had recently been diagnosed with hypothyroidism and was suffering from weight gain, depression, lethargy, fatigue, dry skin, and the desire to sleep all the time. Though her family doctor had prescribed thyroid hormone replacement, Mary saw little improvement in her depression. And despite normal estrogen, progesterone, and testosterone levels, her sexual desire remained nonexistent.

When a woman is experiencing caregiver's burnout, her body is often, quite literally, running on empty. She may have insufficient levels of many nutrients, such as the B vitamins and magnesium, which contribute to her fatigue. And her adrenal glands may be producing too much adrenaline and either too much cortisol or, after years and years of unabated stress without replenishment, too little cortisol. Either way, the end result is physical exhaustion. Sleep, not sex, is what women like Mary find themselves fantasizing about. Interestingly, sleep is often the best way to restore hormonal balance.

I prescribed a program for Mary that focused on her rejuvenation from the inside out. I told her that she needed to get help at home at least two days per week. She also needed to improve her eating habits, cutting way back on refined carbohydrates such as cakes, candy, and cookies and increasing her intake of protein, essential fatty acids, and fresh fruits and vegetables. I also suggested a high-potency multivitamin and told her she needed to go to bed by ten o'clock every night and get at least eight hours of sleep per night— preferably ten! Mary had known all along that her life needed to change, but, she told me, she was relieved to finally have a medical authority supporting her in the changes she would have to make if she was going to resume optimal functioning—which would include the rekindling of her libido. If she didn't stem the chronic draining of her life force by getting adequate rest, exercise, and nutrition, then her libido, like every other aspect of her health, would pay the price. It's too bad that so many women who have taken on the caretaker role need a doctor's "prescription" to give them permission to live more healthfully.

DOROTHY: *Grief, Instant Menopause, and Loss of Libido*

Dorothy and her husband, John, had a solid marriage and a good sex life. They had two children, a girl who was ten and a boy who was five. John was employed as a lawyer, and Dorothy enjoyed teaching at a local university. Everything suddenly changed when their son tragically died in a car accident. Dorothy was thirty-nine at the time. The stress of this loss led to premature menopause and a twenty-pound weight gain—the direct effect of the excess cortisol produced under stress. Her abject grief also caused her to lose all interest in intimacy with her husband. She became "cold and distant," she said. "I was completely shut down and unable to tolerate my husband's touch or his need for mine."

Dorothy just couldn't seem to dig herself out of the depths of her despair, and being intimate with her husband was simply too much for her. Meanwhile, John, who was also grieving, now had to grieve the loss of intimacy with his wife, something that had always been a great source of joy and comfort to him. Eventually, as happens so often in cases like this, the couple divorced and went their separate ways.

Over the next decade, Dorothy was finally able to appreciate what had happened to her—and to her libido. Better yet, she and John were able to forgive each other and move on in their lives. They each eventually remarried other people but still remain friends.

Dorothy's experience is not uncommon. When stress levels and subsequent cortisol levels are high, oxytocin levels tend to fall, and anything pleasurable—including sex—becomes a burden instead of a joy. This can tank a marriage unless both members of the couple realize what is going on. Most women find it more difficult than do most men to compartmentalize their grief. It spills over into every aspect of their lives. Over time—and, often, with the right kind of therapy—the acute grief subsides and oxytocin levels return. But it can take some conscious effort to, as Dorothy put it, "return to the land of the living." It takes patience, compassion, and forgiveness, but it is possible. So if this story resonates with you, take heart. This needn't last forever.

HORMONE LEVELS ARE ONLY
ONE PART OF LIBIDO

One of my colleagues underwent a hysterectomy (uterus removed, ovaries left intact) at the age of forty-eight, a procedure that is associated with measurable declines in estrogen and testosterone because the surgery compromises the blood supply to the ovaries. This is the reason given for the fact that many women experience some sexual problems following hysterectomy. But my colleague, who had started a new relationship just prior to her surgery, couldn't wait to get out of the hospital and back into bed with her new love. She told me, "When you have someone waiting for you whom you're madly in love with, you can bet you're not likely to have much problem with desire or lubrication, or anything else." And that is exactly what research shows. On the other hand, if you are in a relationship that has been problematic for years, a relationship in which you have had little or no interest in sex (perhaps because you didn't know how to get your sexual needs met) but put up with it anyway, you can bet that your body will do anything it can to keep you from having to get back into that position again. It is well documented, for instance, that unassertive women in dysfunctional sexual partnerships experience limited genital arousal and few if any orgasms. Sexually assertive women, on the other hand, report higher levels of sexual desire, orgasmic frequency, and greater satisfaction with both their sexual and marital relationships.[25]

Sexual impulses and desire are controlled, in part, by the frontal lobes of the brain, and anything that changes frontal lobe activity can affect libido—in either direction. Frontal lobes are areas of the brain involved in choosing and directing conscious thought. Frontal lobes can also inhibit unbridled desire, channeling it into socially appropriate behavior. In the frontal lobe dysfunction known as depression, libido is often decreased. But in the frontal lobe dysfunction known as dementia, sexual impulses can run rampant, sometimes resulting in socially embarrassing behavior. An example of this is a nun I once treated who had developed an uncontrollable urge to masturbate all the time. Although she was not distressed by this, her community was. She eventually ended up under the care of a neurologist, for dementia.

Changes in libido can, of course, be triggered by declining hormone levels, especially in women who have undergone medical or surgical menopause.[26] In my professional experience, however, fading life force is equally likely, if not more so, to be at the root of declining sexual desire. Two influences are universally underestimated in terms of their potential impact on libido: the state of a woman's relationship with her sexual partner, and her overall emotional and spiritual love for life. And, interestingly, both of these factors may well have the potential to change hormone levels in and of themselves.[27]

A woman with a strong current of life force, who is in love with her life, who feels sexy, and who knows how to turn herself on, can continue to have a strong libido regardless of what her hormones are doing. This fact is supported by research that shows that the hormonal changes of menopause, per se, are not the cause of decreased libido. In fact, the relationship between hormones and libido may be a chicken-and-egg question, as it seems equally plausible for a faltering life force to be the result, rather than the cause, of a dying sex life.

The late researcher and sex therapist Gina Ogden, Ph.D., has shown in her landmark sex survey Integrating Sexuality and Spirituality (ISIS) that not only is sex not just physical, it's not even mostly physical. When women in the ISIS survey described sexual pleasure and ecstasy, Dr. Ogden reported, they used some 5,000 words from the emotional and spiritual realm (such as *love* or *connection*), while they mentioned their genitals only twenty-three times. "Another finding that tells me sex researchers have been asking the wrong questions," she noted. In her book *The Heart and Soul of Sex: Making the ISIS Connection* (Trumpeter, 2006), Dr. Ogden reported that 47 percent of women say they have experienced God during sexual ecstasy, and 67 percent say sex needs to be spiritual to be satisfying. This is not surprising, given that one of the many regions of women's brains that show activity during orgasm is the pineal gland, the region connected with religious ecstasy and spiritual experiences.

Therefore, I want to encourage every woman to consider the health and vitality of her connection with life—her connection to Source energy—along with the more conventionally accepted hormonal issues as she evaluates her sex life and the possibility that it may need help at this stage of her life. I also encourage every woman to update her thoughts about her sexual desirability. It's important to think of yourself as sexy and desirable, even though you may not even be in a relationship right now. Remember, the vibrational quality of our thoughts creates a magnetic field around us that attracts our circumstances to us. A woman who is tapped into Source energy has the power to transform her body-mind-spirit and sexual experience starting with how she feels about herself.

SECONDARY LIBIDINAL SUPPORT: ESTROGEN, PROGESTERONE, AND HERBS

With all that said, it is possible for a woman to experience a fading libido during and after menopause even if she is involved in a true partnership, one that supports her life force rather than drains it. If a woman is in love with her life, if her life force—a repository for sexual energy—is free-flowing and vigorous, then a weakening libido may be due to secondary, hormonal, or nutritional factors. Factors such as hysterectomy, ovarian removal (or decreased ovarian function), and premature menopause (before age forty) may also have an adverse effect on hormone balance.[28]

As we learn more about the roles of estrogen and progesterone in the maintenance of bodywide functions such as circulation, nerve transmission, and cell division, it becomes clear how declining levels of these hormones may contribute to changes in sexual response in some women.[29]

~ The entire nervous system is surrounded with estrogen-sensitive cells.[30] It stands to reason, then, that a decrease in estradiol levels can have a dampening effect on nerve transmission during sex for some women. Research has shown that estrogen deprivation can lead to actual peripheral neuropathy—a form of nerve dysfunction that makes a woman less sensitive to touch and vibration. Estradiol replacement and/or herbs such as maca or *Pueraria mirifica* can restore this sensitivity to levels that approach those seen in women who are still menstruating.

~ Declining levels of estradiol and progesterone can have an effect on a woman's potential for sexual arousal, sensitivity, sensation, and orgasm, because at optimal levels these hormones increase the flow of blood to the sexually sensitive areas. In other words, a woman's physical response to sexual stimulation may be slower and less likely to build to orgasm because of decreased speed and volume of blood supply to the sexually sensitive areas, which may in any case be less sensitive than before because of the nerve dysfunction sometimes caused by estrogen deprivation.[31] It is also completely possible to learn how to maximize sensation in these areas by consciously spending time learning how to pleasure oneself through genital stimulation.

~ Estrogen levels that are too low can lead to cell atrophy in the genital region, which can cause thinning of the vaginal and urethral tissue, with the result that intercourse becomes painful. Women with estrogen depletion may also experience urinary problems such as recurrent urinary tract infections or even stress urinary incontinence.

~ Vaginal fluid production during sexual arousal and intercourse may be an estrogen-dependent process, although the experience of many perimenopausal women is that this fluid production is also very related to how turned on one is with one's sexual partner.

But if estrogen is low, there may be a reduction of vaginal fluid, resulting in vaginal dryness and painful intercourse. Because a woman's level of sexual arousal tends to be judged by the amount and ease of vaginal lubrication achieved, lack of vaginal fluid can lead to the perception that she has low sexual arousal. While sexual arousal may be negatively influenced by the anticipation of pain, libido is not the real issue in these circumstances. Because of the powerful mind-body connection, some women can teach their bodies to lubricate well just by turning themselves on.

~ Progesterone has additional effects on libido that have not been as well studied as those of estrogen but are no less important. Its effect seems largely to be one of maintenance, valuable in keeping a woman's existing libido from declining. Moreover, as a precursor of estrogen and testosterone, progesterone is important for maintaining high enough levels of these other hormones for optimal sexual pleasure. A normal balance of progesterone also acts as a mood stabilizer and supports normal thyroid function, thereby enhancing the libido both emotionally and metabolically.

The bottom line is this: a deficiency of estrogen and/or progesterone can decrease a woman's libido by orchestrating physical changes that, quite simply, make the sex act less pleasurable. Dryness and thinning of the vaginal wall can result in physical discomfort during intercourse, as can vaginal muscle spasms. Changes in nerve function can numb ordinarily sensitive body parts, and changes in blood circulation can decrease the physical response when stimulation occurs, making it ever more difficult to reach orgasm.

Research has shown that libido-dampening effects are most likely to occur when a woman's blood levels of estradiol (our body's most biologically potent natural estrogen) drop below 50 pmol/l. Salivary estradiol levels can also be used, with 1 pg/ml being the lower end of the threshold for normal sexual function.[32] Blood flow to the vulva and vagina is dramatically increased when supplementation brings estradiol back to these levels, and often this is enough to restore sexual response.

With some assistance, achieving this level is simple. Depending on the individual woman, a transdermal estradiol patch (usually the 0.1 mg strength) or 0.5 to 1 mg oral estradiol taken twice daily is adequate, gentle, and consistent in restoring estradiol levels to that comfortable threshold. And in the early stages of perimenopause, when many women have declines in progesterone levels but estrogen levels that are still within the normal range, ¼ teaspoon of natural progesterone cream massaged into the hands or soft skin twice a day can have a restorative effect on a subtle downturn in libido.

Vaginal estrogen also works well, even for women who are already on HT.[33] While the FDA initially required boxed warnings on these products, the most recent research shows that low-dose vaginal estrogen does not increase risk of heart disease, stroke, blood clots, and cancer and that these products are safe for women.[34] As a result, the North American Menopause Society has called for a removal of such warnings. (The use of high-strength vaginal estrogen creams, on the other hand, should be limited to four weeks.) An ultra-low-dose softgel vaginal insert called Imvexxy (which is available in two strengths) entered the market in 2019. (See https://imvexxyhcp.com for more information about this product.)

It isn't always necessary to rely on a prescription drug for this assistance, however. A recent twelve-week clinical trial that involved postmenopausal women from around the country looked at three groups—women who used currently marketed vaginal estrogen tablets plus placebo vaginal gel, those who took placebo vaginal tablets plus a currently marketed vaginal moisturizer gel, and those who took placebo tablets plus a placebo gel.[35] The results were similar in all three groups, meaning the prescription preparations performed no better than placebo. This is interesting to me not so much because it showed the estrogen products didn't perform any better than placebo gel (since we know estrogen does give better results in longer-term studies) but because it showed that at least in short-term use, nonprescription gel works just as well. In fact, my *Pueraria mirifica* gel very often restores both vaginal moisture and libido. (The pill form also works well; take 80–100 mg twice per day.) Here's what one user wrote to me about this:

> I've always seen myself as very intuitive and empathic. But I was out of touch with what I could call my inner self up until a few years ago. I suffered from anxiety, didn't exercise, and had no sex drive. I was just plain shut down after a lifelong career in healthcare. I guess you could say that I was burned out.
>
> But I finally did enough inner work to discover who I really am, and I then understood something had to change or I would be headed for some kind of illness. I changed my diet, started reading inspirational books, and started to meditate. Now I am spiritually awakened, happy, abundant, and in excellent health. I also have to thank you for your Amata products—both for me and my husband. We are having the best sex we have ever had, and that has spilled over into every other area of our lives. My husband is a new man, and our lives and our marriage are better than ever.

LASER OR THERMAL TREATMENTS FOR VAGINAL REJUVENATION

Carbon dioxide laser or radiofrequency treatments—such as MonaLisa Touch (www.monalisatouch.com) and ThermiVa (www.thermiva.com)—are other options that have worked well for vaginal rejuvenation in some women, although the FDA has not yet approved any such energy-based devices for this use. Still, several studies show promise.[36] The procedures stimulate the production of collagen and elastin, to help restore vaginal thickness and elasticity, and also improve blood flow to vaginal tissue, increasing vaginal moisture. Three treatments are usually suggested, about four to six weeks apart, although some women report success after the first treatment alone. An annual maintenance procedure is also suggested. Inappropriate use of laser treatment on vaginal tissue can cause burns or pain during intercourse, however, so if you do opt for this procedure, go with a practitioner who has a lot of experience with the technique. More studies will undoubtedly be coming soon.

JEANNETTE: *Where Did My Sex Drive Go?*

"Dave and I have been through some rough times," Jeannette said, "but I really feel our relationship has grown along with us—we're better than ever. The trouble is, I just don't have any desire to make love. I love Dave, I really do, but I could go the rest of my life without having sex and I wouldn't care."

Now forty-five years old, Jeannette had noticed some early signs of perimenopause. She hadn't had any hot flashes or vaginal dryness, but her periods, which used to come "like clockwork," were more erratic, and she thought she might have had some night sweats ("either that or I just had on too many covers").

Hormone testing revealed that Jeannette's estrogen levels were still well within the rather broad limits of the normal range, but her progesterone level was on the low side, and her testosterone level was significantly below normal for a woman her age. After some discussion, we decided to boost her progesterone levels with a 2 percent natural progesterone cream, ¼ teaspoon massaged into her hands and wrists twice a day. For her testosterone supplementation, Jeannette opted for an oral testosterone pill. Her prescriptions were filled at a formulary pharmacy. "It made all the difference," she reported. "I find that I'm in the mood more often, and even if I'm not in the mood, I can get aroused a lot faster than before."

TESTOSTERONE: THE HORMONE OF DESIRE?

Although much has been written in the popular press about testosterone's role in sex drive, a deficiency of testosterone is probably the least common cause for a woman's waning libido, coming in at a distant fourth place behind relationship issues and progesterone and/or estrogen decline. Part of the reason testosterone has gotten so much attention, however—aside from the fact that testosterone is universally thought of as a male hormone—is its very specific effect. While estrogen and progesterone play a supportive role in a woman's healthy libido, supplemental testosterone can directly and quickly stimulate the sex drive in both men and women if the reason for the diminished libido has to do with lowered testosterone levels.

Contrary to popular belief, however, testosterone levels do not fall appreciably after menopause. In fact, in most (but not all) women, the postmenopausal ovary secretes *more* testosterone than the premenopausal ovary. Still, testosterone levels do undergo a gradual decline in some women, beginning in their late twenties and continuing through midlife, and it is possible for levels to dip low enough to quash libido.

The Adrenal-Ovarian Connection

Ovarian function is intimately connected to the function of the adrenal glands. Many women reach menopause with depleted adrenals from too many years of unremitting stress, nutrient depletion, and not enough sleep. Recall that the adrenals are the place in the body where the stress hormones cortisol and epinephrine are produced. But they also produce a hormone called DHEA that is a precursor for all the other sex steroids, including testosterone. The body requires B vitamins, magnesium, vitamin C, and a host of other nutrients in order to produce DHEA and adrenal stress hormones. That's why many women who reach menopause with adrenal fatigue find that this is a setup for lower libido and lower testosterone.

Sometimes the decline in testosterone—and hence in libido—is sudden, rather than gradual. This can occur following removal of, or loss of function of, the ovaries. The same can happen if the adrenal glands are exhausted. (See chapter 4.) That's because the ovaries and the adrenals (as well as the liver and the body fat) all produce the steroid hormones collectively known as androgens, one of which is testosterone. If you've had a loss or sudden decrease in ovarian function secondary to chemotherapy, radiation, or surgery, then you may find that your libido dramatically decreases because your body has not had time to shift androgen production to the other body sites that make it. Women with this problem often complain of "not feeling like myself anymore . . . it's as if my life energy has somehow gone." And they lose their libido—their sex energy—as well. The reason this doesn't happen to *all* women who lose ovarian function is that some women's bodies *are* able to make the move to other androgen production sites without much interruption in the hormonal output. But for those whose bodies don't adjust as easily, prescription supplemental hormones may be required to restore their androgen levels.

In women with testosterone levels that have declined significantly, for whatever reason, supplemental testosterone often does have a positive effect on libido. Topical testosterone (both in skin patches and transdermal gels) is particularly effective for improving desire in postmenopausal women. The usual dose is 300 mcg per day. While this drug appears to be safe, its long-term safety isn't yet assured and studies are ongoing. Also, the use of testosterone is associated with some significant side effects, including unwanted hair growth, acne, and sometimes a lowering of the voice. Some studies have shown that 65 percent of menopausal women with depleted testosterone who received testosterone supplementation experienced increases in libido, sexual response, frequency of sexual activity, sexual fantasies, and sensitivity of erogenous zones.[37]

However, in my experience, results are completely satisfying only if a woman has a positive view of herself and her sexuality and a healthy relationship with her partner. This is particularly true at midlife, when a woman is less likely to sweep resentments under the rug. When her significant relationship is in trouble, testosterone supplementation is much less likely to be effective in stimulating her sex drive.

If, however, you think your decline in libido may be related to lowered levels of testosterone or one of the other androgens, you may want to have your unbound (free) testosterone and/or DHEA levels checked. This can be done through either blood, saliva, or urine testing. Ask your physician to prescribe a DUTCH test, which measures cortisol, stress hormones, and sex hormones.

If your levels turn out to be low, your physician can prescribe natural testosterone, available through a formulary pharmacy. Natural testosterone can be used either as a capsule or as a vaginal cream. The usual starting dose is 1–2 mg every other day, gradually increasing if necessary. Transdermal testosterone is another option. A 2008 study of 814 women showed that it does increase sexual satisfaction, although almost half the study group dropped out eventually because of unwanted hair growth and voice deepening, and four developed breast cancer.[38] For women who want to try transdermal testosterone, I recommend starting with less than 300 mcg per day, either as a patch or in a skin cream from a compounding pharmacy.

Yet another option is DHEA supplementation. In some women this hormone, which is a precursor for testosterone, will raise testosterone levels sufficiently to improve a waning sex drive. You can take nonprescription supplemental DHEA at a dose of 5–10 mg once or twice per day. The cream known as Julva, formulated by Anna Cabeca, D.O., the author of *The Hormone Fix* (Ballantine Books, 2019), is a good option (see drannacabeca.com).

If that doesn't work, you might consider asking your healthcare provider for a prescription for prasterone (brand name Intrarosa), a plant-derived form of DHEA approved by the FDA in 2016 as the only vaginal non-estrogen treatment for moderate to severe painful sex due to menopause. The product is designed to be used once daily at bedtime for twelve weeks. Clinical trials showed the drug to be safe and effective, with the most common side effects reported to be vaginal discharge and changes on Pap tests.[39] For more information, see https://us.intrarosa.com.

AIDS TO LUBRICATION

Some women at midlife find that though their libido is fine, they don't lubricate as much as they'd like. This is easy to address. Just use one of the many over-the-counter lubricants, such as K-Y Jelly or *Pueraria mirifica* vaginal moisturizer, which has been shown to restore vaginal epithelium very nicely. Some women may require vaginal estrogen to restore optimal vaginal function. Again, this is a very easy problem to solve.

NATALIE: Sustaining Ongoing Relationships

Natalie first came to see me when she was fifty-two. Her husband, Brad, accompanied her on her visit. Natalie's health was good, but she had been having problems with intercourse. She couldn't seem to get lubricated before intercourse, which made lovemaking difficult. And she had also had a couple of episodes of urinary burning and frequency that felt like urinary tract infections (UTIs).

As I watched Brad and Natalie interact, it was clear that although Brad was uncomfortable talking about the situation, he was genuinely concerned about his wife. He didn't want to hurt her, but he couldn't understand what had gone wrong with their lovemaking. And both expressed fear that their sexual problem could spread into other areas of the relationship, causing them to become distant from each other in general. I performed a pelvic examination on Natalie and found that her vaginal wall was significantly thinned, which would make it less resilient and more sensitive to irritation and discomfort from the stretching and friction that is inevitable during intercourse. Her vaginal thinning also explained the UTI symptoms, given that vaginal thinning is associated with thinning and irritation of the outer third of the urethral passage as well. Natalie's exam also showed an obvious lack of natural lubrication, which would make intercourse more traumatic for her and less pleasurable for both partners. Suspecting that Natalie was in perimenopause, I took a vaginal sample and sent it to the lab for what is known as a "maturation index," a test to see how many cells are well estrogenized and how many aren't. I also had her estrogen, progesterone, and testosterone levels tested. Her testosterone was well within normal range, but her estrogen and progesterone were low. Her maturation index confirmed that she had what is called atrophic vaginitis, a term that simply refers to a lack of estrogen in the cells of the vaginal lining, making it thin and inflamed.

I explained to Natalie her treatment options and ultimately prescribed *Pueraria mirifica* gel for the vagina, plus progesterone cream to be applied anywhere on her skin. In a follow-up visit within a month, Natalie reported that their sex life was "back to normal." This is exactly what I had expected would happen. Treating bona fide perimenopausal vaginal dryness and thinning is safe, easy, and very effective.

GRACE: *Beginning a New Relationship*

Grace was fifty-five when she came to see me for a checkup. Her husband, with whom she'd enjoyed a monogamous relationship for twenty years, had died five years before. Her marriage had been a happy and fulfilling one, and she did not actively look for a new partner after his death. She enjoyed a busy life teaching tennis, gardening, and traveling. But then she was reintroduced to a man who had been one of her boyfriends in high school and whom she hadn't seen for many years. He, too, was widowed—his wife had died several years before. Since he lived in Utah and she in Maine, they began writing letters and calling each other. Her visit to me was prompted by his invitation to come out to his ranch to spend a few weeks. He had told her he wanted her to consider marrying him. Though she wasn't exactly planning on having sex with him during her visit, she wanted to be prepared. Like many women, Grace was worried that her vagina had "shriveled up" from so many years of disuse. I assured her that her vagina was designed to be functional for her entire life, even though it might need some initial help after years of abstinence. (This is not always the case. Women who pleasure themselves in ways that involve vaginal penetration often maintain excellent vaginal function even when not in a relationship that involves sexual intercourse. And of course, many women experience orgasm and good vaginal lubrication without penetration.)

Grace had been postmenopausal for five years and had decided not to take hormone replacement therapy because her bone density was excellent, and she wanted to avoid any increased risk for breast cancer.

On pelvic exam, however, Grace's vagina looked a bit reddened, and the lining, called the vaginal mucosa, appeared somewhat thin. Sometimes this condition is associated with painful intercourse, and sometimes it is not—it depends on the individual. When women are fully aroused, lubrication is often adequate without hormonal assistance. It was entirely possible that Grace would be able to have intercourse with no problem at all, but on the other hand, given the newness of her situation, I felt it was best if she had a couple of options. Grace agreed that she didn't want to take chances. Though she had not experienced any sensation of vaginal dryness or discomfort for the past ten years, she wanted to be sure that she'd be able to have comfortable intercourse.

I offered three options: vaginal estrogen cream, the Estring vaginal ring, or *Pueraria mirifica* vaginal moisturizer. Grace chose the *Pueraria mirifica* vaginal moisturizer so that by the time she got to Utah three weeks later, her vaginal tissue would be very well estrogenized and thicker than it now appeared. She also wanted to come back to see me just before leaving so that I could assess her progress. Had Grace chosen estrogen cream, I would have told her that all conventional estrogen creams, such as Premarin or Estrace—as well as the estradiol in the Estring vaginal ring—also work well for vaginal thinning and dryness, but the estrogen in these can act as a growth factor in breast and uterine tissue, which may be of concern if you've had cancer in one of these organs. However, at low doses they don't appear to cause any appreciable problem, and many, many practitioners recommend them. These creams can also be very helpful in treating urinary incontinence that stems from localized lack of estrogen. (See the pelvic floor rehab section, page 354.)

I prescribed daily use of the moisturizer for one week, to build up what is called the cornified layer of epithelium in the vagina, then one to three applications per week afterward, to maintain the suppleness, resilience, and moistness of her vaginal tissues. I also told her that if she began having regular intercourse, the blood supply to her vagina would increase. This, combined with the repeated stimulation and stretching of her vagina, would result in a much decreased need for the cream—possibly to the point of being able to eliminate it completely, with just a touch of a nonprescription lubricant as needed.

By the way, estrogen vaginal cream or *Pueraria mirifica* vaginal moisturizer is also excellent for women who have suffered vaginal narrowing and drying because of radiation treatments. While the tissues of the body are considered "plastic" and can therefore return to near-normal function with regular use, the estriol cream helps in the meantime.

If you opt for an estrogen cream, don't expect overnight change. It will take a week or so for the vaginal tissue to be restored and a bit longer for the uppermost part of the vagina to dilate. In the meantime, I recommend lovemaking through oral or manual stimulation of the clitoris, which can be very satisfying and is a good way to keep the blood flow optimal in the pelvis.

Nonprescription Help with Lubrication

There are many choices of lubrication available that work just fine for relieving vaginal dryness. Good old K-Y Jelly is available at every pharmacy, though this water-soluble lubricant may not be enough for some, and for others it can form an annoying residue. Other lubricants that work very well are Albolene (available in pharmacies), Emerita's Personal Moisturizer (which contains a number of soothing herbal extracts such as calendula), and Amata Life's vaginal gel. Many herbal remedies taken systemically can also help restore vaginal lubrication: black cohosh, wild yam, *Pueraria mirifica* (as Pueraria Mirifica Plus), dong quai, or chasteberry are good examples. Vitamin E suppositories are effective, too.

Another key to vaginal health is to become aware of your pelvic floor regularly throughout the day and to do Kegel-type exercises to stimulate and strengthen your pelvic floor muscles (see chapter 8). They're easy to do, and they can be done anytime, anywhere; nobody can tell what you're doing. Studies have shown that in addition to increasing blood supply (which will increase vaginal wall thickness as well as lubrication), these exercises can improve libido by increasing clitoral tumescence and sensitivity and increasing the strength of orgasm. As a happy side effect, Kegel exercises also can help prevent, or reverse, urinary incontinence (leakage).

THE MAGIC OF SEX-ATTRACTANT PHEROMONES

In 1986 Winnifred Cutler, Ph.D., a women's health researcher and author, discovered sex-attractant chemicals given off by the female body that greatly enhance a woman's ability to attract love and partnership. These sex attractant molecules are excreted by the exocrine glands of the body (in the armpit and groin areas) during ovulation. And because the human sense of smell is so potent and so connected to the limbic system of the brain, certain smells are highly associated with increased libido and romantic encounters.

In 1993, Dr. Cutler's lab created a synthetic version of these hormones that can be added to perfume or scent. The results of her many studies showed that women who used these had significantly more romantic encounters than did the control group. Here's a testimonial from her website: "Following my divorce this year, I began dating again at age fifty. I began using your 10:13 [pheromone product] six months ago and am currently juggling three attractive men. I haven't had this kind of attention in decades."

I have recommended Dr. Cutler's Athena Institute products for many years and can attest to their efficacy. They can be used whether or not you are single because they enhance your attractiveness and desirability. To read the studies or to order pheromones, go to www.athenainstitute.com.

TELLING THE TRUTH

At midlife, more and more women become comfortable with telling the truth about their sexuality—to themselves and to others. Here are some areas you might want to reevaluate.

⁓ COME TO TERMS WITH YOUR OWN SEXUALITY. All humans are sexual by nature—it's part of being human. Women undergo vaginal lubrication at regular intervals during sleep, and men get erections. But how you choose to express your sexuality when you're awake will depend upon many factors, including your upbringing, your hormone levels, your general overall health, and your level of satisfaction with your sexual partner, if you currently have one. The most important thing I'd like all women to know is that through the power of their thoughts and emotions, they can learn how to turn themselves on and feel more sexually desirable. This change alone can be revolutionary.

⁓ STOP KEEPING SCORE. What is a normal sex life? Only you can answer that question for yourself. To help you find your personal truth about this issue, let me remind you that we live in a society that often confuses quantity with quality. Even the medical profession equates the quality of one's sex life with the frequency of intercourse. This is a gross disservice to couples everywhere, many of whom will inevitably feel they don't measure up. For perspective, you may find it comforting to know that a recent study from the University of Chicago pointed out that it's pretty common for couples to have intercourse three times per month and be completely satisfied with that. Ask yourself the following question, and answer it honestly: if your life were ideal, how much time would you like to devote each week to being sexual—either with yourself or with a partner? You can always improve your sex life by intending to do so!

⁓ RESPECT YOUR INHERENT SEX DRIVE. Sex therapist Patricia Love, Ed.D., notes that people can be divided into three different categories when it comes to innate sex drive: high, moderate, and low.[40] Individuals with relatively high testosterone levels (high T's) tend to have a higher sex drive than those with lower levels (low T's), while those with low T levels often find that after the initial honeymoon period of a relationship wanes, it takes a lot of energy for them to initiate or become interested in being sexual. Because it's not uncommon for a high-T individual to be attracted to a low-T person, there's a good chance that a couple's sexual appetites may differ from time to time. But this doesn't make either of them "wrong" or "abnormal."

And although our culture teaches us there is something wrong with us if we can't keep our sex life at its original fever pitch, the truth is that the initial emotional and physiological high of a new sexual relationship eventually needs to be replaced by a more consciously created and sophisticated form of passion and intimacy.

~ PRACTICE SAFE SEX. All women need to be aware of the risk they face from unprotected sex if they are not in a long-term monogamous relationship. The latest statistics from the CDC show that although new HIV diagnoses are declining among people age fifty and up, about one in six HIV diagnoses are in this age group.

It is all too easy to assume that anyone you would partner with is probably not infected. You may be a good judge of character, but a sexual partner is only as safe as every partner he or she has ever had. Remember also that there are many other STDs out there, including genital herpes, genital warts, and hepatitis B. Perimenopausal and postmenopausal women are at greater risk for contracting all STDs than are younger women.[41] The decrease in vaginal lubrication and the thinning of the vaginal walls make it easier for microscopic tears to occur during intercourse, creating an entry point for bacteria and viruses.

Safe sex means keeping your partner's body fluids out of your vagina, anus, and mouth until you are certain you are safe together. Body fluids include semen, vaginal secretions, blood, and the discharge from STD lesions, such as herpetic sores. Though most people reduce the concept of safe sex to the use of a condom, it is really much larger than that. It includes being honest with yourself about the risk you face from unprotected sex with a partner whose STD status is unknown to you. It also includes waiting to have sex with someone until you know each other well enough to discuss your sexual history, and such issues as using a condom and/or getting a blood test. Though this kind of conversation is rarely easy, it is a good test of the intimacy that is possible between you and your partner.

What About the HPV Vaccine?

Human papillomavirus (HPV) is the most common sexually transmitted infection in the United States. There are more than forty strains of HPV, thirteen of which can lead to cervical cancer. (The other strains lead only to fairly harmless genital warts.) To be clear, the vast majority of HPV cases do not lead to cancer, although most cervical cancer is caused by those thirteen high-risk strains of HPV.

In 2006, the FDA approved the HPV vaccine Gardasil, said to prevent four strains of HPV, those most often associated with cervical cancer. It was replaced in 2014 with Gardasil 9, said to prevent the original four strains as well as an additional five. At the time, Gardasil was approved for use only in males and females ages nine through twenty-six. The CDC noted that vaccination by age eleven or twelve was ideal, since the vaccine is most effective before the recipient is exposed to HPV.

Then in October 2018, the FDA announced Gardasil 9 would now be recommended to men and women up to age forty-five. The thinking was that even if these adults had already been exposed to HPV through sexual activity, they may not have been exposed to all nine strains that Gardasil 9 claimed to protect against. However, the American Cancer Society came out against this decision, noting on its website that the vaccine is "unlikely to provide much, if any, benefit as people get older."[42]

Let's take a good look at the case against vaccination with Gardasil at any age. While Merck, the vaccine's manufacturer, continues to promise that Gardasil is safe, the National Vaccine Information Center (NVIC), an independent organization and vaccine safety group, has documented cases of seizure, stroke, cardiovascular disease, paralysis, autoimmune diseases such as rheumatoid arthritis, and even death connected to the vaccine. (See NVIC's website at www.nvic.org for more detailed information.) In August 2009, an article in the *Journal of the American Medical Association* noted that the government had so far received more than

12,000 reports of adverse events associated with Gardasil immunizations—772 of them considered serious, including 32 deaths.[43]

Researchers around the world have reported problems. The most recent government reports from Australia, for example, show a 16 percent cancer increase in twenty-five-year-olds and a 28 percent increase in thirty-year-olds, several years post-vaccination, while cancer deaths in older (unvaccinated) women have decreased.[44] Japan, France, and India have all either banned Gardasil or filed criminal lawsuits against the vaccine.

Merck's own data reported in the Gardasil 9 package insert says the rate of serious adverse events is 2.3 to 2.5 percent—meaning for every 100,000 people receiving the vaccine, there will be at least 2,300 serious adverse events. Yet only 7.4 women in 100,000 get cervical cancer in the United States.[45] That means 2,300 out of every 100,000 women receiving this vaccine are placed at risk in order to possibly prevent 7.4 cases of cervical cancer (actual prevention statistics are not yet available). Many different experts have even called into question the quality of Merck's initial safety trials on the HPV vaccine.[46]

Note that the vaccine doesn't guard against infection for those strains a person has already been exposed to (an important point for midlife women to consider), nor does it guard against infection for any of the other high-risk strains the vaccine doesn't target. Researchers at Columbia University who conducted the 2012 ATHENA Human Papillomavirus Study, which followed more than 47,000 women, discovered that vaccinated women reduced their chances of becoming infected with HPV type 16 (one of the types Gardasil targets) by only 0.6 percent, while they increased their chances of becoming infected with additional high-risk HPV types that Gardasil doesn't target by 2.6 to 6.2 percent.[47] University of Texas researchers reported similar data three years later.[48]

Now let's look at absolute numbers. Each year, 13,240 U.S. women are diagnosed with cervical cancer and 4,170 die from the disease, according to the American Cancer Society, with somewhere between 90 and 100 percent of those cancers associated with HPV. Gardasil 9 claims to protect against the four most common strains of HPV associated with cervical cancer, plus five other high-risk types that together are implicated in about 90 percent of HPV-associated cases—which means the number of cervical cancer cases that this vaccine may potentially prevent is fewer than 12,000.

Note the use of the word *potentially*. The researchers who did the clinical trials for Gardasil counted the absence of cervical dysplasia (an abnormal Pap test) and precursors for cancer as proof the vaccine was effective.[49] But since most dysplasia does not develop into cancer, preventing an infection leading to dysplasia is hardly equivalent to preventing cancer, making the vaccine's claims misleading.

Here's how Diane Harper, M.D., one of the principal investigators in the initial Gardasil trials who has subsequently come out against the vaccine, explains it. In about 70 percent of all women infected with HPV, the infection will clear on its own in the first year, and in 90 percent the infection will clear within two years. Of the 10 percent who are left with an infection, only 5 percent will develop a precancerous lesion. It takes five years for about 20 percent and thirty years for 40 percent of precancerous lesions to become invasive carcinomas—which would happen only if those women were not followed by routine Pap tests and subsequently treated.[50] So the majority of those women supposedly "saved" from cancer by Gardasil would not have developed cancer anyway.

The bottom line: a far safer and saner approach to preventing cervical cancer at any age would be routine screening, safe-sex practices, and those early treatment measures we already have in place.

⁓ USE CONTRACEPTION IF REQUIRED. I've seen all too many change-of-life pregnancies in women who were absolutely sure they could not get pregnant and who thought diapers and car seats were out of their lives for good. Even if you are skipping periods regularly, you can still be ovulating. The general rule is that you should use contraception for a full year after your last menstrual period. Obviously, you won't know exactly when that is until you have reached the one-year mark.

TEN STEPS TO REKINDLING LIBIDO

The late psychiatrist Helen Singer Kaplan, a pioneer in the field of human sexuality, originated the term "hot monogamy," using it to refer to the potential for enduring sexual passion in a committed, monogamous relationship. Patricia Love, Ed.D., has identified several factors that can help sustain that state of desire. As she explains in her book *Hot Monogamy* (Dutton, 1994), co-authored with Jo Robinson, these factors all interconnect with one another, so progress in one area will have beneficial effects in the others.[51]

1. COMMUNICATION. Even if you and your partner haven't talked much about your sexual relationship until now, being able to talk easily about sexual changes will become increasingly important. Simply letting your partner know what is going on with you is a good first step, and it can pave the way to discussing adjustments you'd like to make. I also recommend that you read *Mama Gena's School of Womanly Arts* (Simon & Schuster, 2002), *Mama Gena's Owner's and Operator's Guide to Men* (Simon & Schuster, 2003), and *Pussy: A Reclamation* (Hay House, 2016), all by Regena Thomashauer. All three books are filled with wonderful, uplifting, and practical advice for accessing your feminine power in a relationship. Chapter 11 of my book *Goddesses Never Age* (Hay House, 2015) is also filled with precisely the information all women need to know to experience the best sex of their lives after menopause.

2. MOOD. At midlife, women must take responsibility for getting in the mood, even if desire doesn't arise as spontaneously as it used to. A fifty-six-year-old colleague told me that for her, "getting older means *deciding* to have a sex life, instead of being *driven* to it." (For help in this regard, see "Sensuality," below.) The good news is that getting in the mood is a choice that begins in your mind! Remember, energy follows awareness. And awareness depends on nothing except your willingness to pay attention.

3. INTIMACY. Take time to make the personal connection. There is nothing more conducive to a good sex life than the ability to share one's thoughts and feelings with one's partner on a regular basis. One of the really nice things about midlife is that we often have more time to spend with our partners than ever before. That time can translate into a second honeymoon. One of my male colleagues and his wife went on a prolonged European vacation—their first significant time

away since their four children were born. When I asked him about the trip, he told me, "We got acquainted all over again. I remembered why I had married her in the first place." Another one of my patients described how rejuvenating it was to be able to make love without children in the house. She laughed and said, "We can be loud!"

I recently saw a good friend, a therapist, at a party. Happily married, he said to me, "I have discovered that compatibility is not what makes a love relationship work—it is the result of loving one another enough so that you become compatible." There is a lot to meditate on here.

4. TECHNIQUE AND AWARENESS. As I already stated, women are orgasmatrons, meaning that by nature we are multiorgasmic and capable of experiencing a great deal of pleasure. Most women haven't even begun to reach the fullness of their pleasure potential because of things such as religious shame, sexual abuse, an uncaring partner, or simple lack of information. Midlife is a great time to change all that! Each of us can learn to turn herself on through regular practice. Remember, energy follows awareness. And just being aware of your erotic anatomy and feeling the tingling or increased blood flow that results from that awareness is a great start. Then add Kegel exercises to that awareness, feeling the increased blood flow each time. Vera Bodansky, Ph.D., co-author of *The Illustrated Guide to Extended Massive Orgasm* (Hunter House, 2002) with her husband, Steve Bodansky, Ph.D., teaches us to "enjoy every stroke." The Bodanskys also teach that the orgasm begins with the first involuntary contraction of the pubococcygeus muscle (the so-called love muscle), which is the same muscle group that you contract with a Kegel exercise.

The Bodanskys' book is actually a biofeedback manual in which you teach yourself how to feel more and more with less and less stimulation. That's right—you can actually train your body, through your awareness, to feel more! This is a practice best done without a vibrator. I have nothing against these devices, but over time, if you don't wake up other pleasure pathways, a vibrator can dull feelings, and you will need increasing amounts of stimulation to feel anything. Your goal is to tune in to your pleasure so exquisitely that you can turn yourself on with a simple touch. Please know that some women are able to have an orgasm simply from nipple or earlobe stimulation! I suggest that you start practicing on your own. In fact, it's completely possible to have a good sex life on your own. And the good news there is that waking yourself up sexually makes you more magnetic and more attractive to a potential partner, if that is your desire.

Learning to pleasure yourself and feel all the different erotic areas in your body is invaluable when it comes to making love with a partner, because you've already discovered, and can teach, what works for you and what doesn't. Believe me, men are not born knowing this any more than you are. And part of becoming a new partner at midlife involves waking yourself up to yourself.

VISITING DIGNITARY EXERCISE

In their book *The Illustrated Guide to Extended Massive Orgasm* (Hunter House, 2002), Vera Bodansky, Ph.D., and Steve Bodansky, Ph.D., share a life-changing exercise called Visiting Dignitary. Here's what you do. You clean and prepare your boudoir or bedroom as if a visiting dignitary were coming to stay and would be using that room. Remove clutter, arrange fresh flowers, and perhaps light a scented candle. You get the picture. You also prepare a favorite juice or other drink and perhaps have a piece of dark chocolate or other snack awaiting you. You might also want to have some favorite massage oil or lotion on hand. Now you have set the stage.

Next, you—as the visiting dignitary—enter the room. By candlelight, in front of a mirror, you slowly undress and begin to admire the parts of yourself that you really enjoy— perhaps your eyes, your shoulders, your skin. Candlelight is very flattering and will allow you to truly appreciate your beauty. If you notice a critical voice in your head, just tell her you love her but you need her to be quiet because you are loving yourself right now. Your job is to feast your eyes on the beauty and wonder of yourself and your body. Now close your eyes and feel the aliveness in your hands, your feet, your abdomen—throughout your entire body. Revel in this for a couple of minutes and notice that this aliveness increases as you appreciate your body. Remember that energy flows where attention goes.

When you feel full of aliveness, it is now time to move your attention to your female erotic anatomy—your breasts, your clitoris, your labia, and your sacred spot. Quite possibly these areas are already humming with energy and aliveness, and chances are good that you have even started to lubricate in your vaginal area and that your clitoral system is becoming engorged. In other words, you are turning on from simply appreciating your erotic nature. Your body is doing its job as a barometer for life force—and your anatomy responds.

Then lie down comfortably and simply begin stroking yourself in your erotic zones. You are not trying to accomplish anything; you are just stroking and appreciating your body—specifically, how your female erotic system is a kind of GPS for your life force. Use plenty of lubricant when you are massaging your genitals. Next, try massaging your clitoris with whatever hand and fingers feel the best. Your goal here—for turning on your female erotic anatomy and making it more responsive—is to give yourself an orgasm within the next thirty minutes. Do this without a vibrator so that you train yourself to feel more with less stimulation. Think of this as biofeedback training, because it is.

But don't get overly goal oriented. With time and practice, you will easily have an orgasm within the thirty-minute window. The Bodanskys teach that an orgasm begins the moment you first feel a contraction in your pubococcygeus muscle. Given that, it's very helpful to think of this entire practice as one prolonged orgasm. It takes the pressure off the situation. Remember, you are playing with your female erotic anatomy and waking it up so that it can better serve you. I recommend a couple of Visiting Dignitary sessions per week, though there is no limit on how much you can enjoy this exercise. You can also add a crystal wand to stimulate your sacred spot, or a dildo, or a yoni egg—or a combination. I know women who self-pleasure daily as a spiritual practice.

But if you are new to self-pleasuring and you want to birth a new, more vital, more sensual you, then practicing the Visiting Dignitary exercise regularly will help immensely because it is so simple, yet so powerful.

5. SEXUAL VARIETY. Both you and your partner need to explore your willingness to add creativity, fun, and novelty to your lovemaking. To help you, I recommend the DVD *10 Secrets to Great Sex* (available on Amazon). I also highly recommend taking workshops as well as online courses or trainings that help increase your life force and aliveness. One especially good resource here is Kim Anami, who

teaches online courses on intimacy and hosts retreats in destinations such as Mexico and Bali (see kimanami.com).

6. ROMANCE. You and your partner need to learn how to show love for each other in concrete ways. Flowers, cards, words of appreciation, special nights out, and so forth are all part of what it takes to keep romance alive. Women also must realize that they need to ask for what they want. Most men long to please you—but they can't read your mind. So you have to make it obvious. You do that by approving of them when they make an effort, and instead of criticizing them for what they didn't get right, you instead say, "You know what would make this even *more* perfect?" And then you tell them. I highly recommend the work of Alison Armstrong and her book *The Queen's Code* (PAX Programs, 2013) if you want to learn more about how to interact effectively with men in a romantic situation.

7. BODY IMAGE. Dr. Love describes body image as "your inner image of your outer self." Many women don't feel good about their bodies because we've learned to compare ourselves with the airbrushed, perfect models we see in the media. This is especially true when our bodies start changing at midlife. When we feel bad about our bodies, it is very difficult to be fully present for lovemaking. Here's the good news: men don't care nearly as much as you think. I've asked dozens of them. They just want a woman who wants them and who is fun to be with. If body image is a problem for you, stand in front of a mirror twice a day for thirty days, look deeply into your own eyes, and say out loud, "I accept myself unconditionally right now." Spend time admiring yourself in the mirror—an exercise that works especially well when the room is lit by candlelight. The more you do this, the more illuminated you will feel. This may sound silly, but it works—and it can instantly point out to you the areas in your life that need love and compassion. The more you enjoy your body yourself, the more erotic you'll feel. Feeling sexy starts as an inside job with your thoughts and beliefs.

8. SENSUALITY. To enhance your libido, you must be willing to relax and involve all your senses in your lovemaking. You also have to give up the "goal" of orgasm and instead just allow yourself to feel. That's what sensuality is all about—coming home to the goodness of your body.

Sight: According to feng shui, the Chinese art of placement, the bedroom should be a place of rest and relaxation, not a place to pay bills or watch television. The bedroom should also be a sensual place. To help make it so, choose bedroom wall and sheet colors with your partner that will enhance the romance of your surroundings.

Many couples enjoy watching sensual movies together. Most women, including me, find that sensual movies need a good sound track, a good story, and good lighting. Some suggestions include *Emmanuelle I* and *II, Delta of Venus,* and *Two Moon Junction.* Many women also like erotic literature, which tends to leave more to the imagination than graphic movies. I personally like the erotic stories compiled by Lonnie Barbach, such as *Pleasures* and *The Erotic Edge.* Anaïs Nin's erotica (*Delta of Venus* and *Little Birds*) has also stood the test of time. Romance novels can help get you in the mood, too. Here are two of my favorites, both of which have great erotic sections: *The Valley of Horses* (Crown, 1982), by Jean Auel, and *Outlander* (Delta, 2001), by Diana Gabaldon. *Note:* Be selective when it comes to erotic material and make sure that the movies, photos, or books you look at are not degrading to women in any way. Nothing is a bigger turnoff. Lovemaking should be an activity that enhances the well-being and self-esteem of both partners. If you are currently with a partner whose sexual demands feel degrading to you, get outside help.

Smell: Women are more attuned to the sense of smell than men are, and we often prefer different odors than men do. You and your partner will need to be honest with each other about odors one of you might find offensive, such as sweat, bad breath, and the like. Aromatherapy can be wonderful—but you must agree on a scent. Speaking of scent, the science of pheromones, though just in its infancy, is fascinating. It has been well documented by the research of Winnifred Cutler, Ph.D., and others that pheromones are important sexual attractant molecules secreted by glands in the armpits and pubic areas. When women are ovulating, they secrete a pheromone that increases their attractiveness to men. Men also secrete pheromones that make them more attractive to women. Women who've had hysterectomies may have a decreased amount of pheromone secretion— and midlife women who are no longer ovulating may have the same thing. But the good news is that commercially available pheromones can be added to your perfume or just applied to your skin. Though more studies need to be done, there's enough information (and anecdotal evidence) on the effectiveness of pheromones that I wouldn't hesitate to give them a try and see what happens with your sex life and sex appeal. (See the Athena Institute at www.athenainstitute .com, or Love Scent at www.love-scent.com.) Just remember, feeling sexy is the most powerful sex attractant there is.

Touch: Practice giving each other foot and shoulder rubs. Learn to *receive.* You'd be amazed at how many women have difficulty lying still and receiving pleasure in this way. Practice telling your partner what feels good and what doesn't. Notice that the lighter the touch, the more you feel. Approve of every stroke! Don't forget the clitoris! Roughly 75 percent of women don't reach orgasm through intercourse. Instead, try oral sex or manual sex, or try the woman-on-top position.

Taste: Many options are available in this area if it appeals to you, such as flavored oils, chocolate, whipped cream, honey, and so on.

Sound: For many reasons, we've all been taught to keep quiet when having sex. But making sounds and keeping our mouths and throats open and relaxed greatly enhance pleasure. So practice making a variety of different sounds when making love, whether alone or with a partner. It's also very useful to give positive feedback to a partner. Vera Bodansky, Ph.D., and Steve Bodansky, Ph.D., teach women to make a list of affirmative words to say to their mates when they are getting it right. Examples include *yes; more, please; oh, that feels great,* and so on. Men want to get it right. And they want positive feedback when they do!

Use sensual music to set the mood. Turn off your cellphones and make sure that others aren't around or that the door is locked. Nothing is more distracting for most women during lovemaking than the fear that one of the children might walk in at any minute.

9. PASSION. Dr. Love notes that it is not possible to be passionately in love with a person you don't know. She describes passion as the "ability to combine intense feelings of arousal with love for your partner." However far we may have strayed from this state, it is certainly a destination to which we can all aspire—an example of what is possible at midlife as our *kundalini* energy rises to our hearts and we achieve a fusion of sexuality and spirituality not just in our genitals, but in our hearts and souls as well.

10. TAP INTO THE POWER OF PLEASURE. Deciding to feel pleasure and take pleasure in your life is an act of courage. It also takes discipline. Nothing is easier than allowing yourself to be sad, depressed, and unhappy. That's the norm. But this needn't be the case. The brain is the biggest sex organ in the body. Your ability to choose how you think about sex and pleasure of all kinds is your most powerful ally in reinventing yourself sexually at midlife. A woman's desire—her ability to get turned on—is one of the most potent aphrodisiacs in the

world. And remember that a turned-on woman who is fun is what turns on a man—and other women. Ultimately, it's not love that keeps couples together. It's fun. At midlife, you have to reinvent the fun. A woman who feels irresistible and desirable has the ability to turn herself on and thus enjoy a far more pleasurable life. Her life force and enthusiasm are contagious. If you don't currently have a partner, cultivate a sensual relationship with yourself. The sexier and more attractive you become (for yourself), the happier and healthier you'll be.

The two things that block us from feeling our natural desire for all kinds of pleasure, including sexual pleasure, are anger and self-doubt. At midlife, when all the unfinished business of the first half of our lives rises up to be cleansed, it takes great courage to own our anger and use it as fuel to burn through years of self-doubt and self-limitation—whether sexual or otherwise. Deciding to see ourselves as irresistible, sexy, beautiful, and deserving of pleasure is an act of power. Deciding to tell our mates and our children what we want without undue anger and resentment is also an act of power. This is an inside job. We don't need a white knight to rescue us, a new job, or breast implants. We need to know, deep in our cells, that we are worthy of the best that life has to offer—and that we have the power to attract it by making time for and concentrating on what brings us pleasure. The crucible of menopause is the ideal time to allow our self-doubts and anger to be burned away so that we may truly re-claim the erotic—the life force—in our lives. In her book *Women's Anatomy of Arousal: Secret Maps to Buried Pleasure* (Mango Garden Press, 2009), Sheri Winston has a section called "Becoming an Erotic Virtuoso." When I read it, I had an aha moment. My body said yes to that idea! Deep inside, nearly every woman I've ever met wants to be in touch with what Sheila Kelley, founder of the S Factor pole danc-ing exercise program for women, calls her "inner erotic creature." We long to express the sex goddess inside us. For many, she got si-lenced in childhood or adolescence. But now, at midlife, we have the skills and the discipline to channel our erotic energy into pathways of health and pleasure that promote the health and happiness of every-one around us. We're not irresponsible teens anymore. So give your-self the space, time, and attention it takes to awaken your full erotic potential. Doing this will enhance your circulation, raise your nitric oxide levels, balance your hormones, and make you more magnetic—*and* it will make you feel wonderfully alive and vital!

10

Nurturing Your Brain:
Sleep, Mood, and Memory

The changes that go on in women's brains at midlife prepare us for living with more wisdom and meaning than ever before. This new wisdom gets wired in our brains as we move from the alternating current of our menstruating years to the more direct current available after menopause. As this natural adjustment takes place, we may find ourselves experiencing disturbing symptoms, ranging from insomnia and depression to forgetfulness. Rather than succumbing to the common cultural view that we are about to begin the long, slow glide into senility and depression, we need to realize that the brain changes we are experiencing are usually normal— temporary bumps in the road that can be alleviated when we have the courage to see them as messages from our inner wisdom. No study has ever shown that menopause per se increases one's risk for any mental disorder, whether depression, forgetfulness, or anxiety, unless we are already predisposed to them. Perimenopause *amplifies* our brain and thought patterns, also bringing up past memories of events that require processing and forgiveness. Perimenopause allows us to upgrade the areas of our lives that need support and change.

Fighting or trying to control mental symptoms with denial, drugs, or even overdependence on mental techniques such as meditation is ultimately doomed to fail. Instead we need to heed the messages behind our symptoms, support ourselves fully with sound information, and, when necessary, be willing to take life-changing action, such as leaving a job or a marriage.

Given our culture's love affair with control, this approach takes a great deal of courage and faith. Some women have to go through painful breakdowns before they are ready to relinquish this struggle for control. I am no stranger to this path myself.

PRUDENCE: *The Anxious Siren*

Prudence, a corporate attorney married to a college professor, first came to see me when she became pregnant with her first child, at the age of thirty-four. Prudence and her husband appeared to be the perfect couple, with the kind of dual-career lifestyle to which many of us aspire. Prudence's pregnancy, labor, and birth were normal, but postpartum she fell into a dark depression that lasted for about six months. During this time she sought help from a psychiatrist and went on antidepressant medication for about a year. She subsequently remained stable except for rather severe PMS symptoms such as anxiety, mood swings, and cravings for sweets that lasted from midcycle through the first day of her period. Prudence was able to control these symptoms with progesterone cream, diet, and exercise. I never pressed her further to see what was going on in her life that might be precipitating her PMS symptoms. Her program was working, she was satisfied, and I intuitively felt that Prudence was not interested in looking more deeply into her life or her psyche. That all changed at perimenopause.

When Prudence began skipping periods in her mid-forties, she couldn't seem to get a handle on her PMS symptoms anymore. She didn't know exactly when to use the progesterone cream, and her former self-discipline when it came to diet and exercise disappeared. In addition to this, she often found herself unable to get to sleep at night. But Prudence had another worry that completely surprised me: every time she skipped a period, she worried that she might be pregnant. Since her husband had had a vasectomy after their child was born, I knew that something had definitely changed in her life.

When I asked Prudence if there was anything unusually stressful going on, she admitted to me that she was having an affair with a coworker. She said, "I don't know what has come over me. I never thought I'd ever do anything like this. But I feel possessed. When I'm with David, I feel young and wild—as though a part of me has awakened that I didn't even know existed. I'm interested in sexy black underwear for the first time in my life. I sit at my desk, and when I should be going over legal briefs, I fantasize about my next business trip with him. I feel higher than a kite when we're together or I'm even just thinking about him. But when I have to be home and we can't see each other for a while, I crash. I feel anxious and depressed and I can't sleep."

At first Prudence simply wanted my opinion about contraception and also whether or not she should go back on antidepressants or start using sleeping pills. She also wanted to know what effect medication might have on her newly recharged sex drive. Though I agreed that drug therapy of some sort might be an option to help her symptoms, I also wanted to help Prudence make the link between her perimenopausal mental symptoms and her life.

Why was she having the affair now? At first she told me that her marriage was fine and that her husband was a good man. But after a few minutes she broke down in tears and told me that he had not been given tenure at his university and had become more difficult to live with over the past year or so. As is so often the case, Prudence's husband was also going through a midlife crisis of sorts, but he preferred not to talk about it. This was especially difficult for Prudence because her own work life was better than ever. In fact, given her husband's discouragement and apparent depression, she increasingly preferred being at work to being at home.

I asked Prudence what the affair had done for her. She thought it over for a moment and replied, "It makes me feel alive, powerful, and sexy in a way I haven't felt before." Prudence's uncharacteristic affair allowed her to move into a part of her brain's temporal lobe—an area that had probably been relatively shut down since her late teens or early twenties but which, as we've already seen, becomes increasingly activated during perimenopause. The temporal lobe is associated with ecstasy, sensuality, transcendent experiences, and creativity. Its messages are always present, but they are often overridden by our frontal lobes—the centers in our brains associated with rules, regulations, childhood programming, and conventional morality.

At midlife our bodies and brains cry out for balance, and the dictates of our souls become increasingly persistent. Those who have been overly intellectualized and controlled need to break free and become more fluid and spontaneous, while those who have lived in the moment, pursuing pleasure and creative self-expression with abandon, now need to rein themselves in with more structure and self-discipline if they are to stay healthy.

Though I don't prescribe midlife affairs, I do recognize how therapeutic a passionate out-of-control experience of some kind can be for women like Prudence. (This is delightfully illustrated in the 2009 movie *It's Complicated* with Meryl Streep and Alec Baldwin.) Regardless of the circumstances that awaken a woman's joy and ecstasy at midlife, she will flourish only to the degree that she relinquishes her need to control her world. Affairs are sometimes just another means of controlling joy by allowing oneself to feel fully only through sex and only within contrived, secretive parameters. Instead, midlife calls us all to learn how to trust bliss, joy, and pleasure within a healthy and sustainable container as part of our daily lives.

I suggested to Prudence that she spend a few months thinking about the following questions, either alone or with the help of a therapist or other professional: Did she love her husband? Did she intend to stay married to him and grow old with him? What were the circumstances that led to the affair? What feelings had it brought up for her? Did she believe that it was possible to feel the ecstasy of the affair in other parts of her life? Was her affair important enough to her to risk losing the life she had built with her husband? Was she willing to see the link between her symptoms and her life?

Prudence told me she'd think about what I had said. She then went to see a psychiatrist for her depression, anxiety, and insomnia. Over the next two years she went through a series of medications, none of which worked for very long and all of which gave her side effects. After having been given prescriptions for Prozac, Celexa, Effexor, Xanax, Valium, Elavil, and Desyrel, Prudence was finally offered Nardil, a monoamine oxidase inhibitor (MAOI), which required her to be on a special diet. After all these attempts at trying to find peace through pills, many of her symptoms were still present.

Prudence did not return to my office for an exam until two and a half years later. Her affair had come to an end, she told me, and she was still married. When I asked her how her husband was doing, she told me that he had found another teaching job but seemed to be just marking time until retirement. Before she left, Prudence began to sob. Through her tears, she said, "I feel as though my body is totally out of control. The more I try to control my symptoms, the worse things get. I have no idea what to do next." I told Prudence that she had finally reached "breakdown to breakthrough"—a place that, while uncomfortable, is usually the first step toward living more fully and joyfully. I also told Prudence the truth: you have to feel it to heal it.

After this, Prudence went to a therapist to work through the aspects of her life that required changing. Prudence's body and mind had presented her with a dilemma that simply couldn't be solved with more control or more information. She finally surrendered and knew that she had to take her life and her health one day at a time. This is true for many.

Midlife teaches us a liberating truth: many aspects of our lives, including our mates, our families, our children, and our jobs, are simply not under our control. True mental health always involves striking a balance between certainty and ambiguity. At midlife the kinds of certainty and control that often served us well earlier in our lives must now make room for another way of being in the world. We must learn to trust our inner wisdom, a reality that we cannot see, taste, touch, or measure—let alone control.

ENHANCING MIDLIFE SLEEP

Midlife women often go through changes in their sleep patterns, not unlike those we experienced at adolescence. Some of us find ourselves needing more sleep than ever, some suffer from insomnia, and some find that sleep simply isn't as refreshing as it used to be.

Unfortunately, insomnia makes the entire midlife transition harder. Insufficient sleep increases our levels of corticosteroids and catecholamines, stress hormones that can, over time, throw off our hormonal balances and depress our immune systems. Studies show that 20 to 40 percent of women have sleep disorders, and women are far more likely than men to have insomnia after the age of thirty-five.[1] Perimenopausal women often need more sleep than do men of the same age.[2]

Sleep restores both physical and mental energy. Laboratory animals have been shown to die from sleep deprivation. Insufficient sleep leaves us obviously drowsy, fatigued, and irritable. We also suffer from decreased concentration, lowered efficiency, decreased work motivation, and a higher rate of errors in judgment. This is why the Federal Aviation Administration has strict rules about how much sleep flight crews require. When we are sleep-deprived, we are more accident-prone, since our brains will fall into "micro-sleeps" that may not be apparent to those around us. A host of recent studies confirm that not getting enough sleep can worsen a number of different health issues, including high blood pressure,[3] obesity and type 2 diabetes,[4] impaired immune functioning,[5] cardiovascular disease and arrhythmias,[6] mood disorders,[7] and neurological disorders and dementia.[8]

Let's look more at how sufficient sleep is related to maintaining a healthy weight. I'm willing to bet that many of you have lost two to three pounds or more overnight after a sound sleep! Sleep quite literally makes you look and feel lighter. A 2005 study done at Columbia University showed that the less sleep subjects got, the more likely they were to be obese.[9] Those who only got four hours or less of sleep a night were 73 percent more likely to be obese than those who slept from seven to nine hours each night, while those getting five hours a night were 50 percent more likely and those getting six hours a night were 23 percent more likely to be obese. Researchers believe that when you don't get enough sleep, your body produces less of the hormone leptin, which signals your body that you're full, and more of the hormone ghrelin, which tells your body you're hungry—leaving you feeling both hungrier and less satisfied.

Insomnia Is Often a Message from Our Inner Guidance

At menopause, insomnia and fatigue are frequently the result of unprocessed and unresolved emotions such as anger, sadness, or anxiety, which often accompany the enormous changes of midlife. The brain chemicals that are important for sleep undergo changes in many women at menopause, and they are also profoundly affected by our feelings.

For example, it is not uncommon to be so exhausted emotionally after a fight with a spouse that despite going to bed early and sleeping for ten hours, you still feel tired. One of my patients realized that her insomnia was associated with chronic worry about her daughter's seeming inability to find a career and a living situation that suited her. Her sleep problem resolved when she decided to stop enabling this twenty-three-year-old by allowing her to live at home without making any contribution to the household. She insisted that her daughter find a job—any job—and learn how to support herself in the world.

One of my perimenopausal patients could not understand why she was having trouble sleeping. She said she was not having hot flashes or sweats, did not drink coffee, and wasn't really stressed. I asked her if she slept better when she was not in the same bed as her husband. She said, "Yes. I've noticed that I do." I told her that this was a sign from her inner wisdom. She replied, "But what am I supposed to do? You can't not sleep with your husband." I told her that although I couldn't tell her what to do about her sleeping arrangements, she still needed to be aware of the connection. She might consider sleeping separately for a while. She would learn a lot by how her husband responded to this suggestion. And a new arrangement could open the door to even more intimacy later on.

How Much Sleep Is Enough?

Our inherent biological rhythms are also taxed by the demands that modern life makes on our sympathetic nervous system, which is responsible for keeping us alert. We forget that the electric lightbulb has only been around for a very short time, evolutionarily speaking, and most of us weren't meant to stay up until midnight every night. Taking naps, sleeping late on dreary mornings, or going to bed at sunset are regarded with disdain in our "sleep macho" culture. Instead, we worship hyperactive individuals who work sixteen hours a day, and we even brag about how little sleep we get! Yes, there appear to be a few individuals who seem to do well with only four hours of sleep a night—or at least they appear to. But the vast majority of us require eight to ten hours of solid sleep each night to function optimally.

In 2018, the University of Western Ontario set out to answer this question by using the internet to recruit more than 10,000 people from around the world for what they called "the world's largest sleep study."[10] Participants, ranging in age from eighteen to a hundred, took a series of twelve online tests to assess how sleep affects different types of cognitive function. The scientists found the perfect window is seven to eight hours a night. Sleeping less than that (as well as sleeping more) negatively affects cognition. This was true for every age group. The further the subjects got in either direction from that ideal of seven to eight hours, the worse their cognition scores were. (If you're curious about why more sleep would be a problem, keep in mind that oversleeping can be a sign of depression or of one of several different sleep disorders, including apnea.)

In medical school, particularly after lunch as I was sitting in lectures, I would fantasize that there was a bed up on the podium, where I could sleep while the lecturer droned on. Some of this fatigue was from low blood sugar; I was eating too many carbohydrates. But even with a better diet, I couldn't have stayed alert on only five to six hours of sleep a night. Whenever I get too little sleep I feel extremely groggy in the morning and have difficulty getting motivated to do my work.

It's important to be flexible and compassionate about our sleep needs when life makes extra demands. Like it or not, what we really need during times of unusual demands is to get into bed and let our parasympathetic nervous system restore us. The much-maligned midday nap can be profoundly rejuvenating. Some corporations have even found that the productivity of their employees goes up when they are allowed to nap.

Sleep is an indispensable bodily function, as important as breathing and eating. It is hands down the most effective way for the body to metabolize excess stress hormones and inflammatory chemicals, which if left unchecked can eventually result in chronic degenerative diseases such as high blood pressure, arthritis, and cancer. Sleep is critical for bodily rest, for consolidation of learning and memory, and also as a way to help us sort out in our minds and bodies the things we have learned and experienced during the day. You've probably noticed how a good night's sleep helps you integrate new information or even new physical skills, such as exercise or dance moves that you may have struggled with the day before. When we allow ourselves to "sleep on" something, we're actually allowing ourselves to make connections in our sleep that we couldn't have made before.

Research has shown that our most restful sleep takes place when we are following our internal biological rhythm. For some that means getting up with the sun and going to bed relatively early, between nine and ten at night. This takes discipline, and it may not be your natural rhythm. Think back on a time in your life when you felt clearest and most rested. What time did you go to bed and what time did you wake up? In other words, synchronize your daily clock with your biological one.

Many menopausal women have been dismayed when they find that the amount of sleep that sustained them a year or two earlier seems inadequate now. I personally found that I needed much more sleep during perimenopause than I did a few years before. I knew that this was my body's way of getting the restoration it needed, given all the changes that were happening in my life. During both adolescence and perimenopause, it is a biological truth that we need more sleep than at other times in our lives. It is important for a woman to recognize this, honor it, and get the rest she needs, any way she can. For many, this means eight to ten hours a night. When I've been traveling or in times of stress, I often sleep for ten to twelve hours. And I no longer feel guilty about it.

Sleep is, quite simply, my go-to healer. Occasionally I find myself being overcome by sleepiness as early as seven o'clock in the evening. When I get this feeling, I get into bed and fall almost instantly into a deep, deep sleep. I sometimes sleep until ten the next morning. (Obviously this was *not* possible for most of my adult life because of my schedule, but it is now.) In the past, allowing myself to sleep this much would have been an unthinkable luxury. I would have beaten myself up for being so "lazy." Not anymore. I now know that when my body needs an unusually long stretch of deep sleep, I am rebooting my entire system, which is undergoing some kind of upgrade. I surrender now and am actually proud of myself for allowing this. This happens perhaps three times a year. But I want you to know about this in case you too need more sleep than our society considers "acceptable." And please note that I am definitely *not* talking about the kind of sleep that is associated with depression, where you simply cannot get out of bed; in these cases it is activity, not more sleep, that can turn things around.

Tips for Better Sleep

The following are some suggestions for better sleep during perimenopause. What works for one person may or may not work for another, so you should expect to go through some trial and error. Experiment with such sleep aids as meditation, deep relaxation exercises, listening to soothing music, or sipping a mug of warm chamomile tea. Whatever your routine, be sure to keep it free of "performance anxiety"—don't think about how few hours of rest you'll get if you don't fall asleep right away, don't look at the clock, and above all don't give in to your mental to-do list and get busy. You might end up establishing a night-owl habit that will be that much harder to break in the long run.

⌐ COOL YOUR HOT FLASHES. Hot flashes and night sweats are by far the most common reasons for sleep deprivation during menopause. Unless you're able to grab a nap during the day, your first priority should be to cool your hot flashes so that you can get the rest you need at night.

   As I've explained, hot flashes and night sweats are triggered by neurotransmitter changes in the brain that result, in part, from erratic estrogen levels or by wide deviations in the balance between estrogen and progesterone levels (even when total estrogen is normal). These are often triggered by excess stress hormones. In addition to maintaining hormonal balance, progesterone has a calming effect on the central nervous system, particularly on the brain.[11] It follows, then, that unbalanced estrogen can be a cerebral irritant, affecting the body in much the same way as adrenaline does.

Sleep disturbances are one of the most common reasons that I recommend natural progesterone cream, estrogen replacement, acupuncture, or herbal remedies (alone or in combination) to help a woman stabilize her hormone levels. But keep in mind that erratic hormones are not the only factor in sleep disturbances. Hot flashes are also exacerbated by underlying unresolved stress and anxiety and the unfinished business that fuels these symptoms.

~ CHILL OUT! Sometimes the only thing necessary to cool hot flashes is a cold pillow. I'm a big fan of the Chillow, a foam pillow into which you put water, which absorbs and then dissipates heat, keeping you cool naturally (see www.chillowstore.com). It keeps your face cool all night, thus helping prevent a hot flash from waking you up.

~ EAT FOR BETTER SLEEP. High blood sugar and insulin are often associated with poor sleep because they result in cellular inflammation throughout the body—including the brain. Following the diet outlined in chapter 7 (and adding foods rich in phytoestrogens, such as organic fermented soy, or taking supplements such as *Pueraria mirifica* or maca; see page 209) will often result in a good night's sleep. The number-one rule of thumb is: do not go to bed on a full stomach. If you lie horizontally when your stomach is full, it can cause gastric reflux, which occurs when pressure from the stomach's contents overwhelms the lower esophageal sphincter and food (or stomach acid) comes back up the esophagus. The result is heartburn, sour stomach, a bad taste in the mouth, and, possibly, asthma-like respiratory distress. The ideal is to wait three hours after eating before going to bed (or reclining on the couch).

On the other hand, a carefully chosen snack before going to bed can be good for you. A snack that is relatively high in protein and low in carbohydrates, or high in complex (unrefined) carbohydrates, is usually well tolerated. This would include fresh fruit, cheese, brown rice, a baked potato, lean meat, tofu, or cottage cheese. Notice what this list does not include: a Ring Ding, cookies, leftover pie, brownies, pizza, ice cream, Oreos, or potato chips. Refined and processed foods simply do not promote rest, relaxation, and the sort of deposits that need to be made in your health bank while you're rejuvenating yourself for the next day.

Taking antioxidant supplements twice a day can also support refreshing sleep.

~ AVOID CAFFEINE. Even one cup of coffee in the morning can disrupt sleep that night. Caffeine is cleared from the system much more slowly in women than in men. In addition to its effects on the central nervous system, caffeine, especially in coffee, is a bladder irritant: it will cause you to wake up at night to urinate.

~ AVOID ALCOHOL. Alcohol is a sedative that will put you to sleep. But it also disrupts the brain-stem sleep mechanism, resulting in rebound insomnia—meaning that you are more apt to awaken in the middle of the night. So that glass of wine that many use as a way to induce sleep is not a good long-term strategy.

~ GET REGULAR EXERCISE. Among a host of other benefits, regular exercise improves one's ability to get a good night's sleep. However, vigorous exercise within three to six hours of bedtime may be counterproductive. The increased activity boosts the metabolism and stimulates the central nervous system, making restful sleep more difficult to achieve. Relaxation exercises, on the other hand, such as hatha yoga and meditation, can be very helpful. Experiment with your own body's response to before-bed activities. As a general rule, the hour or two prior to bedtime is best spent winding down and creating an "electronic sundown."

~ SLEEP IN THE DARK. Electric lights, headlights of passing autos, even moonlight streaming through your window can disrupt a good night's sleep. If lack of pure darkness is disturbing your sleep, pull your shades down and make sure that you can't read the face of your alarm clock. Seeing what time it is can cause anxiety if you have a tendency toward insomnia. Get a bedside clock that is silent and dark but has a button on top that allows you to see the time if you need to. You might also try wearing an eye pillow. I swear by these, and I also travel with one. (For me, the ones made of silk with flaxseeds inside work the best.) For added comfort, I scent mine with calming lavender oil or use the ones that come pre-scented.

~ TAKE A WARM BATH WITH EPSOM SALTS. I often end my day with a warm bath to which I've added a couple of cups of Epsom salts (which I keep in a large container on the edge of the tub). I slip into the water and read until I am sleepy. Then I get into bed and sleep soundly until the next morning. Epsom salts is actually magnesium sulfate, and magnesium calms nerves beautifully. In fact, many perimenopausal women are deficient in this mineral, which can be absorbed through the skin, making soaking in a bath with Epsom salts a great way to get your magnesium. Stay in the tub at least twenty minutes.

REVERSE THE DAMAGE OF ELECTROMAGNETIC POLLUTION WITH VITAMIN G (GROUND)

Electromagnetic pollution (or electropollution) is caused by what is called "dirty electricity"—excess electromagnetic fields (EMFs) from electrical outlets, microwave ovens, cellphones, televisions, computers, and other everyday household appliances. Overexposure can damage our health when these fields clash with our body's own low-frequency bioenergetic fields. In fact, this electropollution is a major cause of insomnia. In the most susceptible individuals, electromagnetic pollution can also contribute to headaches, arthritis pain, anxiety, and even arrhythmia. Children, the elderly, and people with compromised immune systems seem to be at the most risk. And with the rollout of 5G, which is one step below a weapons-grade frequency, many people are suffering from the ill effects of EMFs. To combat this, I recommend placing EMF filters on every outlet in your home that reads above 50 on a device used to measure dirty electricity. I also recommend that you turn off your cellphone at night and never, ever sleep with it near your head. Better yet, remove Wi-Fi from your home altogether and instead use ethernet cables for your devices.

A most effective way to discharge electrical pollution is to connect with the earth—literally. The surface of the earth contains free-flowing electrons constantly replenished by solar radiation and lightning. This subtle electric signal is actually health-giving, helping to keep our bodies in a state of bioenergetic balance. Because modern life leaves us disconnected from the earth, thanks to rubber- and plastic-soled shoes and the fact that we no longer sleep on the ground the way our forebearers once did, that balance can get out of whack. Electropollution exponentially magnifies the problem.

However, the remedy is as close as your back door or your local park or beach. Walking barefoot on dirt, sand, or grass (or swimming in the ocean or a lake, for that matter) will electrically ground you. (Pavement and asphalt won't work.) This practice is called grounding, or earthing, and the idea behind it is that when your skin comes in direct contact with the ground, the free electrons transferred to your body from the Earth's surface neutralize free radicals, reducing inflammation. (Think of those free electrons as natural antioxidants from Mother Earth.) In addition, grounding has been shown to improve chronic muscle and joint pain, reduce overall stress and tension, boost mood, improve heart rate variability, reduce blood glucose levels in diabetics, and improve immune response, among other benefits.[12] Some twenty studies to date have reported significant physiological improvements when the body is grounded compared to not being grounded.[13] For example, researchers at the University of California at San Diego tested grounding on a group of sixteen massage therapists for a six-week period.[14] The subjects practiced grounding for four weeks followed by a two-week period when they did not ground. They reported significant improvements in pain and quality of sleep during the weeks when they practiced grounding. In addition, their biomarkers for inflammation, blood viscosity, and heart rate variability also improved.

For more information, read *Earthing: The Most Important Health Discovery Ever?* by Clinton Ober, Stephen T. Sinatra, M.D., and Martin Zucker (Basic Health Publications, 2010), or visit Dr. Sinatra's website at www.HeartMDInstitute.com. I also recommend the explanation of earthing on the website for an organization called Grounded, founded by Dr. Sinatra (see https://grounded.com/what-is-earthing).

~ COVER YOUR BEDROOM MIRRORS AT NIGHT, OR REMOVE THEM. If you have mirrors in the bedroom that you can see when lying down, they can be a deterrent to sleep. The reflections in them can make you feel jumpy and unsafe. According to the principles of feng shui, the ancient Asian art of working with the environment, mirrors enliven a room and increase the energy flow in it. Obviously, this is exactly the opposite of what you want in a place designed for sleep and relaxation. One solution is to put curtains over your mirrors that can be drawn back during the day.

~ DEVELOP, AND ADHERE TO, A GOING-TO-SLEEP RITUAL. Sleep aids such as melatonin, valerian, and other natural remedies (see page 442) can be great for getting you through several restless nights, but you also need to establish and adhere to a going-to-sleep ritual based on good overall sleep habits. This is known in the trade as "good sleep hygiene."

First, count backward from your preferred wake-up time to establish a bedtime that gives you sufficient sleep. Keep to this bedtime every day, even on weekends, so that your body clock can stabilize. It is quite well documented that most people do their best if they are in bed by 10:00 P.M., thus getting their deepest sleep in the earlier hours of the night.

Get out of your regular clothes and into something more comfortable (even your pajamas) up to a half hour before sleep, to give your body the signal that it's time to start winding down. Do your bathroom rituals at least half an hour before bedtime, too, including brushing your teeth, washing your face, and taking bedtime medications, so you can go straight to bed without reawakening yourself with these tasks.

~ BE YOUR OWN EDITOR. Don't use social media, or watch or listen to anything that might be disturbing to you, before bedtime (especially the 11:00 P.M. news). First of all, it is well known that the light from a computer or cellphone screen is activating and not healthy for the eyes, especially before sleep. The blue light the devices emit suppresses melatonin, the hormone that controls our sleep/wake cycle. (Looking at screens in the dark can also speed up macular degeneration, by the way.) While a blue-light filter on your device can help (as can using the "night" mode if the settings for your phone offer one), it won't eliminate the problem completely. You can also purchase blue-light-blocking glasses that are quite effective.

A computer screen or cellphone can also activate your sympathetic nervous system, thereby taking the rest-and-rejuvenation functions of the parasympathetic nervous system offline. (When I went to see the movie *Titanic* with my kids many years ago, I couldn't sleep that night because of visions of freezing, drowning victims. The same goes for war movies or anything else that is disturbing.) Also, please get the television out of the bedroom. On an energetic level, even having a television hooked up in your bedroom means that you are only a switch away from all the worries of the world. Spending hours on social media into the wee hours is the latest impediment to a good night's sleep. We're all eager to hear and see the latest news from our friends and children, but be sure to disconnect an hour or so before bedtime so you can truly relax.

⌐ AVOID EMOTIONALLY STRESSFUL DISCUSSIONS OR POTENTIALLY DIFFICULT PHONE CALLS NEAR BEDTIME. For some people, an urgent unresolved issue with a loved one will result in a sleepless night. You know the old adage "I need to sleep on it"? Well, there is great wisdom in that. Many times, allowing yourself to get a good night's sleep will help you sort things out and may even provide solutions in the form of dreams. So instead of having a difficult conversation at night, go to bed and see if sleeping on it will help. Of course, if you can resolve the issue before bed, that might also be a good strategy. The point here is to know yourself and consciously decide which approach works best for you.

⌐ GET THE GERBIL WHEEL OUT OF YOUR HEAD. One of the most common sleep detractors is the gerbil-wheel-in-the-head syndrome: stewing over worries, things not said, things not done, or things on the docket for tomorrow. When I get into one of these states, I get out of bed, take a couple of herbal tinctures known as Amantilla and Babuna (see page 442), step into a warm bath, and read a good book. Then, when I am sleepy, I consciously send God's love into my sleep and into my dreams. After about a half hour I go back to bed, and I don't look at the clock.

⌐ PUT YOUR WORRIES TO BED. Another way to get rid of the gerbil wheel is to write down everything that is bothering you just before you turn out the light. Then turn your worries over to the higher power of your choice, asking this power to guide you toward solutions to your problems while you sleep. Then imagine that when you wake up the next morning you'll have a healthier perspective and be inspired to the right action to change your situation for the better.

⌐ IMPROVE YOUR SLEEPING SURFACE. Many people try to get a good night's sleep using mattresses that have lost their support years before. You spend about one-third of your life asleep. Make sure you support yourself well when doing so. I recommend a new mattress at least every ten years. Every five would be far better! Also, get the best mattress you can possibly afford. I purchased an all-organic one several years ago and love it.

Prescription Sleep Medications: Caution

Use prescription sleep medication sparingly. Many healthcare practitioners prescribe sleep medications such as Lunesta and Ambien very freely. Other sleep medications are of the benzodiazepine class of drugs, such as diazepam (Valium), lorazepam (Ativan), and temazepam (Restoril). All of these drugs work in conjunction with the GABA receptors in the brain to produce a calming effect. All are habitforming and lose their effectiveness over time as the brain builds up tolerance, so you need more and more to get the same effect. I've seen many older women who were prescribed Valium for anxiety and insomnia during their perimenopausal years and who were still addicted to it thirty years later. These drugs have their place, but don't use them for longer than seven to ten consecutive days. (They're particularly good on overnight flights for those who can't sleep on airplanes.)

Other medications that can initially help sleep problems include the antidepressants known as selective serotonin reuptake inhibitors (SSRIs), such as fluoxetine (Prozac), venlafaxine (Effexor), and sertraline (Zoloft). Like the benzodiazepines, these can also lose their effectiveness over time.

Over-the-counter sleep remedies such as diphenhydramine (Sominex or Benadryl) interfere with the production of the brain chemical acetylcholine, which is very important for memory. Over time, the use of these drugs can cause serious memory problems and confusion.

Natural Sleep Aids

NATURAL PROGESTERONE: Try ¼ teaspoon of 2 percent natural progesterone skin cream (providing 20 mg progesterone) at bedtime. Natural progesterone binds to the GABA receptors in the brain and has a calming effect. Addiction to its brain effects is very rare but has been reported; I've only seen it in one patient in more than twenty years of practice.

PUERARIA MIRIFICA: One of the things I hear regularly about this herb is that because of its ability to quell hot flashes, women often get a good night's sleep within a week or so of regular use.

AMANTILLA AND BABUNA: Amantilla and Babuna are natural medicines, originating from the valerian plant (*Valeriana officinalis*) and the flower of the manzanilla plant (*Matricaria recutita,* commonly known as chamomile), respectively. In a double-blind, randomized, placebo-controlled multicenter study of these two herbal medicines, patients received 15 drops of each or of both together, administered thirty minutes before sleep. Amantilla was 82.5 percent effective in helping patients sleep, while Babuna was 68.8 percent effective.[15] Take Babuna (15 drops) thirty minutes before going to sleep when keyed up or anxious, and then follow it with Amantilla (15 drops) just before turning off the lights. What I like about these tinctures is that they have no side effects. (See Resources.)

VALERIAN: Studies comparing valerian with small doses of the benzodiazepines and barbiturates have shown that it is just as effective in inducing sleep and preventing nighttime awakening, but without inducing morning sleepiness.[16] If you use a type of valerian other than Amantilla, it often has a very bad taste in tincture form, so I recommend taking it in capsule form. Dosage is 150–300 mg of a product standardized to 0.8 percent valerenic acid at bedtime.

MELATONIN: The hormone melatonin is secreted by the brain's pineal gland in response to cycles of light and darkness. It produces drowsiness. Melatonin is also an antioxidant, and adequate levels help prevent degenerative illness. Our natural melatonin secretion is affected by depression, shift work, seasonal affective disorder, and jet lag, and supplemental melatonin can often help the sleep problems associated with these conditions. The usual dose is 0.5–3.0 mg taken an hour before bedtime. Some people use much more. And it can even be used in suppository form. If you are a shift worker, you can maintain a normal sleep pattern by taking melatonin about an hour before going to bed—even if bedtime occurs in the middle of the day. Melatonin also helps reset your biological clock if you have to go on a new sleep/wake cycle.

5-HTP: Melatonin is made from the precursor molecule 5-HTP (5-hydroxytryptophan), which has also been found to be very effective for treating sleep disorders, as well as PMS and seasonal affective disorder. It is safe and widely available. The starting dose is usually 100 mg three times per day. This can be very gradually increased over several months' time to a dose of 200 mg three times per day.[17] *Note:* Even natural substances such as valerian and natural progesterone may lose their effectiveness over time, because they bind to the same place in the brain as do prescription sleep drugs. It's best to use them sparingly, and only after you've tried other routes to a good night's sleep.[18]

DEPRESSION: AN OPPORTUNITY FOR GROWTH

Twenty-five percent of women will suffer from at least one major depression in their lifetimes. Millions more suffer from low-level anxiety and mild to moderate depression. Women receive the vast majority of prescriptions for drugs such as Elavil and Prozac.

But contrary to popular myth and medical opinion of the past, depression is *less* common among middle-aged women compared to women of other ages.[19] That said, there are still a significant number of women who experience midlife depression or an exacerbation of underlying depression when they enter midlife. Gladys McGarey, M.D., a family physician and friend of mine who has been in practice for over sixty years, told me that before hormone replacement and antidepressant medication, she sometimes saw women who negotiated the change by closing the door and taking to their beds, leaving their families to care for all the details of daily life. Months later, many emerged from the chrysalis of depression rejuvenated and ready to face the second half of their lives. By then, of course, their families' expectations about their roles and duties had also been transformed.

Fortunately, there's now a great deal more that can be done to support women's bodies through midlife depression. If you are depressed, it is crucial that you take action to get help. Depression can rob you of the pleasure of your achievements or the initiative to make changes for the better. It is also an independent and highly significant risk factor for both coronary artery disease and osteoporosis.[20]

Remember that depression, sadness, or anger often accompanies the emotional growth spurt that our psyches are undergoing. Just knowing this is sometimes all that is necessary to get you past the dark days. Sometimes outside help in the form of diet, herbs, or even antidepressant medications is needed. Before you can decide what action to take, you need to ask yourself the following questions.

~ Am I depressed? (Depression often is masked as unexplained symptoms such as chronic pain, constipation, headache, mood swings, or backache.)

~ What is my depression related to? (Depression is very often anger turned inward—not that a depressed person would know this consciously.)

～ Can I allow my body to process the unfinished business of my past? Am I willing to reclaim my own life and my own autonomy and do what it takes to liberate myself from limiting beliefs from my past?

The discussion below may help you to answer them.

The Anatomy of Depression

Depression exists on a spectrum ranging from the blues, which go away on their own, to the normal grief following a loss, to a more persistent and dangerous disorder. In major depression, as defined by psychiatric handbooks, a person not only suffers from depressed mood, but also has changes in appearance, behavior, speech, perception, and thoughts. When you are depressed, your insight and judgment can be affected, as can your ability to work, take care of yourself, and function in society. Depressed people may appear sad or have an expressionless face. Poor posture and grooming are sometimes evident. If you are depressed, you may derive very little enjoyment from normal daily activities, and you may begin to complain about numerous physical aches and pains that never bothered you before. (Statistics gathered at centers for chronic pain show that up to 90 percent of those with chronic pain have emotional stress factors such as depression that contribute significantly to their pain syndromes.)[21] Depression is often accompanied by sleep disturbances: you may be unable to get out of bed, or you may suffer from insomnia or early-morning awakening. Appetite disturbances—either overeating or loss of appetite—can result in significant weight gain or loss. Your thoughts can be affected by depression, and you may have difficulty concentrating and remembering things. (Many midlife women blame their memory loss on aging when it's really caused by depression.)[22] Your mind can go around and around in circles, and you may dwell on thoughts of guilt, self-blame, hopelessness, helplessness, and worthlessness. As depression deepens, thoughts of death and suicide can occur.

If you recognize yourself in this description, please know that there is a great deal you can do. My colleague Kelly Brogan, M.D., a psychiatrist who is also board certified in integrative holistic medicine, has written one of the very best books on the topic of depression and women that I have ever read. It's called *A Mind of Your Own* (HarperCollins, 2016). In it, Dr. Brogan examines the underlying evidence showing that antidepressant medication is highly addictive and often difficult to get off of—with the withdrawal actually creating the same symptoms for which the drug was originally prescribed. She points instead to a large body of evidence that proves that dietary and lifestyle change as well as various supplements, including magnesium and vitamin D, can often radically change a woman's mood. Dr. Brogan also runs an online community in which she teaches women how to manage their mental symptoms through self-compassion, insight, and dietary change. (See www.kellybroganmd.com.) Her results are astounding, with hundreds of women getting their lives back after years and years of failed pharmaceutical treatments.

If you are suffering from a major depressive disorder, it is very helpful to enlist professional assistance to work through the backlog of unfinished emotional business that may be contributing to it. Now is the time to address your unmet needs. In my experience, just getting on medication is not enough, though that might be something you choose.

Treatment can be lifesaving—especially if you also suffer from anxiety, which many women with depression do. In a 2009 study of more than 5,000 healthy Dutch midlife women, those with anxiety were shown to have a 77 percent increased risk of premature death.[23] Depression is also an independent risk factor for both heart disease and osteoporosis, probably because depression is associated with increased levels of stress hormones, which have very potent physical effects. (See chapter 12, on bone health, and chapter 14, on heart health.) Even more concerning is what we've learned from the Adverse Childhood Experiences (ACE) Study, which found that people who experienced serious neglect or physical, sexual, or emotional abuse as children have a markedly higher risk for both psychiatric and medical disorders, including depression, heart disease, stroke, substance abuse, and suicide.[24] The frequency of such abuse was alarming—researchers found that depending on the category, such abuse had occurred for 8 to 25 percent of the 17,000 people they studied.

Depression and Hormone Therapy

All sex hormones, including progesterone, estrogens, and androgens, can affect mood, memory, and cognition in complex and interrelated ways. Receptor sites for these hormones are found throughout the brain and nervous system, and nerve tissue itself has been found to produce them. Estrogen, the hormone that predominates during the first half of the menstrual cycle, has been shown, for example, to increase mood-enhancing beta-endorphins in menopausal women as well as in cycling women.[25] It has also been shown to boost levels of serotonin and acetylcholine, neurohormones that are associated with positive mood and normal memory.[26] Though androgens such as testosterone have not been as well studied as estrogen, they, too, appear to be associated with improvements in mood and vitality in some cases.[27] Given this, it's not surprising that many women report they feel better when they take some kind of hormone therapy. One of my colleagues tells me that she needs just a small amount of estrogen (less than 1 mg of estradiol twice per week) to keep her from getting the blues. As a physician, she swears by this. When the dosage of estrogen or androgen is too high, however, women often report adverse central nervous system effects such as headaches and increased anxiety. Synthetic progesterone is frequently associated with depression in women. Bioidentical progesterone only rarely has this effect. The general consensus at this time, given the WHI study results, is that there's not enough data to recommend HT as a primary treatment for depression. But I feel it is definitely worth considering for many women.

IRIS: A Cloud Descends at Midlife

Iris first came to see me when she was fifty-one. She had not had a period in six months. Iris was a very slim, attractive, healthy woman who exercised regularly, took nutritional supplements, and had a fulfilling career. She told me that starting about a year previously, a cloud had come over her mood, and she couldn't shake it. She couldn't pinpoint any particular life crises or other changes that might have precipitated her dark mood. Since her estrogen and progesterone levels were low, we decided to give estrogen replacement with natural progesterone a try.

When Iris came back two months later, she looked like a different person. She told me, "Within a few days of taking the estrogen and progesterone I felt like the lights went back on in my head."

Iris continued to feel better for the next two years. But then her depression returned despite the hormone therapy. Iris told me that she had begun to have flashbacks and memories of sexual abuse from early childhood. In retrospect, she realized that these memories had begun to surface during perimenopause. Though she had tried to ignore them and get on with her life, she felt that they had finally culminated in depression, which she was initially able to quell with estrogen and progesterone. When even that stopped working, she realized that "the only way out was through." She had to be willing to allow her body to feel and her brain to know what had happened to her as a child so that she could finally release the pain she'd been holding on to for a lifetime.

Iris consulted a skilled art therapist, who helped her work actively with her dreams and the creative process. She also signed up for a series of weekly full-body massages, which helped her release muscle tension. She later told me, "I was so surprised when the tears came the first time the massage therapist touched me. But I felt safe and secure, and she intuitively knew enough to simply let me do what my body needed to do. I just lay there and let myself feel everything. I let myself sob."

Within six months, Iris's depression lifted completely and has not returned. She continues with her hormone therapy because it feels right for her. Many times, depression lifts only when a woman gets in touch with her anger, anger that may have been suppressed by "niceness" for years. Anger is always preferable to depression because it mobilizes us and leads to change. It's a stage, not a destination. But I can assure you, it's a very powerful stage that can be liberating and life-giving!

Antidepressants Do Not Cure Depression

Antidepressant drugs have long been the first treatment offered for women suffering from depression. One popular category of antidepressants, SSRIs, work in part by increasing the availability of the neurotransmitter serotonin in your brain. Popular examples of these drugs include fluoxetine (Prozac), citalopram (Celexa), escitalopram (Lexapro), paroxetine (Paxil), and sertraline (Zoloft). Another commonly prescribed group of drugs are the tricyclic antidepressants (TCAs), which include imipramine (Tofranil) and amitriptyline (Elavil).

While many have found these drugs might initially be helpful, there is strong reason for caution. First of all, data published in 2009 from the more than 136,000 women in the WHI study indicate that both SSRIs and TCAs have been linked with an increased risk of death, and SSRIs have also been linked to an increased risk of stroke in postmenopausal women.[28] Although this risk is indeed small, it may not be a chance you want to take, considering that recent research shows that the benefits of these drugs have been greatly overstated. In a 2008 article published in the *New England Journal of Medicine,* former FDA psychiatrist Erick H. Turner, M.D., reported that 94 percent of studies showing SSRIs have therapeutic benefits were published, compared to only 14 percent of the studies that showed either no benefits or inconclusive benefits.[29] Considering all the medical literature, Dr. Turner determined that SSRIs helped those with severe depression more than those with mild to moderate depression—but the bottom line was that in most patients with depression, they were no more effective than a placebo.

A newer study, published in January 2010 in the *Journal of the American Medical Association,* not only confirmed Dr. Turner's findings about SSRIs, but also found that patients with mild to moderate depression received the same amount of relief from TCAs as they did from a placebo.[30]

You should also know that the side effects of these medications can be quite troublesome. Prozac and other SSRIs can cause nausea, loss of appetite, headache, nervousness, insomnia, restless leg syndrome, and difficulties with libido and sexual dysfunction. The tricyclic antidepressants can cause blurred vision, dizziness, dry mouth, heart rate disturbances, constipation, and difficulties with memory. Those who take these medications often have to try a different drug or dosage level in order to find the one that works best for them.

There are apt to be additional side effects from the long-term use of these drugs. This is certainly true of any drug that alters brain chemistry, and many of the popular psychotropic drugs on the market today are too new for anybody to say with authority that they are safe in the long run. Candace Pert, Ph.D., the scientist who discovered the receptor sites for many important chemicals in the brain associated with mood, commented:

> I am alarmed at the monster that Johns Hopkins neuroscientist Solomon Snyder and I created when we discovered the simple binding assay for drug receptors twenty-five years ago. Prozac and other antidepressant serotonin-receptor-active compounds may also cause cardiovascular problems in some susceptible people after long-term use, which has become common practice despite the lack of safety studies.
>
> The public is being misinformed about the precision of the SSRIs [Prozac, Zoloft, Paxil, etc.] when the medical profession oversimplifies their action in the brain and ignores the body as if it exists merely to carry the head around.[31]

I couldn't agree more, especially in light of a PMS drug that has been heavily marketed to women. This drug, Sarafem, is simply Prozac (fluoxetine) under a new name and with a new indication—an indication guaranteed to support women's continued mistrust of their body's wisdom. This is why I so highly recommend the work of Dr. Kelly Brogan, who has helped hundreds of women get off their medication and walk into a new life.

If your depression is severe enough to warrant trying prescription medications, I recommend you start with a six-month trial to be sure you are giving the drugs a chance to work. Half of those who stop their medication within three months of starting get depressed again. (I also suggest supporting your treatment with the Program for Boosting Mood, on page 452.) Optimally, the medicine will result in a gradual lifting of your depression. This will give you the energy to mobilize your own resources to make positive changes in your life. Think of these drugs as a bridge to help you cross a particularly rough stream in your life, but don't plan to live on that bridge for good. The true cure for depression lies in learning the skills associated with full emotional expression and then taking positive action. I realize that this is a very controversial topic, but my opinion is that psych meds should be avoided if at all possible. The risks are simply too great.

Many experts believe that depression is a recurrent disease. Of the patients who experience a major depression, 50 to 85 percent have additional episodes after they are successfully treated. Studies have shown that about 80 percent of people on antidepressants have a recurrence within three years after stopping medication.[32] Though these statistics seem grim, they would be much less so if all of us were willing to take a good look at what depression really is.

All too often antidepressants are given in a vacuum, as though depression were just a "Prozac deficiency." But depression is not a simple chemical disorder that lands on you when you least expect it. And depression is not a natural human condition. Studies have shown that depression is virtually nonexistent among many indigenous peoples. Depression is a consequence of how we live our lives. To get over it, we must be willing to make some changes that will support healthy brain biochemistry. Otherwise, depression is likely to recur. Antidepressant medication and getting help are associated with a very significant placebo effect. When you feel you are getting help, your body naturally gets better. Antidepressant medication works best when a patient is also willing to enter some kind of therapeutic relationship with a counselor to help her sort out the aspects of her life that need improvement. In other words, we, as a society and as individuals, need to understand that getting on the right medication does not guarantee a cure for depression.

Like all symptoms, depression is one way your body's inner wisdom tells you that something in your life is out of balance. Often its message is that a part of you has ceased to grow or has stagnated, or that you have lost the passion for living that is a natural part of being alive. It may also be a hint that you are angry with someone but do not feel free to express that anger directly. Depression may result from unresolved grief over the loss of a loved one through separation or death.

The best cure for depression that I know is to be completely honest with yourself about everything you are feeling—even, and especially, those feelings you've been told you shouldn't have, such as jealousy, anger, guilt, sorrow, and rage. All of these feelings are part of being human. They will never hurt you if you simply acknowledge them, express them safely, accept yourself for having them—and realize that you're having them for a reason. All so-called negative emotions occur when you don't feel that you're getting your needs met, whether those needs are for closeness, intimacy, validation, recognition, or something else entirely. For a listing of needs and emotions, I recommend the website of the Center for Nonviolent Communication (www.cnvc.org), a nonprofit organization founded by the late Dr. Marshall Rosenberg. Once you can identify your unmet needs, you'll be in a better position to take action to meet them. I've never seen depression lift without the sufferer taking some kind of positive action to help herself. This could be as simple as volunteering at an animal shelter.

In my experience, staying in dead-end jobs and/or relationships is a major factor associated with unremitting, chronic depression in women. So is being sedentary. Sometimes just taking action—which might be as simple as a daily walk—can jump-start a better mood. If you feel depressed and "dead," and if this has been going on for six months or more, it is probable that either you have unresolved grief about an important loss in your life or you have anger, resentment, or resignation about continuing to participate in a relationship or job that does not replenish you at the deepest levels. Many women at midlife finally have enough ego strength, life skills, and support systems in place to safely feel and release the unacknowledged pain of their pasts. For those who are willing to do this kind of work, depression and other symptoms may be alleviated rather quickly. There is no medication, supplement, exercise, or herb that will cure this problem. However, getting your blood sugar stable and making sure your nutrition is optimal can go a very long way in supporting you.

Program for Boosting Mood

The following lifestyle suggestions are excellent whether you choose prescription drugs for depression or whether you're trying to avoid psychotropic drugs and have opted instead to try a nutritional/lifestyle program.

⁓ STOP DRINKING. Alcohol consumption can make depression particularly persistent. This is partly because alcohol is itself a depressant, and partly because women too often use alcohol as a way to suppress their feelings.

⁓ ENGAGE IN REGULAR EXERCISE. Exercise changes brain chemistry by increasing beta-endorphins, lowering catecholamines, and increasing monoamines, and both aerobic and nonaerobic forms have been shown to be helpful in individuals with mild to moderate depression. (In some studies, 50 percent of people with depression were cured with exercise alone.)[33] Exercising twenty to thirty minutes per day four to five times per week can have a significant positive effect on your mood. It doesn't matter what you do—even dancing around the house to the music on your playlist will help—though the longer the exercise and the higher the intensity, the better the effects.[34] One recent study from the German Center for Neurodegenerative Diseases showed that both dancing and endurance training increased the volume of the hippocampus (the region of the brain critical for learning and memory, which is damaged in people who have Alzheimer's).[35] In addition, the popular dance-fitness class Zumba has been the subject of several new studies that show its psychological benefits.[36]

Yet another benefit of exercise is that it increases the amount of neurotransmitters in the brain, specifically serotonin and norepinephrine, which improve information processing and mood.[37] John Ratey, M.D., associate clinical professor of psychiatry at Harvard Medical School, believes that exercise is the single best thing we can possibly do for our brains and that it's at least as good for depression as prescription medication, if not better. Dr. Ratey, the author of *Spark: The Revolutionary New Science of Exercise and the Brain* (Little, Brown, 2008), explains that exercise helps the brain stay young, vibrant, and resilient because it can boost the formation of new brain cells, increase memory and the capacity for learning new things, and improve motor function and auditory attention, among other benefits. (See www.johnratey .com.) Exercise also promotes the production of neurotrophins, proteins that aid neuron survival and function. Having more neu-rotrophins leads to greater brain plasticity, which boosts memory and learning.

⁓ GET OUTSIDE IN THE NATURAL LIGHT AS MUCH AS YOU CAN. Light is a nutrient, pure and simple, and the wavelengths of natural light can help lift depression. Natural light or full-spectrum lighting helps combat seasonal affective disorder (SAD) and raises your brain levels of serotonin naturally. In the fall and winter, you may need a light box or full-spectrum lightbulbs to get enough light. (See Resources.)

⁓ TAKE A GOOD MULTIVITAMIN THAT SUPPORTS YOUR BODY AND BRAIN, AND MAKE AN EFFORT TO EAT WELL. If you are to function optimally, it is important that your brain gets balanced levels of serotonin, essential fatty acids (particularly omega-3 fats), and glu-cose. Avoid refined carbohydrates, eat protein at least three times a day, and be sure to include a source of omega-3 fat in your diet regularly. Eating balanced amounts of complex carbohydrates (with protein) provides the body with appropriate amounts of tryptophan, a building block of serotonin. (See chapter 7.)

⁓ AVOID FREQUENT CONSUMPTION OF CAFFEINATED BEVERAGES AND REFINED SUGAR. There is evidence to suggest that they may play a role in recurring depression.

If mild depression and/or anxiety is your primary problem and you're already taking a good multivitamin plus omega-3 fats and magnesium, then the next thing I'd add is St. John's wort. It has a history of hundreds of years of safe use. If after two months you've not noticed any difference, switch to 5-HTP. Reports on 5-HTP use have been particularly positive from people suffering from weight problems and insomnia in addition to depression. Be sure to get it from a reliable source, because of the possibility of contamination. If you also suffer from symptoms of panic disorder, obsessive-compulsive disorder, or anxiety plus depression, then I'd recommend a trial of inositol. Cannabidiol (CBD) oil can also be very helpful for many. It's been shown to have anti-inflammatory properties and to help with pain, mood, anxiety, and sleep issues.[38] (By the way, CBD oil will not produce a high like marijuana because it contains no appreciable amounts of tetrahydrocannabinol [THC], and CBD that comes from hemp is now legal in all fifty states.)

Remember, each of the suggestions above works well for some people but not others. This is true whether you opt for medication, exercise, psychotherapy, nutritional supplements, or another approach. You need to be willing to experiment in order to find the approach that seems to beckon to you. If you suffer from anxiety, depression, mood, or memory problems, the first place I'd go is to the work of Kelly Brogan, M.D. (www.kellybroganmd.com). I also highly recommend that you read *Unstuck: Your Guide to the Seven-Stage Journey out of Depression* (Penguin Books, 2008) and also *The Transformation* (HarperCollins, 2019), by my colleague James S. Gordon, M.D., a holistic psychiatrist and founder of the Center for Mind-Body Medicine in Washington, D.C. Dr. Gordon is a recognized authority on trauma and how to heal it and has worked in war zones all over the world.

Supplements to Combat Depression

The following vitamins, herbs, and other supplements have proven extremely useful for lifting depression. In conjunction with the lifestyle suggestions presented in the previous section, they work well for many women. *Note:* If you are taking prescription medications for depression, do not combine your drug therapy with any of these supplements without consulting your physician.

VITAMINS AND OTHER NUTRIENTS: Deficiencies of biotin, folic acid, vitamin B_6 (pyridoxine), vitamin B_{12}, and vitamin C have all been linked to depression. Vitamin B_6 deficiency, for example, has been shown to lower levels of serotonin. Vitamin B_6 has a role in the production of the monoamine neurotransmitters, which are important for mood stabilization. Deficiencies of calcium, copper, magnesium, and the omega-6 fatty acids may also relate to depression.

Fish oil may be particularly helpful. A large clinical trial published in 2009 showed that fish oil may benefit half of all people with moderate to severe depression (although not those whose depression was accompanied by anxiety).[39] The omega-3 fatty acids contained in fish oil support the serotonin system by helping serotonin get to the brain, where it's needed. Omega-3s have been shown to lower risk of all kinds of mental illness, and may also help reduce stress.

For preventive and/or therapeutic benefits, consider adding the following nutritional supplements to your program.[40]

~ PYRIDOXINE (B_6). Recommended dose 50–500 mg per day. Pyridoxine should be taken with the other B complex vitamins listed on page 303.

~ VITAMIN C. Recommended dose 1,000–5,000 mg per day.

~ OMEGA-3 FATS. Recommended dose is to start with 400 mg per day of EPA and DHA combined and work up to as high as 5,000 mg per day if needed.

~ MAGNESIUM. The vast majority of the population could use more magnesium, and many have an outright deficiency, which is associated with anxiety in many women as well as heart rhythm problems. Taking 400–1,000 mg a day can often work wonders and is, along with a good multivitamin and omega-3 fat source, the first thing I'd recommend. The most absorbable and effective magnesium supplement on the market is ReMag, formulated by Carolyn Dean, M.D., N.D. I recommend that you take both ReMag and ReMyte to replenish magnesium optimally. (See www .rnareset.com.)

ST. JOHN'S WORT: This herb, which contains the active ingredients hypericin and hyperforin, has been very well researched, with some studies indicating that it is as effective as Prozac in treating mild to moderate depression. The usual dose is 300 mg of herb standardized to 0.3 percent hypericin and 3 percent hyperforin, three times per day.

VALERIAN: If you have an anxiety component with your depression, add valerian to your St. John's wort. The usual dose is 100–300 mg standardized extract containing 0.8 percent valerenic acid.

GINKGO: If your depression is associated with attention and memory problems and you are age fifty or older, consider *Ginkgo biloba* in addition to St. John's wort. The usual dose is 40–80 mg three times per day.

INOSITOL: Inositol is an effective over-the-counter alternative to many commonly prescribed antidepressants.[41] The exact mechanism of action is unknown, but it appears to be linked with the serotonin system, affecting the same pathways of brain chemistry as do the tricyclic and SSRI antidepressants, though without the side effects. I've prescribed inositol for several patients who have tolerated it well. One, a person with a very significant family history of depression, used it following the loss of a loved one. She reported, "In the past, before inositol, I would have gone through my grief and then fallen into a black hole. This time I could still feel all of my feelings deeply, but I was able to move through them without a depression hangover." Usual therapeutic starting dose is 12 g per day; however, inositol has been shown to be well tolerated in doses as large as 18–20 g per day. (See Resources.)

5-HTP: 5-hydroxytryptophan is a compound naturally produced in the body from the amino acid tryptophan, which is an important precursor to serotonin. Although tryptophan is found in many foods, it can be difficult to consume enough tryptophan in the diet to overcome serotonin deficiency. (Tryptophan supplements were once widely used as sleep aids, but they were taken off the market after some products were found to be contaminated.) 5-HTP can be extracted from plants and is now available as a nutritional supplement. It has been used for decades in Europe as an approved treatment for both depression and sleep problems. The side effect of nausea is sometimes reported, but an enteric-coated formulation should help avoid this. The usual dose is 100–200 mg three times per day. (For more information, see *5-HTP: The Natural Way to Overcome Depression, Obesity, and Insomnia* by Michael Murray, N.D. [Bantam, 1998]; also see Resources.)

SAM-E: S-adenosyl-L-methionine has been found to be instrumental in promoting cell growth and repair. On a molecular level, it also contributes to the formation of key neurotransmitters, the basis for its mood-stabilizing activity and the promotion of mental clarity. Additionally, SAM-e has antioxidant and anti-inflammatory properties, and thereby supports immune function and joint health, mobility, and comfort.[42] The usual dose is 800–1,600 mg per day. (See Resources.)

MEMORY LOSS AT MENOPAUSE: IS THIS ALZHEIMER'S?

Many women experience "fuzzy thinking" or "cotton head" during perimenopause. They complain of forgetting names, misplacing objects, or having difficulty balancing their checkbook. This is usually not a memory problem or the beginning of Alzheimer's disease. It is, instead, the result of a shift of attention from the outer world to the inner world, and from the left hemisphere (where words and linear thinking tend to reside) to the right hemisphere (which is associated with music, art, intuition, and spirituality). I have come to see that the brain changes of perimenopause are really our inner guidance attempting to get us to pay attention to ourselves and our innermost world instead of the outer world. As our hormones change and our brains rewire, this fuzzy-headed feeling is common. Some women become terrified because of their need for a high degree of intellectual control—a response that makes the problem far worse. Others find themselves willing to trust the process once they're reassured that it's normal, part of the wisdom of perimenopause that focuses our attention inward. The same thing often happens both premenstrually and during the postpartum period.

Memory problems at midlife are also due to temporary overload from the many external demands on your limited time. It's like trying to call an Uber in New York City during SantaCon, when so many people are running around the city dressed as Santas or elves and being given free drinks; all the bandwidth for cellphones is being used and you can't get through.

If you find that you can't remember something instantly, like the name of a person you know quite well, just relax, do something else for a while, and give yourself the time, space, and respect that allow your brain to retrieve stored information. Getting anxious and putting yourself down for forgetting only makes the problem worse.

But Aren't We Losing Brain Cells?

In medical school, I was taught that we reach peak brain size in our twenties and then our brain shrinks after that. But much newer studies have shown that we continue to add cells to our brains (a process known as neurogenesis) for our entire lives, even if we live into our nineties and beyond.[43] How we eat, how much and what kind of exercise we get, and various other lifestyle factors determine our brain's biological age, which is not at all the same as our chronological age.[44] Research indicates that throughout our lifetime, as we move from naïveté to wisdom, our brain function becomes molded by our experience. Think of your brain as a tree that requires regular pruning if it is to acquire its optimal shape, size, and function. Brain cell loss over the years is akin to pruning the nonessential branches. But the interconnections among various brain cells continue to grow—which is what happens when you learn any new skill.

Eleanor Maguire, Ph.D., professor of cognitive neuroscience at University College London, performed a prospective study of individuals training for their cabdriver licenses. She started by doing MRIs of their brains. After they had gone through the incredible task of memorizing 25,000 streets—which takes several years—she again did MRIs of those who successfully passed the test and got their cab-driver licenses. She found that their hippocampal memory areas had increased dramatically in size and function compared to when they began their training.[45]

Research has conclusively shown that in response to learning, new brain cells continue to form in the hippocampus (the area of the brain associated with memory) throughout one's lifetime.[46] Every single one of us has the same ability to increase the size of our memory areas as we grow older. In fact, our brain connections—created by dendritic and axonal branching—increase with age, as our capacity to make complex associations increases. Some aspects of our memory actually improve in later life, such as the ability to extract patterns and make accurate predictions. In short, the older and more experienced you become, the more efficient and sophisti-cated your brain. It's also worth noting that while learning abilities may decrease during perimenopause, they rebound to premeno-pausal levels afterward, according to a 2009 study of more than 2,000 women.[47]

Dementia of all types, including Alzheimer's, is a different matter. It is associated with free-radical damage to brain tissue, which results from the overproduction of inflammatory chemicals at the cellular level, eventually leading to the damage or death of brain cells. Free-radical damage and the resulting tissue inflammation are the final common pathway by which emotional, physical, and environmental stressors of all kinds adversely affect every tissue in our bodies, in-cluding our brains.[48] We now know that dementia is also caused by chronically high blood sugar and insulin resistance over time. This association between blood sugar, insulin, and dementia is why Alz-heimer's is sometimes called "type 3 diabetes."[49] A 2017 study headed by Mayo Clinic neuroscientist Guojun Bu, Ph.D., showed that while a variant of the Alzheimer's gene called APOE4 (which interrupts how the brain processes insulin) is present in only about 20 percent of the general population, it's present in more than 50 percent of people diagnosed with Alzheimer's.[50] Dr. Bu and his team also found that in those with the APOE4 gene, the insulin resistance caused by diet in turn induced insulin resistance in the brain, speeding up the onset of Alzheimer's. Other recent research shows that even in those who don't carry the APOE4 gene, being insulin resistant is associated with a dramatic increase in risk for the accumulation of amyloid in the brain, a marker of Alzheimer's.[51]

Studies show that those who are well educated, in good health, and financially secure, with above-average intelligence and social status, and who actively pursue their interests as they age have a very good chance of preserving their memory as they grow older. In fact, they may even improve it, whether or not they're on estrogen.[52] In addition, those with a strong sense of purpose in life are almost two and a half times less likely to develop Alzheimer's disease, according to a 2010 study.[53] (The study also showed that purpose in life reduced the risk for cognitive impairment not related to Alzheimer's.)

Given the fact that the brain responds to such factors as a meaningful life, nutrients, exercise, stable blood sugar, community, learning, supplements, and so on, perimenopause is the perfect time to begin a brain health program for prevention of dementia later on. Holistic neurologist David Perlmutter, M.D., an expert in nutritional influences on neurological disorders and co-author of *Power Up Your Brain: The Neuroscience of Enlightenment* (Hay House, 2011), writes that "in reality, we are *all* at risk [of dementia] and that risk is substantial, approaching 50 percent by the time we reach eighty-five years. So implementation of a preventive program is far more meaningful, as it has far-reaching benefits well beyond brain health." I couldn't agree more.

Preventing Alzheimer's: Some Lessons from the Nun Study

Even with reassurance that it's normal to go through some transient changes in thinking and focus during perimenopause, many women still fear becoming demented and unable to live independently as they get older. Alzheimer's disease currently affects about 5.8 million Americans age sixty-five and older—that's one in ten people among this age group. Experts estimate that by the year 2050, that figure will be 13.8 million.[54] Not surprisingly, it's also the leading cause of dependence and institutionalization in the elderly, although—and this is a shock to many—only 4 percent of Americans over sixty-five live in nursing homes.[55]

It appears at an earlier age in women than in men, and up to two-thirds of cases reported have been in women—in part simply because women live longer. According to estimates from the Aging, Demographics, and Memory Study (ADAMS), 14 percent of all people age seventy-one and older have dementia.[56] But that means that 86 percent *don't*. Still, we all know someone with dementia and how burdensome it can be to care for them. And so each of us will want to do everything we can to care for and enhance our brain function at perimenopause—long before memory problems or dementia have a chance to develop.

Alzheimer's disease was named after Alois Alzheimer, a German neuropathologist who, in 1906, looked under a microscope at the brain tissue of a fifty-five-year-old woman who had spent the last years of her life in a mental institution, where she was prone to paranoia and fits of anger. Alzheimer identified two substances in her brain that have come to be associated with the disease: dense *plaques* formed by the protein beta-amyloid outside the brain cells, and stringy *tangles* within the nerve cells themselves. Whether these plaques and tangles are the cause of Alzheimer's dementia is controversial. We do know, however, that there's a great deal of overlap between the senile dementia caused by cerebrovascular insufficiency and stroke and that which is associated with the plaques and tangles of Alzheimer's disease. And we also know, as previously stated, that Alzheimer's is associated with blood sugar instability.

Alzheimer's has a genetic component as well.[57] But even if Alzheimer's runs in your family, that does not mean you will inevitably get it. Brain function is multifactorial, meaning that it is affected by many different aspects of our lives, from the amount of antioxidant-rich vegetables we eat, to blood sugar levels, to the level of education we've attained. It is also shaped by events and behaviors that begin in childhood and continue into old age. That's why there will never be a hormone or magic bullet that can guarantee brain protection for life. However, you can affect your brain health by the lifestyle choices you make.

Nowhere has this been more convincingly demonstrated than in the famous study of a group of hundreds of nuns belonging to the School Sisters of Notre Dame, who donated their brains for study after death.[58] Because these women have spent much of their lives in the order, there is a wealth of data about each woman, often spanning many decades. One surprising finding was that a greater or lesser capacity for complex thought—known as "idea density"—in early life was correlated with the likelihood of developing Alzheimer's disease in later life. Upon entering the convent (usually in her early twenties) each of the nuns was required to write an autobiography. When linguistics experts analyzed these years later, they found a startling correlation between the nuns' language skills and the eventual occurrence of Alzheimer's. The lower their idea density, the higher their risk.

Another fascinating finding from the Nun Study is that the presence of plaques and tangles in the brain does not always predict the mental status of an individual. One of the nuns had strikingly good mental status and attitude before her death in her late eighties; researchers were startled to find severe loss of neurons and multiple amyloid tangles in her brain at autopsy. This evidence supports a great truth: that the physical body and the spirit are inextricably linked. For people who are optimistic, lively, and engaged, as this particular nun was, anatomical limitations often seem not to result in disability. A similar finding was reported in a 2010 study of 1,157 people that showed that mentally stimulating activities delayed the onset of dementia, but if symptoms *do* eventually appear, deterioration is more rapid than normal.[59] It's almost as if the mental activity is strong enough to cover up the signs of the physical changes, holding them off for as long as possible. That means that those who are mentally active end up staying mentally healthy for a greater percentage of their lives, even if they do end up getting dementia eventually.

On the other hand, the Nun Study has shown that small-vessel disease, in the form of mini-strokes, is strongly predictive of dementia. Chronic depression also seems to be correlated with Alzheimer's. When we shut off the circulation of blood to an area of our body, we are shutting off life force. Similarly, depression is a shutting down of the life force within us.

Not surprisingly, researchers have recently found that there's a direct correlation between cardiac index (the amount of blood, relative to a person's size, that is pumped by the heart) and brain volume. Researchers from the Framingham Offspring Cohort, part of the Framingham Heart Study, found that people with low cardiac indexes—and even people with cardiac indexes that were merely on the low side of normal—had smaller brains.[60] The effect shows up even in people who are otherwise perfectly healthy and do not at the present time have heart disease. And because having more brain volume is associated with better brain health, this means that the more you can do to keep your heart and circulatory system healthy, the healthier your brain will be, too.

Another serious challenge with Alzheimer's, of course, is the huge emotional toll it takes on those who care for loved ones with the condition. As poignantly shared in *The Shriver Report: A Woman's Nation Takes on Alzheimer's,* a 2010 report produced by Maria Shriver in partnership with the Alzheimer's Association, women account for 60 percent (about 6.7 million) of the 11.2 million Alzheimer's and dementia caregivers in this country. One-third of these women caregivers are "on duty" twenty-four hours a day, seven days a week, and 60 percent say they've become caregivers because they don't have other family to shoulder the responsibility. Many are stretched in multiple directions—one-third of the women also have children or grandchildren under eighteen living at home with them.

HORMONES AND ALZHEIMER'S

An impressive number of studies have shown an association between estrogen use and the delay or even prevention of Alzheimer's.[61] This wasn't the case with the 2006 WHI study, however, which showed an increased risk with Premarin and Prempro. Nevertheless, estrogen (as well as progesterone and testosterone) has been shown to stimulate the regeneration of damaged neurons. Estrogen also appears to increase the production of the neurotransmitter acetylcholine, which regulates memory, learning, and other cognitive functions. In fact, estradiol (a type of natural estrogen) binds to the areas in the brain that are associated with memory: the cortex, the hippocampus, and the basal forebrain. Estrogen has also been shown to enhance nerve cell branching.[62] Research indicates that women with the highest endogenous levels of estradiol have the lowest risk for Alzheimer's disease.[63]

Despite the results of the WHI study, there is still convincing evidence of the beneficial effect of hormones—not just estrogen—on brain function.[64] For example, as mentioned in chapter 8, women who have their ovaries removed before age forty-five have a fivefold increase in risk of mortality for neurological or mental diseases as well as an increased risk of developing Parkinsonism, cognitive impairment, and dementia later in life, according to a Mayo Clinic study published in 2009.[65] And there is evidence that small baseline amounts of estrogen are essential for certain memory functions. Many women's bodies produce enough throughout life, while some do not. The research of Barbara Sherwin, Ph.D., has shown that women's verbal memory decreases following hysterectomy with removal of the ovaries, but then returns to normal following hormone therapy.[66] Dr. Sherwin used only estrogen therapy, but other studies support a role for progesterone and probably androgens as well.[67] Even transdermal estradiol, if begun soon after menopause, may give at least modest protection against Alzheimer's, according to a 2009 study done at Emory University School of Medicine in Atlanta.[68]

Ovarian hormones also bind to areas of the brain that are important for mood regulation. This helps to explain research findings indicating that estrogen has significant antidepressant effects and that progesterone decreases anxiety and promotes restful sleep. While the research on estrogen and memory is not conclusive, a small amount of bioidentical estrogen (and/or progesterone, testosterone, or phytoestrogens) definitely helps the brain function of some women. If you've had your ovaries removed and are not producing small amounts of steroid hormone on your own, you may well want to consider adding a bit of hormonal support of some kind to your brain.

NONHORMONAL WAYS TO PROTECT YOUR BRAIN

Consider the following brain-health-enhancing practices.

⁓ FEED YOUR BRAIN WITH NUTRIENTS. A diet high in refined sugars and including partially hydrogenated fats is associated with depletion of many nutrients necessary for optimal brain function. For brain function, as for every other aspect of your health, I recommend a diet of whole, organic foods that keep blood sugar stable, including healthy fats and some protein. Studies have shown that demented and depressed patients often have inadequate levels of zinc, B vitamins (especially vitamin B_1 or thiamine), selenium, and antioxidants such as vitamins E and C, compared with patients with normal mental function.

Zinc, for example, is necessary for optimal transport of the B vitamins into the cerebrospinal fluid. This fluid bathes and nourishes the brain and spinal cord. Many women do not get adequate levels of zinc in their daily diets.[69] In one study of severely demented patients, ten patients were given vitamin supplements for two months, while a control group was not. After one month, the patients who received the supplements showed clinical memory improvement.[70] Alzheimer's may also be associated with the inability of some elderly people to absorb enough minerals, vitamins, and essential trace elements from their food.[71] They may have problems with transporting these nutrients from the blood to the brain as well. Since nutritional supplementation improves memory in people who are already demented, imagine the preventive potential of feeding your brain right!

⁓ QUELL POTENTIAL FREE-RADICAL DAMAGE TO YOUR BRAIN TISSUE. Brain health is to a great extent affected by free-radical damage.

And high blood sugar is the number-one cause of free-radical damage because it damages the lining of all the blood vessels in your
body. This is known as "glycemic stress." So you have to get serious about bringing your insulin and blood sugar levels to an optimal level, and also make sure your diet is high in antioxidants such
as vitamins C and E, the B vitamins (including folic acid), and selenium.[72] Another class of powerful antioxidants is the proanthocyanidins (also called procyanidins), found in pine bark and grape
seeds. (The dosage ranges for these are given in chapter 14, page
701.) Studies have shown that the risk of stroke is very low in
those women who eat at least five servings of fruits and vegetables
per day. Clearly, brain protection is yet another reason to eat
plenty of these nutrient-rich foods.

- BOOST YOUR LEVEL OF VITAMIN D. Many, many people have suboptimal levels of vitamin D, which is associated with everything
from multiple sclerosis to depression. In recent decades, researchers have discovered a link between vitamin D levels and Parkinson's disease. A 2010 study following more than 3,000 people
from Finland for twenty-nine years showed that the higher the
subjects' levels of vitamin D, the lower their risk for the disease.[73]
An increasing number of studies also point to a link between suboptimal levels of vitamin D and dementia, including Alzheimer's.
A 2017 study that tracked 916 people in France for twelve years
showed that adults with vitamin D levels less than 20 ng/ml doubled their risk of all-cause dementia and almost tripled their risk
for Alzheimer's.[74] A 2019 study from China showed similar significant associations, with people whose vitamin D levels measured
less than 10 ng/ml having the most risk for Alzheimer's and
other types of dementia.[75] The connection seems to be related to
the immune system, which vitamin D is known to support. With
sufficient vitamin D, the immune system is able to break down
beta-amyloid plaques in the brain and flush them out via the
bloodstream, while with insufficient levels, the immune system becomes dysfunctional and may actually worsen the plaques' effects.

As mentioned in chapter 8, an optimal blood level for vitamin D is 40–80 ng/ml. Everyone should have their blood levels
checked. If yours is low, it generally takes 5,000–10,000 IU of vitamin D_3 per day, plus or minus regular doses of sunlight, to reach
optimal levels. Then you can reduce the dosage to 2,000 to 5,000
IU per day, depending on sun exposure. For more information on
the importance of vitamin D, see www.grassrootshealth.net.

- AVOID SMOKING AND EXCESSIVE ALCOHOL INTAKE. Cigarettes are well-known factors in causing cardiovascular disease and small blood vessel changes that decrease oxygen to your brain, among other areas. And excessive alcohol intake affects the basal forebrain, an area associated with memory.

- EXERCISE. Researchers at the Aging Research Center of the Karolinska Institute in Sweden found that those who exercise at least twice per week reduced their risk of dementia in general by more than 50 percent and of Alzheimer's specifically by 60 percent. The study, which is the first to show a long-term relationship between physical activity and dementia later in life, examined 1,449 participants at midlife and again twenty-one years later at ages sixty-five and seventy-nine. At the follow-up exam, 117 showed evidence of dementia and 76 had Alzheimer's. But those who exercised had a greatly reduced risk of dementia and Alzheimer's even after adjusting for other lifestyle factors. Interestingly, the greatest benefit was seen in those with a genetic susceptibility to dementia and Alzheimer's.[76] Quite a number of newer studies confirm these findings, including a few that show significant improvement in cognitive function after only six weeks of a moderate aerobic exercise program.[77] The meta-analyses are perhaps the most telling—one published in 2019 looking at thirteen randomized controlled trials showed that physical activity and exercise improve cognition in older adults with Alzheimer's.[78] Exercise definitely turns on a whole-body mechanism that helps to keep the brain healthy. It also increases blood flow.[79] Basically, any activity that increases heart rate and results in sweating will work!

- ENJOY MUSIC. Research shows that music may regenerate or stimulate several areas of the brain while it also slows brain cell degeneration. Fortunately, there's no one best type of music for this—the music you like best is what will work best for you. By the way, the studies showed that music with vocals tends to be the most promising for treating those who already have dementia.[80]

- WRITE OR DRAW, BUT NOT USING A COMPUTER. It turns out that handwriting is good for your brain. Writing by hand (as opposed to typing on a keyboard) activates regions of the brain associated with learning and improves memory for new information, according to a 2017 study.[81] The researchers believe that this practice may promote "deep encoding" of new information in ways that keyboarding does not—especially when combined with creating doodles, shapes, arrows, and other symbols. Any practice that enhances learning stimulates the hippocampus.

~ ENHANCE YOUR BRAIN'S ACETYLCHOLINE LEVELS. Many factors can affect your acetylcholine levels and, subsequently, your memory. If you're already on estrogen or other hormones to treat other symptoms, stick with them—though I wouldn't recommend hormones solely for Alzheimer's prevention, be reassured that they are probably helping your acetylcholine levels. And avoid drugs that are known to decrease acetylcholine levels.[82] You'd be amazed by how many of these there are and by how few doctors realize their adverse affect on brain function. Check the label of any medication used for sleep, colds, or allergies to see if it contains diphenhydramine. Examples of such medications include Sominex, Benadryl, Tylenol PM, Excedrin PM, and Tylenol Severe Allergy. The cough suppressant dextromethorphan also affects acetylcholine and has other anticholinegeric effects that can impair memory. It is found in Robitussin DM and a wide range of other cough and cold remedies.

~ BOOST YOUR DHEA LEVELS. Studies suggest that DHEA (and the related hormones progesterone and pregnenolone) act as neurotransmitters in the brain and can promote the same kind of dendritic and axonal branching between brain cells that is seen with estrogen. The best way to enhance levels of DHEA is to follow the adrenal restoration program on page 152.

Other Brain Food Choices

The food supplements listed below have been shown to help memory in many people. Try just one at a time, so that you know if it works for you. Use your intuition to pick one to start with. Your first impulse will usually be the right one.

GOTU KOLA: Widely known as a "memory herb," gotu kola (*Hydrocotyle asiatica*) also increases circulation to the brain. The usual dosage is 90 mg per day. *Note:* Gotu kola is a stimulant and should not be taken at bedtime.

OMEGA-3 FATS: Nerve fibers throughout your body are coated with a fat called myelin. For good brain and nerve function, you need small amounts of high-quality (not partially hydrogenated) fat in your daily diet. Two studies on rats and one on mice have shown that a diet supplemented with the omega-3 fatty acid DHA (docosahexaenoic acid) significantly improves memory—one study showed dramatic improvement after only four days![83] Dutch researchers who tracked more than 1,600 adults between the ages of forty-five and seventy for six years concluded that those who ate more omega-3 fats regularly scored higher on a battery of tests involving brain health, including memory.[84] I recommend consuming fatty fish such as salmon or sardines, ground flaxseed, or fish oil in supplement form. DHA made from algae is a good choice for taking oil in supplement form, particularly for vegetarians (I like the Neuromins brand). I recommend supplementing with a combined total of 400 mg per day of DHA and EPA at first, and working up to as high as 5,000 mg per day if needed. Mercury-free fish oil supplements (including USANA BiOmega and Vital Choice Alaskan Sockeye Salmon Oil) are also available. (See Resources.)

PHYTONUTRIENTS: Many plant foods are very rich in what are known as phytonutrients, which have a beneficial effect on the lining of the blood vessels through their antioxidant effect. In fact, studies have shown that women who eat the most fruits and vegetables daily have a much lower risk of stroke. A meta-analysis done by University of London researchers and reported in the *Lancet* showed that people who ate at least five servings of fruit and vegetables a day lowered their stroke risk by 25 percent.[85] Since small-vessel disease and stroke are inextricably linked, it's clear that plant foods rich in a wide variety of beneficial substances can help preserve good brain function.

The herb *Pueraria mirifica* is another excellent option. A study done in Thailand found that it significantly decreased nerve cell death and was protective against beta-amyloid plaques, which increase risk for Alzheimer's disease.[86] Yet another published study showed *Pueraria mirifica* helps combat brain cell degeneration and is effective in restoring memory in both early and late stages of cognitive impairment (although, not surprisingly, it's most effective when taken in the early stages).[87]

Maca (*Lipidium meyenii*), a plant found in the Peruvian Andes that was considered sacred by the Incas, may also be helpful. Studies on rats show that maca improves learning abilities and memory function,[88] as well as prevents Alzheimer's.[89]

In Japan, where consumption of soy is far higher than it is in the United States, the incidence of Alzheimer's and other dementias is much lower than it is here. Wake Forest University Health Sciences was awarded a patent in 2003 based on their research into the use of soy to prevent Alzheimer's disease.[90] Preliminary research has shown that soy phytoestrogens affect the brain like estradiol, but not as strongly.[91] Soy isoflavones also act as antioxidants in the brain.[92] Several studies indicate soy can help boost memory as quickly as six weeks after adding it to your regular diet.[93] One recent study showed that postmenopausal women consuming 60 mg of soy isoflavones a day for six weeks improved their nonverbal short-term memory, mental flexibility, and planning ability.[94] Another study of postmenopausal women showed that consuming soy isoflavones improved verbal memory.[95] And since soy definitely helps the cardiovascular system, it may also help prevent the strokes that are so common in dementia.

Substances Your Brain Doesn't Need

ALUMINUM: Aluminum has been found in the brains of Alzheimer's patients, and this disease has been associated with increased tissue levels of aluminum along with decreased levels of zinc and selenium. Although the nature of the link is not clear, there is evidence to suggest that aluminum is, indeed, a brain toxin in individuals who are genetically predisposed to Alzheimer's. If you have any Alzheimer's sufferers in your family, I'd recommend that you avoid aluminum cookware; antiperspirants, toothpaste, and cosmetics containing aluminum; soda from aluminum cans; and baking powder containing aluminum (use Rumford's, for example, rather than Calumet or Clabber Girl).[96] The German Federal Institute for Risk Assessment (known in Germany as the BfR) further suggests not preparing or storing especially acidic and salty foods in uncoated aluminum containers or in aluminum foil. They also advise that you vary your diet (good advice for a number of reasons) and alternate the products and brands you use to reduce any risk of high intake of aluminum from individual highly contaminated products. I would also stay away from vaccines that contain aluminum as an adjuvant; the kind of aluminum currently being used in vaccines is not found anywhere in nature and has been shown to cross the blood-brain barrier.[97]

EXCITOTOXINS: Aspartame, with the proprietary names Equal and NutraSweet, is an excitotoxin, which means that it causes nerve cells to overfire. In susceptible people this can lead to the death of brain cells. This is one of the reasons aspartame has been associated with a multiple-sclerosis-like syndrome in some women.[98] The aspartame in diet colas seems to cause the worst problems in susceptible women.

Many women are addicted to diet cola, drinking several liters per day without taking in much else in the way of other nutrients. This is a setup for a wide range of neurological symptoms in susceptible individuals, including headache, dizziness, anxiety attacks, memory loss, slurred speech, numbness, muscle spasms, mood swings, severe depression, personality changes, PMS, insomnia, fatigue, hyperactivity, heart palpitations, arrhythmia, chest pain, hearing loss, ringing in the ears, blurred vision, decreased sense of taste, skin lesions, nausea, digestive disturbances, water retention, and seizures. If you have a history of such problems, avoid this artificial sweetener, especially in the form of diet colas. (Aspartame-induced symptoms go away when consumption is stopped.) The herb stevia is a safe sweetener. MSG (monosodium glutamate) is another excitotoxin that not only adversely affects the brain, but is also added to junk food to stimulate appetite. You don't need it!

SERMS (SELECTIVE ESTROGEN RECEPTOR MODULATORS): Given the role of ovarian hormones in brain function, the antiestrogen drugs tamoxifen (to prevent breast cancer) and raloxifene (to prevent osteoporosis) stir up some legitimate concerns about the whole-body effects of estrogen deprivation over time. Just as tamoxifen blocks the effects of estrogen on the breasts, there is also compelling evidence that it blocks some of the effects of estrogen on the brain.[99] Raloxifene (Evista), a drug prescribed to women to prevent osteoporosis, also affects the brain. This is one of the reasons hot flashes (which are mediated in the hypothalamus) are listed as one of the side effects of SERMs. Depression is also among a host of other side effects. Though these drugs have their place and may be appropriate for some women who are truly at high risk, the very real potential drawbacks of these drugs are not getting enough attention.

If you're currently taking tamoxifen or raloxifene, it's doubly important for you to follow some of the suggestions outlined above to protect your brain function. Many women report alleviation of their tamoxifen-associated depression, for example, when they take high doses of soy. This may be because of soy's hormonal effects. (For a fuller discussion of SERMs, see chapters 5 and 13.)

MAXIMIZING MIDLIFE WISDOM

Your brain is like your muscles. If you want it to stay in peak form, you have to use it regularly. Brain function is also profoundly affected by our expectations and attitudes about life. While there is no formula—hormonal or otherwise—to "cure" aging, there are many things you can do to preserve your mental vitality.

STEP ONE: Catch yourself indulging in any stereotypical thinking about the aging process. For example, if you forget something, don't say "I'm having a senior moment." This phrase and others like it are nothing but ageist, self-fulfilling prophecies. Don't ever allow yourself to make comments such as "I'm too old for this." I've seen this kind of thinking in women who are only in their early thirties! My mother told me that when she turned sixty, her mailbox was suddenly full of ads for all kinds of health aids, ranging from incontinence diapers to hearing aids. She simply tosses this information in the recycling bin at the post office. In 2009, at the age of eighty-four, she trekked to a Mount Everest base camp in Nepal at an altitude of nearly 18,000 feet with my sister Penny. The trek was fifty miles in and fifty miles out over the roughest terrain in the world. Several years before this, my mother had fallen on some ice and injured her back. She slowly made her way back to full physical activity in the next year or so. She told me that the biggest impediment to becoming her usual active self again was not in her body but in her mind. When the invitation came to go on the trek to Everest, she took it as a sign and got on with the training.

Take your cue from my mother and start viewing yourself as a younger person, unfettered by the age-related problems the media tell us all to expect. When I use an exercise machine, for example, I always program in my age as forty! Though "thinking young" may seem simplistic, it is one of the most important health behaviors you can adopt. That's why I don't ever compare myself to "women my age." It's a box I have thankfully stepped out of, since I relate to people of *all* age groups. In fact, I *never* give my age. This is because we co-author each other's biology, for better or for worse. In other words, when we know someone's age, we tend to treat them in a certain way. Age just might be the most boring false identity around. A friend of mine said she hated "being" a certain number. But why bother? You're only infinity itself pretending to be that age. In fact, buying into negative stereotypes about aging (such as "as you age you become useless"), which tends to happen in childhood, actually translates into an increased risk of premature death. I don't want to know anyone else's age either, including for many of my friends and colleagues, because I too have a tendency to place them in a box based on their age. I also do not believe in celebrating "milestone" birthdays. That's because that so-called milestone too often becomes a millstone.

Consider this: a study of 600 people age fifty and older by Yale researcher Becca Levy, Ph.D., showed that those who had a more positive view of aging as relatively young adults lived an average of 7.5 years longer than those with less positive views—even after factoring in such variables as age, gender, socioeconomic status, loneliness, and overall health. How the subjects viewed aging had a greater effect on their longevity than having low blood pressure and low cholesterol (each of which is associated with living up to four years longer) or having a lower body mass index, no history of smoking, and a tendency to exercise (each of which can add up to three years to your life). "Our study carries two messages," the study reports. "The discouraging one is that negative self-perceptions can diminish life expectancy; the encouraging one is that positive self-perceptions can prolong life expectancy."[100]

Mario Martinez, Psy.D., author of *The Mind-Body Code* (Sounds True, 2014) and founder of the Biocognitive Science Institute, suggests changing the verb "age" to "growing older." He says, "Growing older is inevitable. Aging is optional." Dr. Martinez recommends looking at growing older as an opportunity to increase your value and competence. One of the ways that I routinely "program" my own mind for youth and vigor is with affirmations. Here are a couple of my favorites (I say these out loud every morning when I'm working out on the elliptical trainer):

> "My body is now radiantly healthy, beautiful, flexible, strong, and eternally youthful. The spirit of Divine Love and Power now manifests throughout my entire body as radiant health, radiant beauty, and radiant youth."

> "I give thanks that my body, mind, spirit, and behavior now align to easily maintain my ideal size and weight."

STEP TWO: Stay mentally active and socially connected. Continuing to expose yourself to new ideas, new people, and new environments is as necessary to staying mentally healthy as physical exercise is to maintaining the health of your heart, muscles, and bones.[101] Remember that learning causes actual growth of new neurons, even in an older brain.[102] Step outside the comfort of familiar territory. Cultivate a wide social network of individuals from diverse age groups. Take classes, get together with friends, learn a new sport or activity, start a new career or business, engage in volunteer work. Tone your brain cells and neural pathways with new ideas, new connections, and new thoughts every day. I started taking Argentine tango classes in 2008 and was positively terrified to be a beginner at a place where I didn't know a soul. It was a humbling experience that required a lot of courage. But now, after years of regular dancing, I have a whole new circle of friends, and a whole new range of motion in my hips and torso. (For more on the benefits of tango, see "Shall We Dance? The Triumph of Argentine Tango," on page 281.)

I've noticed that some of my older friends tend to get a vacant look on their faces when they are with a group of new people or in an unfamiliar setting. Although they seem fine in their own homes, they can't seem to keep up with the conversation when challenged with a new situation. They've spent so much time screening out any newness from their environment, digging themselves deeper into the safety of their day-to-day ruts, that they've lost the ability to adapt to change. It's tragic to witness what happens to the faces, bodies, and minds of these formerly vital people as they begin this downhill slide.

The famous brain researcher Marian Diamond, Ph.D., says, "There's a very simple principle when it comes to the brain. Use it or lose it." When our nervous system no longer receives new input, it atrophies, a phenomenon that has been demonstrated clearly in the laboratory. In one study of aging rats, Dr. Diamond added new toys and other novel items to enhance the environments of some rats, while leaving the other rats in their familiar surroundings. At the end of the study, the rats in the enriched environments had more cortical brain tissue than those with the standard environments. Interestingly, this change in brain structure occurred even in old rats that were 75 percent of the way through their life span.[103]

STEP THREE: Develop an optimistic attitude toward life. I was once in Toronto at an I Can Do It! conference sponsored by Hay House. The conference was opened by the late Louise Hay herself, who at eighty-four looked more vibrant and alive than she had at her eightieth birthday. She said to the crowd, "At the age of eighty, I decided that this next decade was going to be the best decade of my life. And so far it is!" Talk about inspiring!

Optimism—the ability to perceive the glass as half full instead of half empty—is a natural protectant against depression. Also, an impressive body of research has documented that optimists are healthier and live longer. In one study of individuals with no risk factors for heart disease, for example, depressed people were four times more likely to suffer from heart attacks than their optimistic, nondepressed counterparts; since heart disease is also associated with dementia, you can see the connection between a healthy attitude and a healthy brain.

After doing extensive research on healthy people who are a hundred years old or more all over the world, clinical neuropsychologist Mario Martinez, Psy.D., found they all practice what he calls the "causes of health." This entails maintaining an elevated cognition (thinking positive and uplifting thoughts), experiencing exalted emotions (engaging in things that bring you joy, awe, delight, and inspiration), and allowing yourself to feel righteous anger when your innocence or humanity (or that of another) is threatened—for example, standing up for a waitress who is being treated poorly.

STEP FOUR: Actively work with your thoughts and behaviors to modify those personality traits—such as hostility, pessimistic thoughts, and the tendency to isolate yourself socially—that are known to be associated with premature death and disability. If necessary, seek help from a therapist. Cognitive behavioral therapy (CBT) can make you more aware of your negative, self-limiting thoughts and help you find ways to redirect them in a more positive, empowering direction. This does not mean denial of life's difficulties. CBT teaches you how to accept your situation and validate it, but at the same time deal with it more constructively. As a result, you learn to worry less. To help you use your own power to change your thoughts, I recommend that you read *I Can Do It* (Hay House, 2004) and *Experience Your Good Now!* (Hay House, 2010), both by Louise Hay, as well as *The Amazing Power of Deliberate Intent* (Hay House, 2006) by Esther and Jerry Hicks.

STEP FIVE: Develop and express a healthy sense of humor. Get "humor aids," such as Loretta LaRoche's video *How Serious Is This?* or her book *Relax—You May Only Have a Few Minutes Left* (Villard, 1998). Or watch reruns of comedy programs you loved years ago. I've recently started to watch old Steve Martin and Mel Brooks movies. Comic genius is always in style and never grows old! The many videos of JP Sears are also wonderful, as he does such great send-ups of our current culture in videos like "How to Get Instagram Famous" from his Ultra Spiritual Life series. (Check out his YouTube channel, AwakenWithJP.)

STEP SIX: Eat healthfully and exercise regularly. As already mentioned, a large body of research has demonstrated that almost all dementia is due, in part, to small-blood-vessel disease in our brains. The number-one reason why so many of us get these blood vessel changes is because we eat poorly and avoid exercise. Get moving, every day. This includes walking, aerobics, sports, swimming, or lifting weights. Movement keeps the blood flowing to all your organs, including your brain, and brings more nutrients and oxygen to your tissues. If you want, you can get your movement and social needs met at the same time by taking up a sport with a group of people who are noncompetitive and just enjoy the fun of moving.

STEP SEVEN: Practice full emotional expression and heal your life as you go along. The emotional pattern associated with heart disease, including hardening of the arteries in the brain, is a tendency to avoid feeling your emotions fully—whether those emotions are positive or negative. One of my perimenopausal patients once told me:

> I grew up in a household in which we were taught to be afraid of strong emotions. You weren't allowed to feel too good—or too bad—about anything. If we needed to cry, we were told to go into the basement and bury our face in a pillow so that we wouldn't disturb the rest of the family. If we shouted with joy about a good grade or winning a game, we were told not to "blow your own trumpet." So I learned to distrust an entire range of feelings—basically anything except bland and boring pleasantness. Not surprisingly, dementia, depression, and heart disease run very strongly in my family on both sides. At midlife I feel as though I have to completely relearn how to feel. Often I have to tune in to symptoms in my body and just sit with them until I start to feel the emotion associated with them.

This falls right in line with anecdotal evidence suggesting that the tangles and pathology of Alzheimer's tend to "attack" the area of the brain associated with memories that are painful. Likewise, a 2010 study showed that older veterans returning from Iraq and Afghanistan with post-traumatic stress syndrome had twice the risk for dementia as those without the disorder.[104] The researchers, who studied 181,093 veterans age fifty-five or older at the San Francisco Veterans Affairs Medical Center, noted that stress may damage the hippocampus or cause changes in neurotransmitter and hormone levels that could increase risk. The way I see it, it's almost as if the bodies of people who are faced with extremely painful memories try to protect them by causing them to forget altogether.

A poignant example came from a patient I once had whose father was a convicted pedophile. But his wife (my patient's mother) made sure he got out of jail early, which meant that she lived with him for many, many years in which she was fully aware of his deviant sexual behavior. She eventually got Alzheimer's. When her husband died, she immediately called her daughter (my patient), who brought her home with her to live until other arrangements could be made. "The first thing Mother did was sleep for nearly two days straight," she told me. "When she woke up, my mother was back—it was as if she'd never had Alzheimer's. We sat and talked for about ten hours. She completely understood the implications of my dad's behavior and her role in enabling him. Then she told me that she couldn't stay and was going to 'go away again.' She took another nap and woke up with Alzheimer's." The mother suffered from progressive dementia from that moment on and eventually died. This story has stayed with me for years because it points to the role of the soul and the human will in disorders such as Alzheimer's.

So whatever emotions you are feeling, it's vital that you allow yourself the fullness of your feeling. What you will find is that it dissipates. But if you instead try to make yourself feel something else, and put yourself down for having an "unpleasant" emotion, then that emotion will get locked in your body and may be expressed later as a disease.

Hostility, on the other hand, is a stuck chronic emotional pattern. It can be self-destructive to loiter in this space for very long, and the best way to get out is to find something to appreciate about every situation you are in, no matter how small it is, until appreciation begins to replace hostility as a mental and emotional pattern.

STEP EIGHT: Never retire. Don't allow yourself to start thinking about "retirement" at midlife, the way so many people do. Instead, do what Dolly Parton does: find out what you love to do for work, and you'll never work a day in your life! You may wish to retire from working for a company or for another individual, but you need to have something that you're interested in doing—for pay or not—every day of your life. Jacquelyn B. James, Ph.D., co-director of the Center on Aging and Work at Boston College, says psychological health is as important as financial health in retirement. Her research shows that only people who are truly engaged in their post-retirement activities reap the psychological benefits.[105] These days, many retirees actually find satisfaction in going back to work—for themselves, that is, as entrepreneurs doing work they find both stimulating and meaningful.

In conclusion, consider the following experiment: In a famous study at Boston's Beth Israel Deaconess Hospital, researchers Jeffrey Hausdorff, Ph.D., a gerontologist, and Harvard graduate student Becca Levy (now a Ph.D. and faculty member at the Yale School of Public Health) tested the effect of subconscious beliefs on walking speed. Walking speed often declines with age, and that in combination with balance and coordination problems as well as other factors, such as medication, produces the stereotypical elderly "shuffle." The researchers tested healthy individuals ages sixty-three to eighty-two by first having them walk down a hall the length of a football field. They measured both speed and "swing time"—the time the foot spends off the ground. After that, the participants played a brief computer game. On half of the computers, upbeat words such as *accomplished, wise,* and *astute* flashed across the screen just long enough to register subconsciously. The other group had negative words such as *senile, dependent,* and *diseased* flashed across their screens. The participants then walked down the same hallway again. This time, the positively influenced group walked 9 percent faster and had much more "swing time" and much less shuffling. The negatively influenced group didn't get any worse, perhaps because they, like most of us, had already been saturated by society's negative aging stereotypes.[106]

This study is clearly a wake-up call for becoming conscious of our own beliefs about aging and the physical effects of those beliefs. I've seen far too many women talk themselves into physical deterioration starting as young as thirty! And who hasn't witnessed the black balloons and jokes about being "over the hill" at birthday parties for friends turning forty?

Ellen Langer, Ph.D., a Harvard psychologist who wrote the classic book *Mindfulness* (Addison-Wesley, 1989), observed: "The regular and 'irreversible' cycles of aging that we witness in the later stages of human life may be a *product* of certain assumptions about how one is supposed to grow old. If we didn't feel compelled to carry out these limiting mindsets, we might have a greater chance of replacing years of decline with years of growth and purpose."[107]

Amen.

11

From Rosebud to Rose Hip: Cultivating Midlife Beauty

I'll never forget the last time my former harp teacher, the late Miss Alice Chalifoux, came to borrow my harp for her students to use at the summer harp colony in Camden, Maine, where she taught for more than sixty years, and where I myself first took lessons when I was fourteen.

Though she never paid much attention to diet, exercise, or supplements, her skin was pink, fresh, and smooth, her eyes were bright, she was never sick, and her irreverent and earthy sense of humor was utterly delightful. With a twinkle in her eye, Miss Chalifoux told me that she had cut her schedule way back that summer. She taught only thirty-six hours a week—about half-time by her standards. She was a perfect example of a woman who was beautifully attuned to the power of what I call the late-rose-hip stage of life, sowing her seeds of wisdom and inspiring others wherever she went. Her impish soul shone out through every pore, its youthful effects written all over her face. Miss Chalifoux was ninety-two years old then and lived until she was a hundred.

The late Louise Hay was another example of ageless beauty. Louise founded her company, Hay House, at the age of sixty, after having great success with a self-published book. She then traveled all over the world with her empowering message. And then, in the two years before her death at the age of ninety, she had a great love affair with a man who was much younger. A true ageless goddess.

No one would deny that every season of the year is imbued with its own special beauty and wisdom. The same is true of the seasons of our lives. Most of us know or have seen at least one woman like Miss Alice Chalifoux or Louise Hay who is living proof that beauty is possible at every season of our lives, depending upon how we live them.

Perimenopausal women can be likened to the full-blown rose of late summer and fall as it begins to transform itself into a bright, juicy rose hip—the part of the rose that contains the seeds from which hundreds of other potential roses can grow. These juicy and tasty rose hips are in their glory on the coast of Maine every autumn. Until recently, our culture has worshipped only the rosebud stage of development, thereby rendering relatively invisible the beauty of the other stages. In fact, not so long ago, the dewy rosebud was often used as a prominent symbol for ads selling conventional hormone therapy drugs to women. The subliminal message was clear: if you used HT, you could stay at the rosebud stage of beauty for the rest of your life and never have to go through the process of maturing and ripening into the resilient and potent rose hip. But it's not true.

Once you're on the way to becoming a rose hip, you can't go backward to being a rosebud, though our culture certainly entices us to try. Learning how to maximize the strength and resilience of the juicy rose hip stage is absolutely necessary if you are to look and feel your very best as a woman in the full bloom of midlife! Just remember that when you're becoming a rose hip, any attempt to remain in the rosebud stage tends to look desperate and ridiculous. It's like trying to reglue the autumn leaves back onto the tree and then paint them all green to simulate the spring. It simply doesn't work. Instead, our task is to come to appreciate the beauty and power of the season we are in, instead of longing for what can no longer be. In fact, being present in the moment you are in right now is actually one of the best possible ways to remain youthful—in the same way that young children are very "in the moment" because they haven't yet been indoctrinated into the concepts of past and future. Hence, their life energy and aliveness are maximally available to them.

Staying present with "what is" may be a particularly difficult task if, before menopause, you were the type of woman accustomed to using the power of your looks and body to attract the attention of men or women whenever you so much as walked into a room. If this has been true for you, then you're viscerally familiar with the power of external feminine beauty and have, perhaps, capitalized on it since adolescence. If your looks have charmed people for years, it is quite likely that you will have a harder time with becoming a rose hip than someone who didn't have this experience and therefore had to turn inward at an earlier age to find her sense of worth and beauty. I had an acquaintance like this once. When she turned forty-five, she bemoaned the fact that men no longer turned to look at her when she walked into a room. Since all of her influence and money had always come to her by virtue of her appearance and its effect on powerful men, becoming a rose hip was truly a harsh wake-up call, letting her know that her former wiles would no longer serve her in the second half of life. She'd spent her life swimming in the shallow end of the pool. Her challenge now was to go deeper. Those of you who've never experienced the power of great physical beauty in the first place will probably have a much easier time settling into the rose hip stage. In fact, if you're anything like me—and I know many of you are— you may happily find yourself becoming interested in clothing, skin care, and makeup perhaps for the first time in your life. What's more, you'll also find that the self-confidence and self-esteem from all you've done in the first half of your life have built a solid foundation of self-acceptance that leaves you feeling more empowered than ever before.

But whether or not we were ever raving beauties, all of us want to look our best at every age. During perimenopause, as we heed the call to truly come home to ourselves, we find ourselves lit from within by an inner glow. We find that we may never be rosebuds again, but we can still remain as attractive as possible by paying attention to good skin and body care. And we may even want to avail ourselves of plastic surgery or other cosmetic procedures. More choices are available to budding rose hips than ever before.

MAKING PEACE WITH YOUR CHANGING SKIN

One of the most distressing parts of midlife for many women is watching our skin begin to sag and get "crepey." I began to notice changes in my skin—a tendency toward more dryness and some fine wrinkles around my eyes—starting in my late thirties. When these first became noticeable, I decided to like them, since they reminded me of my father's eyes, which were always surrounded by the crinkles of lots of laughter and smiles. But I also wanted to do everything possible to keep those lines from getting deeper and more unattractive as time went on.

One of my e-newsletter subscribers eloquently shared the common dilemma of midlife skin changes and their potential emotional impact:

> I am forty-eight years old, at my ideal weight, and extremely fit. I work out on a regular basis and lift weights as part of my exercise program. I hike whenever I get the chance. However, it seems like almost overnight, the skin on my legs has become extremely slack. As I look down when I walk, I can see the skin on my thighs shake with each step. I'm sure it's the result of cumulative sun damage along with many years of gaining and losing those stubborn ten pounds. Is there anything that can be done? I now use sunscreen whenever I am outdoors, never bake in the sun, and try to keep my weight stable. Must I resign myself to wearing long dresses? Are there any supplements I can take? Is there anything that would rebuild the collagen? Any surgery that would help? I'm in the process of a divorce after twenty-seven years of marriage and am, naturally, concerned about my appearance. I'd be very grateful for any suggestions.

Fortunately there's a great deal that we can do to both preserve the health of our midlife skin and even heal some of the damage that has already been done. While we're doing this, however, we still have to go through midlife with the courage to live our lives joyfully and fully, despite such things as aging skin and changing bodies. I know both from my practice and from my own life experience that this feels much harder when you're going through a divorce or loss of a life partner.

Nevertheless, it's important to remember that many women find love and happiness at midlife and beyond, regardless of a little sun damage or sagging here and there. This point was brought home to me rather dramatically during an event at which I spent time talking to two different women. One, a stunning woman in her late thirties with flawless skin and an almost perfect figure who was also a very successful businesswoman, was bemoaning the fact that there simply weren't any good men around with whom she could find happiness.

About half an hour later I met another woman. About fifty-five years old, she had a plain but lively face, unadorned by any makeup, and she was at least thirty or forty pounds overweight. Since we were discussing medical topics, she told me about a mastectomy she'd had years before that had left her chest quite disfigured. In the course of the conversation, she said, "I think we underestimate men, don't you? They can be so sweet." It turned out that she was dating three different men, one of whom she felt was the one she was destined to marry! This woman's inner beauty and sense of humor made me feel happy just being around her. When I compared her energy and attitude with that of the showstoppingly beautiful woman I'd met earlier, I realized how transient the impression of mere physical beauty can be when it's not lit from within by a beautiful soul. Since then, I've seen this phenomenon repeatedly: midlife women finding wonderful life partners online, and everywhere else, simply because they've decided to stay in the game.

Remember this when you are tempted to succumb to the cultural and media-driven notion that after thirty-five it's all downhill for women, our best years are behind us, and no one will ever love us again because we are no longer twenty-five. I've come to see that nothing could be further from the truth. In fact, many men have told me that it's a woman's enthusiasm for her life, her self-acceptance, and her sense of fun that they find most attractive.

A Primer on Skin: Our External Nervous System

To prevent unnecessary aging of the skin—which manifests as dullness, sallowness, uneven pigmentation, dryness, and wrinkles—you first need to understand what your skin does for you and how it does it.

The skin is derived from the embryonic layer known as the neuroectoderm, the same tissue layer that becomes the brain and the peripheral nervous system. It functions as a kind of external brain, gathering information about our outer environment through its ability to sense pressure, temperature, pleasure, and pain. The skin is also the largest and most important part of the immune system.

The research of Tiffany Field, Ph.D., on the striking immune-system-enhancing benefits of massage is compelling evidence of just how intimately our skin is connected with and affected by every aspect of our health, from our emotions to our nutrient intake. Our skin is, quite literally, the boundary between us and our environment. As our first line of defense against the vagaries of that environment, including bacteria, viruses, excessive ultraviolet radiation from the sun, wind, air pollution, and secondhand smoke, it is not only vulnerable to what's going on outside of us, it's also affected by our internal environment, both emotional and nutritional.

The condition of your skin says a great deal about how well you're fitting into and feeling supported by your current environment. There's an unmistakable glow emanating from women who are happy and satisfied with their lives that no amount of cosmetic surgery can create. It comes only from connecting with Source energy. If, for any reason, you feel as though you cannot be safe or true to yourself in your environment, and you are not particularly aware of this, then your skin may react for you. That's why it is well known in dermatology that patients may need simultaneous treatment of their skin and their mind and emotions for best results. Dermatitis and hives, for example, are two of the conditions known to be caused by a mixture of psychological and physical factors, while disorders such as psoriasis, hair loss, and eczema may also be affected by psychological factors. Almost everyone has had the experience of developing a large pimple in a prominent area of her face just when she was most concerned about looking her best for some big social event, or breaking out in oral herpes (cold sores) just before going out on a date, or getting itchy hives on taking a new job or moving to a new city. Sooner or later all of who we are and have been shows up on our faces.

The Anatomy of the Skin

The skin consists of three layers: the outer epidermis, the middle dermis, and a fat layer underlying both of those. The paper-thin epidermis is a protective layer of dead skin cells that holds in moisture and oil. It is constantly being shed and replaced as fresh cells push their way up to the surface, get flattened, and then die. As we age, the sloughing process tends to slow down, which is one of the reasons why skin tends to lose its "freshness."

At the base of the epidermis are the basal cells, which contain the melanin-generating cells known as melanocytes. The amount and type of melanin determine the tone of your skin—a trait that is inherited from your parents.

The dermis layer, which makes up about 90 percent of the skin, is where the nerve receptors and blood vessels are located. It also contains sweat glands and sebaceous glands; the latter produce oil and are attached to hair follicles. Blackheads and pimples inevitably arise from clogged sebaceous ducts at the root of hair follicles. The sweat and oil secretions from the dermal layer help protect the skin from infection by creating a protective acid mantle, but this mantle is easily disrupted by using harsh detergents and non-pH-balanced soaps.

Two proteins known as collagen and elastin, which give skin its elasticity and flexibility, are also located in the dermis layer. On average, collagen production starts to diminish at a rate of 1 percent per year starting in our twenties. By midlife we may have lost up to 20 percent of our collagen layer, though there is enormous variation among different individuals and this is not inevitable. The darker your skin tone, however, the more collagen and elastin it has—which is why the skin and bones of dark-skinned women tend to be more resistant to the wear and tear of aging compared to women of Caucasian descent. It is also why black- and brown-skinned women are less apt to have wrinkled skin compared to white-skinned women. The television personality Star Jones put it this way: "Black don't crack." Those with yellow skin tend to fall somewhere in between.

FIGURE 15: THE ANATOMY OF THE SKIN

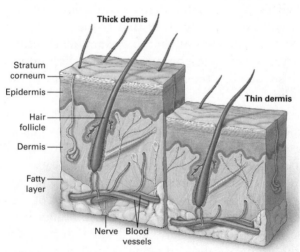

In addition to the thinning of the collagen layer of our skin with age, our oil glands tend to decrease their secretions, resulting in a greater tendency toward dryness. By about age fifty, the capacity of the skin to repair itself tends to slow down, for reasons that aren't entirely clear but may be related to free-radical damage. (See the next section.)

Free Radicals and Skin Aging

If you take a look at the skin on your buttocks and lower back, you'll notice something important: skin that has been protected from environmental pollutants and excessive sunlight is smoother and more wrinkle-free than elsewhere on our bodies. That means that skin aging is related to more than simply chronological age. It's also related to our environment—both inside and outside our bodies.

Premature aging of the skin—and of every other cell in our bodies—is related to the production of what are known as free radicals, oxygen molecules that have become unstable because they have lost an electron in the course of interacting with other molecules in our body during such basic metabolic processes as breathing and digestion. Free radicals are also produced when sunlight hits the skin, by repeated bouts of high blood sugar and insulin (glycemic stress), and by toxins of all kinds, including cigarette smoke and air pollutants. Emotional stress also results in free-radical damage secondary to the effects of cortisol and adrenaline. In the body, these unstable free radicals bounce around, attaching themselves to the cell membranes of virtually any tissue that is available in order to stabilize themselves with an electron from that tissue. If they take an extra electron from collagen in our skin, for example, this can damage the collagen. Over time the skin becomes stiff and discolored and loses its elasticity. It's much like the process by which iron rusts when left out in the open air.

Wrinkles result from the breakdown of elastin and collagen fibers in the deeper layers of the skin. Collagen and elastin are responsible for the resilience of the skin, allowing it to stretch and contract. When collagen gets broken down, skin tends to sag and wrinkle.

Free-radical damage can also harm and break down the fats within our cells and cell membranes, and the DNA of the cells, where the genetic code resides. Over time, cell membranes become stiff instead of fluid and flexible. There's no doubt that free-radical damage is one of the primary causes of aging, including skin wrinkling, and age-related diseases such as heart disease, Alzheimer's, arthritis, and so on. Glycemic stress from eating too many refined foods also contributes to premature aging.

Since some free radicals are produced as an unavoidable part of daily living, it's not surprising that our bodies have developed defense systems for dealing with them. This defense system is based on the effects of molecules known as antioxidants. These include vitamins C and E found in foods, and others produced in the body, such as glutathione, catalase, and superoxide dismutase. Antioxidants work by donating electrons to the unstable free radicals, thus rendering them harmless by preventing them from combining with other molecules and damaging our tissues.

Given this defense system, one might wonder why we age at all. As with all things, it's a question of balance. Though our bodies manufacture antioxidants and we ingest them in foods and as supplements, sometimes our antioxidant systems become overwhelmed by the sheer number of free radicals produced by such things as cigarette smoke, air pollution, sun exposure, diets that are heavy in trans fats or other suboptimal ingredients, high blood sugar, and emotional stress of all kinds. The resulting free-radical damage in our bodies is known as oxidative stress. Hundreds of research studies have now documented that we can keep the oxidative stress in our bodies to a minimum by ingesting antioxidants, applying products that contain them, avoiding environmental toxins, eating a low-glycemic-index diet, and maintaining emotional equilibrium.

How Smoking Damages the Skin

Midlife is the time when the ill effects of smoking become as plain as the nose on your face. Women who smoke heavily have a paler skin tone and more lines and wrinkles than nonsmokers. Some of this effect is from the decrease in circulation to the skin caused by nicotine. Decreased skin circulation results in fewer nutrients getting to the skin and a decreased ability of the skin to release the toxic waste products of cell metabolism. This results in a slowing of skin growth and rejuvenation. A 2010 study done in Italy followed sixty-four female smokers who participated in a smoking cessation program. At the beginning of the study, the researchers gave each woman a score based on the condition of her skin and found that on average, the women had a biological age that was nine years older than their actual chronological age. After nine months in the smoking cessation program, the researchers scored the women again and found that their average biological age had decreased by thirteen years.[1]

In addition to this, smoking directly poisons the ovaries, leading to decreased levels of estrogen, which is necessary to help maintain elastin and collagen fibers.

How Excessive Ultraviolet Radiation Damages the Skin

It is estimated that about 70 percent of the change we see in our skin as we age is the result of damage done to collagen fibers in the dermis. Sun damage, in particular, causes the skin to lose its resiliency and elasticity.[2] Skin that is chronically overexposed to the sun without optimal antioxidant levels in the body to counteract this is in a constant state of mild inflammation. Though we've all been brought up to feel that a tan makes us look more youthful in appearance (not to mention the fact that new evidence shows the use of indoor tanning beds in certain young adults can actually be addictive), these presumed health benefits are an illusion: the mild inflammation and swelling of tanned skin plumps the skin up, temporarily minimizing wrinkles, and gives the appearance of a more youthful look.[3] But once the tan goes away, the wrinkles reappear, and what you're left with is skin that has lost its normal architecture.

Excessive exposure to ultraviolet radiation results in tissue inflammation that begins with free-radical damage to skin cell membranes followed by the release of harmful inflammatory chemicals that ultimately damage collagen and elastin fibers. Eventually collagen and elastin fibers that were originally flexible and fluid become stiff and hard. The aging process that your skin collagen goes through is much the same as what happens to a flexible and clear egg white when you drop it on a hot griddle: the fluid protein in the egg white is transformed into denatured protein, a dense, hard, inflexible type of protein. Ultraviolet radiation also damages the blood vessels in the skin, thus decreasing the flow of blood and other nutrients to this organ. This is in part the reason for those pesky dilated blood vessels on the cheeks and nose. Uneven pigmentation, roughness, and thickening of the skin result from disruption of both immune and cellular replication processes as we age. They are not inevitable but are brought about by DNA damage and oxidative stress from stresses of all kind, in particular UV damage from the sun.

How Excess Blood Sugar and a Nutrient-Poor Diet Damage the Skin

No one doubts the health benefits of nutrient-rich fruits, vegetables, lean proteins, healthy fats, and enough fiber. What most don't realize is that exactly the same diet that prevents diabetes and heart disease also provides you with a radiant complexion. A study of data taken from the first National Health and Nutrition Examination Survey (NHANES I) of 4,025 midlife women showed that women who avoided high-carb, high-glycemic-index diets and ate foods that contained plenty of vitamin C and linoleic acid (an omega-6 essential fatty acid) had fewer wrinkles, less dry skin, and less thinning of the skin.[4] This makes perfect sense because a diet too high in refined carbohydrates raises blood sugar too quickly, and too much sugar in the blood results in a process known as glycosylation (or glycation), in which the sugar actually combines with proteins in the blood and the body—including the skin. When this happens, the collagen becomes stiff and inflexible—like the cooked egg white I mentioned earlier.

New, healthy skin starts with healthy blood vessels. But when your fibroblasts (the cells that make collagen) don't get the nutrients they need and your collagen is damaged from glycosylation, your skin simply doesn't look its best. You also need the right kinds of omega-3 fats to replenish your skin. The effect of a low-glycemic-index, nutrient-rich diet on the skin is the basis for *The Wrinkle Cure* (Rodale, 2000), by Nicholas Perricone, M.D., which provides the sound dietary advice that will also help prevent cancer and heart disease. (See chapter 7.) Another great source of research on this is *The Paleo Diet* (Wiley, 2010) by Loren Cordain, Ph.D.

PREVENTING OR TREATING WRINKLES

The key to younger-looking skin at perimenopause is to avoid smoking and overexposure to the sun (the earlier the better), follow a low-glycemic-index diet, and use antioxidants, both topically and internally. Uneven pigmentation, roughness, and hyperkeratinosis are the direct consequences of disruption of the cellular replication and immunological processes. As discussed above, these are brought about by DNA damage and oxidative stress resulting from absorption of UVR photons. Some women, by virtue of their genes, simply seem to have wrinkle-free youthful skin for a lifetime, regardless of how much sun exposure they get. But most of us have to give our skin a helping hand when it comes to midlife preservation or improvement.

Over the past decade or so, a huge amount of research has been done on the role of antioxidants in both preventing and even reversing the free-radical damage and tissue inflammation that are the root cause of skin aging. Excess sun exposure combined with the effects of a nutrient-poor diet and too much stress are what cause the kind of skin deterioration that we begin to notice during perimenopause. But these same factors can be addressed so that a great deal of the damage that has already been done can be stopped and even reversed.

Midlife Skin Care Regimen

~ CLEANSE YOUR SKIN REGULARLY. The skin has been called a "third kidney" because it removes almost as much waste material from the body each day as the kidneys themselves. If your skin is dry, you need to cleanse it thoroughly once per day. If it's oily, then twice per day may be better. Remove all makeup every night. When you care for your face, don't forget your neck—it's the first place you notice the effects of aging. Cleansing your skin thoroughly will clean out your pores and allow your skin to remove waste products efficiently from your body as you sleep, a time when your body is rejuvenating itself.

Use a cleansing lotion or soap that preserves the acid mantle of the skin, because it's one of your body's natural defenses against infection and breakouts. Look for the term "pH balanced" when shopping for a soap or cleanser. Many good brands are available.

If your skin is oily, be sure to avoid overuse of astringents, which usually contain alcohol. They can actually make an oil problem worse and also damage your skin over time.

~ CLOSE PORES AFTER CLEANING. Use a toner to close the pores after cleansing, especially if your skin is oily. Or simply use cool water to close the pores—it works well for all skin types.

~ RENEW SKIN WITH EXFOLIANTS AND TOPICAL ANTIOXIDANTS. One of the reasons that skin starts to look dull and old at midlife is that the rate of skin growth and cell turnover slows down. As a result, the plumper new skin cells that give your complexion a glowing appearance tend to stay below the surface. In order to help remove old dead skin from the surface, open your pores, and speed up new skin growth, you'll need regular exfoliation. This can be done either mechanically, with a washcloth, or with products that contain fruit acids, which include alpha hydroxy, beta hydroxy, and glycolic acids. (See page 489.)

Avoid using abrasive cleansers such as those made from the hulls of nuts, which is like cleaning your skin with sandpaper. This can lead to breakage of capillaries and microabrasions of the skin that raise the risk of infection and even acne.

If your skin is oily, apply a mild cleanser to a washcloth, and use that to exfoliate each night. Use a clean washcloth each time to decrease the amount of germs that your skin comes into contact with. Follow this with an application of a mild alpha hydroxy, beta hydroxy, or glycolic acid product and/or one of the antioxidant products I recommend below. Many products on the market today contain both antioxidants and fruit acids. If your skin is dry or sensitive, skip the washcloth and simply use an alpha hydroxy acid (AHA) or antioxidant preparation to do your exfoliating for you.

⁓ USE A SUNSCREEN EVERY DAY ON YOUR FACE, NECK, AND HANDS. Make a habit of putting sunscreen with an SPF of 15 or higher on your face, neck, and hands every morning except during the brief early-morning or late-afternoon "sun bath" that I advocate for optimal vitamin D levels. (See chapter 12.) There's been a lot of concern about sunscreen products having exaggerated SPF claims and, even more troubling, potentially hazardous ingredients. The Environmental Working Group (EWG) rates sunscreens and posts an annual guide on its website (see www.ewg.org/sunscreen for the most current guide). EWG's top-rated products all contain either zinc or titanium; none contain oxybenzone or vitamin A. Of particular concern is retinyl palmitate (also called retinyl acetate, retinyl linoleate, and retinol), a derivative of vitamin A that is contained in a significant number of sunscreens currently on the market. Skincare product manufacturers often add vitamin A to their creams and lotions to reduce blotchiness, roughness, and wrinkles, but an NIH study done in 2012 by the National Toxicology Program found evidence that this practice speeds the growth of cancerous tumors in mice when skin is then exposed to sunlight.[5] This happens because the retinyl palmitate, when exposed to UVA and UVB radiation, forms free radicals that damage skin lipids and DNA.[6] For this reason, EWG recommends consumers avoid sunscreens and other skin and lip products with any of these forms of vitamin A included in their ingredients.

⁓ MOISTURIZE. If your AHA, antioxidant, or sunscreen formula is not in a moisturizing base, then finish off your daily skin care regimen with a light moisturizer for day and a richer formula for the evening. This helps much-needed moisture remain in your skin cells, keeping them plumped up. I also recommend that you use some hydrating spray on your skin right after cleansing. Just spritz your skin and press the moisture in with your hands. You can then add a very thin layer of moisturizer or even a bit of skin oil after hydrating.

BOTOX: MUCH MORE THAN SKIN DEEP

Botox (botulinum toxin type A) is the most popular minimally invasive cosmetic procedure right now, with almost 7.5 million procedures performed each year. For these treatments, doctors inject tiny doses of what is actually a neurotoxin into targeted areas on the face to block the signals between the nerves and the muscles in that area. The muscles become immobilized, so the fine lines around them don't move and the skin appears smoother and less furrowed. The effect lasts for three to six months, and the procedure must be repeated to maintain the results. In addition to cosmetic procedures, Botox can also be used for various therapeutic treatments, such as overactive bladder and excessive sweating. Sales of this drug are now more than $3 billion, a figure experts estimate will rise to $4.6 billion by 2024.

However, it's important to realize that this procedure is associated with both major and minor risks, including some you may not be aware of. First of all, you should know that Botox is derived from a bacterium called *Clostridium botulinum*. When ingested in food, this bacterium causes botulism, a type of food poisoning associated with paralysis and even death. While very tiny amounts are used in Botox treatments, the toxin has been known to travel through the central nervous system to other areas of the body where it does cause harm.[7] For this reason, since 2009 the FDA has required Botox to carry a black box warning citing side effects that include muscle weakness, double vision, drooping eyelids, problems swallowing and breathing, and even death.

Botox has some other negative effects that, while seemingly more subtle, could end up affecting many more women in important ways. A popular site for the injections is the procerus muscle between the eyebrows, which is the area known as the third eye, or the Yin Tang (Hall of Impression) point in Traditional Chinese Medicine. This point is associated with cognition, emotion, intuition, and inner visions— so you may want to think twice before you ask a doctor to inject toxins or induce paralysis there. In addition, a host of studies now show that Botox injections can alter how the human brain responds to emotional situations (including the ability to empathize), as well as cognition and the way we process and understand language itself.[8]

A safer route is simply to see facial lines and wrinkles not as something you want to erase but as confirmation that you've had plenty of experience with life and have acquired all the character and wisdom that comes along with it.

Exfoliants and Antioxidants

FRUIT ACIDS: Alpha hydroxy acids (AHAs) and other fruit acids do double duty as exfoliants and antioxidants, boosting the effectiveness of the other antioxidants in your skin care preparation. As exfoliants, they work in three ways: (1) they help dissolve the "glue" that holds dead skin cells together, thus resulting in easier removal, so new and plumper cells can rise to the surface; (2) they increase the hydration of the skin through increasing the production of glycosaminoglycans (GAGs), which are present in the interstices of the collagen matrix, thus boosting the amount of moisture in skin and reducing fine lines and wrinkles;[9] and (3) they encourage the repair of elastin and collagen in the skin and even help thicken it a bit.

Commercial products usually contain from .5 to 10 percent fruit acids, concentrations that are low enough and safe enough for all skin types and tones. It's always best, however, to test any product first, either on the inner part of your elbow or just under your jawline. If your skin is sensitive, start with a 5 percent product. If you can tolerate that, gradually work up to a 10 to 12 percent product. You may experience a slight stinging with some products until you get used to them. Higher-strength AHAs (up to 70 percent) are used to lighten the skin or cause a deeper peel and should be used only by professional estheticians or doctors.

Fruit acids help normalize your skin whether it's dry or oily. If it's oily, they remove the top dead layer of cells, thus allowing oil to flow out of the follicle more easily so that it can be removed without stripping away essential moisture. If your skin is dry, fruit acids remove the dry dead layer and stimulate cell renewal.

It usually takes about two weeks before you'll notice a difference in your skin with regular use of a fruit acid. They can reduce wrinkles and improve roughness, sallowness, and hyperpigmentation at concentrations as low as 5 to 8 percent.[10] Most people start by using AHAs only at night, but once you know they work for you, you can apply them twice per day.

As antioxidants, fruit acids can also alleviate some of the free-radical damage that results from exposure to sunlight and pollutants in the air.

ANTIOXIDANT VITAMINS AND HERBS: An ever-growing number of natural plants, vitamins, and herbs have been found to help the skin resist free-radical damage and inflammation when applied directly. Many can also help reverse the aging process. The effect of antioxidants is synergistic, and they work best when used in combinations.[11] For example, vitamin C and vitamin E suppress the skin's sunburn reaction well when used together.[12]

Differing types of antioxidants exert their antioxidant effects through different pathways. Those that are known as nonenzymatic antioxidants (e.g., vitamins C and E) get depleted as they scavenge free radicals. Therefore they must be replenished regularly, especially under conditions where the free-radical burden is high, such as being under heavy emotional stress or outdoors in the wind and sun. This is why it's best to apply at least one product in the morning for protection during the day, and another at night that is designed to replenish moisture as well as fight free-radical damage. A good antioxidant skin care regimen will improve skin circulation, decrease edema and puffiness (including under the eyes), decrease fine lines and wrinkles, possibly help shrink large pores, and also decrease ruddiness and restore a healthy, natural glow to the skin.

The following is a list of some of the best-studied antioxidants, though there are certainly more.

VITAMIN C: Research has shown that in the proper form, vitamin C, a powerful and ubiquitous antioxidant, can restore a smooth surface and youthful glow to aging skin. Data from the NHANES I study mentioned earlier showed that women who got plenty of vitamin C in their diet were less likely to get wrinkles.[13] This is but one aspect of the very well-documented role vitamin C plays in protecting virtually every organ in our bodies from the effects of aging. In the skin, this vitamin is essential for the production and repair of collagen. It also helps heal inflammation because it blocks the production of some of the inflammatory chemicals.

The problem with using natural vitamin C topically is that it's very acidic, which is irritating to the skin. It is also water soluble and breaks down rapidly, losing its potency within twenty-four hours. That's why most products containing conventional vitamin C aren't effective. But when vitamin C is combined with substances that render it more bioavailable, it becomes nonacidic while maintaining its antioxidant and collagen-enhancing properties. Vitamin C that is rendered absorbable by the cells can penetrate the thin membrane that encases a cell, and it offers maximum protection against free radicals in the place they do the most damage—the outer membrane of the cell. Studies have shown that vitamin C in fat-soluble form, known as liposomal vitamin C, is absorbed much more quickly and achieves levels in the skin that are ten times higher than natural vitamin C (ascorbic acid). Vitamin C in the form of such substances as tetrahexyl decyl ascorbate is stable and can be added to creams and lotions, where it will keep its potency for months.

Vitamin C creams help heal sunburn. And because fat-soluble vitamin C compounds help stimulate the growth of fibroblasts, the cells that help produce collagen and elastin in human skin, it has been shown to help reduce fine lines and wrinkles, firm skin that is sagging because of damaged collagen, and heal inflamed or irritated skin. It also gives skin a healthy glow.

TOCOTRIENOLS AND VITAMIN E: Up until very recently, scientists felt that the tocopherols, particularly d-alpha tocopherol, were the most potent part of the vitamin E complex, and the alpha tocopherols have been widely used in cosmetics and other products for over thirty years. Alpha tocopherol is often used in cosmetics in its ester form on the assumption that a process known as enzymatic hydrolysis in the skin will restore it to an active form. But this isn't the case because, in the stratum corneum of the skin, where vitamin E's antioxidant defenses are most needed, there is only very limited enzymatic activity necessary to change the ester into the right form. The result is that many of these vitamin E products remain largely inactive.

The ideal form of topical vitamin E is a natural blend of the tocopherols and the tocotrienols (another part of the vitamin E complex). The tocotrienols inhibit peroxide formation—a measure of free-radical damage—much more efficiently than alpha tocopherol, and they're better at increasing the levels of the various skin enzymes that help protect the skin from ultraviolet damage. In fact, research suggests that the tocotrienols are forty to fifty times more powerful than other forms of vitamin E.[14] This relatively new type of high-potency vitamin E is made using a special extraction process on rice bran oil or palm fruit oil. The resulting liquid can easily be mixed into creams, lotions, shampoos, or other cosmetics. Topical tocotrienols can help dry, damaged hair, severely dry skin, and brittle fingernails. Look for the words *high-potency E* or *HPE* on the label to be sure you're getting the right products.

When applied topically, both tocotrienols and tocopherols rapidly penetrate the skin and become most concentrated in the superficial stratum corneum layer, right where the threat of UV damage is the greatest.[15] Vitamin E, like vitamin C, has also been found to inhibit collagenase enzymes, which break down collagen following UV exposure.

COENZYME Q_{10}, OR UBIQUINONE: This powerful antioxidant is essential for the health of the entire cardiovascular system because of its ability to help cellular mitochondria produce energy. But it also functions as an antioxidant and helps inhibit collagenase.[16] In one German study there was a 23 percent reduction in fine lines on the face when a cream containing coenzyme Q_{10} was used topically.[17] Creams with coenzyme Q_{10} are readily available in natural food and other stores.

TURMERIC EXTRACT: This ingredient commonly found in curry has powerful antioxidant and anti-inflammatory properties that give the skin a more youthful appearance. (Hindu brides in India traditionally rub this Ayurvedic spice on their bodies for this reason.) For a long time, turmeric couldn't be used in skin cream because of its strong scent and its skin-staining pigment. Research from two studies presented at the 2010 meeting of the American Academy of Dermatology revealed that a new moisturizing cream containing purified turmeric extract (which is white instead of orange) significantly improved the appearance of facial spots, fine lines, and wrinkles.[18] Skin care lines that contain at least some products with turmeric include Juara (see www.juaraskincare.com) and Vicco (see www.viccolabs.com).

MELATONIN: Melatonin is best known for its effect on sleep and diurnal cycles, but it's also a potent antioxidant. Topical application of melatonin has been demonstrated to inhibit UV-induced redness, thus having a powerful anti-inflammatory effect.[19]

PROANTHOCYANIDINS AND CATECHINS: Polyphenolic compounds are found in a variety of plants and have many beneficial effects in humans. For example, the polyphenols in green tea are what give it its beneficial effect on the lining of blood vessels. Proanthocy-anidins and catechins, found in grape seeds, green tea, green apples, and other sources, have substantial antioxidant activity.[20]

ALOE VERA: Many people know what a good moisturizer aloe vera gel can be, as well as about its excellent healing properties for treating sunburn and other minor burns, but what you may not know is that ingesting aloe vera capsules reduces wrinkles. A Korean study published in the *Annals of Dermatology* found that aloe both boosts collagen production and decreases gene activity that causes collagen to become damaged. They concluded that taking as little as 1,200 mg of aloe gel daily for ninety days significantly improved wrinkles and elasticity in women over forty-five.[21] Aloe has plenty of other benefits as well, since the gel contains more than 200 phytonutrients.

RED GINSENG EXTRACT: Yet another study from Korea showed that red ginseng (*Panax ginseng*) extract, which is not to be confused with American or Siberian ginseng, also increases collagen. The re-searchers studied eighty-two women over age forty for six months in a double-blind, placebo-controlled study and found that in the group taking red ginseng, facial wrinkles significantly improved, as did sev-eral biochemical markers of wrinkle damage.[22]

PINE BARK: French maritime pine bark extract (PBE) is rich in proanthocyanidins, which help reduce sun damage to skin. A Japa-nese study of 112 women with mild to moderate photoaging of the skin showed that after twelve weeks of taking at least 40 mg of PBE a day, their skin showed significant decrease in photoaging.[23]

CHOCOLATE: Cocoa is rich in flavanols, and this can be good for skin that's been damaged from too much sun. A German study found that taking high-flavanol cocoa dissolved in water for twelve weeks increased dermal blood circulation and improved the appearance of sun-damaged skin.[24]

Other Skin-Enhancing Substances

PHYTOHORMONES: Many women notice that their skin stays much better hydrated and the collagen layer remains thicker if they use supplements or skin care that contains phytoestrogens. This is partic-ularly true for *Pueraria mirifica* and maca.

MICROCOLLAGEN PENTAPEPTIDES: Fibroblasts are the cells that produce collagen in skin. These cells produce less collagen with age for reasons that aren't clear. We do know that they haven't lost the ability because when aging fibroblasts are placed in cell culture and stimulated by growth factors, they can produce significant quantities of collagen.[25]

One of the factors that stimulates fibroblasts to produce collagen is a small segment of the collagen molecule itself, known as a pentapeptide fragment.[26] Researchers have found that it is an effective stimulator of both collagen and fibronectin synthesis—both of which are important components of the interstitial matrix around skin cells.[27]

Testing of this pentapeptide (3 percent concentration) on a panel of thirty-five subjects for a period of six months demonstrated significant to highly significant changes over a placebo cream as well as a commercial 5 percent vitamin C product.[28]

LIPOSOMES: Liposomes are small, membrane-covered sacs approximately 300 times smaller than the human cell that are very useful for penetrating the effective barrier that the skin provides for protection. They consist of a lecithin-based lipid membrane surrounding specific contents that the cells need. When applied to the skin, the structural similarity of the liposome to the cells, as well as its small size, allows it to penetrate readily into the various levels of the skin.

When it hits skin cells, the membrane of the liposome fuses into the cell membrane, discharging its contents into the cytoplasm of the cell over the course of six to eight hours. Liposomal delivery systems thus dramatically increase the effectiveness of any active ingredient in a skin care formulation, making it approximately ten times more effective than when applied without the liposomal delivery system.[29]

How to Evaluate a Skin Care Formulation

The newest skin care ingredients are so effective that they belong to an entirely new category that has been dubbed "cosmeceuticals," given the fact that they have pharmacologic effects on the structure and function of skin. The FDA regards these products as cosmetics and they are regulated as such.

There are two things to consider about this as a result. The first one is that cosmetics manufacturers aren't allowed to make any claims (whether or not they are true) about a product's or ingredient's ability to make permanent changes in the skin. This very much limits the ability of a manufacturer to provide consumers with independent referenced material about the action of a product or its ingredients.

Second, the labeling requirements for cosmetics do not require the manufacturer to disclose the amounts or percentages of ingredients, although all ingredients must be listed on the label. What that means is that the consumer doesn't know whether a product actually contains an ingredient in any meaningful quantity (i.e., the quantity and percentage that clinical studies have shown to be effective). Labeling regulations require that ingredients be listed in descending order, from greatest to the least, for those ingredients constituting 1 percent or more of the total weight. Ingredients making up less than 1 percent of the total may be listed in any order. The label, therefore, is of limited usefulness in determining the concentration of ingredients that may be highly effective at low concentrations. A product containing 1 percent melatonin, for example, would be indistinguishable from a product containing .001 percent. A product might only contain a few molecules of an effective ingredient that will maximize marketing but minimize effectiveness! Therefore the consumer is forced to rely upon independent reviews of the scientific literature or independent reviews of individual products. In the Resources section, I refer you to the skin care products I have formulated for Amata Life using *Pueraria mirifica* as a base. The Marie Veronique line is also very good.

Also, be aware that the cosmetics industry still puts things such as lead in lipsticks and other makeup products. Though people are waking up to the ill effects of chemicals in skin creams, it's important to check ingredients. Good databases include CosmeticsInfo.org (www .cosmeticsinfo.org) as well as Skin Deep (www.ewg.org/skindeep), an online safety guide for cosmetics and personal care products maintained by the Environmental Working Group that covers nearly 86,000 products from more than 2,400 companies.

The Preservative Dilemma

The law requires that skin care products be preserved in order to prevent bacterial or fungal overgrowth, which is known to be dangerous. (There have been cases of blindness from mascara that was contaminated with pseudomonas bacteria.) Most companies accomplish this by adding traditional chemical preservatives known as parabens and formaldehyde-releasing chemicals. (Check product labels for the following: DMDM hydantoin, diazolidinyl urea, quaternium-15, benzalkonium chloride, benzalkonium bromide, chlorhexidine, cetylpyridinium chloride, or thimerosal.) Though preservatives are effective and give products a long shelf life, they themselves aren't entirely safe—especially when used on the skin over many years.

Some are found in very low levels in nature. Generally more than one paraben preservative is used to give broader germ-killing power. Parabens can cause skin irritation and contact sensitization over time. They may also act as environmental toxins that accumulate in tissue, including the breast. Further studies are necessary to evaluate how much risk is associated with longtime use of parabens and formaldehyde-releasing preservatives.

You may also see claims made for "natural preservatives." These products often use essential oils such as tea tree oil or grapefruit seed oil. These "natural preservatives" do not lend themselves to variations in formulas needed to produce an entire line of products; in other words, they have limited use and at times their effectiveness as a preservative or antimicrobial agent is questionable. It's prudent to consider using products that don't contain potentially harmful preservatives whenever possible to decrease one's total lifetime exposure to these common chemicals.

Skin Care by Prescription Only

If you follow the insulin-normalizing diet I recommend in chapter 7 and institute the skin care regimen I've outlined above, including a good antioxidant product with at least two or three of the antioxidants listed, then you probably won't need anything else for your skin. Nevertheless, it's worth knowing about the popular prescription skin care medications that are available. There are two basic kinds: retinoic acid derivatives and hormone-containing products.

RETINOIC ACID DERIVATIVES: Retin-A and Retin-A Micro are prescription medications derived from retinoic acid, a form of vitamin A that helps prevent or reduce fine lines and wrinkles, reverse sun damage, and heal acne. A similar product called Renova, however, was subsequently found not to remove wrinkles or improve sun-damaged skin.

These substances are powerful antioxidants, and regular use of retinoic acid as prescribed by a physician can result in reduction of fine lines and wrinkles, stimulate blood flow to the skin, even out pigmentation, and help prevent wrinkles and lines from forming in the first place.

But retinoic acid is not for everyone. Side effects include redness, dryness, itchiness, and increased sun sensitivity. It takes anywhere from two to six months to notice a real difference if you're not taking any other steps to improve your complexion, and you must be absolutely committed to rigorous sunscreen use.

I personally used a form of Retin-A prescribed for many women before I discovered other, more effective skin care products. Though the Retin-A worked and was nonirritating, it resulted in excessive flakiness of my skin, which I'd sometimes notice on my cheeks and jawline at the worst possible time—usually looking into the mirror just before leaving for a speaking engagement! Not all women have this effect, but I find I get much better results with the topical and systemic antioxidant program I now use.

TOPICAL APPLICATION OF HORMONE THERAPY: Skin contains receptor sites for hormones, and it is well documented that estrogen, which also has antioxidant effects, helps preserve the collagen layer of the skin. Declining hormone levels are one of the reasons for the thinning of the collagen layer during the perimenopausal years. Many women who've undergone surgical or medical menopause notice skin changes within a few months of the loss of their hormonal support unless they take steps to replace those hormones or take phytohormones.

Research has shown that topical application of estrogen can increase collagen thickness, decrease pore size, and help the skin hold moisture. In Europe, estrogen is often prescribed to help beautify the skin. You can get these same benefits by using hormones topically.

If you are already on bioidentical hormone therapy (see pages 185–187), ask your doctor to prescribe your hormones via a formulary pharmacist so that they can be put into skin lotion. In my experience, most women are delighted with this method of using hormone therapy. It improves the skin, enhances moisture, and provides the benefits of HT, all at the same time. As with any type of hormone therapy, it's always best to use the lowest dose that does the job. Levels that are too high can result in excessive oil secretion, acne, and even excessive growth of facial hair.

TOPICAL ESTROGEN: If you are not on hormone therapy already but want to try estrogen for its skin benefits, ask your healthcare provider to prescribe a small amount of estrogen just for this purpose. A formulary pharmacist can put a small amount of estradiol or estriol in an ointment or cream. Use of the cream is safe and effective, without the adverse side effects of too much estrogen. A 1996 study found that the use of dilute topical estrogen produced marked improvement of elasticity and firmness of the skin along with increased skin moisture, decreased pore size, and decreased wrinkle depth. The dose used in the study was 1 g of an ointment containing 0.01 percent estradiol and 0.3 percent estriol, applied daily to the neck and face. Monthly determinations of blood hormone levels of estradiol, follicle-stimulating hormone (FSH), and prolactin failed to show any significant systemic hormonal changes using these dilute amounts on the skin.[30]

TOPICAL PROGESTERONE: Many of my patients have seen skin improvement, including decreased midlife acne, greater moisture, and fading of age spots, by using a 2 percent natural progesterone cream on their skin. This may be all you need without resorting to a prescription for estrogen cream.

Beautiful Skin from the Inside Out: The Right Foods and Supplements

Good skin isn't just an outside job. The skin is a mirror for the health of your insides as well as your outsides. Take antioxidant vitamins (more about that on page 302–303) and eat at least five servings of fruits and vegetables daily. Many of the hundreds of substances present in these foods, such as lycopene in tomatoes, lutein in dark green and yellow vegetables, and the antioxidants in berries, have been clinically proven to help prevent and heal sun damage to the skin. Since antioxidants work in concert with one another, the greater the variety of fruits and vegetables you eat, the better.

The insulin-normalizing diet I recommend for balancing hormones at midlife also helps keep your skin in good shape. Limit caffeine, and cut down as much as possible on high-glycemic-index foods such as cookies, candies, pies, cakes, and non-whole-grain breads, all of which can cause fluid retention from excess insulin secretion. They are devoid of skin-nourishing vitamins and minerals, and quickly break down into sugar, which, as I explained above, causes collagen to lose its flexibility. (This is one of the reasons why diabetic individuals whose blood sugar is not tightly controlled often develop cataracts in the collagen-rich lenses of their eyes and have difficulty with wound healing. It is also why oral supplementation with antioxidants has been shown to alleviate some of the side effects of diabetes.)

FIBER: Make sure that you're getting enough fiber. Nothing shows up on the skin faster than chronic constipation! I've seen many cases of acne clear beautifully once bowel function is normalized.

One of the most effective ways to do this is simply by eating ¼ cup of ground golden flaxseed each day. In addition to the 11-plus grams of fiber you'll get, flaxseeds are also loaded with skin-beautifying omega-3 fatty acids and phytoestrogens. Fruits and vegetables are rich in fiber, too. You can also use fiber supplements such as psyllium.

HYDRATION: For most women, their hydration level shows up in the skin quickly—for better or for worse. But that doesn't mean drinking eight glasses of water per day, as we've all been told to do. What makes a lot more sense is "eating" your water in the form of moisture-rich fruits and vegetables (which are typically more than 80 percent water). The moisture in these foods is known as gel water and is denser than regular water. For one, it contains fiber, allowing us to absorb the water more slowly so it stays in our system longer. Another benefit is that such foods also contain electrolytes (like magnesium, chloride, sodium, and potassium), which create optimal electrical function in our bodies. Because water conducts electricity, this enhances mood, cognition, judgment, and energy. Thanks to all these various factors, water from plants may hydrate twice as well as drinking plain water, according to internal medicine specialist Dana Cohen, M.D., and Hydration Foundation founder Gina Bria, authors of *Quench: Beat Fatigue, Drop Weight, and Heal Your Body Through the New Science of Optimum Hydration* (Hachette, 2018).

As a rule of thumb, drink (or eat) half your body weight in ounces of water per day. So if you weigh 150 pounds, for example, aim to drink (or eat) the equivalent of 75 oz. of water each day. Another option is to add either a pinch of Himalayan or Celtic sea salt to the water, or a few slices of lemon or cucumber. This turns regular water into gel water, which travels more deeply into your tissues, resulting in better hydration. Other good options for optimal hydration include adding a tablespoon of chia seeds and a pinch of good mineral-rich salt to water. Let it sit for ten minutes or so, until the chia seeds swell, and then drink it. (This is also good for bowel function.) If you drink caffeinated drinks such as coffee, which tend to increase urinary output, just be sure that you drink enough extra liquid to replace the coffee you drank earlier. What this would mean is that for every cup of coffee you drink, you drink two cups of water (with a little salt in it).

FISH: Fish, especially salmon, sardines, and swordfish, is rich in omega-3 fats, which are important for building healthy cell membranes everywhere in the body.

PHYTOHORMONES: One of the most common benefits women notice after several months of supplementing their diets with significant amounts of phytoestrogens (such as maca, *Pueraria mirifica*, or soy) is improvement in their skin tone, hair, and nails. For example, in a study of forty postmenopausal women taking Revival soy, 93 percent showed significant improvements in skin (namely, skin flaking and discoloration were reduced after three months, and wrinkling was reduced after six months). The women also reported significant improvements in hair roughness, dullness, manageability, and overall assessment as well as in nail roughness, ridging, flaking, splitting, and overall appearance.[31] *Pueraria mirifica* works well too because, as research shows, it can both increase collagen production and inhibit collagen breakdown.[32] One woman who takes *Pueraria mirifica* wrote, "Within two months of beginning this supplement, my nails became stronger and more resilient than ever, my hair has taken on more body, and my skin has never looked more radiant. I'm thrilled." The phytoestrogen content of certain herbs and foods helps strengthen collagen everywhere in the body, whether in facial skin, vaginal tissue, or bone, while the isoflavones in phytoestrogens may act as antioxidants to protect skin from free-radical damage.[33]

LINOLEIC ACID: This omega-6 fatty acid, found in nuts, whole grains, most vegetable oils, eggs, and poultry, has been shown in clinical studies to keep skin from drying out and thinning.

SKIN-AIDING SUPPLEMENTS: Though all of the various supplements that I recommend at midlife help the skin (see chapter 7), the antioxidants, such as coenzyme Q_{10}, vitamin C, vitamin E and tocotrienols, and proanthocyanidins, are particularly important.

Research has shown, for example, that proanthocyanidins from pine bark or grape seeds help protect skin from the damaging effects of too much ultraviolet radiation. In one study, this powerful antioxidant was shown to prevent ultraviolet activation of a certain area in the nucleus of skin cells, reducing the inflammation that occurs after a sunburn.[34] Many individuals have reported healthy changes in their skin, nails, and hair as a result. The usual dose is 40–120 mg per day; I personally take 60–80 mg per day and even more when traveling or under stress.

Coenzyme Q_{10}, which is found in every cell of the body, is fat soluble and concentrates in the plasma membrane of cells, where it protects against free-radical damage. This antioxidant is used up when skin is exposed to ultraviolet radiation and other environmental insults, so it makes sense to supplement your diet with it or apply it topically. It is also found in red meat, salmon, and nuts. Coenzyme Q_{10} assists in cellular metabolism. The usual dose in supplement form is 30–100 mg per day.

Vitamins E and C taken as supplements have also been shown to help protect against the UV-generated free-radical damage that can lead to skin changes. The dose of vitamin C used was only 200 mg; for vitamin E, it was 1,000 IU.[35] The results are apt to be even more impressive with the newer, more potent forms of vitamin E—the tocotrienols. The supplement regimen recommended in chapter 7 will give you all the skin-nourishing nutrients you need.

SKIN CARE FROM YOUR REFRIGERATOR

Once or twice per week, if you have the time, you can give your face a healthy dose of antioxidants, fruit acids, and plant hormones by using ingredients that you can find right in your refrigerator. Choose the food that most appeals to your sense of smell; you'll be getting aromatherapy benefits as well as direct benefit to your skin. Plain yogurt applied to your face makes a nourishing mask that gives your skin the benefits of lactic acid and also the hydrating effects of milk proteins. You can add pureed fresh fruit to it. (Don't use sweetened yogurt. The sugar is harmful to the skin.)

I love thinly sliced cucumber applied to my eyelids and cheeks to help me relax and get ready for evening. Green tea bags, moistened and applied to the eyelids, also give your eyes a soothing antioxidant life. And mashed-up fresh fruits such as peaches, strawberries, or apples can all be mixed with finely ground oatmeal to form a nourishing facial mask. You can also use parsley or even fresh basil, rosemary, or thyme. Remember, the skin will absorb the nutrients from these foods in about fifteen minutes, so you don't need to lie down any longer than that to benefit from a rejuvenating facial mask.

MIDLIFE ACNE

Anything that compromises the immune system, whether emotional stress or nutritional deficiency, will tend to exacerbate the underlying conditions that lead to acne. So will hormonal imbalances in which the body produces too much androgen. And too much androgen or testosterone is associated with both hair growth and acne. Anytime you are under stress, your cortisol and insulin balance is likely to be upset, which adversely affects your skin—and the rest of you as well. At perimenopause, the same stormy emotions that were present at adolescence often arise again, along with the hormonal swings that exacerbate the situation. It's no wonder that skin breakouts are so common during this life stage.

Are You Thin-Skinned and in Need of Individuation?

Both adolescence and midlife are key developmental periods of our lives when we go through the process of individuating and defining who we are in relationship to others. The skin is the first contact surface between the mother and the infant, and for our entire lives it represents a boundary between us and other people. Some researchers believe that skin disease may be thought of as an attempt to define who we are in relationship to other people and what a healthy boundary between us should be.[36] I agree. Every single time I've had skin breakouts, it is because my boundaries have not been firm enough and I have been overgiving to others at my own expense.

When I was in my early thirties, a time in life when hormones are relatively stable and skin is usually at its best, I developed a very troubling case of acne. It took me a while to understand what was going on. I'd never had much in the way of skin problems in my teenage years, and since I was exercising regularly, taking vitamins, and eating a whole-food diet, it seemed strange to me that I should suddenly be experiencing acne at my age. However, I was working at the time in an office where my ideas on nutrition, emotions, and the mind-body connection were not well accepted, a fact I dealt with by way of a lot of self-deprecating humor, hoping this would enable me to stay safe and fit in as best I could. I desperately wanted the approval of my colleagues and was so thin-skinned that I was constantly trying to forestall any criticism of my ideas and beliefs. Finally, at the age of thirty-five, I realized that I couldn't continue using so much of my energy to try to blend in, and so after a good deal of soul-searching, I took a leap of faith and left to co-found Women to Women. My four-year-long skin problem cleared up within three months and has never returned, even when I was in the middle of midlife hormonal changes! Years later, when in a new relationship, I once again developed significant skin breakouts that lasted for months. In retrospect, this happened because I had (once again) lost myself and my needs and was overgiving. Things eventually cleared up as my boundaries and self-care became my top priorities.

THE ANATOMY OF ACNE

1 Androgenic hormones such as DHEA and testosterone increase production of sebum by the sebaceous glands.

2. Sebum makes the hardened outer layer of skin (the keratin-rich cells known as the horny layer) turn over faster. This results in pores and hair follicles that are clogged with dead skin cells and oil.

3. Skin bacteria of the type known as *Propionibacterium acnes* feed off the sebum and break it down into free fatty acids.

4. Free fatty acids attract white blood cells and other inflammatory molecules (eicosanoids) from the immune system.

5. An acne pimple or blackhead is the result.

Hormones and Midlife Acne

There are numerous studies showing that sebaceous gland activity is heightened by androgens such as DHEA and testosterone and reduced by estrogen or removal of the ovaries, which reduces androgen levels.[37] This is the reason why birth control pills often help clear up acne. But whether or not higher levels of hormones result in acne is an individual matter. Women with the most severe forms of acne generally have a genetic predisposition to androgen sensitivity in their skin, even at hormone levels that are normal.

When sebaceous glands are small, as in children and the elderly, acne does not occur. It is usually first seen in adolescence, when sebaceous gland development begins to take place. It occurs primarily on the face, back, and chest. Endocrinologists have long theorized that acne is an endocrine disease resulting from abnormal androgen production. Hair follicles and attached sebaceous glands contain a specific enzyme known as 5-alpha-reductase, which can convert estrogen into the androgen testosterone. That's why some women experience an increase in acne when their estrogen levels rise, due either to perimenopause or to being put on overly high levels of HT. But two women who are on identical HT regimens, eat exactly the same diet, and have the same amount of stress in their lives may have skin reactions that are entirely different. That's why all treatments, including prescription medications, have their place and can be useful.

Natural Treatments for Acne

If your acne is mild to moderate, I'd recommend that you use the natural treatment program I outline below. If your acne is severe, you may also want to add one of the medications I discuss below, or follow the advice of a skin care specialist.

- ‿ EAT A DIET THAT LOWERS INSULIN. Follow the high-fiber, insulin-lowering diet outlined in chapter 7, because a diet too high in high-glycemic-index carbohydrates, as I've already stated, is associated with excessively high levels of insulin, which in turn can cause higher-than-normal production of androgens. For many women, this is all that is necessary to completely clear up acne.
- ‿ TAKE SUPPLEMENTS. Take a comprehensive vitamin and mineral supplement daily. (See chapter 7.) It is well documented that zinc, vitamin C, and the B vitamins are essential for healthy skin functioning. A good phytoestrogen can also help. Many women notice that their hair and skin improve dramatically when they start on a good supplementation regimen.
- ‿ LOSE EXCESS BODY FAT. Get your body fat percentage into the healthy range. Excess body fat is associated with higher-than-normal androgen levels. Even a small fat loss of five to ten pounds can make a significant difference in insulin and androgen as it affects the sebaceous glands.
- ‿ FOLLOW THE SKIN CARE REGIMEN FOR THE GENERAL CARE OF MID-LIFE SKIN (pages 488–490). Remember that fruit acids, or phyto-hormones combined with fruit acids, often work very well for acne. A good antioxidant skin care program usually helps reduce or completely eliminate acne scars. Intense pulsed light (IPL) treatments can work wonders for old acne scars, as well as spider veins.

⌐ TRY HOME REMEDIES FOR PIMPLES. When you notice a pimple that hasn't come to a head yet, apply tea tree oil at night. The antibacterial properties in the oil will often result in significant regression of the pimple by morning. Some women use tea tree oil daily.

Another effective treatment is to make a paste of baking soda and lemon juice and apply it to the pimple. Baking soda also makes an excellent exfoliating agent unless your skin is sensitive.

⌐ REMOVE BLACKHEADS. For blackheads, get a professional facial with blackhead removal about once per month until your skin has cleared. After that, you can use one of the readily available blackhead removal strips, such as Bioré. Limit use to once per week to avoid overdrying the skin.

Acne Medications

VITAMIN A DERIVATIVES: Tretinoin (in Retin-A, Retin-A Micro, and Renova, applied topically) and Isotretinoin (Accutane, taken systemically) are prescription medications that increase skin cell turnover and allow sebum to be released more easily so that it doesn't get trapped. Accutane is an oral vitamin A derivative that powerfully inhibits both sebum production and growth of acne-causing bacteria. It is the single most effective treatment for severe acne that doesn't respond to other measures. However, it is very irritating and should never be used by anyone who is pregnant or trying to get pregnant, because it can cause birth defects.[38]

BENZOYL PEROXIDE AND SULFUR-CONTAINING PRODUCTS: Various lotions, creams, or gels containing benzoyl peroxide or sulfur are often used for their antibacterial and drying properties. Benzoyl peroxide penetrates the hair follicle and produces oxygen, thus suppressing the growth of acne-causing bacteria, which thrive in an anaerobic (oxygen-free) environment. Although often effective, these treatments can be very irritating for the skin.

ANTIBIOTICS: Tetracycline or erythromycin work by preventing the acne bacteria from breaking down the sebum into the free fatty acids that result in pimples. I do not recommend the use of antibiotics because they kill off the healthy bacteria in the bowel, which can lead to suboptimal absorption of nutrients, diarrhea, and repeated yeast infections. It can also lead to antibiotic resistance.

BIRTH CONTROL PILLS: Oral contraceptives are often used to reduce sebum production. They do this by decreasing the brain's signal to make hormones from the ovaries. I'd avoid these synthetic hormones unless you feel you have no other choice and are unable or unwilling to follow a healthier diet or use one or more of the topical treatments recommended above.

ROSACEA

Rosacea is a common condition at midlife (forties and fifties) and occurs equally in women and in men. Rosacea is, in essence, a neurological disorder of the facial blood vessels, which makes them hyperresponsive. This results in dilated blood vessels in the blush area of the face and upper chest. It is accompanied by facial flushing, a burning sensation in the face, and also papules and pustules. Rosacea clearly demonstrates the seamless connection between emotions and skin, for it always gets worse when women are under significant emotional stress. Psychological studies have linked rosacea with a disordered blushing reaction. Though blushing is a normal response to the emotions of excitement, shame, or embarrassment, in those with rosacea the body's normal response goes too far because the emotion is held too frequently or too long. Studies have shown, for instance, that people prone to this disorder are likely to be perfectionistic and have a strong need to please others. They also have a predisposition to excessive feelings of guilt and shame.[39] Rosacea "triggers" are numerous and include changes in temperature, certain foods, stress, changes in emotions, exercise, and several skin care products. Rosacea generally begins between the ages of thirty and sixty, though it can start as early as the teenage years or even (rarely) in childhood. I've also seen many cases of rosacea clear up with an insulin-lowering diet.

CHERYL: Rosacea and Shame

Cheryl first came to see me when she was forty-two and having problems with irregular periods. She also had persistent reddening of the skin around her nose and cheeks, which her dermatologist had diagnosed as rosacea. Though she was on various topical antibiotics for the problem, they didn't help much. Her problem always seemed to be exacerbated premenstrually, but with such irregular periods, which sometimes came every two weeks, she never knew when her skin would look good and when it would flare up.

As I worked with Cheryl over the next year, we both noticed what a barometer her skin reddening was for emotional turmoil. And Cheryl had plenty. During the year that her rosacea first appeared, she was in the middle of an affair with a married professional—an affair that took place in his office. Over time she discovered that she wasn't the only woman with whom this man was sexually involved. When she discovered this, she felt deeply ashamed. Her childhood history revealed that she had been the victim of incest by her father, something she had also kept secret for years. But Cheryl had a great deal of courage. She began to go to groups for incest survivors and also started individual therapy. At the same time she committed to improving her diet and lifestyle on all levels. Over the next several years Cheryl became stronger and more independent. Eventually she even had the courage to forgive herself for becoming involved with an unscrupulous man in the first place. As Cheryl connected with her inner wisdom and supported herself physically through diet and exercise, her rosacea cleared up, slowly but surely. She now notices flare-ups only occasionally, and only when she reverts to old emotional patterns of shame and neediness, feelings that she now has the skills and self-esteem to work through effectively.

Treatment Options

The standard treatment for rosacea includes both oral and topical medications that are anti-inflammatory (antibiotics or Accutane) and a topical anti-inflammatory (such as a metronidazole-based product). The treatment protocol is generally followed for four to six months until the rosacea is under control. (Often, antibiotics don't help—there's no evidence that rosacea is caused by abnormal skin bacteria.) After that, just topical treatment is continued. The obvious problem with oral antibiotics is that taking them over so many months can result in an imbalance of normal bowel flora. That's why I always recommend taking a probiotic (for example, acidophilus) if you're on an antibiotic. Cellular inflammation aggravates rosacea (and just about every other disease as well), so if you really want to control rosacea, you must follow a low-sugar diet that keeps insulin levels normal. This means eating minimal amounts or eliminating "white" foods, including white bread, white potatoes, products containing sugar, and soda. It's best to include lots of fresh fruits and vegetables, which are also loaded with antioxidants to help fight inflammation. It's also helpful to use skin care products that are self-preserving and do not contain parabens and other irritants. Be sure to avoid products with alpha-hydroxy acids, as they can be irritating. Hydrocortisone, benzoyl peroxide, and topical retinoids should also be avoided.

Some women report that supplementing their diets with betaine hydrochloride, which increases stomach acidity, helps rosacea, for reasons that aren't entirely clear. If you decide to take this supplement, which is available in natural food stores, make sure you take it with food. Otherwise it creates a sensation like heartburn. The usual dose is 500–1,000 mg with meals. IPL (intense pulsed light) can also be very effective.

MIND-BODY APPROACH TO SKIN PROBLEMS

Did my description of the psychological profile of a rosacea patient or someone suffering from midlife acne strike home? If it did, then the next time you feel yourself becoming overwhelmed by emotions of shame, anxiety, or anger, try the following.

1. Take a slow, full, deep breath through your nose for a count of five. Hold for a count of five. Exhale slowly for a count of five. Hold for a count of five. Then continue breathing fully.

2. Close your eyes.

3. Identify where in your body you are feeling the emotion.

4. Describe what you are feeling. Does it have a shape, a color, or a sound?

5. Don't try to change your feeling. Allow yourself to feel it fully, exactly as it is. Love yourself for it.

6. Keep breathing and moving around while doing this— breathing and moving will help you move the emotion right on through.

Here's what you're apt to notice: the minute you give your emotion a chance to be felt fully, it goes away. You can use this technique anytime you feel any difficult emotion. And guess what? You'll find that you have the ability to deal with it without outside help.

HAIR IN THE WRONG PLACES

Many women notice an increase in coarse or dark hair on their chins and upper lips starting at midlife. Although this can be quite distressing, it is perfectly natural and is the result of the higher androgen-to-estrogen ratio that prevails beginning in perimenopause. Androgen can transform fine peach-fuzz-type hair (known as vellus hair) into coarser hair (known as terminal hair). Sometimes, however, excessive facial hair can be a sign of an underlying hormonal imbalance, such as in the condition known as polycystic ovary syndrome. Coarse facial hair is also common in women whose diets are too high in refined carbohydrates, which shifts the hormones in the direction of androgens. Usually, however, the growth of facial hair at midlife is not a sign of hormonal or nutritional problems, just the normal result of proportionally higher levels of androgens.

The same androgenic hormones that are associated with thickening and darkening of hair on your upper lip and your chin may cause hair loss on other areas, such as the head. Androgenic hormones affect the hair follicles of the scalp by shortening what is known as anagen (the growth phase of the hair growth cycle), which causes the hair to regress to a finer, thinner texture. But how androgen affects the hair depends in part on where the hair is located. The androgen receptors in the hair follicles of other areas of the body vary in terms of numbers and sensitivity. That's the reason why excessive androgen can thin out the hair on your head while increasing the amount and thickness of the hair on your face. Of course, not only are there differences in androgen sensitivity in different bodily sites within the individual, but there are differences between individuals. Thus a relatively low level of androgen may result in facial hair growth in some women and not in others. Amount of body and facial hair also varies among different racial groups. Dark-haired, darkly pigmented Caucasians of either sex tend to be hairier than blondes or fair-skinned individuals.

Hair Removal Techniques

As normal as it may be, excess facial (or body) hair may be something you wish to deal with cosmetically. In general, I don't recommend plucking, waxing, or shaving, because over time this can distort the hair follicle, making permanent hair removal more difficult if you decide on that later. Almost all women, including me, have to pluck chin hairs from time to time—sometimes even before the age of forty! But before opting for permanent removal, you may want to try the insulin-balancing diet suggested in chapter 7. As an interim cosmetic intervention, it's best to simply cut the hair as close to the skin as possible or bleach it. If you do decide on permanent hair removal, keep in mind that fine, non-androgenized hair (the peach-fuzz type of hair that is present everywhere on the body) may undergo androgenization at any time during perimenopause or beyond. So even though you may have had your existing coarse hair removed, you may be producing new hair regularly, especially during times of stress, when androgenic hormone levels increase. Sometimes hair growth will also be encouraged by the hormones you're using or your diet and stress levels.

ELECTROLYSIS: Electrolysis is a procedure done by a trained professional that involves sending an electric current into the hair follicle via a carefully placed needle. It can take several (or even many) treatments per hair follicle to truly destroy that follicle and prevent the hair from regrowing. Electrolysis is uncomfortable, so you may want your doctor to give you a prescription for a topical anesthetic known as EMLA (lidocaine and prilocaine), which must be put on the skin an hour before the treatment. Over time—usually a few weeks to a few months—regular electrolysis sessions will result in far fewer dark hairs. But you'll probably have to continue to go for treatments every month or so, as new vellus hairs are transformed into terminal hairs. Make sure that your electrolysis professional is well trained and certified.

LASER HAIR REMOVAL: Laser technology for hair removal is improving all the time and can be very effective but tends to work best in lighter-skinned individuals with dark hair. It doesn't work on blond hair. Like electrolysis, it is painful, so a topical anesthetic (EMLA) is used before the procedure. Make sure you go to a physician who is well trained in laser technology.

PRESCRIPTION MEDICATIONS: The medications mentioned on page 516 for the treatment of hair loss on the head may also, ironically, be effective for treating hair growth on the face, since both may be a result of the hormonal shifts that occur at menopause. Spironolactone in particular is a potent antiandrogen that is sometimes effective when used topically.

Alopecia Androgenica: Midlife Hair Loss from Hormonal Imbalance

Though some women begin to experience some hair loss at menopause secondary to hormonal shifts in the body, most do not. Saying that significant hair loss is secondary to menopause would be like saying that dementia is a normal part of aging. Nevertheless, hair loss at perimenopause is a relatively common problem that erodes self-confidence and self-esteem and makes it difficult to enjoy yourself fully in a social situation.

Alopecia androgenica, which results in what we call male-pattern baldness, is by far the most common cause of hair thinning and loss in women at midlife. Typically, the hair becomes finer and thinner and may eventually recede, though in women usually the front hairline is preserved. Up to 13 percent of premenopausal women and 37 percent of postmenopausal women suffer from hormone-associated hair loss to some degree.

I recently received the following illustrative letter from Evelyn, one of my e-newsletter subscribers.

> I am writing in an attempt to get some clarification on natural hormone therapy. I had a complete hysterectomy last July at the age of forty-four—fibroids. My doctor started me out on Premarin, and I had no problems that I was aware of. However, I had read many books on natural hormone therapy and decided to go with a formula my doctor prescribed for me. I have been using four drops of the hormone lotion to control hot flashes. I noticed after a while that my skin became oily and I am having problems with acne. Also, and what concerns me the most, is that my hair is thinning quite rapidly.
>
> I have had a blood test for hormones and thyroid—everything was within normal limits. The test showed that my hormone levels were higher than in a young, healthy female. I am trying to lower my dose to see if it will have an effect on my hair. I understand that too much estrogen can cause hair loss. My doctor encourages me to go back on the pharmaceutical alternatives, which he tells me he has used successfully for more than twenty years. At this time I am very confused and would do almost anything to keep my hair from falling out. Please, give me some advice on how to pursue this problem.

Clearly Evelyn is converting estrogen to androgen, and the androgens are having an effect at the level of her hair follicles. That's why her skin is getting oily, she's getting acne, and her hair is thinning.

Although the hormone regimen she is on works well for many women, transdermal hormones go right into the bloodstream and as such can give higher levels with lower doses than when the hormone is given orally. I suggested that Evelyn either switch to an oral estrogen-progesterone preparation or cut way back on her topical estrogen and progesterone. For reasons that aren't entirely clear, some women simply do better with oral hormones. I also suggested to Evelyn that she make sure she is following an insulin-lowering diet so that excess insulin from refined carbohydrates isn't pushing her body toward higher androgen production. She could also use one of the phytohormone preparations mentioned in chapter 6 to help her hot flashes and to keep her bones healthy. This infusion of phytohormones might allow her to cut her dose of estrogen or even eliminate it so there would be less of it around for her body to convert into androgen.

If you have hair follicles that are particularly sensitive to androgen, like Evelyn, any hormone therapy regimen that has too much androgen for your body can result in hair loss. The problem goes away once you stop the drug. Most hormonally associated hair loss is not caused by hormone therapy regimens, however; it is the result of an imbalance in your own body's hormonal production.

Androgen-associated hair loss can be likened to the canary in the mine. It is a symptom that often signals a much more pervasive hormone imbalance that affects many women to one degree or another. Though, as I mentioned, up to 37 percent of menopausal women will have some hair thinning from increased androgen production at menopause, and about 10 to 15 percent of women have full-blown androgen-excess syndrome characterized by facial acne, male-pattern hair loss, upper-body obesity (apple-shaped figure), insulin resistance, increased facial hair, and adverse changes in lipid profile.

This syndrome, which overlaps with insulin resistance, which I've outlined in chapter 7, is associated with polycystic ovary syndrome, a high-sugar diet, adrenal hypersecretion, genetic factors, excessive body fat, or unknown causes. Because all of these factors set the scene for early-onset cardiovascular disease and diabetes, your hormone-associated hair loss needs to be seen as only one aspect of a much larger systemic imbalance that you can do a great deal to help alleviate.

How to Get Your Hair Back—and Improve Your Health at the Same Time

First, have your healthcare provider test you to see if there is a systemic cause for your hair loss. Diagnosing the type of hair loss you have will help clarify which options are most likely to work.

Make sure your hormone levels are normal. Even though the vast majority of women with hair loss will be found to have normal androgen levels, it's important to rule out the occasional rare abnormality and also to remember that it's usually not your body's absolute level of androgen that's the problem, but your hair follicles' heightened sensitivity to androgen. Have your doctor check your TSH (thyroid-stimulating hormone) as well as your free triiodothyronine (T3) and free thyroxine (T4) levels. The TSH should be no higher than 3.0 mIU/l, although many experts (including myself) prefer setting the limit at 2.5. (Higher levels indicate subclinical hypothyroidism; a little natural thyroid replacement, such as Nature-Throid or Armour Thyroid, could help.) Have your doctor check your levels of DHEA and androstenedione as well. I also recommend the DUTCH test to ascertain androgen and cortisol levels. (See chapter 4.) If you do fit the description of someone with full-blown androgen-excess syndrome, have your lipid profile, blood pressure, and blood sugar checked.

Even if your hormone levels come back as normal, do the following.

~ Follow the low-glycemic-index hormone-balancing diet outlined in chapter 7.

~ Lose any excess body fat. If your body fat percentage is above 30 percent, as measured in your doctor's office or fitness center, the excess fat is a factory for androgen and could drive your insulin levels, blood pressure, and blood lipids into unhealthy ranges. Excess body fat caused by a sedentary lifestyle and a diet too high in refined carbohydrates and trans fats is probably the key issue in combating not only androgen-associated hair loss, but also the health problems often associated with it.

~ Take a good vitamin and mineral supplement (see chapter 7) to help your new hair grow in fully.

~ Consider taking additional iodine. This helps balance the thyroid as well as balance estrogen and may be all that's necessary to stop hair loss (see page 143).

~ Reduce stress. Stress hormones skew hormone metabolism into the androgen range, so a regimen that includes meditation, aerobic exercise, regular massage, and a low-sugar, whole-food diet will help you to both dial down the stress and reduce your hair loss.

~ Try Chinese herbs. Shou Wu Pian is a Chinese herbal medicine that often works very well to help restore hair growth. My acupuncturist has used it for years, and I have seen wonderful results, including a reduction in gray hair.

TREATING THE SURFACE—MINOXIDIL AND TRETINOIN SPRAY: Minoxidil is currently the only drug approved by the FDA for its beneficial effect on hair growth. Minoxidil is a potent antihypertensive medication that when taken by mouth lowers blood pressure by dilating blood vessels. It was discovered by accident that it increases hair growth. Though it is not clear how it enhances hair growth when applied topically, it may increase the size of the hair follicle, prolong the growth phase of a hair follicle, increase blood flow to the skin, or enhance DNA synthesis. Side effects are rare but may include skin irritation and a short-lived increase in heart rate. In one study, a 2 percent solution of minoxidil increased the total weight of hair by more than 40 percent over a forty-week period of use.[40] When researchers combined a 2 percent solution of minoxidil with 0.025 percent tretinoin (Retin-A) and used it four times per day as a scalp spray, 90 percent of the women in the study showed visible and cosmetically significant improvement in hair quality after six months.[41]

PRESCRIPTION MEDICATIONS FOR HORMONAL HAIR LOSS: The drugs doctors prescribe to rebalance systemic hormonal imbalances work well for some, though not all, women with hormone-associated hair loss. However, too often they help the symptoms without really addressing the underlying cause—too much body fat, unhealthy diet, sedentary lifestyle, and so on—or helping you learn how to heal yourself by using the body's own internal wisdom. If you use any of the following medications, complement them with appropriate diet and lifestyle changes.

~ Birth control pills with ethinyl estradiol, 30–40 mcg, for twenty days of the cycle. Birth control pills sometimes work to stop androgenic hair loss for the same reason they help acne—they reduce the body's susceptibility to the effects of androgen on the hair follicle and its attached sebaceous gland.

~ *Spironolactone* is an antiandrogen that can be taken orally or applied topically. Taken orally, it decreases total and free testosterone. Applied topically, it reduces the amount of androgen that directly affects the hair follicle.

In some women, an individualized prescription for HT, such as the ones described in chapter 5 and above for skin, can help balance hormone levels and help alleviate androgen excess.

Making the Most of the Hair You've Got

While you're working from the inside out—or the outside in—you'll still want to look your best. Make the most of what you've got . . . and enhance it.

Consult a professional who specializes in hairpieces, hair extensions, weaves, and body perms. You might even want to inquire about hair transplantation for women by a dermatologist or plastic surgeon.[42]

Here are some more tips for making thin hair appear its best.

~ Use gentle shampoos, and don't shampoo more than every other day.

~ Don't brush your hair when it's wet—this stretches out the hair.

~ Avoid teasing your hair—it can break the hair shaft.

~ Chlorine damages hair. Shower with pure water. If your water is chlorinated, use a shower filter that removes it.

~ Ask your hairdresser to recommend professional products for fine hair that will give you extra volume.

WHEN GOOD SKIN CARE ISN'T ENOUGH: DECIDING ON COSMETIC PROCEDURES

Sometimes the results you're looking for will be unattainable with diet and good skin care alone. If you have a "fixable" aspect of your face that bothers you every time you look in the mirror, it may be time to consider getting outside help. Whether you want to enhance your smile with cosmetic dentistry or get rid of the bags under your eyes that always make you look tired even when you're not, there's no doubt that fixing an energy-draining "ding" in your appearance can improve the quality of life. That's why so many women get braces at midlife, or have skin peels to give them a fresher look that simply can't be achieved any other way. Cosmetic surgery of all kinds is growing by leaps and bounds because of vast improvements in technology and increasing demand.

It seems to me that it is almost impossible to go through the normal process of facial aging in this culture and not wish that something could be done about certain parts of your face, especially the eyelids and jawline. If you're one of the lucky ones who really aren't at all bothered by sagging eyelids or jowls, bless you. If, however, you want an appearance-enhancing face-lift, eyelid surgery, skin peel, liposuction, laser surgery, or other cosmetic polishing of your exterior, then bless you, too. Through the years I've referred many patients for various plastic surgery or dermatological procedures. Just about 100 percent of them have been thrilled with the results.

In addition to giving referrals for plastic surgery, while I was still at Women to Women, I even took a course in how to do deep facial skin peels. We did the procedure at the office and then cared for the women at a private home for four days thereafter. I always thought of this service as a kind of "cocoon" experience in which the newly peeled and vulnerable women were kept safe, warm, and healthy while they shed their old skins and prepared to face the world with a renewed countenance. I must admit that the results were spectacular for the women (and one man) who went through with the procedure. I was always thrilled on the last day to witness the "unveiling" as we helped our patients remove their masks of powder and apply makeup to cover their renewed but very red skin. This was especially true for those whose difficult and painful past histories had lined their faces with expressions of anger and depression they had since worked through. Virtually all of the women I treated had done lots of inner work. Now they simply wanted their outsides to match their insides.

One of my patients had her eyes done at the age of forty-one, about one year after a mastectomy. With the bags under her eyes surgically corrected, she looked brighter and fresher than she had in years. And her new look helped her outlook and possibly her immune system as well.

Particularly Effective Cosmetic Procedures

Led by the desires of baby boomers to look as young as possible for as long as possible, a whole new range of cosmetic and skin care solutions is now available to rejuvenate aging skin and keep it looking good for years. These include intermittent laser (called intense pulsed light, or IPL) treatments, which are very effective at reducing wrinkles, evening out skin tone, thickening the collagen layer, and removing spider veins. IPL is generally done as a series of five or so treatments followed by maintenance of once every six months. IPL treatments can be alternated with glycolic peels so that you are having a mini-rejuvenation procedure every three months or so. Fraxel is a laser procedure that thickens the collagen layer of the skin. It must be done monthly (after which the skin is quite red for several days) for about four months. But it's effective. Other acid and laser peels are available that can help remove the effects of sun damage and give you a clean slate that is easier to maintain with a good skin care regimen. I am also intrigued by stem cell facial rejuvenation; according to the research I have done, injecting stem cells into certain areas of the face causes a rejuvenation of facial features that can't be matched by other methods because the stem cells know exactly where to go.

If you decide to consult a plastic surgeon or dermatologist or if you already have a procedure scheduled, I'd recommend the following.

~ Be sure that you're having a cosmetic procedure because it makes you feel better. Don't do it for your husband, boyfriend, or mother. Over the years I've seen that the results of surgeries are always much better when our motivation for having them is clear.

~ Choose the right doctor. When it comes to cosmetic surgery, especially laser techniques, there is a great deal of crossover between the profession of dermatology and plastic surgery. For example, laser skin peels that include the eyelid area (usually done in a doctor's office) give a result that is often as good as a face-lift obtained with a surgeon's knife. Look for a board-certified plastic surgeon or, in the case of laser procedures, a dermatologist or other practitioner with extensive training in laser technology.

~ Don't choose a doctor just because he or she offers the lowest prices. All surgical and laser procedures carry a certain amount of risk. This risk increases if doctors cut corners on care and safety to keep prices low.

~ Make sure you go to someone with whom you feel completely comfortable. (This same criterion goes for body workers or anyone else who will be working with your body in any way—including a dentist.) Ask yourself: "Does this person have the kind of clinical, objective, and healing touch that will allow me to feel comfortable even if I have to stand in my underwear and have him or her look at my body and take pictures as part of my care?" A good doctor will put you at ease even in this kind of situation. If there's any feeling of discomfort, go elsewhere. That's what happened with a friend of mine who went to see a plastic surgeon in order to have both her nose and her deviated septum fixed. (She had had a broken nose since childhood.) The surgeon kept staring at her breasts, which are relatively small, while she kept trying to get his attention back on her nose. She had no desire to have breast implants. Though this man had all the right credentials, had trained at the best places in the United States, and was perfectly competent technically, he also had what I've come to call the sleaze factor. His attitude made her uncomfortable. So she chose someone else to do her surgery. Her feeling of unease was confirmed when she later heard via the grapevine that he had told his wife, also a physician, about some of the surgeries he had done and upon whom. This information had made its way around the community. Such a breach of confidentiality is completely unacceptable, but it happens. You can avoid this kind of situation by trusting your gut as well as a surgeon's credentials.

~ Keep your surgery decision to yourself as much as possible. You'd be amazed at the number of judgments your friends may have concerning cosmetic surgery, depending upon where you live. (The Rocky Mountain and Pacific regions are currently leaders in plastic surgeries.)[43] Some of your friends won't think you're very spiritually evolved, for instance, if you want to remove the bags under your eyes. Frankly, how you look is none of their business.

~ If at all possible, go away to have your procedure done. Too many of my patients have had the experience of being home with a bruised face after plastic surgery, looking like battered women, and then having to answer the door for the plumber, the mail carrier, and everyone else who comes along. If that doesn't bother you, no problem.

~ Give yourself enough time. Recovery from eyelid or facial surgery usually takes a minimum of two weeks before you look present-able. So use this time for reading or taking a much-deserved retreat from your usual routine. It will speed your healing process and help the inside of you as much as the outside.

~ Make arrangements to be waited on for at least the first three days post-op. Though you may feel fine, you're apt to be more tired than usual and perhaps a bit weepy and emotional during this vul-nerable time. Give yourself the space you deserve.

~ Stock up on the Chinese patent herb Yannan Pei Yan and begin taking it, 1 tablet four times a day, as soon as you possibly can after surgery. This herb speeds healing and cuts way down on postoperative bruising. I also recommend taking at least 2,000 mg of vitamin C for two weeks pre-op and four weeks post-op to help build up collagen in your skin. You can also use skin cream con-taining vitamin C ester to speed up healing.

~ Use guided-imagery tapes before and during surgery, and ask your surgeon and anesthesiologist to work with you. (See Resources.)

~ Be realistic. Cosmetic surgery won't change your life, despite what our culture would lead you to believe. If you are beautiful on the outside but ugly, depressed, or unhappy on the inside, your appeal will begin to fade within thirty seconds of walking into a room. I'm sure you've all had the experience of meeting people who be-come more and more attractive right in front of your eyes as you begin to know and appreciate the humor, joy, or fun they bring to every situation.

VARICOSE VEINS

Chances are you don't like the look of prominent blue varicose veins and want to do whatever you can to prevent them or, if you already have a few, minimize them. Appearance isn't the only problem with varicose veins, however. If they get bad enough, they are often asso-ciated with a painful, heavy feeling in the legs, especially at the end of the day. Happily, there are a number of strategies to help you prevent varicose veins in the first place, or keep them from getting worse if you already have a few.

Let's start by going over what varicose veins are and why they develop. The term *varicose* refers to a vein that is dilated, tortuous, and located just beneath the skin. Quite often the valves of these veins, which are designed to keep the blood from flowing backward, no longer work as they should. When a surface vein stretches and loses its elasticity, and the valves don't shut properly, blood flows backward, pooling in the affected vein, which then enlarges into a mass of blue tissue beneath the skin. Varicose veins can be large, having the appearance of blue worms, or they can be very small and purplish blue in color. These small "spider" veins often occur in a fanlike pattern in the thigh area. Varicose veins, whether large or small, are the end result of poor circulation.

Diet and Varicose Veins

It is very clear that the fundamental cause of varicose veins is a diet high in refined carbohydrates and low in fiber—the same kind that is also associated with heart disease, breast cancer, and bad skin. Such a diet often results in subtle nutritional deficiencies, excess weight, and constipation, all of which increase intra-abdominal pressure, which over the years puts too much pressure on the veins in our legs.[44] Chronic coughing does the same thing—and so does excess fat in the abdomen.

Varicose veins are virtually nonexistent in rural Africa, where the diet tends to be high in fiber-rich whole foods and very low in refined foods. But thanks to our own very different diet, almost all of us in this country are at an increased risk for developing at least a few dilated veins in our legs. Varicose veins can also be aggravated by the hormonal changes that women experience during three specific times in our lives: at the onset of our menstrual periods, during pregnancy, and at the beginning of menopause. These are the times when we are most susceptible to subtle changes in our blood flow that put us at increased risk for damage to our vein walls. Because of these hormonal changes, varicose veins can show up as early as age twenty. In men, by contrast, varicose veins develop evenly throughout the life span up until the age of seventy and don't appear to be hormonally related.

Program for Preventing or Treating Varicose Veins

Now that you know what you're dealing with, let's get down to the business of keeping your veins in top shape.

⌒ GIVE YOUR LEGS THE SUPPORT THEY DESERVE. If you already have varicose veins or if you have a family history of varicose veins, make sure that you wear compression or support stockings of some kind whenever you know you will be on your feet for a long time. And elevate your legs as much as possible. I have a family history of varicose veins, so when I was a resident in training, I always wore compression stockings when I was on call at night. Putting those stockings on always gave me a new lease on life. Though I was only in my twenties at the time, I found that when I didn't wear them, my legs ached and my ankles got swollen after being on my feet all night. (I used Jobst brand stockings; another good brand is T.E.D. These are available at your pharmacy. The cost is sometimes reimbursable from your insurance if you have a doctor's prescription.) Avoid standard knee-highs and thigh-high stockings if you have varicose veins, because the elastic at the tops of these impedes venous blood flow and increases the pooling of blood in the veins that is the cause of the problem in the first place. I also recommend support hose when flying or traveling long distances in a train, bus, or car. They keep the blood from pooling in your legs and ankles and you arrive at your destination far more refreshed than you otherwise would. (In these cases, knee-high support stockings are fine.)

⌒ IF YOU TAKE ESTROGEN, MAKE SURE YOU'RE TAKING THE RIGHT DOSE. Low-dose estrogen replacement therapy does not appear to cause varicose veins in women, but occasionally a woman will notice that her legs ache and seem to swell more when she is on estrogen replacement, and existing varicose veins may seem to get worse. If you've noticed that your veins seem to be worse on estrogen replacement, consider lowering your dose.

⌒ AVOID CONSTIPATION. Follow a diet that has adequate fiber, plenty of water, and very few refined carbohydrates.

⌒ USE YOUR MUSCLES TO KEEP YOUR BLOOD MOVING. Rhythmic exercise such as walking, biking, running, rebounding, or swimming keeps your blood moving and uses the mechanical action of your muscles to get the blood out of your veins and back to your heart. I've seen many women cure their symptomatic varicose veins and improve the cosmetic appearance of their legs by starting and staying with a regular exercise program. It's worth noting that my mother had fairly severe varicose veins during her childbearing years. With all of her hiking and a good diet, they have resolved on their own!

⁓ NOURISH AND PROTECT YOUR VEIN LININGS. The herb bilberry (*Vaccinium myrtillus*) contains flavonoid compounds known as anthocyanosides, which are potent antioxidants that improve microcirculation and protect vein linings. Blueberries and currants do the same thing. These same substances also increase blood levels of a hormone known as prostacyclin (an eicosanoid), which prevents platelet aggregation, so blood flows more smoothly through the vessels. This herb has been successfully used to help prevent and treat varicose veins in pregnancy.[45] The usual dose is 160 mg per day for general prevention of varicose veins, and up to 480 mg per day to treat varicose veins that already exist. The flavonoid compounds in berries, particularly blueberries, blackberries, and raspberries, are very helpful for keeping veins healthy. I also highly recommend a supplement known as Cardio Miracle, which increases the production of nitric oxide from blood vessel walls and therefore aids every cell in the body (see www.cardiomiracle.com).

⁓ KEEP YOUR VEIN WALLS SLIPPERY. Research has shown that individuals with varicose veins have a decreased ability to break down fibrin in their vein walls. Fibrin is a protein in blood that is involved in clotting. When it isn't metabolized properly by an enzyme known as plasminogen activator, it coats the inside of the vein, causing it and the surrounding skin to become hard and lumpy. Normally veins have enough plasminogen activator already in their walls to keep fibrin from building up. But when they become varicose, the levels of plasminogen activator decrease.[46] So you have to import your own.

A substance known as bromelain, found in pineapple, has been shown to act in a manner similar to plasminogen activator to cause fibrin breakdown.[47] In supplement form, it can be used to improve varicose veins that already exist or, in smaller amounts, to prevent them.

The usual dose of bromelain is 125–450 mg three times per day on an empty stomach. Use the smallest amount as general prevention, and the larger amount to treat veins that are already present. Bromelain is readily available at health food stores. You can also get bromelain by eating pineapple.

⁓ MAKE SURE YOU'RE GETTING ADEQUATE AMOUNTS OF VITAMIN E. Since vitamin E deficiency has been associated with the exacerbation of varicose veins, you'll want to be sure to get enough of this vitamin every day. An adequate dosage is 100–400 IU per day, the amount I've already recommended for your daily multivitamin/ mineral combination.

When to Consider Medical Treatment—EVLT, VenaSeal, or Sclerotherapy

If your varicose veins are causing you pain of any kind that doesn't respond to the measures I've outlined (and pain includes feeling too embarrassed to wear shorts or a bathing suit), I'd recommend that you look into either of two relatively quick, simple, and effective treatments—endovenous laser therapy (EVLT) and a newer treatment called VenaSeal, both performed by interventional radiologists (specialists who use ultrasound technology to help diagnose and treat).

EVLT has a 98 percent success rate and typically requires only one procedure (although you will need an initial consultation so the specialist can evaluate your veins using ultrasound). Here's how it works: after administering a local anesthetic (usually to the ankle or knee), the doctor makes a very tiny cut and inserts a thin catheter into the damaged vein. A laser fiber is threaded through the catheter and is guided to the end of the problem vein. Additional anesthetic then numbs the whole leg and causes the blood to leave the vein. When the doctor fires the laser, it heats the inside of the vein wall, causing it to collapse and seal shut. The laser is then withdrawn back down the length of the vein to treat the entire problem area.

The doctor checks the vein with ultrasound to make sure it is completely closed, after which the catheter is removed and the leg is bandaged. The patient leaves wearing a waist-high compression stocking to be left in place for seven to ten days. The whole procedure usually takes only ninety minutes, and the patient can resume most activities right away—although lifting anything more than five pounds is discouraged for the first week or so.

The most common side effects are mild swelling and bruising or minor pain, which may worsen during the first week after treatment. Over-the-counter medications such as Motrin or Tylenol easily take care of such problems, and some patients even report that their post-op pain is less than the pain they experienced before surgery! The incision site also occasionally becomes infected, which is treated with antibiotics. Patients typically return for a follow-up exam after two weeks and again after two or three months to make sure that the vein remains closed.

Richard Baum, M.D., an interventional radiologist at Brigham and Women's Hospital in Boston, told me that of all the procedures he does, which include life-saving hemorrhage control, the patients who are the most grateful are those who have this procedure! (For more information, visit www.evlt.com. Also, if you are thinking about having this therapy, consider the Brigham and Women's Hospital Vascular and Vein Care Centers, one of the best clinics in the country; for more information, visit www.brighamandwomens.org /radiology/vascular-and-vein-care-centers.)

VenaSeal is a newer procedure (approved by the FDA in 2015) that is similar to EVLT but uses a special adhesive to close the vein instead of heat. This soft, flexible, medical-grade adhesive is placed in the vein using a small catheter (guided by ultrasound) to glue the diseased vein shut. Blood then naturally reroutes to nearby healthy veins. The procedure requires no anesthesia and involves even less pain and bruising than EVLT. Patients can usually resume normal activity immediately. No compression stockings are necessary, only an adhesive bandage to cover the spot where the catheter was inserted. A vein specialist can determine if you are a good candidate for this procedure, based on the result of your ultrasound exam. (Brigham and Women's Hospital Vascular and Vein Care Centers also do this procedure.)

On the other hand, if your problem is unsightly but painless spider veins, chances are all you need is a simple office procedure known as sclerotherapy—which has been safely used in Europe for the last fifty years and is finally catching on in the United States. After an ultrasound evaluation, the physician (typically a dermatologist) injects the veins with a solution designed to irritate the wall of the vein, causing it to swell and cut off the blood supply. No anesthesia is necessary, although several procedures may be required.

Should you decide to go through with a vein procedure, I recommend that you follow all my suggestions for maintaining healthy veins before and after your treatment. Doing so will lower your chances of having any recurrent problems.

Despite our best efforts to appear youthful, life is full of challenges that sooner or later etch themselves on our faces and bodies. Happily, at midlife most of us are far better equipped to handle this than we were at twenty, when we still believed that our lives would be perfect if we could just lose that final five to ten pounds or if our noses looked different. We can still be beautiful—especially since the crucible of perimenopause removes some of our self-consciousness. We've had enough life experience to be happy that our legs still work, even if they don't look perfect, happy that there are amusing things to laugh at, even if doing so creates crinkles around our eyes. What a relief!

Update Your Personal Style

Few things are more uplifting than a good makeover. I just love watching a woman's face light up and her demeanor brighten when she has a new, flattering hairstyle and the right wardrobe that complements her innate energy. Heck, I like the same thing for myself! Throughout the years, I've had my colors done and worked with several stylists who have helped me find the colors and styles that work best for me. But nothing—and I mean nothing—has compared with finding the work of Carol Tuttle, who developed Dressing Your Truth. Carol has discovered that each of us falls into one of four main energy types, based on our innate energy signature. I'm a type one, which is like bubbling water. We type ones look best in bright playful colors—think Lilly Pulitzer, a fashion line I used to make fun of until I discovered that these styles are often perfect for me! Type twos are like still, calm lakes, and look best in muted colors. Type threes are larger-than-life individuals whose style is in-your-face wild. Type fours look best in tailored, CEO-type outfits. When I found out that I was a type one that looked best in bright colors, at first I didn't believe it. Like so many professional women, I had spent years trying to look "professional." Hot pink and big pearls just didn't seem to fit the image I had of myself. But as soon as I began dressing my truth, something in me came alive, and I realized that I was now wearing the things I had been naturally drawn to in childhood but had rejected for being too frivolous! Dolly Parton once said, "Find out who you are, and do it on purpose." Well, finding out what your energy type is and then dressing to express it will cut your shopping time in half. You won't get caught up in style trends that simply are wrong for you. Your life will become far simpler. No matter what your size or your budget, you'll enjoy finding your style and clothing "truth." So go to Carol's website (my.liveyourtruth.com) and get started.

As with all things during perimenopause—whether it's making choices about supplements, diet, entertainment, or career—you are being asked to remember who you really are, and then live that way. How you dress and adorn yourself is a very direct expression of this. So enjoy the process.

12

Standing Tall for Life: Building Healthy Bones

During the summer before I wrote the first edition of this book, I had the privilege of seeing rock-and-roll legend Tina Turner live in concert. At an age (then sixty-plus) when the majority of women have resigned themselves to slowing down and taking it easy, Tina tore up the stage in her towering heels (an athletic feat in itself), belting out her signature high-energy music for two solid hours while outshining dancers less than half her age. Her awe-inspiring performance laid to rest any notion about the inherent limitations in physical stamina that are supposed to come with growing older. I was thrilled that my two then-teenage daughters were with me, so that they, too, could internalize this icon of female power and health. Watching Tina Turner that night, I was reminded anew that we midlife women can hone our physical strength and skills for years to come if we are willing to continue to move, to work our muscles regularly—and, of course, to unload any Ikes who are holding us back. More recently, I listened to Dan Stickler, M.D., co-founder of the Apeiron Center for Human Potential (a precision genetic nutrition and lifestyle coaching company), talk about his seventy-two-year-old mother, who can deadlift something like 200 pounds; I don't recall the exact figure, but you get the idea.

My own mother has been a perfect example. At the age of eighty-four, she fulfilled a lifelong dream of climbing to a Mount Everest base camp, at an elevation of about 17,800 feet, where the air has half the oxygen it does at sea level. Mom had completed the Appalachian Trail in her late sixties, then climbed the hundred highest peaks in New England in her seventies, all with her friend Anne, who was four years older. But two years before the Everest trek, she fell on some black ice on the steps of the log cabin where she lives, landing on her midback. She was alone at the time and couldn't move her arm. Thanks to her fitness level and bone strength, she didn't sustain a fracture in the fall (or in any of a few other falls she's taken while hiking, or in one particularly bad spill she took down a set of stairs at Christmas when her socks slipped on the polished wood floor).

Even though my mother hadn't broken any bones, she was in such pain for the next three months that she couldn't sleep lying down. It took her quite a while to fully recover. During that time, she was unable to participate in her active lifestyle of skiing and hiking—activities she had always taken for granted—and for a while there, she had to face her mortality and make peace with the fact that she might not be able to continue to do some of the things that had been such a huge part of her life. So her injury was not only physical, it was also emotional.

When she had pretty much given up on her Everest dream, she got a call from Werner Berger, a man who had climbed Everest in his seventies and was taking a group to base camp. He invited my mother. At first she said no. But then my sister Penny and her husband decided to go on the trek and support my mother. As a teenager, my sister had formed a very strong bond with our mother when Mom drove her to countless ski races (my sister made the U.S. Alpine Ski Team and the World Cup circuit at the age of sixteen). On all their drives up the New York State Thruway, my mother had talked about her Himalayan dream. In addition, she had previously been asked to help out with base camp operations for a professional mountain climber named Julie whom she had joined earlier on a skiing trip around the base of Mt. McKinley in Alaska. Julie and her husband were planning to climb K2 the following year, but Julie was killed in an avalanche soon thereafter, and my mother never got to go.

So when our mother turned down Werner's invitation, my sister was determined to change her mind. Penny decided that she would "stand" for my mother and be there for her as she met the incredible challenges of this trek. And that's exactly what happened—they made it to the base camp and back. (When I saw their slide show after they returned, I was stunned. I've never seen anything so rigorous in my life. And I was very glad that I didn't have to do it!) My mother's biggest obstacle turned out to be the willingness to accept help in the form of getting on a horse for part of the route. (Staying on the horse on that terrain was also a huge challenge. As Mom said, "Every muscle that I didn't use for climbing, I had to use to stay on the horse.")

What I found equally fascinating was that my mother returned from the climb feeling stronger than when she left. She was also more flexible and more surefooted. In other words, by meeting the challenge of the climb, she actually developed better coordination and stamina—proof positive that the body has the ability to grow and develop throughout our entire lives. My late colleague Louise Hay wrote to me when she was eighty-four and said, "This has been the best year of my life so far." Talk about a winning attitude!

Tina Turner, my mother, Louise Hay, and thousands of other older women who stand tall in their lives offer a clear alternative to the realities of inactivity and osteoporosis. You don't have to look very far to see women who are bent over or otherwise crippled by this devastating disease. Osteoporosis begins in earnest at perimenopause in susceptible women, but its effects may not appear until twenty or more years later, often when it is too late to do much about it. When it comes to bone health, prevention is absolutely essential. And that prevention needs to start as soon as possible, ideally in adolescence. But it's never too late. Perimenopause is an ideal time to shore up your bones—the part of you that is your foundation for moving forward in your life.

OSTEOPOROSIS: THE SCOPE OF THE PROBLEM

Bone loss starts silently, asymptomatically. In the early stages it is called osteopenia. As it progresses to osteoporosis, the bones become increasingly porous, brittle, and subject to fracture. The National Institutes of Health Consensus Conference defined osteoporosis as a disease of increased skeletal fragility, accompanied by low bone density (a T-score for bone mineral density below –2.5) and microarchitecture deterioration.[1] Make no mistake: this is a potentially fatal disease.

Currently, 10 million people (including 8 million women) in the United States have osteoporosis, and 44 million have osteopenia. This accounts for 55 percent of the population who are at least fifty years old. Half the women in this age group will have an osteoporosis-related fracture in their remaining lifetime, an incidence greater than that of heart attack, stroke, and breast cancer combined. Hip fractures are especially problematic, because after six months, only 15 percent of patients are able to walk across a room unaided. Even worse, 24 percent of Americans fifty and older who fracture their hip will die within a year. (Vertebral fractures are also linked to an increased risk of death.) Women who fracture a hip have a fourfold greater risk of sustaining a second such fracture.

Osteoporosis also increases the risk for wrist and vertebral crush fractures, which can result in pain, disability, and disfigurement. It is the vertebral crush fractures, in which the bone in the spine collapses, that result in the shrunken, hunched-over posture—complete with dowager's hump and pot belly—that is often seen in elderly women. If your mother or grandmother looks like this, you may be seeing your future—unless you act now.

The risk for African American women is less than it is for women of European ancestry, while the risk for Asian American women falls somewhere in between. This difference is related, in part, to the fact that women with more pigment in their skin also have a thicker collagen matrix upon which their bones are built. (Men typically have thicker, stronger bones than women, partly for genetic reasons and partly because of their higher levels of bone-building testosterone.

FIGURE 16: FEMALE VERTEBRAE

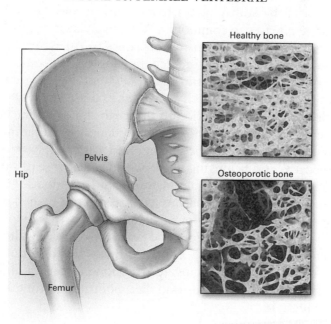

Though men, too, may get osteoporosis, it's often related to alcohol intake or steroid use and shows up at a later age than in women.) The annual costs of treating hip fractures worldwide are an estimated $34.8 billion, a figure that is expected to increase substantially over the next several decades.[2] In the United States, the medical cost of hip fractures averages $50,508 per patient.[3]

Given these discouraging statistics, it is little wonder that so many doctors are quick to prescribe drugs such as alendronate (Fosamax). Please remember, however, that statistics are derived from entire populations and may not have anything to do with you personally. In my practice I saw eighty-year-old women with the bone density measurements of an average twenty-five-year-old. I also saw twenty-five-year-olds with the bones of an average eighty-year-old. And today there are many safe and natural options available to help you either maintain the bone you have or build it to new, healthier levels.

WE'RE DESIGNED FOR LIFETIME STURDINESS

There is nothing inherent in the human condition in general, or the postmenopausal woman in particular, that causes our bones to weaken and break as we age. We were designed to live on this planet well supported by sturdy bones from youth to old age. Like other degenerative diseases so common in Western civilization, such as coronary artery disease, hypertension, and obesity, osteoporosis is either unknown or very rare among indigenous peoples living time-honored, hunter-gatherer lifestyles characterized by a strong connection with the wisdom of the earth as well as regular exercise and a whole-food diet. A deep sense of connection to the earth shores up the health of our first emotional center—the part of our emotional anatomy that is associated with a sense of belonging, and with our basic sense of safety, security, and belonging in the world. This sense of safety and belonging affects our bones, blood, and immune systems.

When an entire culture teaches us to regard our bodies as uncontrollable and unreliable, it is not surprising that so many women have lost their sense of connection and support—with resulting first-emotional-center disease such as osteoporosis. It is also not surprising that so many are beginning to lose bone at earlier and earlier ages, a side effect of a refined-food diet, poor nutrient intake, and a sedentary lifestyle.

The gravity of the earth itself (weight-bearing exercise) and sunlight are two of the keys to bone health, as we will see in this chapter.

HOW HEALTHY BONE IS MADE

If you want to keep your bones strong and healthy, you need to understand the dynamic and effortless way in which your body is designed to build and remodel bone throughout your life. The process that results in osteoporosis is actually a survival mechanism created over millions of years of evolution to help your body maintain biochemical balance. Once you begin to work with that essential body wisdom, even bones that have already weakened can regain strength.

Bone metabolism is a complex process in which construction and demolition crews work side by side. Each of our 206 bones harbors cells that continually deposit a protein framework made from collagen. Minerals from the blood then attach to this matrix and harden into bone. Those same bones also contain cells that can break down that structure. In childhood, as we grow, the bone builders keep ahead of the bone destroyers. But the balance can shift as we get older. A wide variety of conditions—including depression, deficiencies of vitamin D and bone-building minerals, a high-acid diet, and steroid use—can allow the osteoblasts, the cells that make bone, to be outpaced by the osteoclasts, the cells that break down bone. The result is weakened bones.

Osteoporosis and Osteopenia: Scurvy of the Bone

Suzanne Humphries, M.D., a conventionally trained nephrologist who has become well versed in functional and holistic medicine, points out that loss of bone is largely a nutritional deficiency, which she refers to as "scurvy of the bone."

She recommends a regimen of vitamin C, vitamin K_2, vitamin D_3 (in winter months; sun exposure in summer), boron, silica, and magnesium. Though conventional wisdom is focused on calcium and drugs such as Fosamax for treating low bone density, to prevent fractures it is far more important to make sure you're getting enough of these nutrients.

Excess calcium can land in the blood vessel walls, as well as in the muscles and valves of the heart, which becomes a setup for cardio-vascular disease. But if you are getting enough vitamin C, D_3, and K_2, your body will actually direct the calcium you ingest from food to where it belongs. It's a question of balance.

How Vitamins C, K_2, and D_3 Strengthen Bone

Vitamin C helps mineralize bone and helps osteoblasts (bone-forming cells) to grow. It also inhibits osteoclasts (the cells that degrade bone). As an important antioxidant, it prevents free-radical damage (which is mostly what the so-called aging process is all about), and it is vital to the synthesis of collagen, the substance that forms a matrix for bone minerals. But when vitamin C levels are low, osteoblasts stop forming new bone and osteoclasts begin breaking down bone too quickly—hence the phrase "scurvy of the bone."

Elderly patients who suffer from bone fractures have been shown to have significantly lower than normal levels of vitamin C in their blood.[4] And in women who supplement with vitamin C, bone mineral density is higher regardless of estrogen levels.[5]

Humans cannot make vitamin C, and when we are under stress, we need even more than we do normally. I suggest 2,000–5,000 mg per day of vitamin C as sodium ascorbate, liposomal vitamin C, ascorbic acid, or Ester-C. Ester-C is very well tolerated in those who have sensitive stomachs and is very effective.

Vitamin K_2 is also necessary for healthy bones. Do not confuse it with vitamin K_1, which is necessary for blood clotting. Vitamin K_2 has two crucial functions: cardiovascular health and bone resto-ration. K_2 helps remove calcium from the lining of the blood vessels and shuttles it into your bone matrix. In fact, having enough vita-min K_2 in your system helps vitamin D transport calcium into your bones, where it belongs. It also helps prevent hardening of the arter-ies, which happens when too much calcium gets deposited in your blood vessel walls.

Vitamin D and vitamin K_2 work together to produce and acti-vate what is called matrix Gla protein (MGP), which is a part of the collagen matrix upon which bone is built. You can't have strong bones without this key ingredient. Vitamin K_2 is found in abundance in fermented foods and also in animal foods such as eggs and dairy. It's available as a supplement as well. The recommended dosage is 180 mcg per day. Make sure the supplement you take contains vita-min K_2 as menaquinone-7 (MK-7). Vitamin K_2 may lessen the effects of warfarin, the blood-thinning drug sold as Coumadin, although it does not necessarily affect other blood thinning drugs. If you take blood thinners, check with your doctor before taking this supplement.

Bones Are Storehouses for Essential Minerals

Bones are the major storehouses for calcium, phosphorous, and magnesium, as well as other minerals, all of which are necessary for the healthy functioning of every cell in the body. Calcium, for example, regulates processes ranging from the beating of the heart and the clotting of blood to the firing of nerve cells. When blood calcium levels become low, a series of complex and interrelated biological reactions is activated.

~ The parathyroid gland (in the neck) releases parathyroid hormone (PTH).
~ PTH stimulates the kidneys to convert the body's stores of vitamin D into an active form and release calcium from the surface of the bone. It also slows down the mineralization of bone, which uses calcium.
~ Activated vitamin D acts on the intestine to increase the absorption of calcium from food, encourages the kidneys to retain calcium that would otherwise be lost in the urine, and facilitates the release of more calcium from the bone.

As soon as calcium levels in the blood are restored to an acceptable level, all these feedback mechanisms are reversed. Similarly, complex feedback loops are involved in the metabolism of the other essential minerals.[6]

It is the job of the osteoclasts to break down microscopic bits of bone, thus releasing minerals into the blood. Each day more than 300 mg of calcium is dissolved from our bones. Over a year's time 20 percent of our adult bone mass is recycled and replaced as our bones continually undergo breakdown and renewal in response to the overall needs of our bodies. If more minerals are taken out than are replaced, the end result is low bone mass.

It's worth noting that osteoporosis can sometimes be the by-product of a parathyroid tumor. These tumors, which are almost always benign, cause the parathyroid gland to produce excess PTH, leaching extra calcium from bones into the bloodstream. The best place to have the parathyroid gland examined and any tumors re-

moved is the Norman Parathyroid Center in Tampa, Florida (www
.parathyroid.com/parathyroid-surgeon.htm).

Bones Constantly Remodel Themselves
to Adapt to Physical Stress and Strain

Among the amazing properties of the basic bone cell, the osteocyte,
is its ability to act like a strain sensor, evaluating the amount of stress
placed on a bone. Though the exact mechanism by which this happens isn't entirely understood, stress on a bone sets up a tiny electrical current that attracts calcium and other minerals to the site. This
is known as a piezoelectric effect and is similar to the mechanism by
which quartz crystals operate in electronics and clocks.

What is fascinating about this process is that it takes into account
precisely where bone is needed and where it needs to be reduced. The
old song about how "the hip bone's connected to the thigh bone" is
about more than mere anatomical proximity. All our bones, like
every other cell in our bodies, are functionally connected to one another. A strain on a bone in our leg not only helps build that bone but
also helps determine the bone density in our spine and shoulders.[7]
Regular stress on bones is absolutely essential to maintain strong
bone. It's a case of use it or lose it.

One more piece of the puzzle falls into place when you know that
osteoblasts and osteoclasts, the builders and the destroyers, communicate via proteins known as osteoprotegerin (OPG) and OPG-ligand.
As one researcher explains it, "OPG-ligand is like the accelerator of
your car. If you step on OPG-ligand, you lose bone. OPG is the brake
of the system. If you step on OPG, then you have more bone. The
balance between the two determines how much bone we have."[8] Scientists are now finding that almost all the substances that stimulate
bone loss do so by slashing production of OPG, boosting creation of
OPG-ligand, or both. For example, the drug prednisone can set off
quick and dramatic bone loss. In the lab, treating osteoblasts (bone
builders) with prednisone inhibits their ability to make OPG but
heightens their OPG-ligand production. In contrast, estrogen stimulates osteoblasts to produce OPG.

Immune status and bone health are also closely connected—
which is not surprising, given that both are under the influence of
the first chakra. Osteoclasts (the bone destroyers) are derived from
the same bone marrow cells that make white blood cells. This helps

explain why individuals with such seemingly unrelated diseases as rheumatoid arthritis, lupus, diabetes, multiple sclerosis, hepatitis, depression, and lymphoma often have osteoporosis in addition to their other symptoms. Scientists have found that anything that stirs quiescent T cells, a ubiquitous part of our immune system, into action—such as chronic infections and autoimmune disorders—also triggers them to make OPG-ligand, which results in bone loss.

The function of both osteoclasts and osteoblasts is influenced by many other factors as well, including daily movement patterns; levels of estrogen, testosterone, thyroid hormone, and insulin; nutritional status; and hormones (such as norepinephrine and cortisol) produced by emotional stress.[9] There is also some evidence to suggest that OPG-ligand may stimulate osteoclasts or other substances, such as cytokines (one of the inflammatory chemicals), to degrade cartilage. This translates over time into joint destruction and arthritis. But simply moving your body regularly through the earth's gravitational field will also halt this degradation.

FIGURE 17: BONE REMODELING

Bone demineralizing	Bone building
Osteoclast (decreases bone density)	Osteoblast (increases bone density)
Stimulated by:	Stimulated by:
Immune system disorders	Progesterone
Depression	Estrogen
Inactivity	Testosterone
Nutrient-poor, acid-rich diet	Vitamin D and nutrient-rich diet
Steroid drugs	Isoflavones
Depleted hormones	SERMs
	Exercise

Osteoblast

Osteoclast

New bone

Old bone

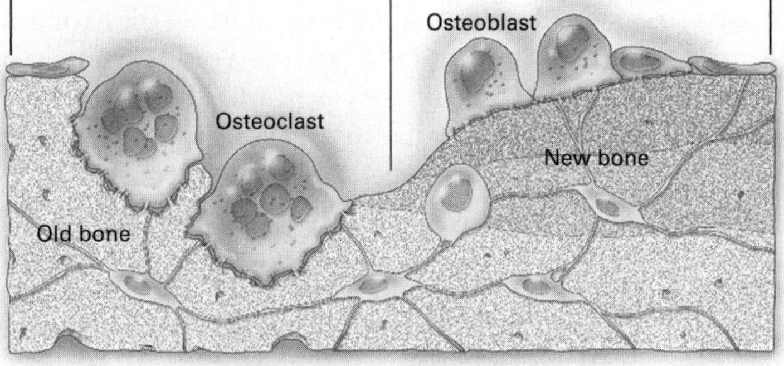

The Ups and Downs of Bone over the Life Cycle

We begin developing our skeleton in utero, and it rapidly increases in size throughout childhood, adolescence, and young adulthood. It reaches its maximum size and density (known as peak bone mass) somewhere between the ages of twenty-five and thirty. Over her lifetime a woman may lose 38 percent of her peak bone mass, while a man may lose only 23 percent of his.[10] But some individuals are resistant to bone loss.[11] One study, for example, showed that 38 percent of men and 2 percent of women age fifty-five to sixty-four lost almost no bone over a period of eleven years.[12] Nevertheless, many women begin to lose bone in their late thirties, long before estrogen levels begin to fall. This loss tends to accelerate perimenopausally. The average Caucasian woman loses 2–4 percent of her bone mass per year in the first five years after menopause. After that, loss slows down markedly or disappears.[13] In men, accelerated bone loss is more apt to begin in the late sixties.

It's important to remember that healthy women can lose some bone during menopause and not be at risk for fracture if their bone quality is good. Thousands of people walk around daily with very low bone density—yet only a small percentage of them experience fractures. It has been shown, for example, that in Japan hip bone density is markedly lower than it is in the United States, but the incidence of hip fractures is two and a half times less than it is here. And the Japanese consume less calcium than we do.[14]

What is the difference between bones that fracture and those that don't? The difference concerns two factors: basic bone architecture and the repair capability of bone. It appears that even those with low bone density still have enough bone mass to withstand the stresses and strains of daily life. Research has shown, for example, that a vertebra that has lost 50 percent of its bone mass is still strong enough to withstand five times the strain load that it would normally be subjected to. If the bone were otherwise normal, in other words, it shouldn't fracture. This means that many women who are diagnosed with low bone density will never go on to get fractures.

Still, we all know that bone fractures do occur in women with osteoporosis, even at very low strain levels—in fact, it has been documented that some women spontaneously fracture their hips and then fall as a result, not the other way around. So osteoporotic fractures must involve more than decreased bone mineral density. There must be something else wrong with the *quality* of the bone and its self-repair process.[15] Poor bone quality results from factors such as nutritional deficiencies, lack of exercise, too little vitamin D, and too much insulin.[16]

The Anatomy of Bone

Bone comes in two types: trabecular and cortical bone. Cortical bone is the tough, protective outer layer of bone. It is more calcified than inner trabecular bone, which is spongy and includes the marrow, where blood cells are made. About 80 percent of all bone in our bodies is cortical and 20 percent is trabecular. The arms and legs are mostly cortical bone; hips are a half-and-half mixture; the spine, ribs, jaw, and lower two-thirds of the wrist are mainly trabecular bone. Because trabecular bone is more loosely packed and porous and has more surface area than cortical bone, it is more susceptible to bone loss, which is one reason why fractures from osteoporosis tend to occur earlier in the spine and wrist, while hip fractures occur later.

Bones have to be strong enough to withstand hundreds of pounds of pressure, but flexible enough to withstand twisting and turning without breaking. This flexibility is provided by the living protein collagen, which makes up about 23 percent of all bone. (This is the same substance that gives skin its elasticity and thickness. Thin skin is also associated with thin bones.) The minerals attached to the collagen matrix are arranged in a crystalline structure that gives bone its rigidity and strength.

We were designed to maintain strong, heavy bones throughout our lives, as do all animals. If we have reached peak bone mass in our twenties, then we can stand a certain amount of bone loss as we age without being at risk for fractures. But because of the vagaries of our modern lifestyle, including lack of exercise or overexercise, smoking, poor diet, lack of vitamin D, or anorexia and bulimia, many women never reach their peak bone mass by age thirty—and it appears that the matrix of the bone that *is* present may not be normal. So many women begin perimenopause with a deficit in their bone banks.

Medical anthropologist Susan Brown, Ph.D., director of the Osteoporosis Education Project, founder of the Better Bones website (www.betterbones.com), and author of the groundbreaking book *Better Bones, Better Body: Beyond Estrogen and Calcium* (Keats Publishing, 2000), points out that the bones of people who are living in Westernized countries are growing ever weaker, and that we now face a virtual epidemic of poor bone health.[17] Research shows that women living several centuries ago had stronger bones than modern women and that Near Eastern populations of some 12,000 years ago had a bone mass that was nearly 20 percent higher than it is today.[18] (And they didn't consume lots of cow's milk!)

Strength isn't the whole story with bone health—body alignment, flexibility, and daily movement patterns play an important role, too. Every time we walk or move, we place what are called "vertical vectors of force" on our bones. As discussed earlier, these forces create a mini-electrical current throughout our bones, but this piezoelectric effect also involves the fascia, connective tissue that encases all your muscles, nerves, and organs—almost as if they were wearing a tight sweater. The tiniest movement in one area of the body is both mechanically and electrically transmitted throughout the entire body instantaneously. If our bones, ligaments, tendons, fascia, and muscles are all properly aligned, then our movement is graceful and pain free and our bones and supporting structures remain healthy.

However, if our posture is poor (for example, if we're hunched over and never fully expand our rib cage), then our shoulders become tight, and we are more at risk for shoulder, neck, and back problems. The same is true for our hips. In fact, the shoulder girdle and hip girdle mirror each other—tight hips, tight shoulders. I am convinced that if women focused on moving with proper alignment, there would be far fewer hip replacements after the age of sixty! For more information about posture and alignment and how to maximize the "primal" posture that we are all born with, I highly recommend the incredible work of Esther Gokhale.

Gokhale studied many people from different indigenous cultures around the world and found that those who do a lot of bending, lifting, and walking (sometimes with as much as eighty pounds on their heads) don't have the same problems with back pain that we in industrialized countries have. The reason, Gokhale discovered, is that their alignment and pelvic position are more natural and don't put undue pressure on their joints and backs. They naturally adopt the posture of "keeping the behind behind" that I described in chapter 8, which means they keep their backs straight except for a curve called the J-spine. The J-spine is located at the segment of the spine between the fifth lumbar vertebra (the lowest vertebra in the low back) and the first sacral vertebra (the highest of the vertebrae in the sacrum, the triangular bone at the base of the spine just above the tailbone). In this more natural posture, the tailbone sticks out a bit, like a duck with its tail out behind it, not like a dog tucking its tail between its legs.

Gokhale used these observations to develop a system of foundational posture training that helps people heal their pain and avoid surgery. I highly recommend reading the book she co-authored with Susan Adams, *8 Steps to a Pain-Free Back* (Pendo Press, 2008), or taking a Primal Posture workshop with one of the many teachers Gokhale has certified throughout the world (see gokhalemethod.com).

I know that I personally would have a chronic right hip problem—and probably an eventual hip replacement—if it hadn't been for Pilates. I started doing Pilates more than twenty years ago because I wanted an exercise program I could do on the road and in a hotel room. Back then I didn't realize how transformational this practice is. Now not only am I taller than I was back then, I am also far more flexible. Most important, my posture and alignment have improved immensely.

Sitting Kills, Moving Heals

It's well documented that the weightlessness experienced by astronauts results in significant bone loss, as does prolonged bed rest. Joan Vernikos, Ph.D., spent seven years as the head of the NASA Life Sciences program that monitored the astronauts in space. She was also charged with overseeing the voyage of the late senator John Glenn when he went into space at the age of seventy-seven. At that time, Glenn was head of the Senate's Special Committee on Aging. He not only trained as hard as the other astronauts but returned from space in good physical condition—better, in fact, then some of the much younger men on that same mission. Still, Vernikos discovered that all astronauts who were exposed to prolonged weightlessness suffered from bone loss. She therefore came to the realization that weightlessness was, in fact, a model for what happens to so many as they grow older—they sit too much! Sitting, she discovered, does the same thing to our bodies as weightlessness. We need to move against gravity if we are to stay healthy. Her book *Sitting Kills, Moving Heals* (Quill Driver, 2011) documents her findings and offers a program for reversing the effects of weightlessness on our bodies and bones. She provides ongoing information on her website, Third Age Health, and in her free e-newsletter (see www.joanvernikos.com). Vernikos authored several studies with William Evans, Ph.D., known for his groundbreaking research at Tufts University's USDA Human Nutrition Research Center on Aging that showed that loss of both muscle mass and strength are the biggest physiological factors associated with aging. Evans's research famously extended to the elderly, show-ing that weight training in nursing home residents who were age ninety and up resulted in far more independence and function.[19] The bottom line is this: we are designed for a lifetime of mobility, but we have to keep moving.

ARE YOU AT RISK FOR OSTEOPOROSIS?

To determine your personal risk for thinning, poor-quality bones, review the following list. If none of the risk factors applies to you, chances are good that your bones are just fine. You can simply con-tinue the healthy lifestyle you are following. If, on the other hand, you can identify with several of them, you need to take steps right now to ensure that you'll be able to literally take steps in the future! Note that some of the risk factors for osteoporosis overlap those for heart disease.[20] As you get a handle on your bone health, you'll also be helping your heart.

- Your mother has been diagnosed with osteoporosis or has had a hip or other osteoporotic fracture. Osteoporosis tends to run in families, but there's still a lot you can do to prevent it.

- You are fair-skinned and blue-eyed. Because of genetic factors, blue-eyed blondes and those with red hair have less collagen in both their bones and skin than do those with brown, black, or yellow skin tones. This gives them less bony matrix on which to lay down minerals. Black women have the least risk for osteoporo-sis because they tend to have thicker bones and more robust colla-gen stores than Caucasian women.

- You are quite thin or tall, or have a slight build and/or less than 18 percent body fat. Tall women, especially those with small bones, may be at risk for purely mathematical reasons: they enter meno-pause with less bone to lose. In addition, body fat is where much of a woman's natural estrogen during and after perimenopause is manufactured. The less fat she has, the less estrogen her body will produce to support her bones.

- You smoke. Chemicals in cigarette smoke poison the ovaries and decrease your hormone levels prematurely. Estrogen, testosterone, and progesterone all have bone-protective effects.

- You spend most of your time indoors. Women who are exposed to very little natural sunlight may be deficient in the natural vitamin D normally produced in sun-drenched skin. Vitamin D is necessary for healthy bone mineralization. Increasingly, we're finding that women who get osteoporotic fractures are the ones with serum vitamin D levels of 20 ng/ml or lower. The link between sunlight and bone health is so important that I've devoted an entire section to it later in this chapter.

~ You are sedentary and spend fewer than four hours per day on your feet. Bones stay healthy only when they have vertical vectors of force placed on them regularly. A sedentary lifestyle provides insufficient weight-bearing exercise to stimulate bone growth. Many studies have shown that bed rest is associated with osteoporosis. In contrast, weight training has been shown to build bone density even in postmenopausal women who aren't on estrogen.

~ You are (or were) a "fitness fanatic," that is, you become irritable and unreasonable if you are unable to get in your daily run or other exercise. The lifestyle of the fitness fanatic includes dieting for weight loss and/or engaging regularly in strenuous exercise such as marathon training. Dietary restrictions and the chronic stress of overtraining can impair mineral intake and absorption. It also messes up what is known as the hypothalamic-pituitary-ovarian-adrenal axis—the exquisite feedback loop between the brain, the body, and our hormone levels. Chronic overexercise without adequate caloric or mineral intake results in stress fractures in ballet dancers, gymnasts, soccer players, and competitive runners, among others. Such fractures are currently on the rise in young athletes and can set the stage for later osteoporosis.

~ You have a history of amenorrhea (no periods) associated with excessive exercise and/or anorexia nervosa.[21] Amenorrhea results in a derangement of the hypothalamic-pituitary-ovarian-adrenal axis similar to that seen in depression. The end result is lower estrogen, androgen, and progesterone, and an eicosanoid profile that favors osteoporosis and other diseases.[22]

~ You drink more than 25 g of alcohol per day. (The following servings each contain about 10 g of alcohol: 12 oz. of beer, 4 oz. of wine, and 1.5 oz. of 80-proof beverage.)[23] Alcohol interferes with the function of both osteoblasts and osteoclasts, thus inhibiting your body's ability to lay down new bone and to remodel old bone.[24]

~ Your liver is overstressed. The liver's ability to produce and metabolize estrogen is essential for the growth and maintenance of strong bones at any age. Drinking more than two alcoholic drinks per day, taking medication known to be hard on the liver (such as certain cholesterol-lowering drugs), and infection with viral hepatitis are among the significant liver stressors that can harm bone health.

~ You drink more than two units of caffeine per day (8 oz. of coffee = 1 unit; 12 oz. of cola = 0.4 units). Caffeine results in increased urinary excretion of calcium; the more you consume, the more minerals you lose. If your mineral intake is relatively low to begin with, regular caffeine consumption could result in significant loss of bone over time. If, on the other hand, your calcium and mineral intake is high, a couple of cups of coffee a day probably won't matter much. *Note:* Even though tea contains caffeine, both green and black tea have been shown to build bone mass—probably because of their phytoestrogen content.

~ You are or have been clinically depressed for a significant period of time. Numerous studies have shown that depression is an independent risk factor for osteoporosis. Depressed people have high levels of the immune system chemical known as IL-6, which overstimulates the osteoclasts (cells responsible for breaking down bone). Depression is also associated with abnormalities in the hypothalamic-pituitary-ovarian-adrenal axis and with elevated cortisol secretion, which predispose one to bone loss.[25]

~ Your diet is poor (little fresh food, few leafy green vegetables, no fermented foods, and lots of processed and packaged food) and you don't take good supplements. Such a diet doesn't provide minerals and other nutrients necessary to support the growth and maintenance of a solid bone foundation.[26]

~ You went through premature menopause (before age forty), have had your ovaries removed surgically, went through menopause as a result of radiation or chemotherapy, and/or have prematurely gray hair. A woman who enters menopause prematurely for any reason is at increased risk for osteoporosis unless she gets adequate hormone therapy during the years when her body would normally have been producing higher levels of hormones. Nonsurgical premature menopause, and the premature graying of the hair that often accompanies it, are the result of an autoimmune reaction affecting the ovaries and hair follicles. The cause of these reactions isn't clear.

~ You take steroid drugs regularly for conditions such as asthma or lupus. Steroid drugs result in accelerated breakdown of tissue in the body—including the collagen matrix for both skin and bone.[27]

Steroids also diminish the sensitivity of the bowel to vitamin D, which in turn reduces calcium absorption.[28] Prolonged steroid use may also significantly decrease estrogen and androgen levels.[29]

~ You've taken high doses or been on a long-term regimen of any of the prescription or over-the-counter drugs known as proton pump inhibitors (PPIs), including esomeprazole (Nexium), omeprazole (Prilosec, Zegerid), lansoprazole (Prevacid), rabeprazole (Aciphex), dexlansoprazole (Dexilant, Kapidex), or pantoprazole (Protonix). These popular drugs, which block the production of stomach acid, are commonly used to treat gastroesophageal reflux disease (GERD), stomach and small intestine ulcers, and inflammation of the esophagus. Recent evidence shows that they may increase risk for hip, wrist, and spine fractures. This makes sense because having some acid in the stomach is absolutely crucial for absorbing bone-building nutrients such as calcium. So when you block the acid with drugs, digestion is also impaired.

~ You regularly use anticonvulsant medication or benzodiazepines such as diazepam (Valium), chlordiazepoxide (Librium), or lorazepam (Ativan).[30] These drugs have been found to interfere with bone metabolism.

~ You've had at least two consecutive bone density tests at least six months apart, done on the same machine, that reported scores more than 2.5 standard deviations below normal for your age.

~ You've begun to lose height. Be sure to have your doctor or other healthcare practitioner measure your height regularly. A study done in Paris on women age sixty and older showed that most of the women did not correctly estimate their current height. Knowing if you've lost height, and if so, how much, is vitally important information, the researchers found, because women losing 4 cm or more have a significantly higher risk for vertebral fracture.[31]

~ You have a thyroid disorder. Women who suffer from hyperthyroidism are at risk because the excess thyroid hormone (thyroxine) that their bodies make stimulates the osteoclasts to break down bone. Those with hypothyroidism may also be at risk if their dose of thyroid medication is too high. If you have thyroid disease, make sure you are on the lowest dose of thyroid replacement possible for your situation, and follow a sound program for maintaining bone health.[32]

Whether or not you are at high risk for osteoporosis, understand that, like the rest of your body, bone is a living work in progress.

That means that there is always something you can do—ranging from drugs to dietary change—to help yourself build bone.

For anyone who is at risk for osteoporosis or low bone density—especially those with fair skin and small bones—I highly recommend *Dr. Lani's No-Nonsense Bone Health Guide* (Turner House, 2014), by Lani Simpson, D.C., as well as her consultation services (see www .lanisimpson.com). Dr. Simpson's work on osteoporosis, including both how to treat it and how to prevent it, is by far the most thorough and accurate approach I have ever found.

MEASURING BONE DENSITY

Women with no risk factors for osteoporosis do *not* need bone density screening. Those who do should get a baseline bone density screening either before or during perimenopause. Though bone density screenings cannot measure the quality of bone, they can measure quantity. And low bone mineral density is statistically associated with an increased fracture risk. Although fractures aren't likely to show up until a woman is in her seventies and eighties, now is the best time to do something about any potential problems. Unfortunately, many insurance plans won't pay for bone density screening unless you've already had documented osteoporotic fractures. This is typical of the Western crisis approach to medicine, which too often neglects prevention. However, I urge you to make this investment in your health.

DEXA Testing

Dual-energy bone densitometry (DEXA) is the current gold standard. It uses a very low dose of X-rays to measure bone density both in the spine and in the hips. A woman's bone density is then charted on a graph to see how it stacks up against normal bone densities for a given age. The World Health Organization (WHO) rates bone density according to a standard curve on which 0 equals the norm. Severity of bone loss is then determined by how far a given measurement falls below that mean.

DEXA is a static test—a snapshot in time. One reading won't tell you whether your bone density is increasing, decreasing, or remaining the same. You need at least two successive tests done at least six months apart on the same machine to determine what the trend is and whether or not you need to make adjustments in your bone health routine. For example, small-boned women may register on the low end of a DEXA test even if their bones are not at risk. Note that a DEXA scan will give you two different types of scores: a T-score and a Z-score. Most doctors pay more attention to the T-score, which compares the subject's bone density to that of a healthy thirty-year-old of the same sex (more or less an apples-to-oranges comparison for midlife women). The Z-score, on the other hand, compares the subject's bone density to that of others of the same age and sex as the person being tested—more of an apples-to-apples comparison. No matter what your score, keep in mind that DEXA scores can't always accurately predict who will suffer a fracture (or who won't) since, as mentioned earlier, bone density is only part of the equation. A Scandinavian study published in the *Journal of Internal Medicine* not only stressed this point but also noted that the majority of fractures in older adults are the result of falls, not low bone density, and that most older people who sustain fractures don't have osteoporosis.[33]

DEXA testing is available at all major medical centers and in many doctors' offices. It requires a doctor's prescription. Because readings vary from machine to machine, try to have your consecutive measurements taken on the same machine. Far too many women have had follow-up testing on a different machine calibrated differently and have been told that their bone density is falling when, in fact, this isn't the case.

BONE DENSITY CLASSIFICATION FOR T-SCORES

NORMAL	−1.0 or above
OSTEOPENIA	−1.0 to −2.5
OSTEOPOROSIS	Less than −2.5

Source: World Health Organization, Assessment of Fracture Risk and Its Applications to Screening for Postmenopausal Osteoporosis, *Technical Report, Series 843 (Geneva: WHO, 1994).*

Skin Thickness Testing

A number of studies have shown that ultrasound measurement of skin thickness (which is dependent upon healthy collagen) predicts

fracture risk as accurately as conventional bone density testing.[34] The
accuracy increases when both skin thickness and bone density are
combined. Skin thickness testing has not caught on widely in the
United States, and it's still the subject of ongoing research. But it's
worth asking your doctor about it; you may be near one of the medical centers that performs it.

Urine Test for Bone Breakdown Products

As bone breaks down, it releases minute collagen fragments into the
urine that can be measured. Because a certain amount of bone breakdown is normal, everyone's urine contains some collagen fragments.
But when the breakdown products in the urine skyrocket, you may
well be losing bone faster than is healthy.[35] Several different types of
urine tests, such as Pyrilinks-D, CTX, and Osteomark, are available.
Unlike the static measurement of the scans, these tests can give you a
day-by-day reading of the metabolic state of your bones long before
a bone density test will register a problem. They also give you a way
to monitor your progress once treatment is initiated. Test kits are
available without a prescription, and results can be mailed directly to
your home. (See Resources.)

The Bottom Line

Bone density screening and urine testing are a marriage made in
heaven. If you are at risk, a simple bone density assessment will give
you a baseline. Normally you have to wait six months to a year to
know if you are gaining bone, losing bone, or staying the same. But
sometimes the subsequent tests continue to read on the low side, even
though you have stemmed the bone loss or begun building new
bone.[36] That's where the urine test comes in. It can tell you immediately whether or not you are losing bone, and if you are, you can repeat it every month or so to make sure that the bone-building program
you're on is working. Your test will show you when you are no longer peeing out your bones! Once your tests indicate that your bones
are stable, I suggest that you retest your urine for bone loss every year
or two.

   These tests can let midlife women know how they're doing in
time to prevent further bone loss and even increase bone density

years before osteoporosis becomes evident. They allow you to create health daily, not wait until symptoms start!

HELGA: Exercise Daily, Bone Loss Daily

Helga first consulted me when she was fifty-seven, five years after her periods had stopped. Active and healthy, she rode horses nearly every day, spent long periods of time outside, and did much of the heavy stable work herself. She had never smoked, and drank only an occasional glass of wine. She wanted to avoid estrogen and wasn't really having any symptoms that bothered her. She simply wanted to be sure that her overall health was good and that her bones were in good shape.

Helga was blond, blue-eyed, and fair-skinned and had always been trim and small-boned, weighing only 105 pounds at her 5'4" height. When her initial bone density test showed that her bones were a bit more than two standard deviations below the mean, I wasn't too concerned, given that her slight build, not significant bone loss, was apt to be the reason for this low reading. I put her on a good supplement regimen (see below) and suggested that we repeat her screening test in six months. When that result came back, it was a bit lower than the first time but not significantly so. To be on the safe side, however, I suggested a Pyrilinks urine test. I was very surprised when this test showed that she was losing bone rather quickly.

Given her reluctance to take estrogen or other bone-building medications, I suggested a whole-soy product that delivers 180 mg of soy isoflavones per day, a dose that has definitely been shown to help preserve and build bone density. I also recommended 30 mg of natural progesterone per day in the form of a skin cream.

I wondered if Helga's ongoing bone loss in the face of a healthy lifestyle could be related to depression or some other loss. Helga had immigrated to this country from Sweden when she was thirty years old and married an American with whom she had three children. She and her family had always enjoyed regular visits to Sweden to visit her mother. But her mother had recently died, leaving Helga without any remaining family in Sweden. Her youngest child had also recently left home. I told Helga that our bone health is often at risk during times when the very foundations of our lives undergo dramatic and irrevocable change. Though emotionally stoic by nature, Helga acknowledged that she had been feeling a great deal of grief in the past year.

Though we can never replace our families or go back to "the way it was," it is possible for all of us to re-create sustaining relationships in our lives. So in addition to adding the soy estrogens and progesterone cream to her regular exercise and supplement program, I suggested to Helga that she seek out some new social ties with other friends of Swedish descent in order to reconnect with her heritage. Within two months, her Pyrilinks tests returned to normal and she stopped losing bone.

LOUISE: Never Too Late

Louise was eighty-six when her son first brought her in for a consultation for osteoporosis. A very slight white woman who weighed no more than 100 pounds, Louise had broken her hip the year before and had twice dislocated the hip replacement that had been inserted. She had been told that she had very severe osteoporosis and her doctors weren't sure there was much they could do for her. One even suggested putting her in a body cast for six months, which alarmed her (and rightly so—immobilization always causes further deterioration of bone).

Louise was mentally very sharp and, up until the hip fracture, had maintained a very active social life, managed a large stock portfolio, lived alone, and took care of herself. She told me the following: "Back in the early 1990s, I was part of the Women's Health Initiative study to determine whether or not calcium was necessary for building bone. I recently found out that during all those years I was on placebo, not calcium or vitamin D. I am furious." Indeed, Louise is the kind of at-risk woman who really needed minerals, an exercise program, and vitamin D_3. She was afraid it was now too late. I told her that nothing could be further from the truth. I put her on a good supplementation program (see chapter 7), as well as 1,200 mg calcium, 2,000 IU of vitamin D_3, and 600 mg of magnesium. I also helped Louise find an orthopedic surgeon who would repair her hip properly and not relegate her to life in a wheelchair just because of her age. Louise had the correct surgical procedure and recovered beautifully. Refusing pain medication, she entered a vigorous physical therapy program. Two months after her surgery, a doctor friend came up to her at church and said, "Louise, you might as well give that walker to me because I need it more than you." The fact is, Louise had been walking around actually carrying her walker in front of her instead of using it. She is now building bone, growing healthy fingernails for the first time in years, and back to her former full social life—as well as driving!

Hormones That Help Build Bone

Supplementing with estrogen (which is far more common than supplementing with DHEA or testosterone) has been shown to help prevent bone loss. But there are so many other approaches that I would not recommend hormone replacement solely for bone preservation. If, however, you are on HT for other reasons, it's helping protect your bones as long as you're on it. In fact, the first FDA-approved indication for estrogen replacement was the prevention of osteoporosis. Some studies have demonstrated a nearly 50 percent decrease in risk of fractures with conventional HT.[37] The 2002 WHI study corroborated this data. But that doesn't mean women need estrogen therapy to maintain healthy bone mass. Those women whose bodies continue to make even a small amount of estradiol or testosterone naturally have been found to have a significantly decreased risk of osteoporosis compared to those whose bodies are no longer able to make these hormones.[38]

Keep in mind, however, that bone mass is affected by far more than just hormones. For example, it has been demonstrated that one-half of the total vertebral bone loss that a woman in the United States will experience during her lifetime occurs before she goes through menopause.[39] I'm certain that a lot of this is related to diet, stress, and activity levels. In addition, some studies have failed to find any significant differences between the spine and hip bone densities between pre- and perimenopausal women and their postmenopausal counterparts. For example, research at the USDA Human Nutrition Research Center on Aging failed to show any accelerated rate of bone loss in the hip or wrist among women close to menopause. Nor did they find any significant change in bone mineral density in the group of women as a whole, a finding that has been duplicated in a Swedish study.[40] Some authorities even hypothesize that only 10–15 percent of a woman's skeletal mass is affected by estrogen.[41] And some women on estrogen therapy still lose bone mass over time.[42] While it is clear that hormones play an important role in bone health, they are just one factor. If you do take estrogen, for example, I recommend taking the lowest dose possible, since bone protection has been demonstrated even at very low doses.

You need a bone-building program if you've had any of the following conditions associated with decreased hormone levels:

~ History of amenorrhea lasting a year or more

~ Premature, surgical, or medical menopause

~ History of steroid use

~ Strong family history of osteoporosis (mother or grandmother with obvious osteoporosis)

~ A diagnosis of osteopenia or osteoporosis

Remember, hormone therapy or bone-building drugs help preserve bone density only as long as you take them. Once you stop, you begin losing bone. The same is true for the effect of exercise on bone.

An alternative to estrogen or androgen is natural progesterone, either as a 2 percent transdermal cream (like Emerita), as a prescription pill (Prometrium), or from a formulary pharmacy. Synthetic progestin (medroxyprogesterone, or MPA) has been shown to stimulate osteoblasts (bone-building cells), and natural progesterone may have the same positive effect on bone density.[43] Double-blind, randomized, placebo-controlled studies show that low-dose MPA with estrogen prevents hip and other fractures.[44] Further controlled studies show low-dose MPA with lower-than-normal doses of estrogen significantly increase spinal bone density.[45]

Endocrinologist Jerilynn Prior, M.D., founder and scientific director of the Centre for Menstrual Cycle and Ovulation Research (CeMCOR) in Vancouver, British Columbia, believes progesterone therapy is just as effective as the bisphosphonates, the strongest bone medicines available. (See "What About Bone-Building Drugs?" later in this chapter.) Dr. Prior recommends dosages of either 10 mg per day of synthetic progestin or 300 mg a day of natural progesterone (taken at bedtime because it promotes sleepiness)—enough to get blood levels up at least 18 or ideally 45 nmol/l.[46]

There is also some solid data that phytoestrogens help with bone density. Studies show *Pueraria mirifica* activates the beta estrogen receptors in bones, making them more flexible, stronger, and resistant to fractures.[47] It seems to have an effect similar to that of estrogen, but without the adverse side effects on breast tissue. The earlier you begin taking this herb, the more bone you will maintain and so the healthier your bone mass will be.[48] A treatment of at least four years is suggested for optimal results.

Calcium: An Overrated Mineral

Doctors have long recommended high-calcium diets and calcium supplements for bone health, based on studies demonstrating that such supplementation helps build bone mass and prevent fractures.[49] However, that connection isn't so clear after all. For example, a 2003 study of more than 72,000 women followed by Harvard researchers for eighteen years showed that a high-calcium diet did *not* reduce fracture risk.[50] And a 2007 meta-analysis also done by Harvard researchers following a total of 170,991 women found total calcium intake was *not* related to risk for hip fracture.[51] Some experts don't find this all that surprising, considering that fracture rates in Africa and Asia are generally 50 to 70 percent lower than they are in the United States, despite the fact that typical African and Asian diets generally include little or no dairy and women in these areas don't usually take calcium supplements. In fact, the highest fracture rates belong to the most industrially advanced countries, where consumption of dairy products is the highest.

In their book *Building Bone Vitality: A Revolutionary Diet Plan to Prevent Bone Loss and Reverse Osteoporosis* (McGraw-Hill, 2009), Amy Lanou, Ph.D., an assistant professor of health and wellness at the University of North Carolina–Asheville, and medical writer Michael Castleman reviewed 1,200 studies on the dietary risk factors for osteoporosis. Of the 1,200 studies, they further analyzed 136 that specifically looked at dietary calcium's effect on osteoporotic fracture risk. Two-thirds of these showed that a high calcium intake does *not* reduce the number of fractures—even in those who took calcium (with vitamin D) during childhood. On the other hand, 85 percent of the studies that looked at the effects on bone density of eating fruits and vegetables showed a positive correlation.

Clearly, calcium is important, but it's not all we need to be concerned about when it comes to bone health. As Castleman explains in a 2009 article in *Natural Solutions,* "Think of calcium as the bricks in a brick wall of bones. Bricks are essential, for sure, but without enough mortar—which comes in the form of about 16 other nutrients—the wall can't hold itself up."[52]

Lanou and Castleman found that the key to preventing osteoporosis is more complicated than just making sure you eat one type of food or take a particular supplement. It actually has to do with the effect of your diet on the acidity of your blood—and for bone health, you want to eat a relatively low-acid diet to maintain a slightly alkaline pH level in your blood. Eating animal protein (including meat, poultry, fish, milk, and dairy), grains, and high-glycemic-index foods (refined carbs) makes blood slightly more acidic. The body tries to neutralize the blood's extra acid content by leaching some of the calcium compounds stored in bone (which are alkaline). Consuming three servings of fruits and vegetables (which make blood more alkaline despite the fact that some of them, such as citrus fruits, taste acidic) neutralizes the acid you'd eat in just one serving of animal protein (roughly the size of a deck of cards), and two servings neutralize the acid you'd eat in one helping of grains. (You might think that eating dairy wouldn't hurt your calcium balance since you'd be adding *and* leaching calcium at the same time, but the calcium in animal food sources such as dairy is actually highly acidic, so it still leaches more than it adds.)

The best rule of thumb is to eat at least five servings of fruits and vegetables for every serving of red meat, chicken, or fish that you eat. I also recommend that one day a week you eat no meat or dairy (essentially a vegan diet), getting your protein instead from beans, tofu, and other plant-based sources. The fact is that for the vast majority of time that humans have been on this planet—over 200,000 years—our main source of food has been nuts, seeds, and fruits foraged in season, plus animal protein. Agriculture, and the grain- and dairy-rich diets that it made possible, has existed for a mere 10,000 years. And recent research into Paleolithic nutrition has found that hunter-gatherer societies—even those in existence today—are healthier on all levels than those whose food sources are primarily grain-based. Plus, they don't have osteoporosis.[53]

According to Robert Thompson, M.D., co-author with Kathleen Barnes of *The Calcium Lie II* (Take Charge Books, 2013), when we supplement with too much calcium, it creates a dangerous imbalance. He points out that calcium is only one of at least twelve minerals in bone tissue, and our intake of all such minerals needs to stay in balance. In his book, he quotes studies showing that taking just calcium supplements alone, without other mineral supplements, can increase arterial plaque (raising risk for heart attack), brain cell dysfunction (potentially leading to dementia), the risk of gallstones and kidney problems, and more. It can also cause bone spurs and unhealthy calcium deposits in non-bone tissue. Furthermore, he says excess calcium can be a factor in obesity, type 2 diabetes, hypothyroidism, gastroesophageal reflux disease, and, ironically, osteoporosis.

Magnesium deficiency is as much a problem in bone health as

inadequate calcium, and because calcium and magnesium work in critical balance, they should be supplemented together. (Among other benefits, magnesium stimulates calcitonin, a bone-preserving hormone that draws calcium out of the blood and soft tissues and back into bones.[54] Magnesium is also critical to assisting vitamin D in its role in protecting bone.)[55] In fact, too much unbalanced calcium can actually decrease the body's ability to absorb magnesium from food. Dietary surveys have shown that 80–85 percent of American women consume less than the RDA for magnesium already. High, unbalanced calcium intake can also block the uptake of manganese, decrease iron absorption, interfere with vitamin K synthesis, and increase fecal phosphorous excretion. Finally, very high doses of calcium carbonate (4–5 g per day), which is the type of calcium in antacids, can cause a serious, kidney-damaging disorder known as milk alkali syndrome.[56]

If you take a calcium supplement, make sure you take magnesium along with it. A 1:1 ratio of calcium to magnesium is ideal, but 2:1 is also acceptable. I recommend ReMag as an excellent magnesium supplement because it is well absorbed; the recommended dose is 600 to 900 mg a day, although you will need more if you take a different brand. (See Resources.) Green leafy vegetables, such as spinach, kale, broccoli, and collard greens, are good dietary sources of calcium.

WHAT ABOUT BONE-BUILDING DRUGS?

Far too many doctors prescribe bone-building drugs as the first line of treatment for women who show any sign of decreased bone mass— even those who are very far from having actual osteoporosis or significant osteopenia. However, there are many safe and effective alternatives that work more naturally with the wisdom of the body.

Here's a brief rundown of the most commonly available bone-building prescription drugs. Like hormone therapy, these work only as long as a woman is on them.

BISPHOSPHONATES: The bisphosphonates are the most widely prescribed antiresorptive agents and are currently considered the first-line treatment for most women with postmenopausal osteoporosis. These drugs interfere with osteoclast function, thus preventing bone breakdown and turnover. That may seem beneficial, but the truth is that this can actually make the bone more brittle, because without the breakdown part of the equation, the bone gets too thick for blood vessels to be able to nourish it. Animal studies show that these drugs also interfere with the normal repair of microdamage to bone, which eventually weakens the very thing the drug was meant to strengthen.

Research on humans confirms that there is indeed reason for caution. For example, in a 2005 study on the bisphosphonate alendronate (Fosamax) done at the University of Texas Southwestern Medical Center, all the patients in the study were found to have severe depression of bone formation.[57] In some cases (up to 50 of every 100,000 patients), spontaneous nontraumatic spinal or atypical femur fractures have been reported.[58] In the fall of 2010, the FDA required all bisphosphonates used to treat osteoporosis (most notably alendronate and risedronate) to carry warning labels disclosing the possible increased risk for these atypical femur fractures, where the thigh bone can crack and may even break from just normal daily activity. Even though these fractures account for less than 1 percent of all hip and femur fractures, a task force investigating the risk reported that 94 percent of the 310 cases under study involved patients who had been taking bisphosphonates, most for more than five years. (The majority of these patients had felt a telltale pain in their groin or thigh weeks or even months before the fracture occurred.) The warning labels also suggest that patients taking these drugs be periodically reevaluated for their need to continue taking them because the optimal length of time for taking the drugs has not been determined.

Bisphosphonates had been initially hailed as a potent way to fight thinning bones because trials showed that in women with osteoporosis, alendronate (Fosamax), risedronate (Actonel), and ibandronate (Boniva) reduced the incidence of hip, vertebral, and nonvertebral fracture by almost 50 percent, particularly in the first year of treatment.[59] But these results are seen only in women who already have osteoporosis; the reduced risk is not seen in healthy women trying to prevent bone loss in the future. An article in the *British Medical Journal* estimated that doctors would have to treat 100 women with these drugs to benefit just one woman.[60]

The side effects of bisphosphonates range from merely bothersome to downright dangerous. Some of the more common side effects of Actonel, for example, include back pain, joint pain, stomach pain, nausea, and vomiting. Fosamax may cause nausea, constipation, and heartburn. In some studies, up to a third of the participants had stomach-acid-related complaints, and one in eight required treatment. Some even developed severe esophageal ulcers.[61] About 50 percent of women stop treatment within a year because of such side effects. Some women on this drug (one in every 100,000 patients) have suffered osteonecrosis of the jaw—death of the jaw's bone tissue, a condition that is not treatable.[62] Others have found that they require root canals soon after beginning alendronate. Both of these serious side effects are likely to be caused by the inadequate circulation problem described above.

Bisphosphonates stay in the body for decades, even after women stop taking them, because they bind tightly to bone. If used at all, they should be reserved for much older postmenopausal women (seventy or older) with major risk factors for osteoporosis. Even in those cases, experts are now calling for a "drug holiday" after five years of treatment for most women who take these drugs.[63]

PARATHYROID HORMONE DRUGS: Drugs in this class, including abaloparatide (brand name Tymlos) and teriparatide (Forteo), build bone. Both abaloparatide and teriparatide require a daily shot for eighteen months to two years but must be discontinued after that. Unlike the bisphosphonates, these drugs don't merely stop bone breakdown but also help build new bone. However, both also carry black box warnings that indicate the drugs can increase the risk of bone cancer.

HUMAN MONOCLONAL ANTIBODY: In 2019, the FDA approved a new osteoporosis drug called romosozumab (Evenity) for women who have a high risk of fracture. It's given as two back-to-back shots once a month for a year (after which point it is no longer effective). Like the parathyroid hormone drugs, romosozumab helps build new bone, but it is much more efficient. Studies show it decreases fracture risk by more than 70 percent and increases bone density in the spine by about 15 percent.[64] However, along with common side effects such as joint pain and headache, the drug is associated with an increased risk of heart attack, stroke, and cardiovascular death, causing such events in about 2.5 percent of those who take it. Because this drug is new, long-term data is not yet available. Another drug in this category is denosumab (brand names Prolia and Xgeva). This drug is also given as a shot, once every six months. Recently concerns have surfaced about patients experiencing an increased chance of spinal fracture after discontinuing the drug if they do not replace it with another osteoporosis treatment, and watchdog groups are petitioning the FDA to call for a black box warning. Like the bisphosphonates, romosozumab and denosumab also carry a risk of osteonecrosis of the jaw and atypical femur fractures.

My opinion of the bisphosphonates, the parathyroid hormone drugs, and the human monoclonal antibody drugs is that they should be used cautiously, but they do have a place, especially in women who are at very high risk for osteoporosis. After all, women who suffer hip fractures show a significant increase in mortality. Still, I prefer maximizing bone health with a regimen that combines vitamin D, vitamin K_2, magnesium, exercise, an alkaline system, and phytohormones or estrogen, rather than taking bisphosphonates. Think very carefully before starting a bisphosphonate or any one of the other bone-building drugs.

CALCITONIN: Calcitonin is a naturally occurring peptide that partially blocks osteoclast activity and regulates calcium loss in the urine. This is an injectable or nasal synthetic form of the parathyroid hormone. It reduces the risk of spinal but not hip fractures and also reduces pain from new spinal fractures. Side effects include nausea and flushing, and there is some concern about an increase in cancer with long-term use. Most experts agree that the bisphosphonates work better.[65]

Bottom line: everyone with low bone density needs to have enough vitamin D, magnesium, vitamin K_2, and calcium, and needs to eat a low-acid diet. Weight-bearing exercise on a regular basis is also essential (see below). Some might also benefit from alendronate or risedronate once weekly (or ibandronate once monthly), but I'd prefer all women try natural methods first.

VERTEBROPLASTY AND KYPHOPLASTY: HEALING PAIN FROM COMPRESSION FRACTURES

Two fairly new and minimally invasive procedures can work wonders for those in pain from a vertebral fracture. Both vertebroplasty and kyphoplasty rely on injecting a special acrylic cement into the damaged vertebra to restore stability. With vertebroplasty (usually an outpatient procedure using only local anesthesia), the doctor injects the cement directly, using imaging technology to guide the needle. With kyphoplasty (which may require general anesthesia and an overnight stay in the hospital), the doctor first inserts a balloon into the fracture and then inflates it to restore the height of the vertebra and to create a space for the cement, which is then injected. After either procedure, patients lie on their backs for about an hour until the cement hardens. Pain relief is immediate and the risk of complications is low.

GET STRONG

Regardless of your diet, supplements, or any drugs you may be on, the big news is that weight-bearing exercise in general and strength training in particular play a crucial role in creating and maintaining healthy bones. If you don't currently exercise regularly, you're not alone. Sixty percent of the U.S. population is sedentary, which is one of the main reasons why osteoporosis has reached such epidemic proportions. Remember, it is not the aging process per se that causes bones to thin—it's the fact that too many women slow down and stop using their muscles.

Weight-bearing exercise helps build bone by stimulating the mineralization and remodeling process. Every major muscle in our bodies is attached to underlying bone by tendons. So each time a muscle contracts, it exerts a force on the bone to which it is anchored. (We know that in tennis players, for example, the bone density in the racket arm is significantly greater than in the other arm.)

Yoga and tai chi can also help build bone mass. For example, a 2009 study from Thailand concluded that weight-bearing yoga training had a positive effect on bone for postmenopausal women, reducing their risk of osteoporosis.[66] (Not surprisingly, the researchers also reported that the yoga training promoted a better quality of life!)

But the most studied method of strengthening bone is weight lifting. Miriam Nelson, Ph.D., known for her groundbreaking research at Tufts University in the 1980s, proved that weight training can slow down and even reverse bone loss. Dr. Nelson studied two groups of postmenopausal women, none of whom were on estrogen replacement, bone-building drugs, or any special supplements. Both groups were sedentary but healthy at the start of the program. One group remained sedentary while the other began a simple exercise program. At the end of one year the women who lifted weights for forty minutes twice per week had turned back the clock in several ways. Their scores on strength tests increased to match those of women in their late thirties or early forties. Without dieting, they trimmed down; muscle is less bulky than fat. Their balance improved greatly, warding off falls. The biggest payoff: while the sedentary control group lost about 2 percent of their bone density during the year, the women who strength-trained gained 1 percent.[67] Dr. Nelson's research also shows that higher-impact activities (including vertical jumping and stair climbing) can help build bone when they're done safely. She recommends a comprehensive exercise program including weight-bearing aerobic exercise, strength training, vertical jumping (when appropriate and for women under fifty), balance exercises, and stretching.

But stronger bones aren't the only benefit of getting strong. Dr. Nelson noted an unexpected but very exciting change in the women who did weight training—a change that I've also seen repeatedly. Within a few weeks the weight-lifting women felt happier, more energetic, and more self-confident. As their muscles began to get stronger, they became more active and daring. In order to control the study, they had agreed not to join other fitness programs. But these former couch potatoes were now going canoeing, inline skating, or dancing because they wanted to. Nelson also confirmed that weight training, like aerobic exercise, lifts depression and helps arthritis.[68]

The joys and benefits of fitness are so numerous that I want to do everything in my power to motivate you to get strong. Of all the ways to stay vital, healthy, and attractive, exercise probably gives the most return for the time spent. Whatever your age and condition right now, physical exercise can improve it and give you a new lease on life—guaranteed. In 1994 researchers proved this by instituting a strength-training program in frail nursing-home patients with an average age of eighty-seven. The exercise group did forty-five-minute strength-training sessions for the hips and knees three days per week. Within ten weeks, their strength increased by over 100 percent. In a nonexercising control group, strength declined by about 1 percent. The improved muscle strength after exercise was unrelated to the age, sex, medical diagnosis, or functional level of the participant. After the strength-training program some of the participants who had previously used walkers required only a cane. Exercise also improved stair-climbing ability, speed of walking, and overall level of physical activity.[69] In a 2009 study, researchers showed that elderly patients who followed a home-based physiotherapy program along with taking high-dose supplementation of vitamin D significantly reduced their rate of falls and hospital readmission.[70]

If these kinds of results are possible in frail octogenarians in nursing homes, think what could happen for a fifty-year-old couch potato. The average midlife woman of today is expected to live until at least age eighty-five, if not a hundred. You cannot afford to let your muscles and bones slip into decline at midlife. There are too many potentially high-quality years ahead. And there's not a single drug, technological breakthrough, or genetic development on the horizon that can or ever will come close to providing you with the benefits you can derive yourself from getting and staying strong. Besides, women who exercise regularly live six years longer than nonexercisers. If you think you don't have time to exercise, I suggest that you reconsider. Slowly shuffling along with a walker instead of striding confidently takes up a lot of time. And dying six years prematurely is truly a colossal waste of time.

Almost every woman I know is too busy to exercise. There are always more things to get done in a day than you have time for. If you wait to exercise until you get everything else done, you are waiting for a miracle. Like muscles that won't get stronger until you reach down and pick up a heavy weight, exercise won't happen in your life unless you make it as much a priority as brushing your teeth or taking a shower. The first thing that must change if you are to exercise regularly is your mind. No excuses.

WHAT WOULD IT TAKE TO GET YOU MOVING?

- Do you enjoy moving your body? Recall a moment in your life in which you were captivated by the sheer joy of dancing, running, swimming, or jumping. When was the last time you felt this way?

- When was the last time you felt that pleasurable sense of complete relaxation that comes from spending a day immersed in the pleasures of some activity—skiing, hiking, sailing, dancing, or inline skating?

- What types of activities did you enjoy as a child? As a teenager?

- If you do not exercise now, why not?

- If you don't exercise now, when did you stop? Why?

- Do you feel that you don't have time to exercise? Why not?

HEALING YOUR FITNESS PAST

When my mother turned eighty a while ago, my whole extended family gathered in my hometown for a big party and other activities that included downhill and cross-country skiing, as well as snowshoeing. My mom kept right up with her grandchildren and still skied beautifully. As already mentioned, she trekked to a Mount Everest base camp at the age of eighty-four. Every summer, she led a group of fortysomethings on a hiking expedition in the Adirondacks that they called Camp Edna. These women loved benefiting from my mother's experience and expertise. So at an age when many women had relegated themselves to the sidelines, my mother was not only coaching the game, she was also actively playing it. Back then she got up at six, mowed the huge lawn on the farm where I grew up, watered all the flowers, then played two sets of tennis with her friends. Sometimes she also played golf.

My mother's physical activity level was way off the charts, and I don't see it as a standard to which I or anyone else should aspire unless they find it as satisfying as she did. As I write this, she is ninety-four. And though she continues to hike regularly, failing eyesight and some balance problems have curtailed her physical activities, though she still lives independently.

My mother's years of physical prowess and strength imprinted me and my daughters with a deep knowing that physical decline and weakness need not be part of growing older. In fact, it's a legacy I received before birth: my mother skied and hiked through all her pregnancies and later carried each of us children in a backpack during these same activities.

Despite this legacy, I had to work through some unfinished business around sports and fitness. In contrast to my mother and siblings, I was not interested in spending every free moment on the ski slopes or hiking up mountains carrying a heavy backpack. I liked to read books—by the fire in winter and sitting up in a tree in summer. As an adolescent, I longed for a Christmas morning in which we could all sit around, relax, talk, and drink cocoa, like they did in the movies. But invariably, as soon as the presents had been opened, everyone rushed out the door to get in a couple of runs at the local ski area before our relatives arrived for dinner. My only chance for having the loving family connection that I longed for was to haul out my gear and join them. So I did. (And yes, I'm a very good skier.)

Still, my overall sports skills lagged behind those of my mother and siblings no matter how hard I tried. During the summer of my thirteenth year, for example, I practiced my tennis strokes daily against the barn door for six solid weeks. My father's only comment was "You're swinging that racket as if it were a broom." This left me with considerable baggage around sports. So at midlife I decided to release this baggage and pick up some barbells—and some insight—instead. When I was forty-five I took tennis lessons, more as therapy to recover from my past than from a desire to play regularly. By the end of the season I realized that I was perfectly capable of playing and enjoying a game of tennis. Later that summer I even played doubles with my mother and brother. What a healing! The truth, however, is that I have about zero interest in sports, except when well edited in movies, like *Field of Dreams*.

John Douillard, D.C., Ph.D., a fitness expert and the author of *Body, Mind, and Sport* (Three Rivers Press, 2001), points out that 50 percent of women experience their first personal failure around organized physical activity in school gym class, and that this sense of being a physical "loser" can stay with you the rest of your life. At perimenopause you have to ask yourself, "Do I really want to continue limiting my health and happiness because of something that happened to me in eighth-grade gym class or with my parents when I was six?"

Get out your journal and write down everything you remember about physical activity and sports from when you were eleven to thirteen years old. What did you love to do? What activities felt good? What are your memories from gym class? What is your family legacy around fitness? What do you honestly believe about the physical capabilities of a woman your age? Age seventy-five? Age ninety? What was the fitness level of your mother? Your grandmother? What happens to you when you walk into a gym or onto a dance floor?

Exercise for Vibrant Health on All Levels

At midlife I finally figured out what type of exercise was right for my body and temperament by realizing that my sports skills, strength, and fitness levels were all about me and my body, not a way to win family approval or measure up to a cultural standard. Regardless of your own fitness past or legacy, you need to know that vigorous regular exercise is an absolute necessity if you intend to live well beyond midlife. Vigorous exercise sends positive signals to your entire body that increase your levels of human growth hormone. Exercise tells your body to stay vigorous, vibrant, healthy, and growing. Sitting on the couch and eating junk food and drinking too much alcohol gives your body the opposite message: get old, deteriorate, and go into decline. It's that simple.

The bottom-line truth is that our bodies respond to the demands of our activities. For example, my mother's Everest trek has left her feeling stronger than ever—even though she'd previously taken two painful falls that resulted in considerable injury. Like all injuries, these too had an emotional component. They brought up persistent self-doubt and messages of "I'm not good enough" from childhood.

The Everest trek opportunity was just the medicine she needed to quell the internal voices of doubt that said, "Maybe I really am too old." She also had to look squarely at her past tendency to use movement and exercise as a way to avoid difficult emotions signaling unmet needs.

Ask yourself what activities you want to be able to participate in for as long as you live. I tried for years to enjoy running. But it never felt good. Though I ran regularly throughout medical school and residency, I never felt that elusive runner's high, no matter how long or hard I ran. In fact, I hated it. I finally gave myself permission to stop. I now go only for those activities that feel right.

RUTH: *Couch Potato No More*

Ruth, fifty-five, came to see me complaining of aches and pains and not being able to sleep well at night. She told me she had raised five children and was now looking forward to retirement from her job as a government secretary. She had never done any regular exercise. Her initial bone density test showed a slight bone loss despite the fact that she had been on estrogen for seven years following a hysterectomy with ovary removal for heavy bleeding. In addition to recommending dietary improvement and a supplement program, I stressed to Ruth that she needed to begin an exercise program: her couch-potato status was putting her at risk for significantly tarnishing her dreams for her golden years.

Ruth decided to start a walking program every morning with some of her friends. Within three months she had lost ten pounds without changing her diet at all, her aches and pains were gone, and she was sleeping better than she had in years. Later that year she and her husband both took up skiing and hiking. Her bone density has stayed steady even without weight training. Fitness and outdoor exercise have become a regular part of her life.

Start Somewhere—Anywhere

If you simply can't see yourself doing something like weight training just yet, commit to doing some kind of physical activity for just ten minutes daily for thirty days. It could consist simply of stretching every day. Here's what I recommend: put on some music you love and dance around your house. Even if you're in a wheelchair, you can sit and move your upper body. No kidding. No excuses. I guarantee that by the end of thirty days or much sooner, you'll be looking forward to your daily dance. Just this simple exercise will wake up the inherent, irresistible desire to move that lies within each of us—albeit more deeply buried in some than others!

Movement is contagious. Today's dancing around your living room will eventually wake up enough of your muscles that you'll want to do more. You can always pick up your cat and dance around with him or her. (This is weight training, after all!) Start very slowly and breathe in and out through your nose—this will expand your lower lungs optimally. It can take a while to create flexibility in your rib cage, so don't get discouraged if nose breathing makes you feel out of breath at first. Don't ever push beyond what is comfortable for your breathing and heart rate. But every day ask your body to move a little faster or bend a little deeper. Simply moving your body begins the bone-building process.

Get Support

After you've done your one month of dancing, you'll have created the movement habit in your life. Now's the time to begin adding some resistance training, weight lifting, or Pilates. I suggest that you go to a Y, an adult education class at your local high school, or a gym and have one of the staff members guide you through a personal strength-training program. This way you'll be learning proper technique, which you can later adapt for home use. Of course, there are also many strength-training programs available online.

Whether you work out at home or in a gym will depend upon your lifestyle and temperament. I've done both and find advantages and disadvantages to each approach. The beauty of the gym is that the phone doesn't ring and no one interrupts you. And the entire environment is dedicated to fitness, so you're more apt to get into the spirit of it. But sometimes taking the extra time to go to the gym is too much. My current personal fitness regimen combines one-hour Pilates sessions in a studio with a teacher and thirty-minute Pilates mat sessions on my own at home, each done two to three times per week, as well as two to three hours of Argentine tango a week. I also take regular forty-five-minute walks. I haven't always been able to get this amount of exercise in. One of the benefits of midlife is that my time is more my own than it was at any other stage of my life. And I find that I love moving in ways that my body has always longed for—and finally found.

Build Strength into Your Day

Here are a few tips for adding some strength training to your day-to-day activities. Try these exercises when you're on the phone or have a few spare moments. They cover all the major muscle groups.

- TOE STANDS. Face a wall and stand twelve inches away from it with your feet shoulder-width apart. Rest your fingertips lightly against the wall for balance. (As you improve you can use the wall less and less.) Now raise yourself as high up as you can; remain on your toes for a count of three, breathing normally, then lower yourself slowly. Breathe. Repeat a total of eight times. Gradually hold each toe stand for thirty seconds as you become stronger.

- HEEL STANDS. Stand facing a wall so that you can put your hands against it if necessary. Slowly raise the toes and balls of your feet until you are balanced on your heels. Remain on your heels for a count of three. Slowly lower. Breathe. Repeat. Try for a total of eight repetitions, and gradually increase the amount of time you balance on your heels so that eventually you're holding each heel stand for a count of thirty.

   Both heel and toe stands use your own body weight to strengthen your legs and to improve balance and flexibility.

- PUSH-UPS. Although many women hate them, nothing beats a push-up for strengthening the upper body. You can ease into this exercise with wall push-ups. Stand with your feet about three feet from a wall. Lean forward with elbows bent and palms touching the wall. Now push off the wall, keeping your back perfectly aligned with your legs, making sure that your head is aligned with your back and not pitching forward. Repeat this wall push-up eight times. Build up to three sets of eight repetitions.

   After this becomes easy, you'll be ready for push-ups on the floor. Start on your hands and knees with arms straight. Now bend your elbows and dip your chest to the floor. Go slowly and keep breathing. Try for four knee push-ups. Gradually build up to two sets of eight.

   When you get strong enough, you'll be ready for full-blown regulation push-ups. Start on your hands and knees. Then straighten your legs out behind you so that you are supported by your toes and your arms. Your body should form a perfectly straight line with your head in alignment with your spine. Don't allow your hips to jackknife up in the center. Now dip down so that your chest almost touches the floor. Push back up. Hold. Repeat. Do four, working up to eight. Eventually you'll be aiming for two sets of eight push-ups.

⌐ WEIGHTS. Place a set of graduated dumbbells (5–20 pounds, depending upon your strength level) in front of your TV. During commercial breaks or even during your favorite shows you can easily do a few sets of biceps curls, overhead presses, bent-over rows, or triceps kickbacks. The point is to keep the weights out where you'll run into them regularly.

Take your time. Your body is very forgiving and very responsive if you approach it with respect and love. Each time you lift weights, ask your body if it is willing to breathe a little deeper and lift a bit more weight. Don't push it. On the days when you feel wonderful, do more. When you feel lousy, cut back. Exercise is a discipline, it is true, but once you've made the commitment to do it regularly, get that abusive coach out of your head. The best motivator is the pleasure, joy, and awareness that come from being in your body.

SAFE PILATES AND YOGA FOR WOMEN WITH BONE LOSS

Pilates is an excellent option for women with osteoporosis because it helps develop a strong core and better balance, reducing the risk of falls. Yoga also improves strength and balance, and weight-bearing yoga has specifically been shown to build bone.

Yet traditional Pilates and yoga exercises should be modified for women with osteopenia or osteoporosis so that they concentrate on movements that involve extension and avoid those that involve spinal flexion, or forward bending of the spine—especially when it is combined with side bending and twisting. A Mayo Clinic study showed that in women who had osteoporosis, doing the flexion exercises actually caused an increase in compression fractures.[71]

For the same reason, women with bone loss should avoid the rolling exercises in Pilates (such as rolling like a ball) and lifting their heads while lying on their backs for exercises that use the same motions as sit-ups or abdominal crunches. Instead, these women should keep their heads on the floor when doing exercises on their backs.

An excellent resource for such women is Rebekah Rotstein's Buff Bones program, which draws upon Pilates, somatics, functional movement, and therapeutic exercise to strengthen bone in a safe way for women with osteoporosis and osteopenia. Rotstein is a former ballet dancer who turned to Pilates to relieve chronic pain after injuries ended her dance career. At twenty-eight she was diagnosed with osteoporosis, and she eventually developed a new career in rehabilitation, applying Pilates principles to sports medicine. For more information on the Buff Bones program, visit Rotstein's website at buff-bones.com.

Preventing Hip, Shoulder, and Back Pain

Many women begin to experience joint problems during perimenopause, including decreased range of motion in one shoulder or in the hip joints. You must maintain your range of motion and also keep your spine well aligned and stretched in order to keep the spinal nerves free from impingement, which can lead to back, hip, and other pain. Pilates does this beautifully, and so does yoga. Esther Gokhale's Primal Posture program, mentioned earlier, is also invaluable (see www.gokhalemethod.com).

Our Beliefs Are Stored in Muscles, Bones, and Fascia

Our emotions play a strong role in joint pain because emotions of all kinds can and do "live" in our muscles, tendons, and joints. If we feel beaten down by life, then our bodies may reflect this. You have only to look at the gait of a depressed person who is shuffling along, head down, in order to see the profound effects that emotions have on alignment and movement. Conversely, changing your alignment and posture instantly makes you feel better even when you are depressed, much the same way as voluntarily smiling elevates your mood.

I can also assure you from my years of Pilates that taking the time to open the chest or move the shoulders in new ways often brings up all kinds of emotions. Massage therapists and yoga teachers can attest to the fact that emotional releases of all kinds are very common when people have the courage to consciously open up new spaces in their bodies.

Skilled body workers can in fact often "read" the traumas and blockages that are "stuck" in the muscles and fascia. For example, I once had a session with Melanie Ericksen, a gifted massage therapist and body worker who was able to help me move an energetic blockage that had resulted in intermittent right hip problems for more than twenty years. This hip problem was related to my masculine (right) side and the men in my life. For many years I, like so many women of my generation, felt that I had to lead with my masculine "get 'er done" side in addition to not getting a lot of support from the men in my life. This pattern was not sustainable in my body and needed to be balanced with my feminine (left) side, which is about receiving. Melanie and I were able to release my outmoded beliefs around needing to do it all by myself, which encouraged me to allow myself to be more supported. As we were working, I literally felt a huge amount of energy flow into my left hip and leg, and the hip issue pretty much went away from that moment on. (For more information about Melanie, who can do energy work via phone, check out www.soulplay.us.)

Interestingly, my session with Melanie was right after I danced a tango with my dance partner Jim at Men's Night at Mama Gena's School of Womanly Arts in New York City. Regena Thomashauer (a.k.a. Mama Gena) had previously suggested that I dance there as a way to fulfill my desire to learn tango better and also to demonstrate the dance of male/female energy to the group. There's nothing like having a scheduled performance as an incentive to practice! So for the next eight months, I practiced "following" in tango—a skill that requires surrendering to a leader, usually a man. Talk about learning to receive! The follower part in tango is all about being present, being yourself, and standing in your feminine power and center while also responding to the masculine lead. Being willing to dance a tango in public after only about a year of dancing required courage and willingness on my part. I had absolutely no dancing skill when I started, but I knew that putting myself on the line like this was a very practical way to learn how to be in my feminine energy consciously and on purpose.

Another example of how emotions get stuck in our bodies is a condition commonly known as "frozen shoulder." About six years ago, like so many other midlife women, I developed the beginning of this condition when my right shoulder began hurting so badly that I once fell to the floor in pain after picking up a piece of wood to load into my woodstove. Believe me, the pain was *very* real. On the other hand, I realized that such severe pain seemingly coming out of no-where *had* to have an emotional component. Shoulder issues tend to be about feeling burdened or as though you're carrying the weight of the world. (Back when I first started doing Pilates and I was doing lots of work on my shoulders, I used to joke that the world as we know it would fall apart if I were to relax them!)

Studies have actually shown that frozen shoulder, like much back pain, begins with what is called "tension myositis syndrome," a term coined by the late John Sarno, M.D., who treated thousands of indi-viduals with conditions ranging from sciatica to severe back pain and frozen shoulder. Dr. Sarno pointed out that these painful conditions are related to painful emotions that we can't allow ourselves to feel—usually anger. Hence the emotion goes into our soft tissues and cre-ates tension, which shuts off the blood supply and pinches nerves. Pain is the result. The solution involves acknowledging the probable emotional basis for the problem. You can do this with the Emotional Freedom Technique (EFT). Once the emotion is acknowledged and expressed, the stuck energy can move out of the body. My colleague Larry Burk, M.D., has an entire program for frozen shoulder (and many other conditions) using EFT along with understanding the symbolic meaning of a symptom. Larry's work has helped many peo-ple resolve the problem promptly (see www.letmagichappen.com).

While you're working on this, it's important to keep moving the joint. What usually happens to women who develop this kind of shoulder pain is that they do exactly the opposite. But not moving the joint is the worst thing you can do, because then everything congeals, and you do, in fact, get a frozen shoulder from then on. I was deter-mined to avoid this, so I worked on actively stretching the area twice a day—just to the point of pain, and then a bit beyond, to a slightly painful place, where I'd hold the shoulder until the fascia, ligaments, and muscles relaxed a bit. After I did this for several weeks, while working on identifying the metaphoric "weight" I was carrying on my shoulders, the shoulder pain gradually began to fade, and I even-tually regained full range of motion.

I wish that more women would realize the degree to which their musculoskeletal problems—be they with shoulders, hips, neck, or back—have an emotional basis. Simply acknowledging this possibil-ity opens up huge vistas of healing.

I have worked regularly with Hope Matthews and Chris Renfrow on fascial realignment and have learned firsthand that most of what we call "aging" in joints, muscles, and posture is the result of chronic postural patterns and restriction of movement associated with unprocessed emotions in the fascia. (For more information, read *The Emotion Code* [St. Martin's Essentials, 2019] by Bradley B. Nelson, D.C.)

THE SUNLIGHT–BONE HEALTH CONNECTION

Everywhere we turn, we are warned about the dangers of exposure to the sun, from premature skin aging to fatal skin cancer. Though these risks are well documented, they are overstated, especially for those of us who live in northern climates, where sunlight isn't a glaring issue for most of the year. Women past menopause lose up to 3–4 percent of their bone mass every winter if they live in northern latitudes, above a line approximately from Boston through Chicago to the California-Oregon border.[72] Even on a bright sunny day in December in northern Maine, you cannot get enough ultraviolet exposure to produce vitamin D unless you expose a great deal of your skin to the sun at midday for thirty to fifty minutes or so, a level of exposure that is uncommon. The problem is compounded if your diet is already low in calcium and vitamin D. Forty percent of individuals with hip fractures in northern latitudes are vitamin D deficient. In women whose diets are adequate in calcium and other nutrients, however, bone mass can be regained in the summer months with regular sunlight exposure.

The truth is that sunlight can help you become healthier and can literally save your life. That's because ultraviolet rays from the sun help your body manufacture necessary vitamin D. As with just about everything else, the key is moderation.

Vitamin D is a hormone that helps your bones absorb calcium. If you don't have enough vitamin D circulating in your blood, you won't be able to use the calcium from your diet or from supplements. Therefore, it is an important factor in preventing osteoporosis. Right now the RDA for vitamin D is based on the amount you need to prevent rickets. Rickets is a disease where vitamin D levels are too low, resulting in the body's decreased ability to produce new bone. In adults, this is called osteomalacia, a gradual softening or bending of bones secondary to failure of bones to calcify.

To prevent rickets, you need just a minimal level of vitamin D (200–400 IU per day). But prevention of rickets isn't the only benefit of optimal vitamin D levels. For example, adequate vitamin D can decrease hypertension, so people with higher vitamin D levels enjoy lower blood pressure.[73] It can slow the progression of osteoarthritis and also decrease the prevalence of multiple sclerosis.[74] According to the Vitamin D Council (a nonprofit educational organization; see @VitaminDCouncil on Facebook and Twitter), current scientific research shows that vitamin D deficiency is a major factor in the pathology of at least seventeen varieties of cancer as well as heart disease, stroke, hypertension, autoimmune diseases, diabetes, depression, chronic pain, osteoarthritis, muscle weakness, muscle wasting, birth defects, periodontal disease, Parkinson's disease, and more. In fact, suboptimal levels of vitamin D may be one of the reasons why breast cancer incidence is higher in the northern latitudes than in the South. Research from Austria published in the *Archives of Internal Medicine* shows that those with low levels of vitamin D have more than double the risk of dying (from heart disease, among other causes) over an eight-year period.[75] (For more information about the importance of vitamin D, go to the website for GrassrootsHealth Nutrient Research Institute at www.grassrootshealth.net. This nonprofit group has a wealth of information about vitamin D, including the latest research on its benefits and information on at-home testing.)

In order to decrease your risk for diseases like breast, ovarian, and colorectal cancer, you need much higher serum vitamin D levels than you can get with a teaspoon of cod liver oil or the usual vitamin D supplement. Your safest and most effective route for this is routine sun exposure.

Sunlight Versus Vitamin D Supplementation

Our bodies were designed to get vitamin D from the sun. Our ancestors ran around the plains of Africa for millennia with large surfaces of their bodies exposed to sunlight. Exposure to outdoor sunlight is a much more reliable predictor of vitamin D levels in your body than your dietary intake. In fact, vitamin D intake in your diet correlates poorly with the amount of vitamin D in your blood. This is partly because oral vitamin D requirements have been found to vary tremendously between individuals. And while it is possible to take in toxic levels of vitamin D from supplements, it is impossible for sun exposure to result in too much vitamin D. That's because our bodily wisdom contains a built-in mechanism whereby we manufacture exactly what we need from the sun—no more and no less. The vitamin D that your body makes on its own from exposure to the sun's ultraviolet rays (specifically ultraviolet B, or UVB) is superior to oral supplementation for helping your body absorb calcium.[76]

Sunlight alone can bring your vitamin D levels into the healthy range. If you expose your body to sunlight without sunscreen for about twenty to thirty minutes three to five times per week (which you must work up to gradually so that you don't burn) for four to five months per year (between April and October in northern latitudes), you probably will get enough UVB rays to keep your bone mass intact, because your body has the ability to stockpile vitamin D for use during low-sunlight times. This is nature's wisdom at work, because not all regions of the country are equal when it comes to ultraviolet exposure. If you have very dark skin, you need to be in the sun longer—even an hour or two hours to get the same result.

The more skin you expose, the quicker you make vitamin D, which is why some experts recommend full-body exposure regularly. In fact, full-body exposure for fifteen to thirty minutes is the equivalent of an oral dose of 10,000 IU vitamin D. (But UV exposure beyond this does not give you higher vitamin D levels.) However, as we age, our bodies become less efficient at making their own vitamin D. So if you are older than sixty-five, you may need more time in the sun to get the same benefit. Here's a general rule: if there's enough sunlight to cause a reddening of your skin when you're outside for any length of time, then there are enough UVB rays to assist your body in making vitamin D.

How to Have Your Sun and Be Safe, Too

Everyone can get the amount of sunlight she needs safely by getting outdoors regularly. The benefits of small amounts of UVB light are so striking that endocrinologist Michael Holick, M.D., Ph.D., and his colleagues at Boston University Medical Center are studying the effects of providing artificial UVB light to seniors. At one time, NASA even contracted with Dr. Holick to put this special light into spaceships for long missions to counteract the effects of weightlessness on bone.[77]

I recommend ten to twenty minutes of exposure without sunscreen (except on your face) per day, more if your skin is dark. Early-morning or late-afternoon sun exposure is the safest. I personally take a forty-five-minute walk about four mornings per week during the warm months, wearing shorts and a tank top to ensure adequate sun exposure. When I can't get out in the morning, I try for late afternoon or early evening, when there is still some sunlight available but when the risk of overexposure is minimal. Other than these "vitamin D–enhancing times" I wear sunscreen.

Avoid midday sun and sunburn. Almost all skin cancers are associated with the harmful effects of sun overexposure without adequate antioxidant protection. In fact, UV exposure beyond pre-erythema levels (reddening of the skin) doesn't enhance your vitamin D levels. In other words, vitamin D reaches maximum levels in light skin twenty minutes after exposure.

Other easy ways to get a little vitamin D enhancement are rolling down the window in your car as you drive, riding in a convertible, or even opening the windows in your house. Why not create a sunroom or sun corner—a place where you can easily open a window and expose yourself to warm sunlight without even having to go outside? This is a good option for city dwellers.

What to Do When You Can't Get Enough Sunlight

Vitamin D is an essential hormone. In the absence of sunlight, you must get it in your diet. While it is nearly impossible to get the high levels of vitamin D you need in your blood without adequate sun exposure, vitamin D supplementation has definitely been shown to help women build or maintain bone mass.[78]

People should take 2,000–10,000 IU per day. Depending on what your current levels of vitamin D are (see discussion on optimal levels below), you may need to "push" the vitamin into your cells with high doses for a while (e.g., 50,000 IU per week for eight weeks) under a doctor's supervision. Then you can take 5,000–10,000 IU per day thereafter to maintain optimal levels.[79] (A 2010 study of women age seventy and older showed that taking one superdose of 500,000 IU per year actually increased falls and fractures, so stick with a daily supplement, and take it along with a meal that contains some fat, to increase absorption.)[80] You may need more or less vitamin D than the amounts suggested here. The point is that sunlight is more reliable than any supplement. Good food sources of vitamin D are liver, cod liver oil, and egg yolks. Also remember to add vitamin K_2.

Why Fortified Milk Isn't the Vitamin D Answer

Though all of us have been taught that it's possible to get all the vitamin D we need from fortified dairy foods, that's not always the case. When Dr. Holick studied the vitamin D content of fortified milk, he found that there's often not enough vitamin D present because of processing problems. In fact, up to 50 percent of the milk tested had less vitamin D than noted on the label. Fifteen percent of the milk had no vitamin D at all! And in skim milk there is a problem getting vitamin D into solution because vitamin D is fat soluble and requires some fat to blend with the product. That's why skim milk products may have little or no vitamin D whatsoever.[81]

Check Your Vitamin D Level

Every woman should have her vitamin D level checked. This is a simple blood test available through your doctor (and now you can also order it yourself through My Med Lab at www.mymedlab .com; see Resources). You can also get an at-home vitamin D test kit from GrassrootsHealth (www.grassrootshealth.net). A vitamin D blood level of 20–25 ng/ml (50–62.5 nmol/l) or lower indicates a severe deficiency. We're now finding that women with osteoporosis have vitamin D levels of 20 ng/ml (50 nmol/l) or lower! Be sure to ask your healthcare provider what your actual vitamin D level is, because having "normal" levels is not the same as having optimal levels. The level of this vitamin that's considered optimal continues to creep upward. Currently, an optimal level of vitamin D is 40–100 ng/ml (100–250 nmol/l), although expert opinion varies somewhat about the higher end of this range. Levels greater than 40 ng/ml (100 nmol/l) have been shown to decrease hypertension.[82] Levels of 30 ng/ml (75 nmol/l) and above slow the progression of osteoarthritis. Studies of lifeguards and farmers—people who are out in the sun all the time—show that they have vitamin D levels of around 40 ng/ml (100 nmol/l). Get your serum levels checked! If your levels are low, get more sun exposure to prevent later problems, even if your bones seem healthy now.

I once did a consult for a woman in her mid-forties who summered in Maine and ran regularly for exercise while covered in sunscreen and clothing. Though she lived most of the year in the Southwest, an area with abundant sunshine year-round, she avoided the sun at all costs because she was worried about skin cancer. When I ordered a serum vitamin D level, it came back at 10 ng/ml (25 nmol/l), indicating severe deficiency. Since then, she has been taking daily fifteen-minute early-morning sun baths in her backyard. Within two months her serum vitamin D level had increased to a very healthy range, and both her mood and her immune system improved dramatically. Within six months her bone density had also improved. She discovered some other benefits as well: she completely recovered from a tendency to catch colds and have aches and pains.

Should You Use a Tanning Salon?

Though dermatologists cringe at tanning salons because of the danger of overexposure, I recommend them for those who are at high risk for osteoporosis, depression, or certain cancers and who have no other way of getting UVB radiation.

A short five- to ten-minute sun bath in a facility once or twice per week in the winter months can boost your brain serotonin levels, lift depression, help build bone, help calm arthritis, and maybe also help prevent some cancers. The key, as with natural sun exposure, is to be sure you never burn or get red skin, and also that your body is fortified with antioxidants. Any longer than this amount can cause more harm than good. We've all seen those people with leathery dark skin hanging around tanning booths, addicted to the high they get from the process.

Take Antioxidants

Increasing numbers of studies have shown that antioxidants such as vitamin E, vitamin C, proanthocyanidins, and beta-carotene help protect the skin from sun damage, and also help it heal more quickly. (See chapter 11 for further information.)

Beware Drug-Induced Sun Sensitivity

Remember that many very common drugs actually increase sun sensitivity and will therefore increase your chances for getting a sunburn if you stay out too long. These include the following: antibiotics such as azithromycin (Zithromax), minocycline (Minocin), tetracycline, and sulfa; diabetic medications of the sulfonylurea family; skin treatments such as Retin-A and Renova; and diuretics of the thiazide family. It's always best to check with your pharmacist.

SHORE UP YOUR EARTH CONNECTION WITH PLANT MEDICINE

Traditional herbalists teach that when we consume plants regularly, our bodies take in their energetic qualities as well as their vitamins and minerals—a perfect way to help us connect with nature and shore up our first emotional centers. Oats (*Avena sativa*) and oat straw (the grass, leaf, and flower of the oat), for example, thrive in chilly, wet climates characterized by harsh winds and sudden storms. These hardy plants are rich in calcium, iron, phosphorous, B complex, potassium, magnesium, and vitamins A and C.[83]

The noted herbalist Susun Weed has found that regular consumption of herbal infusions with their highly bioavailable nutrients helps increase bone density as well as providing other benefits. One of my nutritionist colleagues also recommends them. Using infusions regularly is a very inexpensive and effective way to increase mineral intake.

How to Make an Herbal Infusion

Infusions are stronger than herbal teas. Use 1 oz. (30 g) of dried leaves (two handfuls of cut-up leaves, or three handfuls of whole leaves). Put in a quart or liter jar. Fill jar with boiling water, put the lid on, and steep for four hours at room temperature. This can be kept in the refrigerator.[84] Use 2 cups daily.

When using oat straw or other plant medicines, open yourself to the wisdom of the earth and nature as they have manifested in the plant you are taking into your body. Be patient and persistent. Feel your bones becoming as strong and sturdy as the mountains and rocks that form the backbone of the planet.

STRAIGHT, STRONG, AND FLEXIBLE FOR LIFE: MASTER PROGRAM FOR HEALTHY BONES AND JOINTS

Taking care of your bones and joints—supporting the structures that support your body—is a vital part of midlife health. Fortunately, there's a lot you can do to ensure that your joints maintain or even improve their range of motion and that your body stays in proper alignment. The same is true of shoring up your bones. No matter how many risk factors you identified, it's never too late (nor too early) to build your bones—even if you are ninety or already have osteoporosis. As long as you're alive, your bones are dynamic, living organs that respond daily to every aspect of your life, from your emotions to your diet.

Following this master plan for bone and joint health will go a long way in helping you flourish on all levels, including the ability to move fluidly and stand tall in every way—both physically and emotionally.

- ⌐ CUT BACK ON OR ELIMINATE ALCOHOL AND CAFFEINE. As noted earlier, alcohol interferes with bone remodeling, and caffeine increases the excretion of calcium in the urine.

- ⌐ QUIT SMOKING. Acupuncture can help you a great deal with this.

- ⌐ FOLLOW THE PERIMENOPAUSAL DIET PLAN OUTLINED IN CHAPTER 7. Eat five servings of low-glycemic-index fruits and vegetables per day. These are all high in potassium and boron, which help protect your bones by reversing urinary calcium loss.[85]

- ⌐ MAKE SURE YOUR DAILY SUPPLEMENT PROGRAM INCLUDES THE FOLLOWING (even if your diet is good):

Magnesium	400–1,000 mg (because of farming practices, many foods are low in this key mineral, so it must be supplemented)[86]
Calcium	500–1,200 mg[87]
Vitamin D_3	2,000–10,000 IU (see discussion below)
Vitamin C	1,000–5,000 mg
Boron	2–9 mg[88]
Zinc	6–50 mg
Manganese	1–15 mg
Copper	1–2 mg
Vitamin K_2	0–180 mcg (see discussion below)

- ⌐ GET YOUR VITAMIN D LEVEL CHECKED. Research shows that women with the lowest levels of vitamin D were 71 percent more likely to have a hip fracture than women with the highest levels, so be sure you get enough of this important vitamin.[89] To find out what your blood level is, have your doctor order a 25-hydroxyvitamin D test.

If your levels are very low, start with eight weeks of high-dose vitamin D supplement (between 5,000 and 10,000 IU per day). Once you're in the optimal range, between 40–100 ng/ml, you can take between 2,000 IU and 5,000 IU a day (depending on how much sun exposure you get). I also recommend limited sunbathing, working up to ten to thirty minutes of exposure (the darker your skin, the more time you need) during early morning or late afternoon, three to four times per week—but never enough to burn the skin. In the winter, you can use a tanning booth for five to ten minutes once or twice per week. (See the section on vitamin D earlier in this chapter.)

~ TAKE VITAMIN K. Vitamin K_2 (menaquinone-7), as already mentioned, plays a big role in bone and cardiovascular health. Many human and animal studies from Japan have shown that this vitamin can both increase bone mass and reduce bone loss.[90] Some particularly intriguing studies show that vitamin K boosts the positive effect of vitamin D on sustaining bone density in the lumbar spine and preventing fracture.[91]

Vitamin K_2 is found in meat, fermented products, cheese and other dairy products, broccoli, Brussels sprouts, cauliflower, chickpeas, kale, and seeds. The most robust studies on vitamin K_2 recommend 180 mcg per day of MK-7 (menaquinone-7).[92] *Note:* If you are taking the blood-thinning medication warfarin (sold as Coumadin), you may want to consult with your doctor before supplementing with vitamin K because it may lessen the effects of the drug.

~ IF YOU SUFFER FROM JOINT PAIN, SUPPLEMENT FURTHER. NSAIDs such as ibuprofen (Advil, Motrin) have been implicated in the destruction of cartilage over time. Though these popular OTC drugs definitely decrease joint pain, they do more harm than good over the long haul. Alternatively, many women get significant relief from joint pain and arthritis with the following supplements, taken in addition to a good multivitamin:

- *Pueraria mirifica* (PM): Miroestrol, a potent phytoestrogen found in certain formulations of this herb, is great for bones. Two published studies from researchers at Chulalongkorn University in Bangkok have shown that PM increased bone density in rats that had their ovaries removed. A randomized, double-blind, placebo-controlled study done by researchers at Bangkok's Mahidol University and published in the journal *Menopause* concluded that PM may have the same effect on

humans.[93] PM is also very effective at relieving a host of menopausal symptoms, including vaginal dryness, hot flashes, insomnia, and irritability. Take a brand that contains standardized
miroestrol (approximately 20 mg of miroestrol per 100 g). My
own company, Amata Life, makes Pueraria Mirifica Plus and
Pueraris Mirifica Pure (see www.amatalife.com). The usual
dose is 2 tablets per day.

- Glucosamine sulfate: 1,000 mg twice per day.

- Turmeric: 250 mg twice per day.

- Omega-3 fats (particularly DHA): These healthy fats, found
  not only in fish oil but also in walnuts and flaxseed oil, are
  indispensable for bone health and enhance bone density.[94]
  (Omega-6 fatty acids, on the other hand, weaken bones.) I recommend you start with 400 mg per day of the omega-3s (DHA
  and EPA combined) and work up to as high as 5,000 mg per
  day if needed.

- Proanthocyanidins (OPCs), made from grape seeds or pine
  bark: start with a loading dose of 1 mg per pound of body
  weight, daily in divided doses. Take this for ten to fourteen
  days. After that, you can decrease to a maintenance dose of
  60–200 mg per day. (See Resources.)

~ EAT PHYTOESTROGENS. Soy, ground flaxseed, and *Pueraria mirifica*
are particularly potent in this regard. Several studies have suggested that regular intake of soy protein has a bone-protective effect that is equivalent to that provided by estrogen. A six-month
double-blind study at the University of Illinois found that postmenopausal women on a diet that was high in soy isoflavones were
protected from spinal bone loss.[95] A study of more than 24,000
Chinese women reported in the *Archives of Internal Medicine*
noted that those consuming 13 g or more of soy protein every day
were half as likely to incur a bone fracture as those eating 5 g or
less per day.[96] This is pretty exciting, especially when you consider
that you can get this amount of soy protein simply by drinking two
glasses of soy milk.

In a Danish study, half the participants were given two glasses
of soy milk with isoflavones; the other half drank the same quantity without the isoflavones. Bone loss was measured after two
years, and then four years. The first group of postmenopausal
women had virtually no bone loss at either interval! The second
group saw a decrease in bone mass by a little more than 4 percent,

which is still lower than what many postmenopausal women experience. Researchers concluded that although the soy milk they drank didn't have isoflavones, the daily intake of soy protein still provided some protective benefits for these women's bones.[97]

Yet another study followed fifty postmenopausal women who consumed three servings a day of soy milk (about 7.5 oz. each) or three handfuls of roasted soy nuts, for a total daily dose of 60–70 mg of isoflavones. In twelve weeks the study noted a 13 percent increase in osteocalcin, a marker of bone formation, and a 14.5 percent decrease in markers for osteoclasts, cells that cause bone loss. The benefits of soy were not compared side by side with hormone therapy in this study, but soy protein revealed a bone-forming benefit that estrogen does not provide.[98] A study in the *British Journal of Pharmacology,* however, concluded that the phytoestrogen genistein, found in soy, is superior to alendronate (Fosamax), raloxifene (Evista), and estradiol in preserving bone mineral density and strength.[99]

Studies done at Chulalongkorn University in Bangkok and published in the journal *Maturitas* show that the phytoestrogen-rich herb *Pueraria mirifica* (PM) increases bone density in rats who've had their ovaries removed—a sign that this herb might be very promising in treating bone loss in humans.[100] However, not all PM on the market is the same. I recommend brands that contain miroestrol (see full discussion in chapter 6).

⁓ DRINK GREEN TEA. Green tea is especially rich in phytohormones and antioxidants. Research has shown that women who drink either green or black tea regularly have stronger bones than those in a control group.[101] I keep a pitcher of naturally decaffeinated green tea in my refrigerator and drink it regularly throughout the day.

⁓ CONSUME POMEGRANATE. A number of studies have shown that eating pomegranates or drinking pomegranate juice is extremely helpful for bones. A French study published in the *European Journal of Nutrition* reported that this antioxidant-rich fruit boosts the action of osteoblasts (our bone-building cells) while also lowering the activity of osteoclasts (which break down bone).[102] A Japanese study published in the *Journal of Ethnopharmacology* found that rats with accelerated bone loss were able to return to normal bone density after two weeks of eating pomegranate seeds and drinking pomegranate juice.[103] And a 2013 review of eight studies (including some on animals, some in vitro, and one on humans) reported that they all showed a positive effect of pomegranate extract or juice on osteoporosis (as well as on osteoarthritis and rheumatoid arthritis).[104]

~ DO REGULAR WEIGHT-BEARING EXERCISE. You need three exercise sessions per week, minimum. If you are lifting weights, two sessions per week are sufficient—but activities such as walking, yoga, and Pilates are also good. Basically anything that places force on ligaments, bones, and fascia will help promote healthy bones.

~ IF YOU ARE DEPRESSED, GET PROPER TREATMENT. Regular exercise and exposure to natural light are sometimes all that is necessary. If you work under fluorescent fixtures, replace them with full-spectrum lightbulbs. Though most full-spectrum lights don't provide the UVB light necessary to stimulate vitamin D and calcium uptake, they definitely can help relieve depression and seasonal affective disorder. Interestingly, the nutritional supplement St. John's wort, which has proven antidepressant effects, also lowers a cytokine known as IL-6, which is one of the chemicals that cause cellular inflammation and is involved with immune system activation. When its levels are normalized, bone density may be positively affected. It is unclear whether standard antidepressant medications also have this effect.

~ GET YOUR HORMONE LEVELS CHECKED. Many postmenopausal women have testosterone levels that are normal even for premenopausal women, making them much more resistant to osteoporosis without additional hormones. Some women also have estrogen levels that remain in the low-normal premenopausal range long after menopause. If this is the case, you won't need to worry about taking a drug to support your bone mass.

13

Creating Breast Health

Iremember the many evenings I sat in the labor-and-delivery area of the hospital with one of my midwife colleagues. Though her own children were nearly grown, this woman would sometimes clutch her chest when she heard a baby cry or saw a particularly adorable newborn. "My breasts are tingling so much, I feel as though I could nurse this child myself," she would say at such moments.

Breasts are both literally and symbolically a source of nurturance and pleasurable bonding. Their dual role is in part the result of two brain hormones known as prolactin and oxytocin. These hormones, which are activated during birth, keep the breasts full of milk and also enhance the process of bonding, so that when a mother breast-feeds, both prolactin and oxytocin facilitate the flow of both milk and love to the child. The mother in turn is rewarded not only with pleasurable physical sensations, but with the emotional fulfillment that comes from providing for a being she deeply loves. Prolactin and oxytocin have such powerful effects that many women experience the letdown reflex, which fills the breasts with milk, even when they're not actually nursing. Merely thinking about their child or hearing the child's cries can set the reflex in motion.

But prolactin and oxytocin secretion doesn't occur only during breast-feeding. These two hormones have been found to increase in both men and women when they are involved in pleasurable, mutually beneficial relationships. Not surprisingly, the emotions of love and compassion, which nourish our very souls, are often accompanied by the same tingling sensation in the breasts that nursing mothers feel—and which my midwife colleague described so eloquently.

I like to think of that tingling as proof that the "milk of human kindness" is more than a mere metaphor. Love is hardwired into our biology. That's why nurturing and supporting others feels so good to most women, and why we so often find ourselves "mothering" others. When the emotion of love can flow freely, our bodies are filled with the same hormone that sustains all human bonds, and our breasts are bathed in the energy of health.

OUR CULTURAL INHERITANCE: NURTURING VS. SELF-SACRIFICE

Love has a healing, life-enhancing effect if our relationships are truly reciprocal, allowing us to receive as much as we give. But this ideal is not so common. Most women have been brought up to nurture others in ways that often require us to put our own well-being at risk. Throughout history, we women have been revered for our ability to sacrifice ourselves for the good of those around us. It is no wonder that the late Tammy Wynette's song "Stand by Your Man" is one of the bestselling country songs of all time. But as it turns out, the man Tammy was standing by for much of her married life was beating her, which brings home very powerfully the degree to which our nurturing tendencies can tip the balance toward dangerous self-sacrifice.

Our breasts are the part of our anatomy most identified with nurturing—but also with sexuality. And they are also perhaps the most highly charged area of our bodies, flagrantly exploited by the culture we live in as our most potent weapon in the battle to win the love and approval of a man. Powerful symbols, these breasts. In the movie *Erin Brockovich* the sassy legal-assistant heroine is asked by her astounded boss how she has managed, without any experience or training, to accumulate so much sensitive, damning information concerning a large utility company's environmental pollution practices. Looking resplendently voluptuous in her overflowing bustier, actress Julia Roberts replies, "They're called boobs, Ed."

No wonder one of my friends, when she heard I was getting a

divorce, asked if I was going to get breast implants. Our culture leads us to believe that without a stunning new set of breasts, it would be impossible for a woman at midlife to attract a new man. What more vivid proof could we find of our need for love—and the lengths to which we are willing to go to get it?

The Midlife Breast Challenge

Midlife is when we hear the wake-up call that demands that we start honoring our own needs if we are to stay healthy and joyful. Our children are leaving home or long gone, the time for the kind of self-sacrifice demanded by raising a family may be coming to an end, and we now have the opportunity to reexamine our lives. If we are involved in relationships that are getting in the way of self-realization, we need to think about how we can change them. Perimenopause challenges us to get real, to create relationships that are true partnerships with people who will love us for who we really are. Of course, if you had your children in your late thirties or early forties, you are likely to be going through the need for self-realization at the very moment when your children are most dependent upon you. And that creates its own set of challenges.

Learning to form such mutually nurturing relationships, as part of a commitment to love and nurture ourselves on every level, will improve the health of every organ in the body. But the breasts are particularly likely to be affected, because the breasts are located in the fourth emotional center, which is associated with the ability to express joy, love, grief, and forgiveness, as well as anger and hostility. If those emotions are blocked, then the health of all the organs in the fourth emotional center, which include the lungs and heart as well as the breasts, may suffer.

Forming loving relationships that nurture us, and nurturing ourselves directly through the choices we make about how we live our lives, can help us to create breast health. Such nurturing is not selfish; in fact, it allows us to have within us something that is worth giving to others. Here again we can look to breast-feeding for the wisdom inherent in our bodies. Both the quality and quantity of a mother's milk are improved when the mother herself is well rested, well nourished, and happy. We need to remember this lesson at midlife, when the opportunity for transformation is boundless and the costs of turning our backs on it may be very high.

Midlife Breast Pain

Because of the hormonal changes associated with perimenopause, many women experience breast pain, especially during the second half of the menstrual cycle, from ovulation through the onset of menses. Often because of skipped ovulations and overstimulation by estrogen, breast pain comes and goes seemingly at random. This problem often subsides on its own and is not a sign of cancer. Dietary improvement, taking a good multivitamin, and adding iodine supplementation often quell the inflammation that causes the pain. (See chapter 6, "Foods and Supplements to Support the Change.") Also, eating foods such as cruciferous vegetables and flax can help. Breast expert Dixie Mills, M.D., finds that a sonogram or thermogram is often very reassuring for women who are really worried.

Many times breast pain is a sign that a woman needs to do some emotional updating. The following story is a wonderful example of the power of mind-body breast healing at midlife.

CATHERINE: Fibrocystic Breasts

Catherine had fibrocystic breasts that had hurt premenstrually for as long as she could remember. Around the time she turned forty, the pain and lumpiness increased to the point where she had only one pain-free week a month. She quit drinking caffeine, took every supplement she had heard might help, used castor oil packs, and regularly went for acupuncture treatments. She also saw an herbalist who created an herbal remedy just for Catherine. "My breasts were taking over my life!" she told me. Her doctor was sympathetic but said he wasn't sure what else she could do that she wasn't already doing and, trying to be reassuring, told her that as fibrocystic breasts go, hers weren't all that bad.

Then she went to visit her family for two weeks over Christmas. She was in such a rush taking care of last-minute shopping and errands before she left that she forgot to pack her supplements. "Without having to focus on pill-popping, rushing around to practitioners, or figuring out how to tactfully ask my friends about their breasts, I found that mine started hurting less," she discovered. "But I knew that the fact that I wasn't taking any supplements and was spending less time worrying about my breast pain was not causing the pain to go away. What I realized was that I needed to pay more attention to this problem on a different level." She decided to take an inventory.

In so doing, she realized that the pain had first come on strong during another family visit about four years ago. The trigger was a comment her uncle made in jest about her grandmother complaining about her breasts hurting all the time. "I was very close to my grandmother," Catherine told me, "and my uncle and mother regularly made comments I perceived as negative about her, many of them in the context of how she and I had a special relationship—the subtext being that those negative comments they made about her were also meant to apply to me."

Catherine realized that while she had recognized her emotions on an intellectual level, she hadn't really allowed herself to feel them completely. Remembering that one of her yoga instructors used to say, "In order to heal, you have to feel," Catherine decided to dedicate her yoga and meditation practices to those emotional elements that might be contributing to her breast pain. "I literally dedicated my practices to my breasts!" she told me, and also to the practice of forgiveness, which is a wonderful tonic for all fourth-emotional-center manifestations (including breasts, lungs, heart, and shoulders). For the next several months, she let go of a lot of unspoken anger toward her family, much of it anger she had held in her whole life. And it worked. "While my family needs a lot more support from me lately due to my uncle going through the last stages of lung cancer and an incredible amount of drama surrounding this," she reports, "my breasts are fine—no matter what I put into my body, caffeine included. Since I started letting go of the emotional baggage through forgiveness, my breasts have, in effect, forgiven me. It is truly a miracle."

BREAST CANCER RISK FACTORS

Midlife is also the time when, statistically speaking, your chances of getting breast cancer are on the rise. In fact, for women living in industrialized societies, age is first on the list of established risk factors for breast cancer.[1] But that's only because age is generally associated with the cumulative risk of unhealthy lifestyle patterns. Remember—the vast majority of women *don't* get breast cancer.

~ Age (over fifty years old; risk increases with age until eighty)

- Early onset of menstruation (before age twelve)
- Family history of breast cancer, in either a first-degree relative (mother, sister, daughter) or a second-degree relative (maternal or paternal aunt, grandmother)
- Late menopause (after age fifty-five)
- Giving birth to a first child after age thirty
- No full-term pregnancies
- Long-term hormone therapy (greater than five years)
- Benign breast disease with biopsy showing atypical hyperplasia
- Significant weight gain after menopause
- Regular alcohol consumption
- Low levels of vitamin D
- History of high-dose radiation to the chest
- Not getting enough sleep at night

Note: Early or surgically induced menopause decreases the risk for breast cancer.

THE EMOTIONAL ANATOMY OF BREAST CANCER

Like all diseases, cancer has an emotional component as well as a physical one. Many women with breast cancer have a tendency to hide their emotions behind a stoic face and to stay in relationships where they give much more than they receive. The core belief at the heart of this behavior is that we have to earn love through acts of service because we're not worthy of anything better. And we're willing to stay rather than risk being alone.

The refusal to honor and express our own emotions can sometimes reach pathological extremes. A woman once came to see me because she said she was having trouble breathing. She arrived alone and unsupported, and the tests I had done on her soon confirmed my fear that her breast cancer, which had been diagnosed a year before, had spread to her lungs. She had never sought treatment for her condition because she had not wanted to "inconvenience" her husband or her children. In fact, she had not even let them know about her illness. I told her as gently as possible that her choices, though made in the spirit of generosity and self-sacrifice, were not really helping anyone, least of all herself. She needed support and nurturance, and her family needed to be included in what was happening to her.

In my experience, many women have been denying their needs for so long that they do not even know they have them. One of my friends recalled growing up with a mother whose automatic response to any desire she ever expressed was "Don't ask, don't even think about it." Imagine what that does to a person's ability to ask for what she needs, to express her feelings honestly or to even know what they are! No wonder so many women will do almost anything to avoid appearing self-centered—to the point of putting themselves at risk of dying of a terminal illness.

There are now many scientific studies confirming the idea that our emotional style may influence both the incidence of breast cancer and our ability to recover from it. One study, for example, involving 119 women between the ages of twenty and seventy who were referred for breast biopsy because of suspicious breast lumps, looked into the impact of adverse life events on the likelihood of the breast lump being cancerous. Severe crises such as divorce, death of a loved one, or loss of a job in the five years preceding the breast lump did indeed increase the chance of its being cancerous. But, interestingly, the *way* in which a woman dealt with adversity was also a significant factor in whether she developed cancer. Those who had allowed themselves to experience their grief fully when they confronted devastating losses were three times *less* likely to suffer from breast cancer than those who hid their emotions behind a brave face or submerged their grief in various forms of activity.[2]

Clinical psychologist Lydia Temoshok, Ph.D., shares similar ideas in the book *The Type C Connection* (Random House, 1992), which she co-authored with Henry Dreher. Drawing on hundreds of case histories, she identifies what she calls the Type C behavior pattern: those who are unfailingly pleasant, self-sacrificing, compliant, and appeasing—and also unable to express their emotions, especially anger. This behavior pattern, Dr. Temoshok discovered, is associated with various cancers, including breast cancer.

"The most common comment of this kind of cancer patient with breast or gynecological cancer is, 'I'm not worried about me, I'm only worried about my family,'" notes Dreher. "Those patients with thicker and far more aggressive and life-threatening cancers were more severely self-sacrificing and nonexpressive of their needs and feelings."[3]

Not allowing ourselves to grieve or express anger uses up vital energy, depriving us of the resources we need to heal. No wonder the late Lewis Thomas, M.D., president of Memorial Sloan Kettering Cancer Center in New York City, wrote, "I have come to believe that cancer is the physical metaphor for the extreme need to grow."

At times of loss we must go through the painful and difficult process that I refer to as radical surrender: we must surrender to a power and order that is bigger than we are. Call it what you will—God, the universe, whatever—we must allow this power to heal our lives, and this can happen only through cleansing our physical vessel through the full emotional expression of our grief and anger. In fact, the full expression of anger is often a pathway to truly healing grief.

Another study showed that a woman's feelings about the communication between her and her family, and about the availability of help from her family, affected the function of her immune system and therefore her ability to recover. Women with breast cancer who perceived a lack of social support were found to have immune system depression and a poorer prognosis.[4] On the other hand, social support doesn't have to be from your family to have a positive impact on survival. Studies have shown that breast cancer or other support groups characterized by open and honest sharing of experiences are associated with increased longevity and decreased rate of tumor recurrence.[5]

MARY: *The Ten-Year Plan*

Mary was forty-one when she called a medical intuitive for a reading. Married to a fiercely competitive businessman who spent more time on the road than he did at home, Mary longed for the day when her husband's business would finally be self-sustaining enough to allow him to stop traveling so much. She herself had once been a high-powered executive in the computer industry but was now a stay-at-home mom with two children, ages six and nine. As part of the ten-year plan for work, finances, and family that she and her husband had developed, she had left her career in order to devote herself full-time to rearing the two children they had and the two they were planning to have in the time remaining on that plan.

The problem was that only five years into the plan, Mary was exhausted. She was putting off having a third child until she could get a handle on why she felt so terrible all the time. She wanted to know what her body was trying to tell her through her fatigue. That was why she had scheduled a reading with an intuitive.

Her intuitive reading revealed an energy pattern that was like that of "a widow pacing back and forth on a widow's walk, forever looking out to sea, waiting and pining for her husband to return." This kind of yearning and longing pattern, if held long enough, tends to manifest in the organs of the fourth chakra—and especially the breasts.

At this point, Mary revealed that she had, in fact, been diagnosed with breast cancer four years earlier. The surgery, chemotherapy, and radiation seemed to have successfully eradicated the cancer, but she still felt completely drained by the experience.

Mary knew that something was painfully out of balance, but she didn't know exactly what. She missed her old job and was aware that staying home didn't suit her temperament, but she felt that she should just suck it up and learn to make the best of it in the interest of the plan she had agreed to. She was also aware of how much she longed for her husband to share in the raising of their children, but felt she couldn't voice this longing because it would interfere with his ability to complete his part of the ten-year plan.

So many women can relate to this. We need to know that all illness is a hologram that contains genetic, environmental, physical, nutritional, emotional, spiritual, and behavioral aspects simultaneously. For Mary, the understanding of that hologram required her to question the validity of the plan that had locked her and her husband into a way of life that was in fact unsatisfactory to both of them. Her breast cancer had been a signal to her, and the fatigue that had enveloped her ever since then was another signal. Both were persistent indicators of unrecognized and unmet needs. Her task was to articulate her needs first to herself, and then to her husband and family. One of her unmet needs was for the intellectual stimulation of work outside the home. She had to admit that she was not temperamentally suited to be a stay-at-home mother. Some women would, of course, thrive in such circumstances if, like Mary, they had the economic wherewithal to support that lifestyle. Mary just didn't happen to be one of them.

Up until her reading, Mary hadn't allowed herself to truly feel her level of dissatisfaction with her life. Not realizing that she had a choice, she had fallen into a very common trap for all of us—a trap in which we talk ourselves into putting up with our circumstances because we have been taught that we ought to be able to just grin and bear it, to stuff our emotions and needs and get on with it. Sometimes this is the case—and being able to sit with discomfort for a while is an important life skill. But many times, if we speak up about a need, we have choices we didn't realize we have. And we have needs that we don't even recognize until they manifest in our bodies. Both Mary and her husband were wedded not just to their plan but to an outdated view of gender roles: the woman is to be the full-time nurturer, the man the good provider. At first Mary blamed herself for her own unhappiness and inability to "get with the program." She beat herself up for wanting to get out of the house and thought it meant that she was not a good mother. She thought she needed to squelch these feelings, not use them to articulate and act on her legitimate needs and desires. Mary's unhappiness seemed to her to be her own fault, a sign that she was not a good mother—so it was something she thought she needed to fight against, not act on.

Though the particulars of Mary's story are unique, the basic dilemma is not. But there's a way out. Own your feelings—all of them, including the unpleasant ones like anger, guilt, sadness, and resentment. Connect those feelings with the unmet needs they signify. And get professional help if necessary.

PROGRAM FOR CREATING BREAST HEALTH

Breast health is achieved through the energetic influence of self-nurturance, releasing resentments, and participating in relationships in which we both give and receive wholeheartedly. As with every other bodily organ system, however, our breasts are also greatly affected by what we eat and by other lifestyle choices. This comprehensive program addresses all these factors and will help you achieve maximum breast health throughout your life.

~ BE HONEST ABOUT WHAT YOU'RE FEELING. I highly recommend the website for the Center for Nonviolent Communication (www.cnvc .org), founded by the late Marshall Rosenberg, Ph.D., on which there is a list of emotions and a list of the needs they signal. Go through your own circumstances and have a trusted friend listen for the unspoken "need" that that emotion is signaling. You'll be amazed at how freeing this can be.

Consider the previous story about Mary. Like many women with breast cancer, Mary appeared to be too sweet and nice, despite being in a very difficult situation. She'd say things like "It's not that bad. It's okay, I can handle it," and then two seconds later mention how frustrated she actually was with her situation. Her response reminded me of an episode of the old TV sitcom *Golden*

Girls, in which Blanche was trying to come to grips with her son's decision to marry a much older woman who was pregnant with his child. When a friend of hers asked her what she planned to do, she replied, "Do what mothers always do. Tell my son I love him and that anything he does is fine with me, then complain like hell to anyone else who will listen." This pattern, though funny in a sit-com, is exactly what creates disruption in the energy of our fourth emotional center.

Creating health instead of havoc in your emotional centers requires you to extinguish those "I'm fine" phrases from your vocabulary when they are covering up real and painful emotions that need to be expressed. You may need to work with a therapist to help you learn how to be honest first with yourself and then with your mate or other family members.

You also need the courage to be honest with yourself about any aspect of your life that you aren't ready to change. Given our cultural inheritance about our breasts, it is little wonder that women's fear of breast cancer far overshadows our risk for those things that are more likely to kill us either directly or indirectly, such as heart disease or being battered by a husband or boyfriend. *I've come to believe that the fear of breast cancer serves to numb us to what we're really afraid of—being abandoned and left alone while continuing to pine for true love and the improvement of the relationship we're in.* (When my colleague, breast expert Dixie Mills, M.D., read this, she said, "This sentence is so important, I wish there were a way to make it stand out.") One of my patients, a woman with breast cancer who was also supporting her husband financially and had the means to change her life, finally admitted to me that she continued to stay in her loveless marriage because it felt so much easier for her to die than to risk being the one to be abandoned or left alone first.

⁓ CREATE A LIFE PLAN. You have the power to improve your relationships and love life right now! This process begins with improving your relationship with yourself. Draw up a one- or two-year life plan just for yourself (not for your mate or family members). Spend at least thirty minutes dreaming about how you'd like to fill your time, where you'd like to go, whom you'd like to be with, and so on. When we went over the life plan concept with Mary, she admitted that even the thought of having a third child exhausted her. Gradually she began to come to terms with the fact that the two additional children called for in their infamous ten-year plan might not be right for her. Clearly Mary's body in general, and her breasts in particular, had been trying to tell her this for a long time.

~ CREATE AN ENERGY BUDGET. Draw up a balance sheet with one column listing the activities that rejuvenate you and the other listing the activities that drain you. Then make a daily expenditure plan that tips the balance in favor of rejuvenation. (If you have young children, for example, I'd suggest that you trade off childcare with other mothers or grandmothers in your neighborhood.) Commit to engaging in at least one activity per week that is pleasurable to you—regardless of what your family members think of it. Understand that this is a process, not a destination. Believe it or not, it took me four years to tell my then-husband that I was getting massages every month. Until then, even though I had made them part of my regular schedule, I didn't have the courage to admit to him that I was actually spending time and money on something so nurturing and pleasurable that didn't have an immediate, tangible payoff. I look back on who I was then, and I'm astounded by how much of my power I donated to him. Now, years later, I enjoy a massage every week, and I cannot even imagine having to run my expenditures by anyone but myself. What a huge revelation!

~ MAINTAIN A RELATIONSHIP WITH YOUR OWN CREATIVITY, PLEASURE, AND NEEDS. My colleague Regena Thomashauer, founder of Mama Gena's School of Womanly Arts, points out that daily doses of pleasure are as life-sustaining for women as vitamin C was for sailors in order to prevent scurvy. She insists that if we fail to consciously bring pleasure into our lives, we are at risk for scurvy of the soul. I completely agree. Don't allow your creative pleasure to wither or permit your true self to get lost in the daily grind of living. If you're not working a regular job, consider taking a class or engaging in some other stimulating activity on a regular basis. I've found time and again that the very act of having a schedule tends to help us conserve and direct our energies. (I always practiced my harp with much greater focus when I knew I had a performance coming up.) There is no substitute for having some order, discipline, and structure in your daily life. Just be sure that you are creating the structure, not the other way around.

~ PERIODICALLY REEVALUATE YOUR GOALS AND PLANS. I do this each year around my birthday, and also during the solstices and equinoxes of the year—times when the creative energies of the earth are maximally available to us. Let go of anything that is clearly obsolete and incompatible with your emerging inner wisdom. Mary told me later that when she asked her husband how *his* body was responding to their ten-year plan, he told her that his old ulcer had been acting up lately. But he hadn't wanted to share that with her, because he felt that he needed to show his love and support for his family by remaining a "good provider." This is an example of how a basically good marriage can change and grow when people are honest with each other—and themselves—about their needs.

‾ CONCENTRATE LESS ON A DIET THAT AVOIDS FAT AND MORE ON AVOIDING SUGAR AND REFINED CARBOHYDRATES. For many years, doctors (including myself) recommended a low-fat, high-fiber diet, especially for women at high risk for breast cancer. Such a diet increases the excretion of excess estrogen, making it less likely that estrogen-sensitive breast tissue will be overstimulated. However, the connection between fat and breast cancer is not as straightforward as previously thought, according to data from the famous Nurses' Health Study, which included an analysis of the diets of 88,795 women, ages thirty to fifty-five, who had completed detailed questionnaires about their eating habits every four years from 1980 to 1994. This phase of the study focused on fat because it was known that Asian women, who eat a diet much lower in fat than ours, also have a much lower rate of breast cancer. However, breast cancer was found to be no more common among the women in the Nurses' Health Study who ate a lot of fat than among those who consumed less than 20 percent of their calories in the form of fat. Furthermore, there appeared to be no difference in breast cancer incidence among those who ate saturated fats, or even the infamous trans fats, versus those whose fats were derived mainly from vegetable sources or from fish.

In response to these surprising results, the study's lead author, Michelle Holmes, M.D., an instructor of medicine at Harvard, said, "Our research indicates it's highly unlikely that women who consume a low-fat diet are protected against breast cancer. Equally, it appears that a high-fat diet also poses no increased risk for the disease."[6]

Though I would have been surprised by this study back in the 1980s, I'm not surprised now. Breast cancer is multifactorial, with nutritional, emotional, and genetic aspects. Nutritionally, it's becoming clear that sugar and refined carbohydrates are a far bigger risk factor for breast cancer than dietary fat content, but unfortunately they weren't taken into account in this study. Nor were other factors that may help account for the low rate of breast cancer in Asian women. The different micronutrient intake, the high intake of plant hormones such as the isoflavones found in soy, and a lower amount of refined carbohydrates in their diet may all turn out to be factors that lower breast cancer risk.[7]

On the other hand, a diet that is too high in refined carbohydrates causes higher insulin levels, which in turn raises levels of a substance known as insulin-like growth factor (IGF-1). This substance affects the growth of breast cells in utero, during puberty, and during adult life. Breast cancer is definitely associated with abnormal IGF-1 activity. High insulin levels also trigger a metabolic cascade that results in cellular inflammation, and inflammation is a precursor for cancer. (See chapter 7.) High insulin levels also suppress sex-hormone-binding globulin (SHBG), which ordinarily circulates through the body binding estrogen and lowering its activity. With less SHBG in the bloodstream, more biologically active estradiol reaches the breast tissue and stimulates its growth. Over the course of many years, this relative excess of estrogen may increase the risk of breast cancer.[8]

A 2005 study conducted in Italy found a direct association between breast cancer risk and consumption of sweet foods with high glycemic index and load (including biscuits, brioches, cakes, puffs, ice cream, sugar, honey, jam, marmalade, and chocolate), which increase insulin and insulin growth factors.[9] A later study following data from more than 334,800 European women for eleven and a half years found that those women who ate a diet high in sugars and carbohydrates had up to a 41 percent increased risk of developing ER-negative breast cancer (the deadliest kind).[10]

I would like to make it clear that I have a fundamental problem with any approach, dietary or otherwise, that promises to "prevent" anything. Although there is an extensive body of evidence supporting the hormone-balancing and health-enhancing effects of the nutrient-dense, insulin-balancing diet I've suggested, here's the problem: even women who eat perfectly sometimes get breast cancer. If you make food choices only out of the desire to "prevent" something, then by the law of attraction, you'll actually be carrying the energy of the disease you're afraid of right into your body along with the healthy food!

In the Nurses' Health Study mentioned above, for example, the nurses who ate the lowest amount of fat (less than 20 percent of their daily calories) actually had the highest rate of breast cancer in the group. Though surprising at first glance, these data support a link between breast cancer and self-sacrifice, an association that has been scientifically documented. If you are afraid of breast cancer, it will not be helpful for you to become a dietary martyr, always depriving yourself of the foods you love and find nurturing. Imagine eating a small green salad, all the while craving something more substantial, and thinking, "Well, I'll deprive myself because I'm preventing breast cancer." Does this feel nurturing or healthy to you? It doesn't to me. (Personally, I can't imagine living well without some high-quality chocolate!)

Above all, I urge you to nurture yourself fully every day by eating food that is delicious as well as healthy. Eat well, because doing so is a way of reaching your full potential.[11]

⁓ EAT LOTS OF VEGETABLES, FRUITS, AND FLAXSEED, CHIA, OR HEMP SEEDS. Research has shown that women who excrete the highest amount of lignans—which are formed in the intestinal tract from plant materials—have the lowest risk for getting breast cancer.[12] The food source with the highest known concentration of health-promoting lignans is flaxseed. I suggest that you consume ¼ cup of freshly ground flaxseed daily. Diets high in plant materials also tend to be higher in fiber, which has been shown to help the body excrete excess estrogen in the stool.[13] Start with 1 tablespoon per day and work up. (I have a small coffee grinder that I use only for flaxseed.) Chia seeds come already milled in a product called Mila that I also use. Hemp comes ground as well.

Numerous studies have also demonstrated that fruits, vegetables, and seasonings—such as broccoli, kale, collards, cabbage (the cruciferous vegetables), tomatoes, turmeric, garlic, and onions—contain antioxidants and other phytochemicals that protect against cell damage and mutation caused by free radicals. They may also block carcinogens from reaching or reacting with critical target sites throughout the body.[14] Indole-3-carbinol, the active estrogen-modulatory ingredient in the cruciferous vegetables, is also available in supplement form.

Two recent large-scale studies are particularly telling. The first of these is a 2017 study using data from more than 60,000 midlife women in the Netherlands who were followed for more than twenty years. Researchers found that those who ate a Mediterranean diet (based on fish, fruit, nuts, whole grains, and olive oil) had a 40 percent reduced risk of ER-negative breast cancer (considered the deadliest form).[15] The second is a 2018 analysis of data from the Women's Health Initiative Observational Study, which followed more than 161,000 postmenopausal women diagnosed with breast cancer in the 1990s.[16] In this new analysis, researchers compared the outcome of women who didn't change their diets after receiving their diagnosis to those who reduced their intake of dietary fat by 20 percent by eating significantly more fruits and vegetables. Ten years later, 82 percent of the women who made dietary changes were still alive, compared to 78 percent of the control group. This is not a huge difference, but it is significant. The bottom line is that diet can make a truly remarkable difference.

— EAT FOODS RICH IN PHYTOHORMONES. Foods such as soy, flaxseed, hemp, or chia often help women with breast tenderness and pain, and they may even offer protection for women with breast cancer, or with high risk for it, thanks to isoflavones, which protect estrogen-sensitive tissue against overstimulation by estrogen.[17]

Some women have expressed concern about the phytoestrogens (estrogens from plants) in some herbs recommended in menopause. None of the breast cancer risks associated with estrogen replacement apply to the consumption of these plant hormones. The plant hormones found in whole soy foods, dong quai, maca, *Pueraria mirifica*, chasteberry, and black cohosh have never been associated with the promotion of breast cancer in any study. In fact, many studies have shown that they are protective because of their adaptogenic qualities, meaning their ability to modulate the activity of estrogen in our bodies in a healthful, balanced way. The Shanghai Breast Cancer Survival Study, published in 2009, reported that the more dietary soy women eat—whether soy protein or soy isoflavones—the lower their risk of death and recurrence of breast cancer.[18] (This held up whether or not the cancer was estrogen-receptor-positive or estrogen-receptor-negative and whether or not the women took tamoxifen.) A 2010 study on postmenopausal breast cancer patients receiving adjuvant endocrine therapy showed that those with estrogen- and progesterone-receptor-positive cancers who had a high dietary intake of soy had a lower risk of recurrence.[19] Yet another study, this one from the University of New Mexico, looked at more than 500 postmenopausal breast cancer survivors. Those who reported taking phytoestrogens had lower levels of serum estrogens than those who didn't take them.[20]

The herb *Pueraria mirifica* has actually been found to stop the growth of breast cancer cells in vitro.[21] Multiple studies in both Thailand and in South Korea report that the miroestrol in this potent phytoestrogen increases the expression of the beta-estrogen receptor, and thus the ratio of the beta-estrogen receptor relative to the alpha-estrogen receptor, resulting in an antiproliferative effect. This effect is even stronger at higher concentrations of the herb.[22]

~ EAT OMEGA-3 FATS. Studies have shown that women whose diet is high in omega-3 fats have a lower risk for developing breast cancer. Research has also shown that supplementing the diet with omega-3 fats can create a healthier ratio of omega-3 to omega-6 fats in breast tissue within three months.[23] I've had several patients who have had significant softening of firm scar tissue around their breast implants when they've supplemented their diets with omega-3 fats daily. A diet that contains adequate amounts of omega-3 fats also helps prevent inflammation and tumor growth throughout the body. The 2010 Vitamins and Lifestyle (VITAL) cohort study of more than 35,000 postmenopausal women showed that those who took fish oil supplements had a lower risk of ductal breast cancer.[24] Omega-3s are so powerful that they are even helpful for those already diagnosed with breast cancer. A French study published in 2009 showed that breast cancer patients whose cancer had spread and who had an expected survival time of about fourteen months boosted their survival an average of eight additional months if they took daily 1.8-gram DHA supplements for two to six months. Half the women in the study were able to boost their survival time for an average of nearly three full years on this regimen.[25]

You can get enough omega-3 fats by eating salmon, sardines, or swordfish two or three times per week. Or you can take 200–2,500 mg per day of DHA or fish oil supplements with both DHA and EPA (start with 400 mg per day combined and work up to as high as 5,000 mg per day if needed). Another convenient source of omega-3 fats is ground flaxseed, chia, or hemp seeds. These seeds are true perimenopausal superfoods, and I recommend ¼ cup per day to all women.

~ GET ENOUGH VITAMIN D. Clinicians are increasingly finding low serum levels of vitamin D in women with breast cancer (and other cancers as well). Those with the lowest levels (less than 25 ng/dl in blood) have the highest risk. Studies by Cedric Garland, Dr.P.H., of the University of California, San Diego, School of Medicine and other prominent vitamin D researchers show that if women in the United States could keep their blood levels of vitamin D at 40–60 ng/ml year-round, it would prevent 58,000 new cases of breast cancer (and 49,000 new cases of colorectal cancer) each year.[26] Dr. Garland's research also shows that women with vitamin D levels above 52 ng/ml can cut breast cancer risk in half.[27] A 2018 study showed a 78 to 82 percent lower risk of breast cancer for women fifty-five and older who had vitamin D levels of 60 ng/ml or higher compared to women with less than 20 ng/ml.[28] The same group of researchers had shown two years previously that even levels of 40 ng/ml or higher in the same age group reduced risk by 67 percent.[29]

Women already diagnosed with breast cancer can benefit from optimal levels of vitamin D as well. Breast cancer patients with very low levels of vitamin D are more likely to have aggressive tumors and are 73 percent more likely to die, according to research presented at the 2008 annual meeting of the American Society of Clinical Oncology.[30] A study published the following year showed breast cancer patients with low levels of vitamin D were almost twice as likely to have their cancer spread and were also 1.7 times as likely to die.[31]

We've been brainwashed into avoiding the sun, and women don't get nearly enough vitamin D in food or supplements. There are vitamin D receptors on all the immune system cells and optimal amounts of this hormone/vitamin are essential for proper immunity. In addition to moderate sunlight exposure (about ten minutes or so per day), most people need 5,000–10,000 IU of vitamin D_3 per day to maintain optimal blood levels. This will also help to increase bone density. Be sure to get enough vitamin K_2 as well. (See chapter 12.) It's interesting that a thirty-minute sunbath over most of the body in a light-skinned individual will produce about 10,000 IU of vitamin D under the skin. The body will never produce a toxic level of vitamin D from sunlight alone.

You can order a kit to test your own vitamin D levels by joining the D*action Breast Cancer Prevention Project, the world's largest project designed to solve the problem of vitamin D deficiency (see https://daction.grassrootshealth.net). Members receive information on specific health topics as they relate to vitamin D as well as access to an online health portal that allows them to track their test results and any lifestyle changes they make along with the outcome. The project gives you the option of taking just one vitamin D test or enrolling in the full five-year project, which involves filling out an extended health questionnaire and having your vitamin D levels checked every six months for the five-year period.

~ INCREASE YOUR IODINE INTAKE. Iodine is vital for breast health because it reduces breast pain when taken in adequate amounts—

and at high enough levels, it may even prevent breast cancer. But most American women consume only a fraction of what they really need of this nutrient. The RDA for iodine in adult women is 150 mcg, but current research shows that for optimal health of the breasts, ovaries, and uterus, women need significantly higher amounts. I recommend a dose of 3 to 12.5 mg daily—some women require even more.

In one U.S. study of women with breast pain, more than half those who took 6 mg of iodine daily reported a significant reduction in their symptoms, with relief starting after three months of treatment.[32] In a Canadian study, 72 percent of women with fibrocystic breast disease (FBD) who took iodine therapy reported improvement.[33] (Although the vast majority of breast lumps are indeed benign, studies have shown that 30 percent of the 25 million women in the United States who suffer from FBD have a two- to tenfold greater risk for developing breast cancer, so this is clearly *not* a condition to ignore.)[34]

Compelling evidence also exists for a strong relationship between iodine levels and breast cancer. A 2005 study done in Mexico showed that rats taking iodine treatments exhibited a "strong and persistent reduction" in incidence of breast cancer, possibly because of iodine's antioxidant nature.[35] Even more impressive is a 2006 study from India reporting that molecular iodine causes programmed cell death in human breast cancer cell cultures.[36]

Not surprisingly, in populations with low iodine intake, breast cancer rates are higher, and in cultures where iodine intake is higher, breast cancer rates are lower.[37] For example, the lowest rate of breast cancer in the world is in Japan, where the average iodine intake is about 45 mg per day. By comparison, the average intake in the United States is more than 180 times lower—only 240 mcg—and is continuing to decline.

Iodine works in part because it decreases the ability of estrogen to adhere to estrogen receptors in the breast.[38] The ductal cells (the breast cells most likely to become cancerous) actually have an iodine pump in them, which shows that they have the ability to actively absorb iodine. Iodine can also stop excess cell growth in the ovaries and uterus.

Iodine provides antiseptic mucosal defense in the mouth, stomach, and vagina, which boosts the immune system, protecting cells from environmental and chemical toxins. Low levels of iodine can increase the amount of circulating estrogens in breast tissue, making the breasts a target for toxic estrogens.[39] This nutrient is easily one of the most powerful antiviral and antibacterial substances we know of, although, unfortunately, most doctors think of iodine only in terms of thyroid health and remain vastly unaware of its many additional advantages. (For further information on iodine, read the book *Iodine: Why You Need it, Why You Can't Live Without It,* 5th edition [Medical Alternative Press, 2014] by David Brownstein, M.D.; if you have Hashimoto's thyroiditis, however, you may need far less iodine than Dr. Brownstein recommends in his book because iodine can exacerbate Hashimoto's and accelerate thyroid cell destruction.)

Several options exist for boosting iodine levels. You can eat sea vegetables or take supplements such as kelp, Lugol's solution (which is made up of molecular iodine and potassium iodide), or Nascent iodine drops (see www.thyroidnascentiodine.com, which has a great deal of good information), based on the work of the psychic Edgar Cayce, who channeled a way to make the iodine work better. The drops make it very easy to titrate your dose so you can take exactly the right amount for you.

You can also boost your iodine levels by applying a tincture of iodine to your skin. To do this, paint a quarter-size dot of iodine directly on your skin (you can opt to apply it to a painful spot on your breast or on the nipple, for more direct relief) once a night for two weeks. (If you get a reaction from iodine—usually seen as a skin rash or a bad taste in your mouth—just decrease your dose and proceed more slowly. This reaction, known as iodism, happens when iodine compounds cause the release of excess bromide, fluoride, and other toxins from the system, so it's really more of a detox reaction than an iodine reaction per se.)

Before you start supplementing, it's a good idea to take a twenty-four-hour urinary iodine loading test to accurately gauge your iodine levels. I recommend the one from Hakala Research Laboratory, which is available at LifeSpa, the website of John Douillard, D.C. (see www.store.lifespa.com/product/iodine-deficiency-test).

Be aware that if you are taking thyroid medication, increasing your iodine intake may decrease or even eliminate your need for thyroid drugs. Too much thyroid hormone can cause heart palpitations, so be sure to discuss your iodine supplementation with your healthcare provider, and even then, increase your iodine levels very, very slowly.

~ TAKE COENZYME Q_{10}. Coenzyme Q_{10} (also known as ubiquinone) is present naturally in the body and in organ meats. It has been shown to improve immune system functioning. Hundreds of studies have also demonstrated its ability to help those with congestive heart disease. Several studies have demonstrated that women with breast cancer have deficiencies in coenzyme Q_{10}. Taking coenzyme Q_{10} in relatively high doses, 90–350 mg per day, has been associated with partial or complete remission of breast cancer.[40] In chapter 7 I recommended that all perimenopausal women take 50–100 mg per day. If you are at high risk for breast cancer, I'd increase the dose to 70–200 mg per day. Since statin drugs (prescribed to lower cholesterol) decrease levels of coenzyme Q_{10}, all women on these drugs should take this supplement.

A WORD ABOUT UNDERWIRE BRAS

Medical intuitive Julie Ryan reports that she is consulted by many women who get breast cysts right along the area of the breast where the underwire of a bra goes—particularly near the arm. This makes perfect sense because most of the lymph nodes that drain the breast area are in the underarm area, where a part of the breast known as the tail of Spence is located. When you wear an underwire bra, you are cutting off the flow of lymph, blood, and also life energy to that part of the body. I wouldn't go so far as to tell you that wearing an underwire bra causes breast problems, but it certainly doesn't help anything.

There's a reason why so many women take off their bras the minute they get home from work or an evening out. We intuitively know that the breasts and chest area need to be free from constriction. There is also absolutely no research that proves that wearing a bra prevents breast sagging over time.

That said, put wearing underwire bras into the same category as wearing high heels: reserve them for special occasions and short periods of time. They should not be everyday choices. And if you must wear an underwire bra for some reason, take it off as soon as it is feasible.

I also recommend that you massage the area underneath your breasts and up into your armpit as soon as you remove the bra, as a way to enhance blood and lymph circulation and energy flow to this area of the body.

MULTIVITAMINS AND BREAST CANCER RISK

For overall good health, including breast health, I recommend taking a good multivitamin daily—in part because the antioxidants contained in them (as well as in fresh foods) help to quell cellular inflammation. Chronic cellular inflammation in women diagnosed with breast cancer may also increase the chances of cancer recurring, according to a 2009 study published in the *Journal of Clinical Oncology*. Researchers found that elevated levels of C-reactive protein (CRP), which is a marker for cellular inflammation, even when present as long as seven years after the women were successfully treated for early-stage breast cancer, were associated with reduced survival rates.[41] Even in women not yet diagnosed with breast cancer, elevated CRP levels might be an important warning sign, according to a 2015 metanalysis conducted by Chinese researchers looking at fifteen studies on a total of more than 5,000 breast cancer patients.[42]

~ MODERATE ALCOHOL CONSUMPTION. Many studies have linked the consumption of alcohol with increased risk for breast cancer, with the latest research showing that alcohol use is more strongly associated with hormone-sensitive breast cancers than hormone-insensitive cancers.[43] The risk increases with the amount of alcohol consumed. In the Nurses' Health Study, for example, researchers found that the risk of breast cancer in women who had one or more drinks per day was 60 percent higher than the risk in women who did not drink.[44] In addition, a 2009 study by researchers at the Fred Hutchinson Cancer Research Center in Seattle who looked at breast cancer survivors showed that those who consumed an average of one drink per day had a 90 percent increased risk of cancer recurring in their other breast.[45] Part of the alcohol-breast cancer connection is due to alcohol's effect on the liver's ability to process estrogen effectively.

For women who are taking oral estrogen replacement therapy, the risk of drinking alcohol may be even higher. In one study, women on oral estrogen and synthetic progestin replacement who drank the equivalent of half a glass of wine experienced an increase of 327 percent in blood estradiol levels, a rise that didn't happen in women not on oral hormone therapy. Significant rises in estradiol were noted within ten minutes after drinking the alcohol.[46] In the Nurses' Health Study participants this was prevented in those women whose average intake of folic acid was at least 600 mcg per day. (I recommend 800 mcg per day as methylated folate for everyone.) Alcohol is a known inhibitor of folic acid, and folic acid (especially in methylated form) is required for DNA repair mechanisms. High folic acid intake may therefore prevent some of the gene mutations that lead to cancer.[47]

Another part of the alcohol–breast cancer link is that women too often use alcohol as a way to stay out of touch with the painful feelings of sorrow, anger, and pining for love and relationship that may be associated with increased risk for disease in the fourth chakra organs.

⁓ DON'T SMOKE. A study published in the *Journal of the American Medical Association* in 1996 noted that a flawed enzyme present in millions of Americans (in half all white women and in an even larger number of those of Middle Eastern descent) may raise the risk of breast cancer in women who smoke. Of those with the flawed enzyme, heavy smokers who had reached menopause had about four times the risk of breast cancer as nonsmokers. Postmenopausal women who had the flaw and who had smoked any amount at or before age sixteen also ran a similar risk, which supports the theory that exposure to certain toxic substances adversely changes the way DNA gets expressed during the stages of life when breast tissue is developing.[48] The researchers from the 2009 Fred Hutchinson Cancer Research Center study mentioned above also found that breast cancer survivors who were current smokers had a 120 percent increased risk of developing a second breast cancer.

Smoking, like alcohol consumption, also tends to shut down the energy of the fourth emotional center, rendering us numb to the situations we're in and less capable of doing anything to change them for the better.

⁓ EXERCISE REGULARLY. As many studies have shown, regular exercise decreases the risk of breast cancer considerably, along with all its other well-documented benefits.[49] This is because it normalizes insulin and blood sugar levels and also tends to decrease excess body fat, all of which keep estrogen levels normal. A *New England Journal of Medicine* study showed that women who exercise for about one hour four times per week reduce their breast cancer risk by at least 37 percent.[50] The same study showed that in women who exercised the same amount but whose body mass index was less than 22.8, the risk of breast cancer is cut by 72 percent! You don't need to do strenuous exercise to get this benefit. Walking, gardening, and dancing will all do fine. And it's never too late to start. According to the National Institutes of Health–American Association of Retired Persons Diet and Health Study, published in 2009, postmenopausal women who maintain a regular exercise program of moderate to vigorous intensity reduced their breast cancer risk even if they did not exercise in the past.[51]

~ GET ENOUGH SLEEP. Women who consistently sleep nine hours or more a night have less than one-third the risk of breast tumors compared with those who get seven or eight hours of sleep nightly, according to a 2005 Finnish study of more than 12,000 women.[52] Several studies have shown that exposure to light late at night may increase the risk of breast cancer. The reason is that nighttime light (if it's bright) interrupts the production of the hormone melatonin.[53] Harvard researcher Eva Schernhammer, M.D., Dr.P.H., showed that women with above-average melatonin concentrations are less likely to develop breast cancer.[54] (Dr. Schernhammer's previous research found that female night-shift workers have about a 50 percent greater risk of developing breast cancer than other working women.)[55] So be sure to get plenty of sleep in a dark room every night. (Using a night-light, if it is dim, is not associated with higher risk.) I personally always sleep with an eye pillow filled with flaxseed and scented with lavender. Not only is this deeply relaxing, but it also keeps out ambient light.

~ PRACTICE MIND-BODY TECHNIQUES. It's no secret that many different mind-body practices improve health on all levels, including for those with serious health challenges. A 2015 study done in Canada found that cancer patients who attended support groups that encouraged meditation, yoga, and sharing their feelings instead of suppressing them had a greater chance of survival.[56] The researchers divided eighty-eight breast cancer survivors into three groups. One group attended eight weekly sessions where they received instruction on mindfulness meditation and gentle hatha yoga (while also practicing at home daily). A second group attended twelve weekly sessions where they were encouraged to talk openly about their concerns and their emotions. A control group attended a single six-hour stress management seminar. The researchers measured the subjects' telomeres before and after the study. Telomeres are protein caps on the end of chromosomes that determine how fast a cell ages; shorter telomeres have been associated with cellular aging and disease, while longer telomeres seem to be protective.[57] After three months, the women in the two support groups maintained their telomere length, while the women in the control group who received no mind-body support had shorter telomeres.

BREAST CANCER SCREENING

Most women have been taught that regular mammograms and breast self-exams are the key to breast health. And while there is indeed heartening evidence that the mortality rate for breast cancer is decreasing, this decrease is most likely due to overdiagnosis, because we're now diagnosing more pre-cancers that never would have resulted in death in the first place.

It is also generally accepted that the drop in breast cancer incidence itself is secondary to the decrease in the use of Premarin and Provera (or Prempro) following the termination of the Women's Health Initiative in 2002.[58]

Though screening may be an important part of early detection, keep in mind that mammograms, breast exams, sonograms, and MRIs do not actually *prevent* breast cancer. At best, they diagnose it at an earlier and presumably more treatable stage. This has been the basis of the conventional approach to breast cancer for the past thirty years or so. Unfortunately, this approach is not nearly as clear-cut as we once thought it was. I'm also concerned that the massive national campaigns aimed at getting women to have regular mammograms have taught an entire generation that breast cancer screening is synonymous with creating breast health. Participating in disease screening is no substitute for learning and practicing the preventive, health-building thoughts and behaviors that can transform us.

Every perimenopausal woman needs to know about the limitations of screening and take responsibility for creating healthy breast cells daily by nurturing herself with healthy food and supplements, avoiding excessive alcohol, stopping smoking, and engaging in mutually satisfying relationships.

The Pros and Cons of Early Detection

The idea that breast cancer can be cured by early detection and prompt treatment rests on the belief that all breast cancers grow at the same rate. They don't. Some cancers grow rapidly and others slowly, which is one of the reasons why just about every one of us has heard about or knows a woman whose regular mammogram screening was normal but who was diagnosed with breast cancer several months later. One possible explanation for this is that mammography screening is far more likely to detect slow-growing, nonaggressive tumors than the kinds of cancers those women had. A study conducted at Yale–New Haven Hospital of all the women who received their first treatment for breast cancer in 1988, for example, showed that those women whose cancers were detected via mammography screening alone had an excellent prognosis, not just because of early detection, but because the cancers so detected were relatively slow-growing or even dormant, thus requiring minimal therapy. Many of the women, for example, had a condition known as ductal carcinoma in situ (DCIS), a type of breast pathology that can often remain completely dormant for a woman's entire life.

In fact, autopsy studies of women who died of other causes, such as accidents, have shown that 40 percent have some degree of DCIS in their breasts.[59] Other studies have confirmed that the incidence of DCIS has increased more than fourfold since 1980; this type of cancer now accounts for a quarter of all cancers detected by mammogram. The main reason for this dramatic increase is the widespread use of mammographic screening. H. Gilbert Welch, M.D., a researcher at Dartmouth-Hitchcock Medical Center and author of the must-read books *Should I Be Tested for Cancer? Maybe Not and Here's Why* (University of California Press, 2004) and *Overdiagnosed* (Beacon Press, 2012), puts the dilemma well when he writes, "Our ability to detect subtle forms of breast cancer is a two-edged sword. On the one hand, it offers the hope of preventing some cases of advanced breast cancer through early detection and treatment. On the other hand, it fosters increased worry and labels more women as having disease, many of whom would never develop invasive cancer."[60]

Additional striking research adds more weight to Welch's findings. A study published in the November 2008 edition of *Archives of Internal Medicine* indicates that some breast cancers regress on their own, without any treatment.[61] This important study followed more than 200,000 Norwegian women between the ages of fifty and sixty-four over two consecutive six-year periods. Half received regular, periodic breast exams or regular mammograms, while the others had no regular breast cancer screenings. The study reported that those women receiving regular screenings had 22 percent more incidents of breast cancer. The researchers (as well as another team of doctors who did not take part in the study but who did analyze the data) concluded that the women who didn't have regular breast cancer screenings probably had the same number of occurrences of breast cancer, but that their bodies had somehow corrected the abnormalities on their own. This makes complete sense given that our bodies routinely produce abnormal cells that are then destroyed by our immune systems before becoming a problem.

Because of just such evidence, the American Cancer Society finally shifted its position about cancer screening, admitting that early detection—especially for breast (and prostate) screening—has been overstated. For every hundred women who are told they have breast cancer, for example, as many as thirty have cancers that are so slow-growing that they are unlikely to be life-threatening.[62] "The health professions have played a role in oversimplifying and creating the stage for confusion," Barnett S. Kramer, M.D., associate director for disease prevention at the National Institutes of Health, told *The New York Times* in 2009. "It's important to be clear to the public about what we know and be honest about what we don't know."[63]

And yet, major medical organizations such as the American Cancer Society and the American College of Obstetricians and Gynecologists continue to support the regular use of mammography for women starting in their forties. When the United States Preventive Services Task Force (an influential government-appointed group giving guidance to doctors, insurance companies, and policymakers) revised their guidelines in 2009 to say mammograms should begin at age fifty, the American College of Radiology was so opposed to the change that it even went so far as to ask the task force to reverse its recommendation! I, for one, applauded the new guidelines, knowing full well the limitations of mammography and the fact that mammograms have consequences that are far from benign.

The DCIS Dilemma

DCIS, or what is now erroneously being called stage 0 breast cancer, presents a real dilemma for women and doctors alike. Although our increasingly sensitive technology keeps improving our ability to detect early forms of breast cancer, our understanding of what to do with this knowledge is lagging behind.

What is clear is that in the majority of women DCIS does not go on to become invasive cancer. Recall the fact that in autopsy studies, 40 percent of healthy women in their forties who died in accidents were found to have evidence of DCIS. The fact is that 98 percent of the time, DCIS doesn't spread—and women don't die from it, which means that only minimal treatment (if any) is necessary. Yet many women with DCIS are told that they have breast cancer and are then subjected to very aggressive treatment: surgery (often mastectomy), sometimes followed by radiation, tamoxifen, or both. Because conventional screening modalities cannot identify which types of DCIS or which women are likely to progress, doctors feel obligated to treat everyone as though they are cancers waiting to happen. Given the fear of breast cancer, many women with DCIS understandably decide to be treated. The Yale investigators in the study above, for example, noted that of the thirty-one women with DCIS in their study, all of whom survived without recurrence, fully 48 percent underwent mastectomies. The authors noted, "Since none of these patients had cancer death or recurrence, regardless of the extensiveness of treatment, the need for aggressive forms of therapy might be reconsidered."[64] That's one of the understatements of the decade. The high rate of DCIS that is picked up on mammograms may also be a factor in the much-celebrated reduction in breast cancer mortality that we've seen over the past twenty years; the women so diagnosed would not have died in any case. They'd die with their so-called disease, not from it.

Breast-Screening Concerns

Several years ago I gave a lecture in California to a group that included physicians, allied healthcare professionals, and others interested in a more holistic approach to health. I presented the data on mammograms and DCIS and suggested that women may want this information when making decisions about if, when, and how often to have mammograms. I was dismayed by the reaction.

In the ladies' room during a break, women from the audience were confused and upset. They deeply believed in mammograms and felt safe when they had them. I had introduced doubt. I couldn't help wondering if, by telling the truth about the diagnosis and treatment questions raised by our improved technology, I had inadvertently broken my Hippocratic oath: "First, do no harm." But I decided that confusion is often the first step on the road to clarity and personal power. If a period of uncertainty and questioning was required for these women to rely more on their inner wisdom, then I figured that over the long haul I'd done more good than harm. After all, there is nothing benign about surgery, radiation, and drug therapy, with all their well-known side effects, when they aren't absolutely necessary.

When I came back from the ladies' room I was met onstage by an infuriated radiologist who ran a breast screening center. "You're dangerous. Do you know that?" he spat at me. "I cannot believe that you're telling women this stuff. I am so disappointed in you. You're putting women's lives at risk." He wasn't interested in the scientific reasons for my statements, and it was clear to me that we weren't about to have a balanced discussion about the mammogram issue. His mind was made up. Then and there I learned directly and painfully that when it comes to breasts and mammograms, emotions run very high, and this has nothing to do with science.

In January 1997, the National Institutes of Health convened a panel of prestigious experts who spent six weeks reviewing more than a hundred scientific papers and hearing thirty-two oral presentations on this issue. When they concluded that there wasn't enough evidence to recommend routine mammography screening for all women ages forty to fifty, they, too, were met with vicious attacks.[65] In an editorial on the subject, which also included a reply to one radiologist's particularly vehement objections, Kenneth Prager, M.D., the chair of the Ethics Committee at Columbia-Presbyterian Medical Center in New York, wrote, "Could it be that the radiologist who vilified the panel's conclusion has not only the welfare of women in mind but radiologists' own wallets, in view of the millions that would be spent in the wake of an official recommendation for all women in their forties to undergo mammography?"[66] Nothing much has changed over the past fourteen years. The first time some organizations' mammogram guidelines called for a reduction in mammography for women in their forties (in 2009), there was the same hue and cry. So much for science.

I have long agreed with Cornelia Baines, M.D., professor emerita at the University of Toronto and former deputy director of the Canadian National Breast Screening Study, who wrote in 2005, "I remain convinced that the current enthusiasm for screening is based more on fear, false hope, and 'greed' than on evidence."[67] This remains true today.

The argument isn't just over whether or not annual mammograms are cost efficient or even whether they save lives. The debate is also bringing to light the fact that routine annual screening may actually cause harm. First of all, the procedure itself isn't always benign. A 1994 study in the *Lancet* showed that the breast compression required by mammograms may cause small, in-situ tumors to rupture, spreading cancer cells into surrounding tissues and possibly resulting in more invasive cancers and metastases.[68]

But the most frequent harm done by routine screening involves the incidence of false positives (saying that there's something abnormal when there isn't), which occur in about 10 percent of mammograms. And this risk increases over time. In 2000, the *Journal of the National Cancer Institute* pointed out that the cumulative risk of having false positive mammograms is quite significant in many women. By the ninth mammogram, the study reported, the false-positive risk can be as high as 100 percent in women with multiple high-risk factors.[69] Another study estimated that after ten mammograms, about half of all women (49 percent) will have had a false positive result, which will have led to a needle biopsy or an open biopsy in 19 percent.[70] A Danish study found that false positive diagnoses can cause long-term psychosocial consequences equivalent to those seen in women who did indeed have breast cancer.[71]

In two reviews published in the *Lancet,* Danish researchers Ole Olsen and Peter Gotzsche examined seven randomized, controlled mammography studies and found that the screening tool not only didn't save lives but also often led to needless treatments and were linked to a 20 percent increase in mastectomies—many of them unnecessary.[72]

A groundbreaking *New England Journal of Medicine* article published in 2012 concluded that 1.3 million women over the previous thirty years had been overdiagnosed (and so overtreated), accounting for nearly a third of all newly diagnosed breast cancers.[73] The researchers reported that "screening is having, at best, only a small effect on the rate of death from breast cancer." A study published the following year showed that for every 2,000 women receiving mammograms over the course of ten years, only one would avoid dying of breast cancer and ten healthy women would be treated unnecessarily.[74] And still another study published in the *Journal of the American Medical Association* found that women age seventy and older benefited very little from mammography.[75] The cancers detected at this age would never have killed them.

The most extensive collection of DCIS data analyzed so far is a

2015 study conducted in Toronto that followed more than 100,000 women who had been diagnosed with DCIS for twenty years.[76] Researchers found that these women had nearly the same chance of survival whether they had lumpectomies or mastectomies—proving that more aggressive treatment isn't helpful or needed. Less than 1 percent of the women in the study died of breast cancer, with death rates higher mostly for women under age thirty-five and for African American women. Those who died of cancer did so despite receiving treatment, not from the lack of it. Interestingly, their chance of dying from breast cancer (about 3.3 percent) was the same as it is for women in the general population. In other words, DCIS is not a death sentence.

It's clearly time for the medical profession to change its approach to DCIS. Breast surgeon Laura Esserman, M.D., of the University of California, San Francisco, has been instrumental in this effort. Since 20 to 25 percent of breast cancer diagnoses today are DCIS, she notes, we would see the number of invasive breast cancers drop as more DCIS is detected with screening if this condition were truly the precursor for a more deadly form of breast cancer—yet that's not what's actually happening.[77] Esserman believes DCIS should therefore be seen as a risk factor for invasive cancer, not a precursor, so we can instead concentrate on helping reduce their risk, possibly with hormonal or immunological therapies designed to make breast tissue less hospitable to cancer cells.[78] Not seeing DCIS as true carcinoma, Esserman has called for this diagnosis to instead be called "indolent lesions of epithelial origin," or IDLE.[79] I wholeheartedly concur.

Esserman is currently leading the Women Informed to Screen Depending on Measures of Risk (WISDOM) study, a multicenter trial begun in 2016 that is evaluating the effectiveness of a more personalized approach to screening.[80] This randomized trial of 100,000 women is comparing the outcome of risk-based screening (screening at intervals based on each woman's risk as determined by her genetic makeup, family history, and other risk factors) to simply receiving annual mammograms.[81] Women deemed at high risk will receive recommendations to start screening at an earlier age, have more frequent mammograms, and continue screening until they are older. Those with the lowest risk profile will be advised to begin having mammograms later, screen less frequently, and stop having mammograms at an earlier age. No one in the trial will receive less than the recommended level of screening in the current United States Preventive Services Task Force guidelines, For more information on this study and how to participate, see www.thewisdomstudy.org.

Shelley Hwang, M.D., chief of breast surgical oncology at the Duke University School of Medicine in Durham, North Carolina, is another champion for this cause. "Because [DCIS] is a pre-invasive or pre-cancerous lesion," she noted in a 2018 *Medscape* article, "it really does not have the ability to spread to any other part of the body. If you catch it at that stage, women are almost 100 percent cured. I think we can make the argument, and many of us do, that many women are cured of a diagnosis that would not have caused them any harm during their lifetime."[82]

Hwang, like Esserman, believes active surveillance may well be the best course of action to take after a DCIS diagnosis, rather than aggressive therapy. She's one of several researchers involved in the Comparison of Operative to Monitoring and Endocrine Therapy (COMET) trial, which started in 2017. COMET is the first large phase III randomized clinical trial in the United States to look at different management strategies for DCIS. The researchers are following 1,200 women at about a hundred cancer centers across the country. Half are receiving the current standard treatment, while the other half are being closely monitored with more frequent follow-up exams and tests, progressing to biopsy and surgery only if these tests show changes that require further evaluation. COMET is also considering quality of life along with cancer outcome.

Remember, surgery is not a cure for anxiety. To me, the DCIS dilemma for women is similar to what men diagnosed with early-stage prostate cancer face. Active surveillance is the widely accepted management strategy for low-risk prostate cancer since the vast majority of men so diagnosed will die with this cancer, not from it (as is true for women with DCIS). Far fewer men opt for surgery or radiation to "cure" their condition, knowing they would risk erectile disorder, urinary incontinence, and bowel issues. Men don't sacrifice their organs nearly as much nor as willingly as women do. A recent study from Memorial Sloan Kettering Cancer Center in New York City showed that while one in three men pursuing active surveillance for low-risk prostate cancer is anxious at first, most adjust rapidly.[83] After five years, only 20 percent reported anxiety, and after ten years, the figure dropped to 10 percent. So if men can do well with active surveillance, I believe women with DCIS can do the same.

MRIS AND BREAST CANCER DETECTION

Magnetic resonance imaging (MRIs) are becoming increasingly popular methods of breast cancer detection, and at least 27 percent of women diagnosed with breast cancer opt for pretreatment MRIs to gather information for deciding what treatment they want to pursue. But research suggests that these MRIs may do more harm than good. A 2009 study from the prestigious Fox Chase Cancer Research Center in Philadelphia found women diagnosed with breast cancer who got MRIs delayed their treatment by an average of three weeks and increased their rate of mastectomy by 80 percent (thanks to the high rate of false positives with MRIs), although the pathology reports done after the mastectomies indicated that many of these women would have been good candidates for lumpectomy.[84]

THE PROMISE OF THERMOGRAPHY

Thermography (infrared imaging) is a noninvasive, safe technology that records the amount of heat emanating from breast (or other) tissue, thus detecting inflammation long before the appearance of a tumor. This technology certainly isn't new. It dates back to World War II, when U.S. planes used it to identify active enemy missile silos. Its first medical application was in the 1950s, more than a decade before the introduction of mammography.

According to thermography expert Philip Getson, D.O., when used as part of a comprehensive multifaceted approach, thermography can lead to early detection of 95 percent of early-stage cancers, which increases the long-term survival rate by as much as 60 percent. He adds that when it's done properly, thermography has an average sensitivity and specificity of 90 percent, meaning that 90 percent of the time, scans do not indicate problems that don't really exist nor do they fail to indicate a problem when one really does exist. Some studies show an even better track record. For example, a 2003 study of 769 women who had suspicious mammograms followed by thermograms showed that the thermograms were 97 percent correct in detecting breast cancer.[85] Thermograms can generally detect abnormal activity eight to ten years before any other screening test.[86]

Dr. Getson, an associate professor of medicine at Drexel University College of Medicine in Philadelphia, has been a medical thermographer since 1982, the year the FDA approved thermography as an adjunctive breast-cancer screening test. Certified by four thermographic boards, he lectures extensively on thermography and has interpreted more than 10,000 images. I asked him to share his thoughts on the benefits of thermography, and here is what he had to say:

> Thermography detects the physiologic changes in the breast tissue that have been shown to correlate with cancerous or precancerous states. It is widely acknowledged that cancers, even in their earliest stages, need nutrients to maintain or accelerate their growth. In order to facilitate this process, blood vessels remain open, inactive blood vessels are activated, and new blood vessels are formed (a process known as neoangiogenesis). This vascular process causes an increase in surface temperature in the affected regions, which can be viewed with infrared imaging cameras. Additionally, the newly formed or activated blood vessels have a distinct appearance that thermography can detect.
>
> Since thermal imaging detects changes at the cellular level, studies suggest that this test can detect activity eight to ten years *before* any other test.[87] This makes it unique in that it affords us the opportunity to view changes before the actual formation of the tumor. Studies have shown that by the time a tumor has grown to sufficient size to be detectable by physical examination or mammography, it has in fact been growing for about seven years, achieving more than twenty-five doublings of the malignant cell colony. (At ninety days, there are two cells; at one year, there are 16 cells; at five years, there are 1,048,576 cells, which is still undetectable by a mammogram; at eight years, almost 4 billion cells.)
>
> Thermography is unaffected by breast density, implants, or scars from surgery. It allows for the avoidance of potentially harmful radiation, a known carcinogen. Radiation from routine mammograms poses significant cumulative risk of initiating and promoting breast cancer. In fact, a mammogram results in a thousandfold greater radiation exposure than a chest X-ray. Additionally, each rad (radiation absorbed dose) of exposure in-

creases breast cancer risk by 1 percent annually, an extremely worrisome statistic for premenopausal women whose breasts are more sensitive to radiation. Premenopausal women who get annual mammograms for ten years are exposed to a total of ten rads for each breast. Over a thirty-year time frame (from ages forty to seventy, for example), that amounts to a cumulative dosage of 30 rads of radiation per breast. By comparison, Nagasaki atomic bomb survivors absorbed an average of 32 rads of radiation.

Breast thermography is a noncontact test. Conversely, mammography involves placing the breast between two plates and subjecting the breast to painful compression. The recommended force to be used for the compression of breast tissue in a mammogram is 300 newtons, the equivalent of placing a fifty-pound weight on the breast.

All of this information became even more important on November 16, 2009, when the U.S. Preventive Services Task Force Breast Cancer Screening Recommendations for the General Population was released, changing a long-standing position regarding mammography. Prior to that, in April 2007, the American College of Physicians issued new guidelines that urged women in their forties to consult with their doctors about whether to have a mammogram. These guidelines were then quickly endorsed by the U.S. Preventive Services Task Force, which issues the federal government's official recommendations on preventive medicine.

According to the 1998 *Merck Manual*, for every case of breast cancer diagnosed each year, five to ten women will needlessly undergo a painful breast biopsy. Therefore, statistically, each woman who undergoes annual screening mammograms for ten years has at least a 50 percent chance of undergoing a breast biopsy.

Compare that to breast thermography, which has been researched for more than forty years with a database of more than a quarter of a million women. There are more than 800 peer-reviewed thermographic studies. This research has concluded that a persistently abnormal thermogram is consistent with a twenty-two-fold increase in the risk of developing breast cancer. An abnormal thermogram is ten times more significant as a future risk indicator for breast cancer than a first-order family history of the disease. An abnormal infrared image is the single most important marker of high risk for developing breast cancer.[88] Because of the safety inherent in the test, thermography can be performed on an individual of any age, including those who are pregnant or breast-feeding.

It is true that not all thermographic equipment is the same, nor is every center backed by qualified, board-certified physicians who are specifically trained in the interpretation of these images. Women (and men) seeking to have infrared imaging should ask the following questions:

1. What is the "drift factor" in the apparatus? Anything over 0.2 degrees Centigrade leads to poor reproducibility.

2. What are the credentials of the interpreting physician?

3. Is the room in which the study is performed free of outside light and the temperature always kept at 68–72° F with a proper cooling system in place?

4. Are the images marked up for future comparison?

5. Are the studies read on-site or sent by email to a distant interpreter?

6. Is the physician available to explain and discuss all findings?

In my opinion thermography is the best screening method currently available. Although it is not a diagnostic procedure, one of its great strengths is that it allows a woman and her healthcare practitioner to be proactive about breast health. Because thermograms show subtle changes that occur long before the formation of a tumor, a woman whose scan indicates inflammation can take several steps to decrease the inflammation before returning for a follow-up thermogram to determine if she has been successful. Only when the thermographer deems a scan to be highly abnormal and suspects cancer would a patient need to follow up with a mammogram to confirm the diagnosis. Further, a woman diagnosed with DCIS can use a thermogram (in conjunction with advice from her healthcare providers) to help decide if her treatment should be aggressive or conservative. Thermograms are also better than mammograms for telling the difference between harmless fibrocystic masses and more suspicious lumps.[89]

Here's the empowering story of how one woman is using a combination of thermography with mammograms to avoid overtreatment:

Fifteen years ago, a routine mammogram revealed microcalcifications along the milk duct in my right breast. I had a biopsy that, fortunately, showed the microcalcifications were benign. Five years later, a few more showed up. Both years the microcalcifications appeared had been particularly stressful years when I was doing a lot of caretaking for others but not a lot for myself. Intuitively, I knew this stress was connected to what the mammograms were picking up. I decided to refuse a second biopsy, which unlike the first was not fully covered by insurance and would have cost me $8,000 out of pocket. Instead, I chose to monitor the condition with annual mammograms.

In the meantime, I also did some energy work on myself after I noticed a dark, heavy spot in the energy field above the breast with the calcifications. I imagined drawing in pure love and exhaling it into the dark spot until I felt it dissolve. I consulted an energy healer, who basically saw the same thing (without me sharing any information with him about my condition) and who also did energy work on me.

The following year, my mammogram showed one new microcalcification, and I again refused a biopsy. I have sometimes skipped my annual mammogram since then, but I haven't had any more microcalcifications show up—not a one. Two years ago, I decided to have thermography done to establish a baseline. There were some mildly warm spots around the edges of my breasts but nothing near where my microcalcifications are.

Next, I scheduled a free annual mammogram. I had no issues. I waited a year to get a mammogram again and learned it would now include an ultrasound, something I'd never had that was now included for free. The mammogram showed no new microcalcifications. However, I was told that the ultrasound showed I have an "architectural distortion." These are usually, but not always, benign. I was told that to be sure that the ultrasound wasn't "picking up on something," I should get a diagnostic mammogram [basically the same procedure as a regular screening mammogram but with extra images for a more thorough look]. How about just a repeat ultrasound? I suggested. After all, I knew they usually cost $100 or $200 out of pocket compared to $800 for a diagnostic mammogram. No, I was told, that wasn't possible.

With no baseline ultrasound for comparison, I immediately went for a second thermogram. It showed no hot spots in my breasts. In fact, the new thermogram looked even better than the baseline one had! That made me feel quite confident in skipping a diagnostic mammogram and second ultrasound. I just can't see the point of testing beyond what I've done! I have no history of breast cancer in my family, and I maintain an optimal vitamin D level.

I'm happy to say that my team of doctors and technicians honored my choice. I didn't get the "be afraid, be very afraid" vibe from them. This was in stark contrast to when I had the diagnostic mammogram after the last microcalcification was found, when the technician actually said to me, "I know you have really bad breasts that are dense because they're big." I gently suggested that might not be the best way to think or talk about a woman's breasts!

I've decided to continue having regular thermograms and free screening mammograms with ultrasounds, too. If something new shows up that needs further testing, I'll consider my options. I'm glad I had the courage to do my homework, ask good questions, use alternative screeners, and listen to my instincts.

Thermography can be used on any area of the body—not just the breasts—to identify and track inflammation and to improve overall health. While it is not usually covered by insurance (and can cost anywhere from $90 to $250 for a scan), this has more to do with politics and economics than science. (To find a practitioner in your area who does thermography, visit www.breastthermography.com; www.breastthermography.org; or the websites for the International Academy of Clinical Thermology, www.iact-org.org, or for the American College of Clinical Thermology, www.thermologyonline.org.)

Yet another method of breast cancer screening that doesn't involve radiation is currently being studied. Diffuse optical tomography (DOT) uses near-infrared light to create images that determine blood flow to the tissues and measure changes in the amount of oxygen in them.[90] While this method (which first emerged in the 1990s) is still being perfected, many researchers believe it has much promise. One 2011 study predicted DOT "will completely change our method of breast cancer screening and therapy monitoring in the future."[91]

My Breast Screening Suggestions

~ TRANSFORM THE REGULAR BREAST SELF-EXAM (BSE). For decades, women have been encouraged to examine their breasts regularly as a way to find breast cancer at the earliest possible stage, get it treated early, and thus save their lives. This has led to a "search-and-destroy" approach to breast exams that encourages you to make your hands into mine sweepers in search of something that may kill you. No wonder so many women skip this routine but end up feeling guilty as a result. As the late Francis Moore, M.D., of Harvard Medical School wrote, "What man would enjoy lowering his trousers in front of a mirror once a month and examining his testicles carefully, by rigorous palpation, looking for testicular tumors?"[92] Still, no one seriously questioned the advisability of doing regular BSEs until 2002, when the results of a large randomized trial of BSE were released, showing that the practice didn't change breast cancer mortality.

The study involved over 260,000 women in Shanghai, who were divided into two groups and followed for five years. Half the group was trained in BSE and had that training reinforced at the workplace, while the other half, the control group, had no training in BSE nor were they encouraged to perform BSE of any kind. At the end of five years, the study found that those women in the BSE group found more benign breast lumps than the control group, but their breast cancer mortality was not reduced at all. The death rate from breast cancer was the same in both groups. The study authors concluded that "women who choose to practice BSE should be informed that its efficacy is unproven and that it may increase their chances of having a benign breast biopsy."[93] A smaller but still substantial 1999 study done in Russia followed 57,712 women who did BSE and another 64,749 in a control group, reporting similar results.[94]

In November 2009, the tide turned for good when new breast cancer screening guidelines from the United States Preventive Services Task Force recommended that doctors no longer teach this practice.[95] This guidance was reaffirmed with the latest recommendations in 2016.[96] The American Cancer Society, the American College of Obstetricians and Gynecologists, the Canadian Cancer Society, the Canadian Task Force on Preventive Health Care, the World Health Organization, the U.S. Preventive Services Task

Force, and the U.K. National Health Services all no longer recommend routine BSE.

But even if you don't perform monthly BSEs (and I, for one, don't recommend them), that doesn't mean that you shouldn't get to know your breasts. It simply means that a paradigm shift is called for. When a woman attends to her breasts with loving care and a loving consciousness on a regular basis, it is entirely possible that she will be influencing her breast cells in a positive, health-enhancing way. That's why I recommend a monthly breast self-massage as a healthy and viable alternative to the outmoded BSE. (Do not do this if you have been recently diagnosed with breast cancer, because it may increase tumor spread; it's fine once treatment is finished.) Many women never touch their breasts with love or tenderness, having been led to believe that their breasts are the property of their mates and not really part of their own bodies. Invite your breasts into your life by getting to know them and touching them regularly. Then your regular breast self-exam becomes an opportunity for healing. Breast massage activates lymph drainage, increases blood flow, and oxygenates tissue—all good ways to help create breast health. After all, for millions of years of human evolution, women nursed babies for most of their re-

FIGURE 18: THE LYMPH SYSTEM

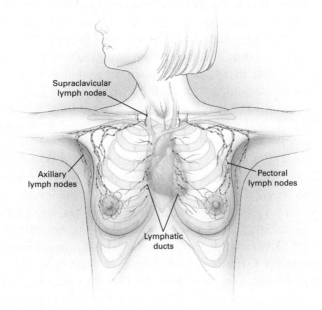

productive years, a process that provides a great deal of breast stimulation. This massage can also be done by your partner in a nonsexual, supportive way.

Here's a technique developed by Dana Wyrick, who practices lymphedema therapy at Mesa Physical Therapy/San Diego Virtual Lymphedema Clinic in San Diego, California.[97]

Self-Massage of Chest and Breast

I recommend doing this massage in the most pleasurable environment possible—for example, in a rosewater-scented bath with your favorite music playing. Do each side of your chest independently. Instructions below are for the left side; simply reverse "hand" instruction to do your right side. Use a light touch. Your object is to *move the skin,* not to massage the muscles. The following routine, when done properly, will assist the lymphatic capillaries in removing toxins and impurities from the body tissue. The stroking will also accelerate transport of impurities to the lymph nodes, where they will be processed and rendered harmless. Finally, cleansed lymph will be returned to the bloodstream, where the now-harmless impurities may be carried to the lungs, kidneys, and colon for elimination.

1. With the first three fingers of your right hand, locate the hollow above your left collarbone. Stroking from your shoulders toward your neck, lightly stretch the skin in the hollow. Repeat this movement five to ten times.

2. Now cover the hairy part of your left armpit with the fingers of your right hand held very flat. Stretch the skin of your armpit upward five to ten times.

3. Next, again using a flat right hand, lightly stroke ("pet") the skin from the breastbone to the armpit. Do this above the breast, over the breast, and below the breast, repeating each path five to ten times.

4. Finally, using a flat right hand, lightly stroke from your waist up to your armpit on your left side, repeating five to ten times.

Now change hands and massage the right side of your chest.

⁓ MAMMOGRAMS FOR WOMEN FIFTY TO SEVENTY-FOUR. The U.S. Preventive Services Task Force guidelines released in 2016 confirm their 2009 recommendation that most women start regular mammograms at age fifty instead of forty (which had been the previous standard).[98] The guidelines further suggest that women between ages fifty and seventy-four have mammograms only every other year. Ideally, mammograms should be done at a multidisciplinary breast center, where your film can be read immediately and where you can also get additional diagnostic procedures or treatment if necessary. Most major medical centers now have these centers. However, I continue to be concerned about the cumulative effect of yearly radiation on breast tissue health. (By the way, the guidelines do not recommend routine screening for women older than seventy-four because the risks and benefits remain unknown.)

The task force cited evidence that women in their forties are less likely to have breast cancer but nonetheless have a 60 percent greater chance of getting a false-positive result from a mammogram because of denser breast tissue, making the risks of routine mammograms for this group outweigh the benefits (a 15 percent reduction in breast cancer mortality).[99] The denser breast tissue is perfectly normal, although it often makes mammograms difficult to read and interpret because the X-rays can't penetrate it. About fifty out of a thousand women with dense breasts will require further diagnostic procedures, such as additional mammograms, sonograms, and even biopsies, to determine whether or not they have breast cancer. Of these, it is estimated that only two will have breast cancer.[100] The others will often go through a great deal of anxiety, which could be avoided if we were to use functional technologies such as thermography. Breast surgeon Dixie Mills, M.D., says, "I often recommend a woman get a baseline mammogram and see how dense her tissue is (a factor that cannot be determined by feel) and add this information into her choice of manner of screening. Women should not be made to feel that they are to blame for their breasts being dense; it is a factor of mammogram pictures being limited to shades of black and gray and white on a flat photo." (In older women this dense tissue is often replaced with fat, making mammograms more accurate.)

I have always individualized the mammogram recommendation depending upon the woman's risk factors and desires. I've also had many patients (and a number of good friends) who avoid mammograms altogether—as I myself have (full disclosure). I have respected this position for over thirty years, and with today's data on the limits of mammography, I respect it more than ever now. If you choose this option, let your doctor know that you're willing to be a partner in your healthcare and release her (or him) from liability for your decision to avoid mammography. Tell him or her that you're willing to put this in writing and sign it as a legal release form. Failure to diagnose breast cancer is one of the most frequent reasons for lawsuits against doctors!

The current guidelines do not apply to women at high risk for breast cancer because of a gene mutation that makes breast cancer more likely or because of previous extensive exposure to radiation. I recommend annual or biennial mammograms and/or sonograms or other screening if you have a positive family history for breast cancer or if you find that getting this screening puts your mind at ease. (Peace of mind produces very positive biochemical changes in the body.) If you have a first-degree relative who got breast cancer before menopause, consider annual screening mammograms starting five years before the age your relative was diagnosed.

In an ideal world, breast health screening would be done via thermography, using the right kind of equipment, and read by a professional who is fully trained in this area and who knows when a mammogram, ultrasound, or MRI would provide more information. I predict that this will be the medicine of the future when it comes to breast health. And it's all good!

Still undecided about what you should do? Try the National Cancer Institute's Breast Cancer Risk Assessment Tool (www .cancer.gov/bcrisktool), consisting of eight simple questions. The tool calculates both your risk of getting invasive breast cancer in the next five years as well as your lifetime risk, and it compares each to the risk for the average U.S. woman of the same age and race or ethnicity. This can be useful in helping you decide if mammograms are right for you, and how often you want to have them.

Let me also suggest another way that is not based on intellect and statistics, and which is not honored in any way by Western medicine: tuning in to your innate body intelligence. There are many ways to do this, including intuitive training, use of oracles, or consulting a medical intuitive.

If You Find a Breast Lump

⌒ IF YOU FIND A LUMP, GET A DIAGNOSIS. It's important to see a practitioner who can help you through the process of finding out whether your breast lump is benign or cancerous. Waiting and imagining the worst are obviously not healthy. Dr. Dixie Mills says, "Many women who come to see me have already reviewed their wills."

~ ALWAYS TAKE SOMEONE WITH YOU. Many women who have found a breast lump are too frightened and overwhelmed to ask questions and explore all their options with their doctor or other medical professional. Having a companion can help you focus; if he or she takes notes, you can review them together later.

~ DON'T LET ANYONE RUSH YOUR DECISION. Many options are available for the diagnosis and treatment of breast lumps, ranging from breast cyst aspiration to needle biopsy to open biopsy. Most breast lumps or thickenings actually turn out to be benign. Many are simply fluid-filled cysts, which can be aspirated right in the office. If the fluid is clear, you have both your diagnosis and treatment at the same time. I've watched women who are scared to death and even wind up having MRIs and mammograms for breast cysts that could have simply have been drained in the office. Nothing further needs to be done. Oftentimes breast lumps or thickenings are the result of hormonal stimulation and will go away after you get your period. This is particularly true during perimenopause, when estrogen overstimulation of breasts is so common. One of my patients developed large, painful lumps in both of her breasts throughout her perimenopause. This really scared her and also made it difficult to tell what was really going on in her breasts. After she finally had her last period, however, her breasts returned to their normal consistency, and her lumps went away for good.

~ GET A SECOND OPINION IF YOU'RE NOT COMPLETELY COMFORTABLE WITH THE FIRST. Even if you do have cancer, in the vast majority of cases your treatment will not be compromised if you take a couple of weeks or even months to find a doctor and a treatment plan you trust and feel comfortable with. Don't assume surgery followed by chemotherapy is your only choice. This was an important conclusion of the groundbreaking Trial Assigning Individualized Options for Treatment (known as the TAILORx trial), one of the first large-scale trials to examine methods for personalizing cancer treatment. TAILORx followed more than 10,000 women from several different countries (including the United States) who were diagnosed with early-stage breast cancer. The results, published in 2018, showed that for 70 percent of these women who have the most common type of breast cancer—hormone receptor (HR)-positive, HER2-negative, axillary lymph node–negative—chemotherapy resulted in no benefit, even after nine years.[101]

IF YOU HAVE BEEN DIAGNOSED WITH BREAST CANCER

Join a breast cancer or other support group in your area. Studies have shown that support groups characterized by open and honest sharing are associated with increased longevity and decreased rate of tumor recurrence. Besides, a support group is a very safe place to learn how to ask for what you need—or even discover those needs in the first place.

The following books and other resources provide powerful support for your inner wisdom during this time, as well as a wealth of practical information.

Radical Remission: Surviving Cancer Against All Odds (HarperOne, 2014) by Kelly A. Turner, Ph.D.

The Cancer Report: The Latest Research in Psychoneuroimmunology (How Thousands Are Achieving Permanent Recoveries) (Change Your World Press, 2005) by John Voell and Cynthia Chatfield

The Moss Reports by Ralph W. Moss, Ph.D., at www.mossreports.com

PUTTING BREAST CANCER RISK IN PERSPECTIVE

Most women grossly overestimate their risk for breast cancer. Surveys of women between the ages of forty-five and sixty-four show that 61 percent feared cancer (predominantly breast cancer) more than any other disease. Only 9 percent feared heart disease the most, despite the fact that it is the leading cause of death in women, claiming more women's lives each year than the next fourteen causes combined.[102] Breast cancer isn't even the leading cause of death from cancer in women. That distinction goes to lung cancer.

Though every one of us probably knows a woman with breast cancer, and though breast cancer is the second-most-common cancer among North American women (surpassed by lung cancer in 2012), the lifetime risk for breast cancer—the widely touted one-in-eight (or one-in-seven for Caucasian women) figure[103]—is a cumulative lifetime risk that applies only if you live beyond the age of eighty-five.[104] According to BreastCancer.org, a woman's risk of getting breast cancer is one in 1,732 at age twenty, one in 69 at age forty, and one in 29 at age sixty.[105] In addition, the one woman in eight who does develop breast cancer has a 60 percent chance of dying from another cause.

Kelly-Anne Phillips and her colleagues at Princess Margaret Hospital in Toronto, Ontario, Canada, have constructed a very helpful chart based on the 1995 incidence and mortality rates in the Ontario Cancer Registry. Here's what it shows.

Out of 1,000 females born healthy and alive:

~ *Ages 35–39:* 986 will be alive. Of these, 1 will get breast cancer, 0 will die from it, and 2 will die of other causes.

~ *Ages 40–44:* 983 will be alive. Of these, 5 will get breast cancer, 1 will die from it, and 4 will die of other causes.

~ *Ages 45–49:* 977 will be alive. Of these, 8 will get breast cancer, 2 will die from it, and 6 will die of other causes.

~ *Ages 50–54:* 968 will be alive. Of these, 11 will get breast cancer, 3 will die from it, and 11 will die of other causes.[106]

Here's another compelling reason not to let your fear run wild. In late 2020, Winnifred Cutler, Ph.D., of the University of Pennsylvania, along with a team of researchers from two other universities, published a meta-analysis of twenty-one previous breast cancer studies.[107] Of the more than 2.4 million pre- and postmenopausal women in their analysis, 99.7 percent of those who had no prior diagnosis of invasive breast cancer remained free of the disease after follow-up exams in subsequent years. Twenty-five years later, 93.41 percent of the women were still free of the disease.

The irrational fear of breast cancer creates a great deal of suffering for women and prevents many from enjoying the benefits of perimenopausal treatments—such as high-dose soy, bioidentical progesterone, low-dose bioidentical estrogen, and testosterone—that can relieve symptoms and help prevent diseases that are far more apt to be a threat to longevity or quality of life.

THE BREAST CANCER GENE: SHOULD YOU BE TESTED?

Fully 95 percent of all breast cancers have little or nothing to do with genetics. The rest are associated with inherited mutations in two different genes: BRCA1 and BRCA2. Women who inherit a BRCA1 mutation have a higher risk than those with a BRCA2 mutation. The most recent research shows that about 72 percent of women who inherit a BRCA1 mutation and about 69 percent of women who inherit a BRCA2 mutation will develop breast cancer by the age of eighty.[108] The same study showed that twenty years after receiving a diagnosis of breast cancer for the first time, about 40 percent of women with the BRCA1 gene and about 26 percent of women with a BRCA2 gene will develop cancer in the remaining breast. Though less is known about the BRCA2 mutation, it is estimated that it will account for an additional 40 percent of hereditary breast cancers.[109]

The implications of breast cancer gene mutations are difficult to determine, in part because the BRCA1 gene is very large and many different mutations have been found within it. One particular BRCA1 mutation has now been detected in approximately 1 percent of Jews of Eastern European descent (Ashkenazi Jews). Different mutations have been found in other populations. In addition, there are other gene pathways besides those governed by BRCA1 and BRCA2 mutations that may lead to breast cancer. When you add to this the technical problems of sequencing an entire gene, it is clear that genetic testing for breast cancer risk is an incomplete science. A negative test for the gene may have little meaning in a setting of a strong family history of breast and ovarian cancer.[110] On the other hand, if there is only one individual in the family with breast or ovarian cancer, the chances of this cancer occurring due to a mutation in either BRCA1 or BRCA2 is quite small.

Francis Collins, M.D., Ph.D., formerly of the National Center for Human Genome Research in Bethesda, Maryland, summarized the current dilemma associated with testing positive for the breast cancer gene.

> We are still profoundly uncertain about the appropriate medical care of women with these mutations. Despite the general usefulness of mammograms for the early detection of breast cancer in women over the age of fifty, there are no data to instill confidence that regular mammography at a younger age, in concert with self-examination and examination by doctors or nurses, will reduce the risk of death from metastatic breast cancer among very-high-risk women with BRCA1 mutations. We do not yet know the appropriate use of more drastic measures, such as prophylactic mastectomy, especially given the anecdotal evidence that cancer can still occasionally arise in the small amount of epithelial tissues remaining after surgery. . . . Clinical research is urgently needed to address all these uncertainties.[111]

However, a 2018 study of 2,733 women in the United Kingdom that's the largest to date comparing survival rates of breast cancer patients with and without BRCA gene mutations showed that having the mutation didn't influence survival, even after ten years, and that having a bilateral mastectomy did not improve the chances of survival.[112]

One more consideration before you opt for testing: though the Genetic Information Nondiscrimination Act (GINA) now protects those who test positive from health insurance discrimination and employment discrimination, the law grants no protection from life and disability insurance discrimination.

EPIGENETICS: THE SCIENCE OF THE FUTURE

In the documentary *The Living Matrix—The Science of Healing* (www.thelivingmatrixmovie.com), leading-edge scientists, physicians, and physicists, including Bruce Lipton, Ph.D.; former Apollo astronaut Edgar Mitchell, D.Sc.; and intention experiment originator Lynne McTaggart, convincingly demonstrate that we are far more than biochemical machines—and, most important, that there are energetic and electromagnetic force fields (which are related to thoughts and emotions) that profoundly affect our health and healing. These quantum fields of energy and information heavily influence our states of health and determine the environment in which a gene functions and how it gets expressed. Dr. Lipton cites data, for instance, that demonstrates that a baby who is adopted into a family in which many members get cancer will end up with the same risk of cancer as her adopted family, despite very different genes. The reason has to do with epigenetics—the science of how genes and the environment interact. It turns out that it is the cell membrane that is the brain of the cell, telling it what to do and what to let in. The genes in a cell, which reside in the nucleus, are more like gonads. They simply help the cell divide. The environment is what actually tells the cell what to do. Hence, even those with positive breast cancer genes (or any other genetic condition) need to realize that they are not mere victims of their genes—and that they have far more impact on their genes than they realize.

Here's the bottom line: genetic testing has great limitations and should be approached very cautiously. Though a negative test for the breast cancer gene can be a great relief for an individual with a positive family history for breast cancer, it's not a guarantee against getting breast cancer. I do not recommend being tested unless you have at least two or more close family members who've had breast or ovarian cancer.

You should also undergo thorough genetic counseling from a professional with extensive knowledge and training in the field, both before and after getting your test results. If your test is positive, seek medical care from a professional who is actively engaged in research protocols to further our knowledge of these disorders. The National Cancer Institute Cancer Information Service (1-800-4-CANCER) can supply information about genetic services at cancer centers supported by the institute.

A third option is genomic testing done by a physician skilled in nutritional and functional medicine, which may help you decrease your risks further through identifying lifestyle changes that may be of particular benefit to you. (See the website of the Institute for Functional Medicine at www.ifm.org.) It's also crucial to remember that many, many women have healed their lives—and their cancers— through lifestyle changes, which include updating old, outmoded, self-destructive childhood programming!

THE EFFECT OF HT ON BREAST HEALTH

Despite the fact that most women, with or without supplemental hormones, will not get breast cancer, the documented link between hormones and breast cancer is worrisome for everyone concerned. Nearly every woman asks, "What is the effect of hormones on my risk for breast cancer?" The answer depends on which hormones she is taking, what her dosage is, and what her inherent risk factors are to begin with. These issues were raised by a letter I received from a man concerned about his wife's hormone supplementation program.

My wife has recently switched from taking Premarin, which she originally took to quell hot flashes, to taking natural progesterone in the form of a skin cream. As a result, her breast pain and tenderness have gone away and so have her headaches. What's more, my wife has had almost complete relief from her hot flashes, too. But, as a result of some things I have read about the possible connection between progesterone and breast cancer, I want to be reassured that my wife is on the right track—and that no unscheduled trains will be coming down that track which could cause her harm in the future.

The experience of the woman described in this letter beautifully illustrates the side effects that often result from taking Premarin, which used to be the most regularly prescribed estrogen drug for perimenopausal symptoms. Breast pain is one of the most common adverse reactions to estrogen replacement of all kinds, with anywhere from 20 to 35 percent of women complaining of it when given standard, non-individualized doses.[113] This is especially frightening for women who have a personal or family history of benign breast disease (also known as fibrocystic breast disease), which, in the past, was felt to be associated with an increased risk for breast cancer. Newer research, however, has failed to show any consistent association between benign breast disease and increased risk of breast cancer.[114] And, as already stated, breast pain is often a sign of suboptimal iodine levels (see page 164).

Headaches are also a common side effect of taking Premarin, since estrogen can be metabolized into a substance that is similar to adrenaline and can result in pounding temporal headaches. Bioidentical progesterone, on the other hand, has been shown to stop hot flashes and has none of these side effects.

Many people, however, are uncertain about potential long-term health problems resulting from progesterone, because of studies from the National Cancer Institute and the Women's Health Initiative, both of which documented an increased breast cancer risk for those women on long-term estrogen/progestin hormone therapy. A reanalysis of the WHI data published in 2011 showed that such risk increases only for women who began taking HT either before menopause or within five years of it. Those who started HT five years or more after menopause had no increased risk.[115] Furthermore, what most people (including doctors) do not understand is the difference between the synthetic hormones at non-individualized doses used in the NCI and WHI studies and bioidentical estrogen and progesterone used at low, individualized doses.

Here are the facts: the National Cancer Institute study was a large epidemiological study involving 48,355 women who were on both estrogen and progestin for varying periods of time between the years 1980 and 1995. Women of normal weight who took this hormone combination for five years had a 40 percent increased risk for breast cancer compared to those who were not on hormone therapy. (Intriguingly, women who were overweight did not have this increased risk, although overweight women are at higher risk in any case because body fat makes estrogen.) They also had a greater risk for developing breast cancer than those on estrogen alone.[116]

The 2002 WHI study showed that out of 10,000 women on Prempro, there would be an additional 8 cases of breast cancer compared to placebo. A 2010 analysis of the data confirmed that after eleven years of follow-up, those who took Prempro who developed breast cancer were diagnosed with more advanced tumors and had higher rates of mortality—yet in terms of absolute rates, the risk of breast cancer mortality was fairly low (2.6 deaths from breast cancer per year per 10,000 women on combination HT compared to 1.3 breast cancer deaths per year per 10,000 women taking placebo—or 1.3 extra deaths from breast cancer per 10,000 women per year attributable to HT).[117]

Though the 40 percent increased-risk figure in the National Cancer Institute study sounds very scary, here's what it really means: if you take 100,000 normal-weight women, ages sixty to sixty-four, who are not on hormone therapy, you could expect 350 cases of breast cancer to develop over a five-year period. If all these women took a combination HT consisting of conventional estrogen with progestin, then the number of cases would increase to 560. As you can quickly see, the vast majority of women would not get breast cancer, with or without hormones.

Here's another way of saying this: statistically speaking, out of 1,000 women who have never taken conventionally prescribed hormones, 77 will get breast cancer by age seventy-five. For women who have taken hormones for five years, that figure climbs to 79; after ten years, it is 83; and after fifteen years, it is 89. Again, the vast majority of women who take hormone therapy (even what I consider a suboptimal form) do not get breast cancer.

The other key point to keep in mind is that virtually all the women in the NCI study—and in most of the other studies that link hormone therapy with breast cancer—were using non-individualized doses of conjugated estrogens (most likely Premarin) in combination with the synthetic progestin Provera. Premarin has been the most-prescribed estrogen in this country for decades, and it is almost always given together with a synthetic progestin such as Provera, often in the combined preparation known as Prempro. In the WHI study, *all* the women were taking Prempro. Each of these non-bioidentical hormones has its own risks.

Studies have shown that when Premarin is metabolized in the body, its breakdown products are biologically stronger, and therefore potentially more apt to promote cancer, than the breakdown products of bioidentical estrogens.[118] It has also been demonstrated that there can be a greater than tenfold variance in blood levels of estrogen among women on the *same* standard dose of Premarin—usually 0.625 mg.[119] What is more disturbing is that many of the women in these studies are on even higher doses, 1.25 mg per day.

Synthetic progestins present their own set of problems. They can bind to both estrogen and androgen receptors in cells and thus stimulate unhealthy tissue growth. They can also *increase* the biological activity of estrogen. This may explain why women in the National Cancer Institute study who were on both estrogen and synthetic progestin had an even greater risk for developing breast cancer than those women who were on estrogen only.[120] This same association has been found in the Million Women Study in the United Kingdom[121] and also in the Women's Health Initiative study. If you are on hormone therapy, you may want to check to see whether or not you are taking anything containing the following synthetic progestins: medroxyprogesterone acetate—MPA (brand names Provera, Amen, Prempro); norethindrone (brand names Femhrt, Activella); or norgestimate (brand name Levlite). If you are, I suggest a change to bioidentical hormones.

A study from Australia that analyzed several studies on HT and breast cancer risk suggests that breast cancer risk linked to estrogen is not as high as assumed. They estimate that the use of HT for about five years starting at age fifty hardly affects the cumulated breast cancer risk up to age seventy-nine. Extended use for ten years increases risk by 0.5 percent and for fifteen years by 0.9 percent. Upon stopping HT, the relative increase in risk quickly declines to zero.[122] The same researchers found the same thing with HT use in California.[123]

What it boils down to is this: HT appears to slightly increase the risk for breast cancer, but not as much as previously thought. It's probably safer to use bioidentical hormones at individualized doses if you're going to use HT.

BIOIDENTICAL HORMONES AND CANCER RISK

There is good reason to believe that the long-term use of bioidentical low-dose estrogen, balanced with bioidentical progesterone, would result in a very limited increase in breast cancer risk, if any.[124] A 2017 review study is the latest to show that hormone therapy containing micronized (natural) progesterone has a significantly lower breast cancer risk than therapy with progestins (synthetic hormones).[125] A much larger study from 2008—one of the largest studies done so far, in fact, following more than 80,000 postmenopausal women for more than eight years—showed that the women using natural bioidentical hormones had significantly less risk of breast cancer than those taking synthetic hormone therapy.[126] When the same group of French researchers looked at the data to see if the timing of HT made a difference, they published another study the following year that showed no significant increase in breast cancer risk among women using estrogen plus bioidentical progesterone for short durations, no matter when HT use was begun.[127] A comprehensive analysis also published in 2009 examined 200 physiological and clinical studies, finding that bioidentical hormones were associated with lower risk for breast cancer and cardiovascular disease than were synthetic hormones.[128] The study further showed that bioidentical hormones were better than their synthetic counterparts at alleviating symptoms such as insomnia, cognitive problems, depression, anxiety, and more.

Estrogen

The breasts are glandular organs that are exquisitely sensitive to cyclical hormonal changes in the body. In the first half of the menstrual cycle estrogen tends to increase breast tissue growth; in the second half progesterone stabilizes and refines this growth. During our menstrual periods our breasts are at their smallest, with both hormones at their lowest levels. During perimenopause, which is characterized by estrogen dominance and a relative lack of progesterone, a woman's breasts may become larger and more tender with no cyclical waxing and waning to keep breast tissue more stable.

For decades numerous studies have demonstrated that, with the exception of phytoestrogens in whole foods, estrogen of all kinds, even that produced by our own bodies, can promote breast tissue growth. In susceptible individuals, this may be associated with an increased risk for breast cancer.[129] It is this sensitivity to long-term, uninterrupted estrogen exposure that explains breast cancer risk factors such as early menarche, late menopause, no children, and obesity. Eating a diet that increases insulin also increases hormonal stimulation of breast tissue. Therefore, to preserve breast health, use the least amount of bioidentical estrogen that gives you the results you seek. And get your hormone levels tested when necessary to make sure you're not getting overdosed.

If you have a family history of breast cancer (grandmother, mother, sister, or maternal aunt) or have the gene for breast cancer, you will probably want to avoid estrogen replacement despite its known benefits.

Opting not to use estrogen doesn't mean you have to suffer in silence. Many alternatives can relieve your symptoms, improve your health, and also protect your breasts: exercise, dietary improvement, whole soy, herbs, and natural progesterone. These alternatives are very effective.

ESTRIOL: Preliminary studies have shown that women who excrete the highest levels of estriol in their urine appear to have a lower risk of breast cancer. One study from the Hebrew University of Jerusalem showed that estriol actually has an antiestrogen effect when given in sufficient dosages, preventing estradiol from binding to estrogen-sensitive tissue, including the breast and endometrium, so tumors don't form.[130] In one study from Berkeley, rats receiving a three-week treatment of estriol along with progesterone had a significantly reduced incidence of breast cancer.[131] Because of such evidence, many physicians have sometimes used estriol, a non-patentable bioidentical estrogen, in their patients' hormone therapy regimes. Estriol is biologically weaker than estradiol and estrone, the two other estrogens produced naturally in the body; as already discussed in chapter 9, it works very well when applied locally to estrogen-sensitive tissue such as the vagina. Estriol is widely used in Europe and gives good relief of menopausal symptoms. It is important to note that estriol has been linked with otosclerosis in some women, a genetically linked condition in which three small bones in the middle ear fuse together and thus fail to transmit sound to the brain. Exercise caution with estriol if you have a family history of otosclerosis. *Note:* The studies on estriol have not been replicated—most likely for financial reasons. Therefore, despite its promise, estriol requires more study.

Progesterone

Though the widely publicized NCI and WHI studies mentioned previously proved synthetic progestin is not protective against breast cancer and may even promote it, their conclusions cannot be applied to the natural, bioidentical progesterone found in such preparations as Pro-Gest cream or Prometrium capsules. In fact, it makes biologi-

cal sense that adding bioidentical progesterone (which has no androgenic or estrogenic activity) to estrogen replacement regimens may
actually help protect the breasts against overstimulation from estrogen and thus further decrease the risk of breast cancer as long as the
dose is low. Bioidentical progesterone has been shown to reduce
estrogen-receptor production on breast cells and also to decrease the
production of estrogen within breast cells. Some women experience
transient breast tenderness in the first week or so of bioidentical progesterone use, since it initially increases estrogen receptors in the
breasts. However, this effect is very short-lived and goes away after
several days. There is no convincing evidence that low-dose bioidentical progesterone causes continued growth of breast tissue. In fact, it
appears to do just the opposite.

Recent research underscores the difference in risk between synthetic and bioidentical progesterone. A 2009 study published in the
New England Journal of Medicine concludes that postmenopausal
women who take both estrogen and progestin (such as in the form of
Prempro) for five years or more have twice the risk of developing
breast cancer.[132] When the women in the study stopped taking the
combination hormone formula, the incidence of breast cancer
dropped about 28 percent within the first year. This study was a
follow-up to the landmark WHI study, which was stopped in 2002
when researchers concluded that Prempro caused a higher incidence
of heart problems and breast cancer. It's interesting to note that the
number of breast cancer cases dropped significantly after 2003.
Rowan Chlebowski, M.D., Ph.D., a medical oncologist at Los Angeles Biomedical Research Institute at Harbor-UCLA Medical Center,
conducted a study to determine if this drop in breast cancer cases was
due to women halting their hormone therapy or if the drop was due
to more vigilant mammography practices. His research indicates that
getting regular mammograms didn't affect the numbers at all, so the
effect was indeed related to the hormone therapy—but not to *all* hormone therapy! Those women who took only estrogen (usually in the
form of Premarin) *without* the progestin were no more likely to develop breast cancer than those women who took no hormones at all.
(Women without a uterus typically aren't given a progestin because
it's deemed unnecessary; these women don't need to protect their
uteruses from uterine cancer.) The synthetic progestin, then, is clearly
what accounted for the higher levels of cancer.

It amazes me that nine years have passed since the WHI study,
and people are *still* lumping synthetic progestins and progesterone
together without understanding the difference. Most of the medical

literature does not even make this distinction! I've recommended progesterone instead of progestin for more than twenty years because it matches the hormone made within a woman's own body far better than any synthetic hormone could. And, as the medical literature now shows, it does *not* increase the risk of breast cancer.

Genes, Hormones, and Breast Cancer: The Cell Growth–Cell Death Cycle

If we were to do a very large, long-term study on natural progesterone, we would probably find that it offers some protection to the breast, especially when used without estrogen during perimenopause, when estrogen dominance is so common. The reasons for this have to do with the fact that progesterone plays a role in cell death. Let me explain why this turns out to be a good thing.

Nature in all her wisdom has created a balance between breast tissue cell growth and breast tissue cell death. Breast cancer is one of the health problems that arises when there's an imbalance between these two processes. Breast cancer—like all cancers, actually—is characterized by two processes: (1) excessive and uncontrolled cell division, and (2) a lack of normal, healthy programmed cell death.[133] The signals that direct cell growth, cell development, and programmed cell death (called *apoptosis*) are directed by the interaction between our genes and our environment. Though this process is extraordinarily complex, we are beginning to understand it, thanks to advances in molecular biology. For instance, we now know that a gene known as the BCL2 gene blocks cell death. This function is appropriate for the times when breast cell tissue needs to grow (such as at puberty and at the ovulatory stage of the menstrual cycle).[134] However, when the BCL2 function is not modulated by other factors, it can cause inappropriate cell longevity and possible uncontrolled growth, which can lead to an increased risk of breast cancer. BCL2 is known as a proto-oncogene, which means that it promotes cancer if its expression goes unchecked. (And that depends on its environment.)

Another gene that influences breast tissue is p53. The p53 gene, in contrast to BCL2, is a tumor suppression gene; it halts uncontrolled cell division by increasing apoptosis (cell death). Activation of this gene helps to prevent cell overgrowth and subsequent cancer.

As it turns out, the p53 and BCL2 genes are influenced by sex hormones in ways that either favor cancer or protect against it. Estrogen increases the expression of the BCL2 gene and thus promotes breast cell growth. As I already mentioned, this isn't necessarily a bad thing. But unabated expression of the BCL2 gene due to excessive amounts of estrogen can result in increased growth of estrogen-sensitive tissue in the breasts, uterus, and ovaries. It is well known that the risk of cancers in these organs is associated with excessive estrogen stimulation.[135]

In contrast, progesterone decreases the expression of the BCL2 gene while increasing the expression of the p53 gene, leading to an increase in programmed cell death at an appropriate time and thus to a decreased risk of cancer in estrogen-sensitive tissues.[136]

Estrogen and progesterone also differ in the *kinds* of breast tissue they stimulate. Estrogen causes breast cells known as ductal tissue to divide and grow. Unopposed estrogen has the capacity to create un-controlled growth of breast tissue—including cancerous growth. Pro-gesterone, on the other hand, causes the breast cells to differentiate into lobular cells—nature's preparation for milk production if preg-nancy happens. If a woman does not get pregnant, these lobular cells simply undergo programmed cell death, dying off naturally at the end of their life cycle. In other words, a well-differentiated lobular cell is not capable of growing into a cancer.

A very helpful analogy was given to me by David Zava, Ph.D., a researcher with years of experience studying the effects of hormones on breast tissue.[137] Dr. Zava likens the different parts of breast tissue to the different parts of a tree. The ductal tissue, whose growth is promoted by estrogen, is like the trunk and branches of the tree. The lobular cells, whose growth is promoted by progesterone, are compa-rable to the leaves that grow from the ends of the branches. Once a tree cell becomes a leaf, it can never go back to being a trunk or a branch. It simply grows up, matures, and eventually dies at the end of its programmed life cycle. This is not true with the trunk or branches, however. Their cells can grow at any time and make an infinite number of branches or growths on the branches or trunk itself—just like the infinite cell proliferation of a breast cancer.

Given the processes I've just outlined, it makes sense that women subject to excessive estrogen stimulation—whether the estrogen is produced in their own bodies (e.g., during periods of estrogen domi-nance, so common during perimenopause, or from excessive produc-tion of estrogen in body fat cells) or is taken in from the outside (through estrogen replacement or through environmental agents with estrogen-like activity)—would be at increased risk for getting breast cancer. But if they take enough progesterone to balance this estrogen, the risk would diminish. And that is precisely what the scientific literature suggests.[138]

Research by endocrinologist Jerilynn Prior, M.D., founder and scientific director of the Centre for Menstrual Cycle and Ovulation Research (CeMCOR) in Vancouver, British Columbia, shows that women's estrogen levels are significantly higher than normal during perimenopause. In an effort to counterbalance this, Dr. Prior, also the author of *Estrogen's Storm Season: Stories of Perimenopause* (Centre for Menstrual Cycle and Ovulation Research, 2005), successfully prescribes progesterone to her patients with menopausal symptoms. Quelling any concerns that the progesterone will increase risk for breast cancer, Dr. Prior points to studies showing progesterone opposes the effects of estrogen and so may decrease the risk of breast cancer.

For example, a study of women with progesterone *deficiency* from anovulation, who were being followed at an infertility clinic, has shown those women to have a risk for premenopausal breast cancer 5.4 times greater than those in a control group. And in a 1995 study in which transdermal bioidentical progesterone was placed directly on the skin of the breast, researchers found that the progesterone was able to inhibit breast cell proliferation. The dosages used were approximately the same as when a woman is using a transdermal cream such as Pro-Gest or PhytoGest—in other words, a 2 percent progesterone cream twice per day at recommended dosages. These levels are about equal to those found at ovulation in most women.[139]

Another study showed that those women who had physiologically adequate levels of progesterone at the time of breast cancer surgery had a decreased risk for recurrence, compared to women whose progesterone levels were low.[140] This study has been repeated with the same results, which has led some breast cancer surgeons to suggest that women use 2 percent progesterone cream on their skin for a week or so before breast biopsy or surgery. It appears that bioidentical progesterone can enhance immune response. It also seems to make any tumor cells that may be released during surgery less apt to attach to other sites and grow. This may be why women with breast cancer who are operated on during the luteal phase of their menstrual cycles—when progesterone levels are the highest—have a significantly decreased rate of recurrence.[141]

A 1996 review of the evidence on progesterone and breast health concluded that bioidentical progesterone not only reduced the rate of spread of breast cancer, but may even be responsible for reducing the incidence of new cases.[142]

Though no one has done a definitive long-term clinical trial of bioidentical progesterone, my clinical experience and that of many of my colleagues, including the late John Lee, M.D., a pioneer in bio-identical hormone research, has led me to believe that bioidentical progesterone can benefit many women, especially if used during peri-menopause, and will very likely be found to decrease the risk for breast and other estrogen-responsive cancers that may well get their start during this time of life.

Progesterone Preparations and Progesterone-Receptor-Positive Breast Cancer

One of the questions I'm frequently asked is whether a woman whose breast cancer has tested positive for progesterone receptors can safely take progesterone. There is a great deal of confusion about what it means to have a breast biopsy that shows that the tumor is positive for progesterone receptors, especially in those women who have been using bioidentical progesterone at the time of their diagnosis.

Here are the facts. All breast cancers that are positive for proges-terone receptors are also estrogen-receptor-positive. Because estrogen is known to stimulate growth of these types of cancer cells, many people automatically assume that progesterone must do the same. Just the opposite is true. Positive progesterone receptors indicate that a cancer is receptive to the balancing and anticancer effects of proges-terone.

To understand this apparent paradox, remember that hormones in the bloodstream and the fluid surrounding cells work by uniting with receptors on the surface of the cell. The hormone fits the recep-tor like a key in a lock. If the right receptor is there, the hormone message makes its way to the chromosomes and turns on the appro-priate gene to produce a specific cellular effect. Progesterone signals the cell to stop multiplying, while estrogen signals the opposite. For that reason, bioidentical progesterone is probably beneficial for women with progesterone-receptor-positive breast cancer.

In general, women with estrogen- and progesterone-receptor-positive breast tumors have the best prognosis, since the presence of both these receptors means that the tumor is well differentiated and slower-growing than more poorly differentiated tumors.

Though I'm convinced that bioidentical progesterone is safe and even beneficial for women with estrogen- and progesterone-receptor-positive breast cancers, this is a controversial area. Use your inner guidance and consult with your doctor.

My Advice About Progesterone

~ If you are currently perimenopausal and using a progesterone cream or another form of bioidentical progesterone such as Prometrium or Crinone, you are helping your body create hormonal balance that may well protect your breasts from overstimulation by estrogen and androgen. I recommend that you continue to use it until after menopause, unless your inner guidance tells you otherwise.

~ If you are at risk for estrogen or androgen dominance, consider adding bioidentical progesterone. Conditions associated with estrogen dominance are the following: irregular periods, body fat percentage greater than 28 percent, sedentary lifestyle, polycystic ovary syndrome, fibroid tumors of the uterus, breast tenderness, a low-fiber diet high in refined carbohydrates, heavy menstrual periods, and hormone therapy with estrogen only. Androgen dominance is associated with acne, polycystic ovary syndrome, and male-pattern baldness.

~ Though not all women's health experts agree on the progesterone question, I personally would recommend that every woman who is concerned about her breast health avail herself of the substantial benefits of bioidentical progesterone, especially during the perimenopausal period, when it is well known that she is likely to start skipping ovulations and therefore to have low progesterone levels. Substantial doses of soy protein, or the phytoestrogen found in *Pueraria mirifica* (see page 229), would be a reasonable alternative to progesterone. Use progesterone for two to three weeks out of the month and then take a week off. This is the most beneficial and physiological way to use it. If you are postmenopausal, get a blood or saliva test done to be sure you're not converting progesterone to estrogen.

What About Testosterone?

Androgens such as testosterone and even DHEA can be converted into estrogen in the body, which means that taking testosterone could theoretically increase your risk for breast cancer. Use the lowest dose that gives you the results you need, or try alternatives first.

Here's the bottom line: it is in our best interest to make the wisest choices we can if we opt for hormone therapy—which means using bioidentical, individualized HT regimens when needed at the lowest doses that give us the results we want. Once we've done that, we simply have to let go of our illusion of control and realize that there are no perfect solutions. We all do the best we can with the information we have at the time. But that information, like us, keeps evolving and changing. This year's best solution may differ from next year's. Nevertheless, most of the time our bodies and our cells maintain their health—which is why the vast majority of women, either on or off hormone therapy, do not get breast cancer.

THE TAMOXIFEN DILEMMA

Tamoxifen (trade name Nolvadex) is commonly prescribed to women with certain types of breast cancer and also to prevent breast cancer in high-risk women. It is one of a class of drugs called selective estrogen receptor modulators (SERMs). Other SERMs include raloxifene (Evista), which is used to prevent and treat osteoporosis and is also now recommended as an alternative to tamoxifen in postmenopausal women. Tamoxifen's antiestrogenic effect on breast tissue has been shown to prolong the disease-free interval and overall survival rate in women with estrogen-receptor-positive breast cancer. It has been prescribed for hundreds of thousands of women, making it the most commonly used anticancer drug in the United States. Tamoxifen became a generic drug in the early part of this century, thus reducing its cost and the profits made from it. As a result, attention has turned to newer, more expensive drugs.

Tamoxifen has significant risks, sometimes due to its estrogenic properties, other times due to its antiestrogenic effects. Some researchers are concerned that its antiestrogenic effects on brain tissue may put women at increased risk for dementia or depression.[143] It has been my experience that many women who are taking tamoxifen suffer from depression but don't tell their doctors because they don't want to bother them. This is particularly true for women who no longer have periods. In its estrogenic mode, tamoxifen results in changes in the endometrial lining of the uterus, ranging from atypical hyperplasia (abnormal thickening) and polyps to invasive cancer. The longer you're on it, the greater the risk.[144] This means that any woman on tamoxifen needs to have regular uterine screenings by ultrasound or other means to make sure she doesn't develop uterine cancer. Another problem with tamoxifen is that if a woman continues to take it beyond five years, it may stop acting like an antiestrogen in her breasts and start to act more like an estrogen.[145] In other words, a woman may develop resistance to it, and, if she does get breast cancer again, it may even increase the chance of the cancer being resistant to treatment.[146] Tamoxifen is also associated with increased risk for stroke, cataracts, and blood clots.

Tamoxifen for Breast Cancer Prevention

Tamoxifen has proven to be controversial at best. Even before placebo-controlled, randomized clinical trials were done to evaluate its effectiveness at preventing breast cancer, it was approved for and marketed to healthy women considered at increased risk. While such a trial has finally been done, showing the drug did improve the five-year survival rate, many women had to stop their participation in the study early because of toxicity.[147] In a highly publicized study done by the National Cancer Institute, the drug reduced the rate of expected breast cancers in a group of 13,000 women in the United States and Canada from 1 in 130 women to 1 in 236 women. Statistically, this represented a 50 percent reduction in the risk of breast cancer in those women who took tamoxifen prophylactically—a figure that certainly got everyone's attention. Though other studies, including two done in Europe, have not shown any breast-cancer-decreasing benefits, the drug was approved for prevention of breast cancer in women at high risk for the disease.[148]

After its approval for prevention in 1998, many ads for Nolvadex appeared in mainstream magazines. One read, "If you care about breast cancer, care more about being a 1.7 than a 36B. Know your breast cancer risk assessment number. You can call 1-800-898-8423 to learn more about Nolvadex and the Breast Cancer Risk Assessment test."

The NCI tamoxifen prevention trial included women with a 1.7 percent risk. This "risk number" is based on what is known as the Gail model, which was developed by a group of statisticians at the National Cancer Institute in the late 1980s. Its purpose was to try to assess the theoretical risk of breast cancer using data developed on only 28,000 white women. Those who came up with this assessment tool admitted that it represented only a "best guess," not the last word in scientific proof.[149] The updated Gail risk assessment that was developed to promote tamoxifen has been controversial from the start, with critics contending that it tended to overstate risk. Even the original creators of the Gail model cited "three major sources of uncertainty" about their risk model. However, these uncertainties, as well as the risks of the drug itself, tended to be underplayed.

For example, women taking tamoxifen for prevention are two to three times more likely to develop uterine cancer or blood clots in the lung and legs than controls. Stroke, cataracts, and cataract surgery are more common with the drug, too. Most postmenopausal women also experienced hot flashes and bothersome vaginal discharge. Quite a few healthy women knew intuitively that the risks outweighed the benefits and decided to take their chances without tamoxifen. And it turns out that their inner wisdom was correct.

In 2006, a study reported in the journal *Cancer* showed that women at the lower end of the risk range did not, in fact, live longer as a result of taking tamoxifen. The study, which was based on a hypothetical population model of a group of fifty-year-old women considered at high risk (1.7 percent or higher), took into account the calculated incidence of breast and endometrial cancers, end-result statistics, and non-cancer-related outcomes of those on tamoxifen. Researchers found that tamoxifen actually *increased* mortality in women with a uterus whose risk was under 2.1 percent. For those with a very high risk number, 3 percent or more, however, there was a potential benefit in terms of decreased mortality. This beneficial effect was especially strong in women who'd had hysterectomies.[150]

The pendulum has now swung back to center when it comes to SERMs and breast cancer prevention. In an article on *Medscape* news, V. Craig Jordan, Ph.D. (dubbed "the father of tamoxifen" by the media), the scientific director for the medical science division at Fox Chase Cancer Center in Philadelphia, said, "This drug has got to be used very specifically. It is not one that should be added to the water supply, and it calls for a huge amount of physician discretion."[151] I couldn't agree more.

In 2009, a study of more than a thousand women with ER-positive breast cancer clearly showed that women who take tamoxifen for at least five years after having a lumpectomy or mastectomy more than *quadruple* their risk of developing ER-negative breast cancer—a rare but more aggressive and more difficult-to-treat cancer—in their healthy breast.[152] Using tamoxifen for less than five years was not linked to the ER-negative breast cancer, but because women don't get the full benefit of tamoxifen until they've taken it for five years, that finding didn't do much to assuage anxiety about the drug.

The bottom line is that while most women with breast cancer will lower the risk of cancer recurring by taking tamoxifen, 25 percent of them will actually *increase* their risk of getting an even more deadly form of breast cancer. I'm not at all comfortable with those odds, especially because of the added risk of blood clots, stroke, and uterine cancer associated with tamoxifen.

My Advice on Tamoxifen and Other SERMs

- If you are already on tamoxifen, feel good about it, and are having no side effects, then I'd recommend that you stick with it for up to five years.

- If taking tamoxifen reduces your fear of breast cancer significantly and brings you peace, then by all means take it. This is especially true if you've watched your sister or mother die of breast cancer. In this case, the overall benefits of tamoxifen—including the sense that you are doing something to protect yourself—may well outweigh the risks.

- If you're offered raloxifene, remember that it is a "same doll, different dress" drug. Though it is touted as having a lower incidence of serious side effects than tamoxifen, they are still significant. Remember, too, that it is recommended only for postmenopausal women.

- If you've had breast cancer, discuss with your doctor whether your type of cancer has shown a response to tamoxifen, and, if so, how long you should take it. Remember that neither tamoxifen nor raloxifene decreases your risk for breast cancer that is estrogen-receptor-negative—the type of breast cancer that tends to be more aggressive.

- If you are at increased risk for breast cancer, decrease that risk by following the suggestions I've given earlier in this chapter. Discuss taking a SERM with your doctor if your risk is 3 percent or greater, but let your inner guidance have a voice in your decision.

- If you opt to take tamoxifen or raloxifene, get regular medical care, including screening for endometrial abnormalities and cataracts.

- You can decrease some of the side effects of tamoxifen by taking soy or *Pueraria mirifica,* using supplements, and following the dietary guidelines given on pages 597–607.

~ Maintain positive expectations for what you choose. A 2016 study of 111 women at the University of Marburg's Breast Cancer Centre found that those patients who expected to suffer more from adjuvant hormone therapy experienced nearly twice the number of side effects as did women who had more positive expectations and thought the side effects wouldn't be too bad.[153]

~ Don't take tamoxifen for longer than five years unless you and your doctor feel strongly that your individual situation warrants it.

OTHER DRUGS FOR TREATING BREAST CANCER: HERCEPTIN (TRASTUZUMAB) AND ARIMIDEX (AROMATASE INHIBITORS)

Two extremely promising drug treatments for breast cancer are helping make some strides against this disease. One, the antibody trastuzumab (the generic name for the drug Herceptin), specifically targets a protein called HER-2/neu that is present in 20 to 30 percent of breast cancer patients. In effect, this drug blocks the ability of the cancer cells to receive chemical signals telling the cells to grow, thereby slowing or stopping the growth of the cancer. It also works by alerting the immune system to destroy the cancer cells the drug attaches to. Although traditionally reserved for treating women with advanced breast cancer, trastuzumab has been proven to delay the growth and spread of tumors in women who are in the early stages of the disease as well. Evidence presented at the May 2005 meeting of the American Society of Clinical Oncology showed that trastuzumab reduced the risk of breast cancer recurrence in this group by about 50 percent and the risk of death by about 33 percent. (The FDA has approved this drug in combination with chemotherapy for treating advanced HER-2/neu-positive stomach cancer as well.) Yet this drug is not a silver bullet—it was also associated with a small but real increase in the risk of developing weakening of the heart muscle. It is the first of what researchers hope will be other, more targeted drugs. It is now standard to check for the HER-2/neu gene and others. The current science on breast cancer is far beyond the scope of this book, and so I urge you to consult a physician who is well schooled in this area.

Aromatase Inhibitors

The aromatase inhibitors are another class of drug (including anastrozole, the generic name for Arimidex; letrozole, the generic name for Femara; and exemestane, the generic name for Aromasin). These drugs inhibit the adrenal glands, fat stores, and breast and other tissues from converting precursor steroids into estrogen, thereby lowering estrogen levels in the body. When given to postmenopausal women with early-stage breast cancer, these drugs reduce the rate of cancer recurrence and lengthen the time between bouts for those who do have recurrences. In one of the early trials, Arimidex delayed tumor progression for an average of 11.1 months (tamoxifen delayed tumor progression for only 5.6 months). While initial evidence showed that aromatase inhibitors cause an increased incidence of heart problems, joint pain, and broken bones, as well as osteoporosis, a 2010 study showed that side effects were worse than previously believed (which has certainly been borne out by my discussions with women who are on these drugs). The study, presented at the annual conference of the American Association for Cancer Research, showed that women taking these drugs were five times more likely to report having hot flashes, breast sensitivity, and chest pain; four times more likely to report night sweats, cold sweats, and hair loss; and about three times more likely to report leg cramps, weight gain, sleep disturbance, tendency to take naps, and forgetfulness than were healthy women.[154] However, the side effects may turn out to be good news for some. A 2008 study done in London of almost 4,000 breast cancer patients showed that women who developed joint symptoms within the first three months of taking anastrozole were 10 percent less likely to suffer from a recurrence of the cancer, while those who reported vasomotor (hot flash) symptoms were 6 percent less likely to have their cancer return.[155] Women who reported *both* joint symptoms and vasomotor symptoms within three months of starting the drug were 11 percent less likely to have a recurrence. Additional research has also shown that these drugs are indeed effective against DCIS, but since 99 percent of DCIS doesn't become invasive cancer, the risk of the drugs is most certainly worse than the risk of invasive breast cancer.

In conclusion, please realize that the problem of breast cancer can't be solved only at the physical level. Don't be fooled into believing that you must always take a drug to help your body stay well. To create healthy breast tissue, each of us needs to be willing to participate in creating a life that is healthy in mind and spirit as well as body. We need to learn how to fully receive as well as give. We must open our hearts and learn how to bring more sustainable pleasure into our lives on a daily basis. Yes, sometimes we may need drugs or surgery; at other times we need only the natural strategies. And at all times, we need to be open to the greater learning that is always part of a difficult diagnosis. As I've emphasized in this chapter and throughout this book, true healing involves eating healthfully, getting exercise, stopping smoking, cutting down on or eliminating alcohol, expressing your feelings, loving and forgiving others, and most importantly, allowing yourself to be loved.

14

Living with Heart, Passion, and Joy: How to Listen to and Love Your Midlife Heart

The years around menopause are the time when women's risk for heart disease, hypertension, and stroke rise significantly as our hearts and the network of blood vessels that carries nourishment to every cell in our bodies call out to us more loudly than ever, demanding that we listen well and allow ourselves to feel the exquisite joy of life more fully than ever. Because heart disease in all its guises claims more lives than any other illness, midlife is a time when a change of heart may save your life.

Despite the fact that seven times more women die of heart disease than breast cancer, failure to diagnose heart disease in a timely manner is rarely the subject of lawsuits, whereas suits for failure to diagnose breast cancer are very common. Statistics (which need not apply to you) show that one out of three deaths in women is a result of heart disease (either a heart attack or a stroke—a stroke is just a "heart attack" of the brain), but only one in every thirty-one deaths in women is due to breast cancer. That's roughly one heart disease death per minute!

Many women never realize that they have a heart problem until the disease is well established. Breast cancer, on the other hand, is seen as an invader from outside ourselves, so we tend to take a fighting stance toward it, for better or for worse.

When it comes to your heart, however, you can't fight it—you must instead follow its dictates if you are to achieve the vibrant cardiovascular health that will nourish and rejuvenate every organ in your body for the rest of your life. Indeed, the latest research shows that keeping your cardiovascular system healthy also leads to healthier brain function—no kidding![1] The heart teaches us directly and persistently. And it is quite forgiving if we will simply heed its messages.

THE HEART HAS ITS SAY AT MENOPAUSE: MY PERSONAL STORY

In chapter 3 I wrote about my first experience of the "empty nest": how I had picked up my younger daughter at camp, taken her to Dartmouth for a college tour, driven the three long hours home with her sound asleep in the car—and then found myself face-to-face with the realization that her physical presence wouldn't heal my emptiness. There is a sequel to that story. The next morning I went for a walk. About halfway through I began to experience an ache in my throat that radiated up into my jaw. No matter what I did, I couldn't make the pain go away. It felt as though a fist were squeezing my esophagus. I kept walking, wondering what this symptom was all about. When I got home the pain was still there and impossible to ignore. So I called a physician friend well versed in mind-body medicine, who came right over. (She would have called an ambulance or driven me to the ER immediately if she had felt that I was having a heart attack.)

The throat is in the fifth emotional center, which has to do with communication, so I wondered if there was something I needed to say. But my friend reminded me that I've never had any trouble expressing myself. Instead, my family legacy of stoicism and heart disease pointed to challenges in the fourth emotional center.

Together we sat down and took out the Motherpeace tarot cards to try to get some clarity. My intuition, which was reflected in the cards, suggested that my throat and jaw pain had in fact originated in my heart. I was also reminded that the classic symptoms of heart attack in women are often located in the neck, jaw, and upper chest. As I reviewed the events of the prior twenty-four hours, I came to see that my literal "heartache" stemmed from my disappointment and grief over my reunion with my daughter—a reunion in which my own needs for partnership and companionship had not materialized at all. That same pain has recurred a couple of times since then, despite the fact that I didn't then, nor do I now, have any evidence of cardiovascular disease (I had a normal EKG, optimal lipid profile, optimal blood pressure, and good cardiovascular fitness). Each time, the message has been the same: feel your grief (or your fear) and open your heart to yourself. The pain was the direct result of constricted blood vessels in the heart, a result of constricted feelings that needed to be released in order to live in a more openhearted way. That wasn't the last time it happened. But in the subsequent years, I knew what it was signaling.

Setting Myself Up for Heartache

Looking back, I see now how I had set myself up for heartache. For several days before going to pick up my daughter, I had fantasized about how loving and warm our reunion would be. I anticipated her every emotional and physical need as I prepared for the trip. I thought that her return would help me heal from the heartache of my divorce. In retrospect, I see that by trying to truly be there for her, I was actually treating her the way I wished someone would treat me. In addition to the drive together, I had hoped that she'd want to spend some time shopping and having a meal with me. I didn't ask for this outright. I've never wanted to be the kind of mother who manipulates her children into taking care of her needs by staging after-all-I've-done-for-you-at-least-you-could-have-dinner-with-me kinds of scenes. Knowing that this approach confuses love with guilt and obligation, I went to the opposite extreme. It never occurred to me, for instance, that it was okay to ask my daughters to spend an evening or a day with me now and then. Instead, I had led my daughters—and myself—to believe that I didn't have any needs that I couldn't fulfill on my own. No wonder my heart was forced to speak up! And in the years since, it still has been forced to speak up if I find that I have slid into that old pattern of overgiving and underreceiving, which is a direct result of feeling as though I have to earn love through service—something many can relate to.

The Stoic Heart: My Legacy

By asking for so little, I was unconsciously carrying on a legacy I had inherited from my stoic maternal line, a legacy that is a setup for heart disease: if you don't ask for much, you won't be disappointed. Instead, you can earn love by providing service. And if you become strong enough and capable enough to meet your needs for yourself, you'll never have to feel vulnerable, never have to face possible rejection, never have to experience how brokenhearted that unhealed child inside you actually feels.

My frenzied redecorating in the three weeks prior to my younger daughter's return was not motivated purely by the desire to create a living space that was pleasing to me, though that was part of it. It was also meant to please and delight my daughters. I had envisioned the newly decorated family room as a space in which they could stay up late and watch movies with friends with no fear of keeping me awake. I wanted their approval.

After my daughter and I arrived home, I eagerly showed her the new rooms, anticipating oohs, ahhs, and praise. She looked around briefly, said she liked it, wondered why I had chosen those particular couch cushions, and then settled down to phone the six friends who had left messages for her.

As I unpacked the car to the background of her enthusiastic conversations, I felt as though I had just provided a very nurturing taxi service. When my children were little, providing a warm, safe place for them to grow up was enough. Now I wanted more. But I didn't know that yet. I was simply aware of vague discontent within me. After all, my daughter's behavior was completely normal for a healthy sixteen-year-old with a burgeoning social life.

Why was I so heartsick? Why did I get chest pain the next morning? My daughter certainly wasn't responsible for that. What was my heart trying to tell me? Over the next few days I began to unearth and let go of a big heartache-inducing legacy that was now obsolete.

Keeping the Peace at Any Price Is a Big Pain in the Heart

Like my mother before me, I had been brought up to believe that it was my job to keep the peace in the family and make a comfortable home for my husband and children. I did this—mostly single handedly—

for most of my marriage. After my husband and I separated, I characteristically plowed ahead, believing that my good-natured efforts would make it okay for the children. The truth is that I was heartsick about putting them through the pain of my divorce and also about stepping down from my position as cheerful emotional buffer for the family. In all this I had neglected the fact that I, too, had emotional needs and that I, too, was hurting and grieving over the loss of my marriage.

In trying to protect my children from their own inevitable pain, I had been doing everything in my power to maintain the illusion that our lives hadn't changed. I shielded them from the reality of bills to be paid and a household to be maintained, and never asked for their help. But my heart was giving me the painful message that this coping style wasn't working.

Intellectually I knew that staying healthy on all levels was far and away the biggest help and support I could provide for my daughters during this difficult time. My chest pain was a sign that I needed to tend to the needs and desires of my own heart if I was going to accomplish this. As soon as I began this process my upper chest and neck pain went away completely—and on the rare occasions when this pain has returned, I immediately know that my heart is talking to me.

At midlife I came face-to-face with an unconscious, deeply buried sense of unworthiness that had, for as long as I could remember, motivated me to prove myself to others through service. In the case of my family, this giving was laced with unconscious guilt for having and loving my career while simultaneously thinking that maybe I really should be spending more time as a stay-at-home mom. I made up for the time I spent on the job—or at least I told myself I did—by becoming as efficient and cheerful as possible, my nurturing providing steady background music in the lives of those closest to me. It was simply expected.

Part of my legacy of stoicism and unworthiness was that I had almost no "receptor sites" in my own body and psyche for the experience of someone actually anticipating and making space for my personal emotional needs. In other words, even if someone had wanted to be there for me in the way I was there for my children and husband, I would not have been open to attracting or even recognizing it. The music may have been playing, but my personal radio dial was always set on another station.

My divorce awakened me to the presence of those friends who had always been there for me—and who always would be. But I first had to open my heart and feel vulnerable and needy enough to allow myself to ask for help and then accept it when it was offered. This didn't come naturally or easily. But it was preferable to the old pattern, and with practice, opening my heart to myself and accepting help and support has become much easier.

Over the years I've observed that many women use pleasing behaviors to make themselves acceptable to others. One of my friends told me that whenever she feels that she doesn't belong or fit in, she does what she did in her family of origin to relieve the tension: she cleans, she buys food, and she makes meals for others.

When we first recognize the patterns within us that shut down the energy of our hearts, our tendency is to beat ourselves up for them—which simply closes our hearts further. The first step we each must take is to acknowledge that the patterns that are causing us heartache in adulthood began as successful adaptations to difficult childhood circumstances. They worked for us then, and they have allowed us to become who we are. So the first thing we want to do when we recognize these patterns is to congratulate ourselves—and also take a moment to give that hurt little child within a hug. Over time, once you realize that it is a hurt little kid (often a seven-year-old) who has been running your endocrine, immune, and central nervous systems, you can "grow" that child up by vowing to now be the adult in the relationship. You gently ask that inner child what she needs, and over time those childlike patterns will leave your body—and your heart. Now, in retrospect, I can't imagine living a life in which I put my desires on the back burner. Now I know that my desires are an important part of my inner guidance and that ignoring them is a health risk. This took a number of years to figure out—and it took even more years to refine it thoroughly, especially in intimate relationships. I highly recommend the Heart Power Recovery online course by Belinda Womack to help you get started (see www.belinda womack.com).

Yearning for Connection: Needing to Be Free

I'm not suggesting that at midlife we need to give up serving others. Participating in true service—where you're not in it for love and approval—is good for the heart. Most women, however, don't get to true service until we learn to balance our need for connection with our need to be free. Like the parasympathetic and sympathetic aspects of our autonomic nervous system, which so exquisitely control the minute-to-minute caliber of our blood vessels, we need both free-dom and connection. Nanna Aida Svendsen, a writer and teacher originally from Denmark, eloquently articulates this balance.

The heart, it seems, yearns for connection. A great grief arises when connection to others seems to come at the cost of connec-tion to ourselves. I notice how dead I become inside, even if only subtly, when I try to conform to other people's idea of who and how I should be and forgo my own feelings—my connec-tion to myself. When the natural generosity, compassion, and caring of the heart becomes distorted or usurped, then all sense of aliveness, generosity, creativity, and true self-expression seems to go and I am left feeling empty and drained. It takes a great deal of energy to shape oneself to fit someone else's needs and expectations, to conform to their demands, to be codepen-dent. And no matter how tempting it is in the hope of gaining love, or of being kept safe, it always costs. Just as it always costs to demand conformity to our needs by others—to be in a hier-archy when the heart is yearning for partnership. You can see that cost in the faces of so many couples. You can see the sup-pressed anger or the deadness that resides there. Though the heart may long for connection and love, it also, it appears, longs to be free.[2]

CARDIOVASCULAR DISEASE: WHEN THE FLOW OF LIFE IS BLOCKED

Cardiovascular disease results, in part, from an accumulation of ox-idized fat that sticks to the inside of blood vessels that have been in-jured by glycemic stress, lack of nutrients, and the effect of elevated stress hormones. This process—known as atherogenesis—is what ends up causing blood vessel and heart damage. Strokes, which kill 84,000 women per year, can be likened to a heart attack in the head. Both heart attacks and strokes are caused by clogged and inflamed blood vessels; what differs is their location. In addition to arterioscle-rotic plaque deposits, emotions such as depression, anxiety, panic, and grief have been shown to cause constriction in blood vessels, thereby impeding the free flow of blood.[3]

Your heart beats 100,000 times per day and 36 million times per year. Anything that causes constriction in your blood vessels makes your heart and your vessels have to work harder to do their job. Clearly both emotional and physical factors are involved in creating or maintaining heart health. Over my years in practice I've seen happy, joyful women with high cholesterol counts live healthy lives into their eighties and even nineties, while much younger women whose lives were characterized by depression, anxiety, or hostility might have their first heart disease symptoms in their early fifties despite normal cholesterol levels. (Fully 50 percent of all heart attacks occur in people with normal cholesterol levels.)[4]

Cardiovascular disease in any one area means that it is also present throughout your entire body. Though most of us wait until midlife to take steps to prevent or treat it, heart disease actually begins in utero. It is well documented, for example, that low-birth-weight babies have a significantly greater risk for heart disease decades later, perhaps because stresses in the womb have contributed to underdeveloped cardiovascular systems.[5] In the famous Bogalusa Heart Study, for example, the beginnings of heart disease were discovered in children as young as age nine.[6]

Regardless of any overt risks we may have for heart disease (such as poor diet or lack of exercise), the seeds for potentially developing heart disease later on are sown the minute we learn to start shutting down our hearts to avoid feeling disappointment and loss. Whether or not heart disease eventually results has a lot to do with how well we learn how to feel and express our emotions fully and name the needs they signify. This is especially true given the inevitable disappointments and losses of life.

At midlife our hearts ask us to wake up and live our personal truth so that there is a seamless connection between what we say we believe and how we actually live our day-to-day lives. As astrologer Barbara Hand Clow writes: "The heart does not open if one is lying to oneself or others, is manipulating or controlling others, or is separated from other people." She goes on to explain, "The heart chakra is experienced very physically, and it is possible to actually feel the heart opening at mid-life as the kundalini energy flows in: Many of my clients, for example, report a burning in their heart areas." If we don't follow our body's lead and fuel our hearts and lives with the energy of full emotional expression, full partnership, and heeding our desire for more pleasure in our lives, then heart attack, hypertension, stroke, and dementia are more likely to result.

When we have the courage to open our hearts at midlife, however, we are opening ourselves up to the possibility of living more fully and joyfully than we have since we were young children—only now we have the skills and power of an adult with which to direct our openhearted energy. Clow writes, "The heart chakra opening is the signal of 'radical embodiment'—the soul totally in the body— which is the most exquisite experience available on Earth. The integrity of a person with an open heart is always astounding."[7]

HEART DISEASE FACTS

- Heart disease actually begins in childhood but often doesn't manifest until around menopause.
- Heart disease (including hypertension and stroke) is the most frequent cause of death in men and women over the age of sixty-five.[8]
- One in every 3.3 deaths in women is caused by cardiovascular disease (and one in every 8.3 is due to coronary heart disease), while only one in every 31.5 deaths in women is attributed to breast cancer.[9] According to the American Heart Association, a woman dies every minute from heart disease in the United States.[10]
- Although more men used to die of heart disease each year than women, by 2017 the numbers were about equal for the first time.

PALPITATIONS: YOUR HEART'S WAKE-UP CALL

There's no question that heart palpitations at menopause are related to changing hormones. However, my experience has been that in many midlife women heart palpitations are primarily from increasing heart energy trying to get in and be embodied in a woman's life. At midlife our hearts and bodies often become increasingly sensitive to those things that don't serve us, including caffeine, refined carbohydrates, aspartame, alcohol, or monosodium glutamate, all of which may overstimulate our hearts. You also might need to avoid scary, violent, or emotionally draining news, movies, books, or individuals.

The following letter from Terri, one of my e-newsletter subscribers, is typical of how midlife heart palpitations often present.

I am a forty-eight-year-old female with no major health problems. I do not take any prescription medicine. I walk five times a week and go to the gym about twice a week to do some light weight lifting. My periods are still fairly regular. I have a fairly healthy diet, although it could be better. I drink about a cup of coffee a day but usually don't drink soft drinks. About a month ago, after a fatty fast-food meal and a large cup of coffee in the early evening, I started experiencing heart irregularities. I felt like my heart was skipping a beat and was going to beat out of my chest! This went on for a couple of days and I went to see my doctor. She did an EKG, which was slightly abnormal, and scheduled me for a stress echocardiogram and Holter monitor. Of course, by the time I had these tests, the palpitations had stopped and the results were normal. Then about a week later, they started again. I have cut out drinking coffee and started doing more yoga. I have also started taking more magnesium in addition to my multivitamins. I have monitored what is going on with my life and I can't seem to find any pattern to when these occur. Most nights when I lie down in bed they usually start up, especially when I lie on my left side. My doctor wants to start me on a low dose of a beta-blocker. I told her I would like to start using natural progesterone cream routinely for a couple of months because I feel these palpitations may be related to hormonal changes. I would really like to avoid taking heart medications. However, these palpitations can interrupt my sleep and are very uncomfortable. Are these palpitations hormonally related?

My suggestion to Terri was that she go through the program for creating heart health I outline in this chapter. Her midlife heart was obviously becoming very sensitive, alerting her to the need to balance freedom and connection and to nourish her heart fully. I concurred with her intuitive desire to start on some natural progesterone as a way to balance potential estrogen dominance. Besides, progesterone is known to be very calming to the nervous system. It may well help her with sleeping, given that it binds to the brain's GABA receptors—the same receptors that Valium binds to. In addition, her heart is telling her to stop caffeine. The caffeine in one cup of coffee can take up to ten hours to be metabolized in some women, so it exerts a stimulatory effect on the central nervous system and the nerves of the heart for quite some time. One's environment is also crucial in this regard. Women have told me that when vacationing in Italy or Spain, a shot of espresso before bed doesn't bother them in the slightest, but it's not true at home.

For many women, heart palpitations stop as soon as they begin to take progesterone cream or estrogen, stop caffeine, and also normalize blood sugar and insulin levels through dietary change. (See chapter 7.) But it's also important to find out what your heart is yearning for. One of my patients with heart palpitations found that they stopped soon after she asked for a promotion at work, something she hadn't had the courage to do before. She got the promotion and finds her work more fulfilling than ever. Her heart no longer has to speak so loudly.

FIGURE 19: THE HEART-EMOTION CONNECTION

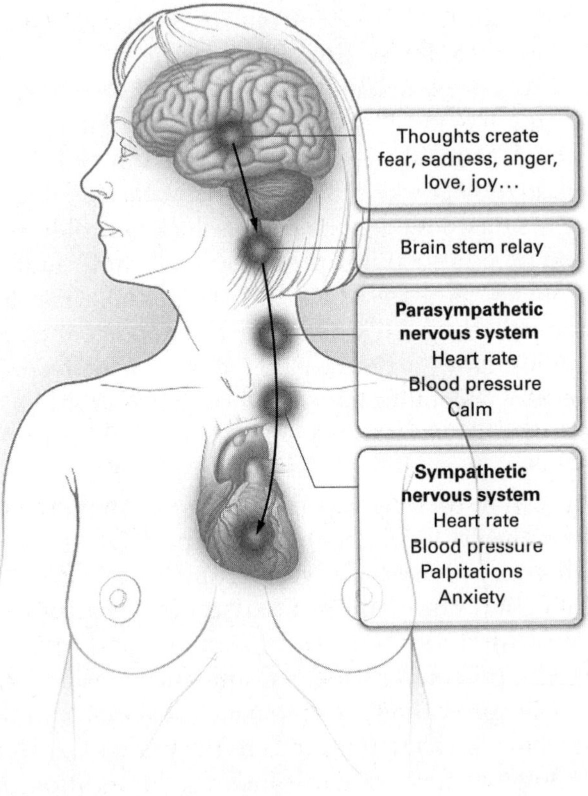

Emotions have direct physical effects on the heart and cardiovascular system, via the sympathetic and parasympathetic nervous systems.

The Brain-Heart Connection

Recall that the emotional and psychological changes of the perimeno-pausal years are to the entire life cycle as the week before one's period is to the monthly cycle. All the issues that have been occurring pre-menstrually and which perhaps had been avoided previously—"Should I quit my job?" "Should I stay in this relationship?"—now come up and hit us between the eyes rather relentlessly, demanding that they be dealt with. Though women with palpitations often tell me that they have examined their lives and there don't appear to be any personal issues bothering them, my experience has been that our bodies speak to us only when we can't seem to "hear" them any other way. When issues of love, issues of the soul, or issues of a woman's unmet passions cry out for attention, they often take the form of heart palpitations. If we are willing to be open to their mean-ing, we will be giving our hearts a chance to be heard. If we act on what we hear, the symptom often goes away.

In his foreword to the book *The HeartMath Solution* (Harper-Collins, 1999), Stephan Rechtschaffen, M.D., writes that "the heart is a physical object, a rhythmic organ, and love itself."[11] We need to think of our hearts as all these things simultaneously and care for them with this perspective in mind. Because of the intricate connec-tions between our brains and our hearts, our thoughts and emotions can and do have a powerful effect on the heart's rhythm.

Let's take the dramatic example of sudden, unexpected cardiac death. This condition claims the lives of more than 325,000 adults per year in the United States, and research into this phenomenon, which focuses on the physical condition of the heart itself, has made relatively little headway in decreasing this number. Sudden cardiac death is caused by a fatal arrhythmia known as ventricular fibrilla-tion (VF), a disorganized, self-perpetuating electrical instability of the heart muscle that results in a failure to pump blood.

VF can occur spontaneously in a completely normal heart and is usually seen when there is some pathological hindrance to the flow of blood in the heart vessels, a condition that often happens in humans in association with some psychosocial stress, such as bereavement, job insecurity, or marital strife. Whether or not a stressor affects the heart physically is dependent on the meaning that stress has for a given individual.[12]

APPRECIATION AND GRATITUDE ARE TONICS FOR THE HEART

The HeartMath Institute, a nonprofit research and education organization in Boulder Creek, California, has been on the forefront of demonstrating and applying the intimate connection between our emotions and what is called cardiac coherence. Cardiac coherence refers to the beat-to-beat variability of the heart—a measure of the balance between the parasympathetic and sympathetic nervous systems. I like to think of the parasympathetic nervous system as the brake and the sympathetic as the gas; too much of either one causes irregularity of the heart rhythm. This can also happen when the activity between the two gets out of sync, which can happen when we get angry or emotionally upset. Over time, this irregularity can lower cardiac coherence, which is highly predictive of heart attack even when there are no other risk factors. But when the beat-to-beat variability is ordered and balanced, the resulting harmonic activity in the heart rhythms translates into optimal cardiac function.

It is now well documented that the electromagnetic field of the heart is 5,000 times more powerful than the electromagnetic field of the brain.[13] And that is why, no matter what we think, what we actually feel is what matters most. Every time. No exceptions. You might be able to fool your brain, but you can't fool your heart. HeartMath has developed an ingenious biofeedback system that displays your heart rhythm patterns (including a measurement of your heart's beat-to-beat variability) and, more important, teaches you how to stabilize and optimize this variability by learning how to cultivate positive emotions in your heart area. You do this by activating the feelings you have toward someone or something that you love unconditionally. Over time, and with practice, you will be able to see how profoundly your emotions affect your heart. This technology comes in two main formats: the emWave 2 and emWave Pro, to be used with your computer, and the Inner Balance Trainer, to be used with a smartphone.

But HeartMath goes further than helping to cultivate and sustain positive emotions. The function of the heart actually influences the function of hormones. Rollin McCraty, Ph.D., HeartMath's director of research, has demonstrated that fifteen to twenty minutes of cardiac coherence practice per day is associated with increased levels of the hormone DHEA.[14] DHEA, which is produced mainly in the adrenal glands but also in the ovaries, is the building block of the sex steroids. With enough DHEA, your body can then produce the right amounts of estrogen, progesterone, and testosterone. This is very significant proof that our thoughts have powerful physical effects on our bodies and that we can't afford to ignore them.

There have now been more than 300 studies, many of them conducted by independent researchers and published in peer-reviewed journals, on the various uses of HeartMath techniques and technologies. While everything HeartMath teaches is designed to reduce stress and improve health and well-being, specific applications cover such diverse areas as sports performance, improved sleep patterns, addiction recovery, trauma interventions, academic performance, and even increased intuition. For more information on Heart-Math, to order HeartMath's emWave or Inner Balance system, or to purchase HeartMath's ninety-minute online video program (*The HeartMath Experience*), visit HeartMath's website, www.heartmath.org.

GENDER BIAS AND HEART DISEASE: OUR CULTURAL INHERITANCE

For thousands of years our culture has valued male hearts more than female hearts. The heart-strengthening dreams, desires, and aspirations of women, as well as the vulnerable and tender hearts of men, have all suffered as a result. Here are the facts.

- The vast majority of research on both heart disease and its treatment has been done on men, even though the female's cardiovascular system is different from the male's.
- Women's brain connections to the heart are different from men's. Men's brains are more lateralized than women's, which means that

in general most men use only one hemisphere at a time, usually the left, which is associated with linear, logical thinking. Women, on the other hand, use both hemispheres simultaneously, and they have more frequent access to their right hemisphere. The right hemisphere is associated with music, emotions, intuition, and a deep experience of oneself. Here's where things get interesting. There are more neuronal connections between the heart and the right hemisphere of the brain than between the heart and the left hemisphere. So in any given moment a woman has a greater neurological and emotional connection to her heart than do most men. Access to one's right hemisphere and more "feminine" side is how we connect with our spirit and with our inner child. This is one of the reasons why it is so crucial that women learn to connect with their hearts—and also assist the men in their lives in doing the same.

~ Given the difference in their brain-heart connections, women with heart problems have different symptoms than men.[15] Men who are having a heart attack typically present with chest pain that begins under the breastbone and spreads to the jaw and the left arm. Women with heart attacks may not have chest pain at all. Instead, they may experience primarily jaw pain and indigestion. (By the way, a study by critical care nurse Martha Mackay at the University of British Columbia School of Nursing reported that during non-emergency angioplasty procedures, men and women were equally likely to report chest discomfort, but women were significantly more likely to report discomfort outside the chest, such as pain in the neck, jaw, or throat.)[16] The first sign of a heart attack in women may also be congestive heart failure, with no evidence of the heart attack preceding it except for telltale changes on an electrocardiogram. They may die from this "silent" heart attack.[17] Women who do have chest pain often experience more functional limitation than men, but fewer women are referred to cardiologists for a complete workup.

~ Until recently, most doctors have not appreciated this difference. Consequently, serious heart problems more often go underdiagnosed and undertreated in women. According to a study of 180,000 heart attack survivors in Sweden who were followed for ten years, women are up to three times more likely to die following a serious heart attack than men due to receiving unequal care and treatment. The researchers further found that when women do receive all the recommended treatments, this difference decreases dramatically.[18] U.S. research backs this up. A 2016 study from Harvard of almost 50,000 people age sixty-five and up who were hospitalized for heart disease showed that women were less likely than men to receive potentially beneficial medications or even to receive advice about the importance of quitting smoking.[19]

~ In 2016, the American Heart Association released its first-ever scientific statement about heart attacks in women. The statement highlighted the fact that within a year of having a first heart attack, survival rates for women are lower than they are for men (even after accounting for age): within five years of a first heart attack, stroke, or diagnosis of heart failure, 47 percent of women will die, compared with only 36 percent of men.[20]

~ When a woman with chest pain or a racing heart shows up at a doctor's office or emergency room, she may appear anxious and depressed, and an affective disorder rather than heart disease may be the first diagnosis considered. While it is true that affective disorders, including depression, phobias, and panic and anxiety, are twice as common in women as in men, they aren't "just in women's heads"—they affect the body as well. One of my most vivid memories of my maternal grandmother is how she often wrung her hands at night. Though she always maintained a wonderfully friendly and cheery demeanor, her hands belied her outward peacefulness. She died of a sudden heart attack at age sixty-eight.

~ If a man shows up who appears to be under stress, his symptoms are more apt to be correctly associated with heart attack—even if he acts hostile.

~ Women's blood vessels are smaller and have a different organization from men's. This is one of the reasons why coronary bypass surgeries and angioplasties don't work as well in women as they do in men and also why more women die after these procedures. More women than men with so-called normal coronary arteries also have heart attacks, angina, and myocardial ischemia. As a result, a normal angiogram (blood vessel study) in a woman with symptoms doesn't necessarily mean that she is free from heart disease.

~ The rate of early death after heart attack is higher for women than men, even if the women receive treatment. Researchers don't know if this difference is caused by older average age at diagnosis, narrower vessels, greater frequency of coexisting illnesses, or inadequate or delayed medical care.

~ The thought patterns and behaviors that are associated with heart disease in women are different from the patterns associated with heart disease in men. In research on men, sudden death from heart attack is related to hostility—so-called type A behavior. This hasn't yet been demonstrated in women. This doesn't mean that men are inherently more hostile than women. In women, hostility just gets expressed differently. Recent studies have shown a correlation between hostility and hardening of the arteries in both men and women starting as young as age eighteen.[21] But men tend to act out their anger and frustration physically in the outer world, whereas women are taught that this is unacceptable and unladylike. Therefore women learn to hold these feelings inside, where they ultimately can set the stage for a great deal of heart trouble.[22]

Let's use the analogy of two pots of water on a stove. The pot on the right—the woman—is on simmer, with a lid on top. The pot on the left—the male—has no lid, and the heat is on high. The heat of the male's anger will cause the water in the pot to boil vigorously, with a lot of steam and noise. In a typical male heart attack, the pot boils over. The woman's pot will never boil over, but the heat is there nonetheless, and the next thing you know, the water has evaporated and the pot has cracked. But because there was no noise and steam, no one was alerted to the problem. The same thing happens with a woman's cardiovascular system.

In the past fifteen years, healthcare providers have been warned about these differences and have been urged to do a full cardiac evaluation of women with symptoms such as anxiety and chest pain. As we move toward a partnership society, our awareness of gender bias in heart disease treatment is becoming stronger. It is encouraging to know that the National Institutes of Health and the FDA now include women in cardiac-related clinical trials. And in 1990, the government also founded the Office of Research on Women's Health (ORWH), which sponsored the Women's Health Initiative, as part of the National Institutes of Health. The mission of ORWH covers not only ensuring that women are included in NIH-funded research and setting research priorities at NIH to include conditions that primarily affect women, but also supporting the advancement of women in biomedical careers.

REDUCING YOUR RISK FOR HEART DISEASE

It's quite easy to reduce your risk for heart disease. The first step is to understand what it is and how it develops over time. Let's start with the anatomy of an artery. Arteries carry blood away from the heart to all the organs and tissues of our body. They are lined with endothelial cells, all of which produce a gas known as nitric oxide (also discussed in chapter 9). When nitric oxide is produced in the lining of healthy blood vessels, it travels virtually instantly to all parts of the body simultaneously. Nitric oxide dilates blood vessels, thus increasing circulation. But it does even more than that. Nitric oxide is the über-neurotransmitter, influencing and balancing the levels of all the other neurotransmitters, including serotonin, dopamine, and beta-endorphin, to name just a few. Neurotransmitters, as you will recall from chapter 2, are the molecules the brain makes when it thinks. But these same chemicals are made throughout the body. In fact, the bowel makes more neurotransmitters than the brain does. The nitric oxide connection is yet another reason why the heart is such a powerful regulator of mood and behavior. (Note that the role of antidepressants such as Prozac is to increase serotonin. Nitric oxide from your blood vessels is designed to do this naturally under the right circumstances.) Nitric oxide levels are increased by regular exercise, healthful pleasures of all kinds, antioxidant supplements, fruits and vegetables, and positive thoughts and emotions. In fact, one twenty-minute episode of aerobic activity in women has been found to increase nitric oxide levels for up to twenty-four hours thereafter. The connection between nitric oxide and health is so powerful that I wrote an entire book about it, called *The Secret Pleasures of Menopause* (Hay House, 2008).

In addition to nitric oxide, the endothelial lining of blood vessels also secretes anticoagulants (molecules that prevent blood clots, coronary occlusion, heart attacks, and embolic strokes) as well as pro-clotting proteins (which prevent bleeding and hemorrhagic strokes). If this endothelial lining is damaged and can't produce adequate amounts of nitric oxide or overproduces the pro-clotting factors associated with stress and subsequent cellular inflammation, the risk for heart attack or stroke rises.

As already mentioned, the entire cardiovascular system, including all the arteries, is influenced starting in the womb and in childhood by diet, genetic tendencies, and ease of emotional expression. The following describes the three stages of development of arteriosclerosis.

1. DEPOSITION OF FATTY STREAKS. These can be found in children. Immune cells called macrophages on the surface of the blood

vessel endothelial cells swallow LDL cholesterol as it floats by. The fat droplets accumulate, causing fatty streaks to develop in the coronary arteries and the aorta. LDL cholesterol and other components of arterial plaques won't stick to the endothelial lining of vessel walls unless there is some kind of damage to these walls in the first place— usually the result of free-radical damage to cells from a refined-food diet, the wrong kind of dietary fat, environmental toxins (such as cigarette smoke), chemicals caused by stress, a nutrient-poor diet, or a combination of all these.

2. FORMATION OF FIBROUS PLAQUES. Over time, the fatty streaks enlarge, causing scarring in the underlying endothelial lining, and these scars can eventually grow into plaques, which are elevated areas of scarred or fibrous fatty tissue in the aorta, the coronary arteries, and the carotid arteries in the neck that bring blood to the brain and are often involved in strokes. These domelike bulges have a central core of cholesterol crystals.

3. COMPLICATED LESION. In time, the dome of the lipid plaque grows large enough to significantly narrow blood vessels, which eventually results in decreased blood flow and thus decreased flow of nutrients and oxygen to tissue—in the same way that mineral buildup clogs plumbing. The calcified plaque may begin to ulcerate. When this happens, there is a much greater risk for blood vessel rupture and bleeding, resulting in a stroke or hemorrhage. Bits of calcified artery can also break off and be propelled by the flow of blood into distant areas where they lodge in a vessel and further cut off blood flow, thus resulting in stroke (dead brain tissue), heart attack (dead heart tissue), or dead tissue in other areas of the body.

Disorders that are characterized by arteriosclerosis include diabetes, insulin resistance, hypertension, a diet too high in refined carbohydrates and too low in antioxidants, decreased thyroid hormone, and a genetic tendency toward producing too much homocysteine.

How Do You Know If Your Vessels Are Healthy?

Only rarely will a doctor be able to diagnose arteriosclerosis from hearing an odd sound (known as a *bruit*) in the carotid artery, or from hearing a click or abnormal rhythm in the heart. If you have diabetes or high blood pressure, are significantly overweight, never exercise, follow a poor diet, or are a smoker, I can virtually guarantee that you already have arteriosclerosis.

Most of the time, arteriosclerosis is not diagnosed until an individual has a cardiac event of some kind, such as a stroke or heart attack. Individuals with chest pain or difficulty walking because of vascular insufficiency often undergo an X-ray test known as an angiogram, which visualizes blood vessels that are injected with dye. Sometimes an ultrasound technology known as a Doppler device will be used to diagnose vessels that are blocked.

Those who don't currently have any symptoms of heart disease but who have several risk factors may choose to have a coronary calcium scan (also called a heart scan). This test uses computerized tomography (CT) to look at the level of calcium buildup in the coronary arteries. Some people with early heart disease have no calcium buildup, however, so a good score is not an absolute guarantee. Nevertheless, the information can often be valuable for assessing risk and avoiding overprescription of statin drugs (see section later in this chapter on statins). For example, in a 2015 study published in the *Journal of the American College of Cardiology,* 5,000 people age fifty and older were screened for ten years. Seventy-seven percent fit the criteria to be on statin drugs, yet half of that group had a coronary calcium score of zero, meaning they were actually at low risk for heart attack and would not benefit from taking a statin.[23] This test is not generally recommended for women under age fifty (because they typically don't have much calcium buildup yet), those with no family history of early-age heart attack, and those already known to be at high risk or who have already been diagnosed. Currently, most health insurance plans don't pay for this test, which can cost anywhere from about $100 to $400.

The good news is that arteriosclerosis can be largely prevented or reversed by diet and lifestyle factors. In fact, the famous Nurses' Health Study, which has followed more than 84,000 women for over fourteen years, has demonstrated that the risk of arteriosclerosis is very low in those women who exercise regularly, abstain from smoking, and follow the kind of diet I recommend in chapter 7.[24] I'll discuss selected risk factors in more detail below. It's important for every perimenopausal woman to get a complete checkup from a healthcare provider who is qualified to evaluate her cardiovascular status. This evaluation should include, as a minimum, a thorough history and physical exam, EKG, blood pressure check, and lipid profile.

FACTORS ASSOCIATED WITH AN INCREASED RISK FOR CARDIOVASCULAR DISEASE

~ You are/were a habitual smoker.

~ You have a strong family history of heart disease (especially before the age of sixty).

~ You have high LDL ("bad") cholesterol (greater than 130 mg/dl).

~ Your HDL ("good") cholesterol is low (less than 46 mg/dl).

~ You have high triglycerides (greater than 150 mg/dl).

~ You have high blood pressure (greater than 130/85).

~ You have high levels of the amino acid homocysteine in your bloodstream.

~ You are overfat (body mass index greater than 25) with an apple-shaped figure (a preponderance of body fat above the level of the hips).

~ Your waist measures 33.5 inches or more.

~ You have a hypertrigliceridemic-waist phenotype—for women, that means a waist circumference of 85 cm (about 33.5 inches) or more *and* a triglyceride level of 1.5 mmol/L (about 133 mg/dl) or more.[25]

~ You have periodontal disease.

~ You have diabetes.

~ You are sedentary and don't exercise.

~ You have a history of significant clinical depression.

Cholesterol

A lipid profile is a measure of your total cholesterol, LDL cholesterol, HDL cholesterol, and triglyceride levels. Here are the numbers to shoot for on the lipid profile. Please note that the American Heart Association keeps lowering these numbers. I believe that this is a direct result of pressure from the pharmaceutical industry, which seeks to increase prescriptions for statin drugs (see page 682).

TOTAL CHOLESTEROL: Below 200. (*Note:* If your cholesterol is slightly higher than 200, don't worry about it if your HDL is sufficiently high.)

HDL (HIGH-DENSITY LIPOPROTEIN): HDL—the "good" cholesterol—should be 45 or higher; 67 or above is ideal. Low HDL cholesterol has been shown to be a more potent risk factor in women than it is in men. Women with low levels of this cholesterol subtype (a reading of 35 or less) have a sevenfold increase in heart disease risk compared to those whose HDL levels are normal.[26] Low HDL is one of the first indicators of insulin resistance.

LDL (LOW-DENSITY LIPOPROTEIN): LDL—the "bad" cholesterol—should be 130 or below. LDL cholesterol rises after menopause in many women, a fact that was the basis for promoting estrogen replacement, which decreases LDL levels. If your LDL is greater than 150 mg/dl (some doctors use even lower numbers), you're considered at high risk for coronary artery disease. LDL cholesterol undergoes free-radical damage and forms plaques in the arteries.

TRIGLYCERIDES: This number should be 150 or lower. Triglycerides are an independent risk factor for women. An ideal triglyceride level for a woman is around 75. A woman with a triglyceride level of greater than 200 has a 14 percent risk of developing coronary artery disease. High triglycerides are associated with toxic abdominal fat and glycemic stress in part because the liver, as well as other areas of the body, stores excess blood sugar as triglycerides.

RELATIONSHIP OF TOTAL CHOLESTEROL TO HDL: Neither type of cholesterol is inherently bad or good. Both are necessary for good health. They need to be balanced in the body. Divide your total cholesterol by your HDL cholesterol. If the resulting number is 4 or less, you are at low risk, regardless what your total cholesterol number is. The ratio of total cholesterol to HDL is a much better predictor of risk than simply your total cholesterol number. Ask your doctor to give you a copy of your lipid profile so that you can get to know your numbers. It's very motivating to watch your lipid profile improve every year when you commit to becoming healthier than ever before at midlife.

Currently 38 percent of American adults have elevated cholesterol levels.[27] Though interpretation of lipid profile results will vary from lab to lab, a total cholesterol level as high as 225 to 240 does not necessarily indicate that a woman is at increased risk for heart disease if her HDL cholesterol is also high (45 or above). Because most of the studies of heart disease and blood lipid levels have been done on men, we still don't know exactly what levels of blood lipids are optimal for women. What we do know is that women can have higher total cholesterol levels than men and not be at increased risk for heart disease.

Get your lipid profile repeated at least every five years if it's normal. If your blood sugar is high, get the test repeated more frequently.

If your cholesterol levels are high, know that dietary change and a good supplement program can lower cholesterol significantly and quickly. There are a number of ways to do this. The Keto-Green diet by my colleague Anna Cabeca, D.O., works very well in that it creates ketosis (fat burning) but also keeps the blood pH alkaline. Many women prefer this to the meat- and fat-heavy approaches that are so popular these days. There is also the Bulletproof diet created by Dave Asprey, the Always Hungry? approach by David Ludwig, M.D., Ph.D., and the Grain Brain diet by holistic neurologist David Perlmutter, M.D. And cardiovascular surgeon Steven Gundry, M.D., has produced groundbreaking books on dietary approaches that heal heart disease. On the opposite end of the spectrum is the low-fat vegan approach by the Medical Medium, Anthony William. This has helped many, many people.

We are each individuals with unique dietary preferences and needs. There is no "one size fits all" diet for heart health. What all of these approaches have in common, however, is that they use whole foods, without preservatives and additives, and they concentrate on plant foods. What varies is the amount of fruit and fat. There are individuals who are so sugar sensitive, for example, that even eating a medjool date causes symptoms. One of my friends gets cracking of the skin on her feet when she eats dates, and the same goes for mangos. That is how sugar sensitive she is.

Oftentimes the positive changes that occur with changes in lifestyles are so motivating that they spur permanent lifestyle changes that not only result in healthy cholesterol levels, but also prevent adult onset diabetes and a host of other chronic degenerative diseases. Permanent fat loss is a most rewarding benefit as well.

If you cannot or will not institute lifestyle improvements, at least take omega-3 supplements and make sure your vitamin D levels are optimal (see page 349).

REFINING CARDIOVASCULAR RISK FACTORS

Newer research shows that a few additional numbers can be very important for assessing risk. According to cardiologist Michael Ozner, M.D., medical director of wellness and prevention at Baptist Health South Florida in Miami, traditional testing that measures only LDL, HDL, and triglycerides uncovers only 40 percent of people at risk for heart attacks. Also checking blood levels of C-reactive protein (an inflammatory marker), apolipoprotein B (apoB, the number of LDL particles in the blood), and lipoprotein (a) (LP(a), a type of small, dense LDL that is more dangerous than other cholesterol-carrying particles) can boost that figure to 90 percent because these tests catch people who are at risk even though they have normal levels of LDL. (For further information, read Dr. Ozner's book *The Great American Heart Hoax: Lifesaving Advice Your Doctor Should Tell You About Heart Disease Prevention (But Probably Never Will)* [BenBella Books, 2008] or visit his website at www.drozner.com.) An alternative way to test for the number of LDL particles in the blood that is gaining much attention is to test for the level of LDL-P using nuclear magnetic resonance (NMR).

These newer tests have been determined to be so important for assessing risk that the updated American Diabetes Association and American College of Cardiology expert consensus guidelines for treating cardiometabolic patients now call for measuring levels of apoB as well as non-HDL cholesterol (total cholesterol minus HDL cholesterol).[28] For those with highest risk (those with known cardiovascular disease or those with diabetes plus at least one additional risk factor for cardiovascular disease), treatment goals are a non-HDL cholesterol level of less than 100 mg/dl, an apoB level of less than 80 mg/dl, and an LDL-P level of less than 1,000 mg/dl. For those considered to be high risk (which includes diabetics with no other risk factors for cardiovascular disease as well as those who have not been diagnosed with cardiovascular disease or with diabetes but who have two major risk factors for cardiovascular disease), the treatment goals are a non-HDL cholesterol level of less than 130 mg/dl, an apoB level of less than 90 mg/dl, and an LDL-P level of less than 1,300 mg/dl.

Not all doctors order such detailed blood analyses, and not all labs do them. However, I think these tests can be very useful because they can determine risk long before symptoms develop. One lab I recommend that offers them is Boston Heart Diagnostics (https://bostonheartdiagnostics.com).

What About Statins?

I am very concerned about the overuse of statin drugs, such as Lipitor, Crestor, and Zocor, among others, which are prescribed to millions of women in the belief that because they lower LDL cholesterol levels, they will prevent heart disease. Adding more fuel to the fire were the results of a large, long-term, double-blind, placebo-controlled, randomized clinical trial called the Justification for the Use of Statins in Primary Prevention: An Intervention Trial Evaluating Rosuvastatin (JUPITER). Published in 2009, JUPITER looked at the effect of a statin called rosuvastatin (sold as Crestor) on 17,802 healthy men and women with normal LDL cholesterol levels but elevated C-reactive protein (CRP) levels, a sign of inflammation. The study was halted after just two years by an independent review panel that saw that the placebo group was having more heart attacks, strokes, angina, and death from cardiovascular disease. Data showed that those taking Crestor reduced their risk of heart attack by 54 percent and their risk of stroke by 48 percent—and the risk of dying from all causes by 20 percent.[29]

Despite this evidence, I still feel strongly that prescribing statins to healthy women to prevent heart disease misses the mark because it's the same line of seriously flawed reasoning that led doctors to prescribe Premarin to millions of women back in the 1980s and '90s because it was shown to raise HDL (good cholesterol) levels. The high LDL cholesterol that statins are prescribed to reduce is not a disease, and lowering levels won't prevent disease—as already mentioned, half of all people who get heart disease don't even have high cholesterol! The cause of heart disease is cellular inflammation and arterial wall damage, which oxidizes LDL and causes it to stick to damaged blood vessel walls and build up plaque. This is what JUPI-

TER showed us—when you reduce inflammation, heart disease risk drops. The researchers happened to be focusing on statins as the means of reducing LDL, but statins are not without serious side effects and risks. (For example, JUPITER also showed that more people taking Crestor developed diabetes than did those on placebo.) Further, because the study was halted prematurely, long-term safety data on taking Crestor were not gathered. Yet there are perfectly safe and very effective ways to lower LDL that don't involve taking statins, such as proper diet, exercise, stress reduction, and supplementation with the right nutrients. *That* is where I think we ought to be putting the attention.

I think it's important to add that, as already mentioned, the bar for what is considered "normal" keeps getting harder to reach. The level of LDL cholesterol that is considered "normal" has been continually reduced over the years, largely because of the behind-the-scenes influence of the pharmaceutical industry, which supplies the majority of research grants to academic medicine. The American Heart Association's 2004 recommendations for "normal" LDL for people with very high risk for cardiovascular disease were lowered to 70 mg/dl, which I consider ridiculous.[30] (The rest of the guidelines range from a recommended LDL level of under 100 for those with high risk to below 160 for those with low risk.) In fact, a 2016 review of the medical literature turned a lot of heads when it showed that in people age sixty and older, those with high LDL cholesterol live as long or longer than those with low LDL.[31] In their conclusion, the researchers actually urged a reevaluation of current guidelines calling for older Americans with high LDL to take cholesterol-lowering medication. The bottom line: I believe that if your cholesterol level is lower than 240–275 mg/dl and your HDL is 60 or above, you don't need a statin.

Here's what all women should know about statins: despite all the hype, JUPITER included, many large studies involving statins have failed to show much benefit. Here's a partial list.

- A study designed to determine whether there was a relationship between statin use and death from coronary heart disease in twelve European countries found that despite tens of millions more people being prescribed statin drugs, there was no evidence of lower death rates from heart disease over a twelve-year period.[32] The researchers noted that among other factors, media attention and pharmaceutical industry marketing may have been behind the large increase in statin use.

~ In a 2015 systematic review of statin drug trials, the average increase in life expectancy for those with established heart disease who took statin drugs for five years was only four days.[33]

~ The ALLHAT clinical trial (announced in 2002) was the largest study in the world using Lipitor.[34] Ten thousand participants with high LDL cholesterol were treated either with statins or lifestyle changes. Though the subjects in the group that took Lipitor did, in fact, lower their LDL cholesterol significantly compared to the control group, there was no difference in death rate from heart attack between the two groups!

~ The Heart Protection study supposedly conferred "massive" benefits to participants who took Zocor for five years compared to controls who didn't take the drug.[35] After five years, those on the drug had an 87.1 percent survival rate compared to an 85.4 percent survival rate for those who didn't. But the survival rates were independent of the lowering of cholesterol, so there was no difference between the two groups in reduction of death from heart disease.

~ The Japanese Lipid Intervention Trial of 2002 was a six-year study of 47,294 patients treated with Zocor. The drug lowered LDL cholesterol dramatically in some participants and moderately or not at all in others. After five years, there was no correlation between LDL cholesterol levels and death rate.[36]

~ A 2003 meta-analysis of forty-four clinical trials involving 9,500 patients found that the death rate for those taking statins was identical to those taking no drugs. More worrisome is that 65 percent of those taking statins experienced adverse side effects that caused many to withdraw from the study. The bottom line: statin drugs showed no benefit in reducing the overall number of deaths.[37]

~ The 2003 ASCOT-LLA (Anglo-Scandinavian Cardiac Outcomes Trial—Lipid Lowering Arm) study compared the benefits of Lipitor versus placebo in patients with normal LDL cholesterol but with high blood pressure and other risk factors for heart disease.[38] After three years, Lipitor was credited with decreasing the risk of heart attack and stroke. But no reduction in deaths occurred. And there were actually more deaths in the women taking Lipitor than in those who didn't take it!

~ The 2003 University of British Columbia Therapeutics Initiative Study found that statin drugs did not prevent heart disease in women.[39]

~ A Canadian study on the effectiveness of different countries' guidelines for statin treatment showed that to prevent one cardiac death, 154 people who had been recommended statins would have to take them for five years. To prevent one cardiac death among people with low risk for heart disease (who had not been recommended these drugs), 23,000 patients would have to take statins for the same length of time.[40]

WOMEN AND STATINS

Just as heart disease can have different symptoms in women than in men, statins affect women differently than they do men. Looking at total mortality figures in major clinical trials, it's clear that the risk-benefit balance of statins is less favorable in women than it is in men.[41] Plenty of evidence now exists to show that low cholesterol, especially in women older than fifty, is associated with higher levels of cancer and early death. For example, a meta-analysis of thirteen studies published in the *Journal of the American Medical Association* showed that for women who do *not* have cardiovascular disease, lipid lowering does not lower mortality. For women who *have* been diagnosed with cardiovascular disease, statins were shown to reduce coronary heart disease events and deaths from heart disease, but they did not reduce total mortality.[42]

A prospective study from Austria comparing cholesterol levels and health outcomes for more than 80,000 women and 67,000 men over a fifteen-year period found that high cholesterol in women over age fifty was not a predictor of cardiovascular problems or stroke (although it was for women under age fifty). The study found that low cholesterol levels in people older than fifty was associated with higher death rates from cancer, liver disease, and mental illness.[43] Another prospective study from Italy of 3,120 women age sixty-five and older who were followed for twelve years found no health benefits from having low LDL levels. For most of the subjects, elevated LDL was associated with greater longevity and fewer cardiac events.[44]

Statin Drugs Deplete Vital Nutrients

If statins were wildly effective in decreasing the mortality rate from cardiovascular disease, then their benefits might outweigh their risks. But this is clearly not the case. And the risks, though vastly under-reported, are considerable. The serious side effects resulting from statins are the result of how they work. Statin drugs block cholesterol production in the body by inhibiting an enzyme called HMG-Co-A reductase. This is the same pathway that the body uses to create coenzyme Q_{10} and substances called dilochols, both of which are absolutely essential for proper cell health. By blocking cholesterol production, statins also block production of these vital nutrients.

Dilochols direct proteins to the areas of the cells that need repair. Without them, the cells can't carry out their genetic programming for cellular functioning and restoration. Statins therefore potentially wreak havoc with cellular repair. Coenzyme Q_{10} (ubiquinone or CoQ_{10}), which is far better known than the dilochols, is a critical cellular nutrient that is necessary for producing energy in the form of ATP in the part of the cell known as the mitochondria. ATP is a molecule that carries energy for cellular function much like gasoline powers the engine of a car. Without it, nothing can run. The heart, in particular, requires an enormous amount of energy and CoQ_{10} to function efficiently. CoQ_{10} is also necessary for the vital role played by cell membranes (the actual "brain" of the cell) and also for the formation of collagen and elastin that make up the connective tissue in skin, muscles, and blood vessel walls. Because every cell in the body requires coenzyme Q_{10} to function properly, depletion of this enzyme from statin drugs causes problems throughout the entire body.

Statins reduce the production of vitamins A and D as well—two other anti-inflammatory nutrients. Statin drugs also negatively affect the omega-3-to-omega-6 ratio, raising the risk of inflammation.[45] (It should come as no surprise, then, that seven clinical trials in recent years show that patients taking statins had better results when they also took omega-3 fats.)[46]

SIDE EFFECTS OF STATIN DRUGS

~ *Muscle weakness, pain, and fatigue.* This is the most common side effect of statins and it is the direct result of depletion of CoQ_{10} in the muscles and heart.[47] Beatrice Golomb, M.D., Ph.D., has studied statin side effects and has reported that nearly all patients taking Lipitor and about one-third of patients taking Mevachor have experienced muscle problems.[48] This side effect is even more common for statin users who are hypothyroid.[49]

~ *Brain and nerve damage.* Cognitive problems are the second most common side effect reported with statin use.[50] CoQ_{10} is essential for normal brain and nerve function. When it is depleted, dementia can result. This is why many people on statins have difficulty with memory, mood, and clear thinking. In a study in Denmark of 500,000 people, researchers found a significantly higher incidence of neuropathies, including peripheral neuropathy, in those taking statins.[51] Another study showed a fourteenfold increased risk of neuropathy after two or more years on statins compared to controls.[52] A study from the University of Mississippi Medical Center suggested that cognitive impairment and dementia should be considered potential adverse effects associated with statin therapy.[53] Even more telling was a study from the University of California, San Diego, reporting that 75 percent of people who took the statins experienced cognitive problems that were determined to be probably or definitely related to statin therapy. Of the people who then *stopped* taking statins, 90 percent reported improvement in their cognitive problems—sometimes within a matter of days. (In some patients, even the diagnosis of dementia or Alzheimer's disease was reversed.) The study also reported significant negative impact on quality of life in people taking statin drugs.[54]

~ *Heart disease and heart failure.* CoQ_{10} levels fall naturally as we age, decreasing by about 50 percent between the ages of twenty and eighty. This is one of the reasons why heart attack, stroke, and cancer increase with age. Statin drugs deplete this nutrient even further, thus increasing the risk of cardiomyopathy and heart failure. The heart is the worst place in the body to deplete CoQ_{10} because it requires so much energy that must be constantly replenished. Cardiologist Peter Langsjoen, M.D., has reported on the adverse effects of Lipitor among twenty patients who started on the drug with completely normal hearts. After six months and a low dose of Lipitor (20 mg per day), two-thirds of the patients started to show signs of heart failure.[55] Dr. Langsjoen credits this effect to CoQ_{10} depletion. While the heart attack rate has decreased somewhat over the last twenty years, cardiomyopathy and heart failure incidence have increased. I'm concerned that this problem will increase even more in those taking statins.

⁓ *Liver damage.* The liver constantly detoxifies the blood and carries out a huge number of enzymatic reactions. So it, too, requires a good supply of CoQ_{10}. Even a modest deficiency can cause liver problems, reflected in increased liver enzymes on a blood test. People on statins need to get liver enzymes checked regularly. Liver damage can begin the moment one begins taking statin drugs.

⁓ *Psychiatric problems, including depression.* A 2007 study from New Zealand reported an increase in reports of suspected psychiatric adverse reactions (including depression, memory loss, confusion, and aggressive reactions) associated with statins, as well as with other lipid-lowering agents.[56] A Norwegian study noted that psychiatric disorders (including aggression, nervousness, depression, anxiety, sleeping disorders, and impotence) represent 15 percent of the adverse reactions to statins in that country.[57] It is well documented that low cholesterol is associated with depression and may even increase the risk of suicide. This all makes sense because cholesterol is an essential building block of brain and nerve tissue. It is like the coating on the wires that govern nerve conduction and function—including maintaining a stable mood. It is fairly common for women to begin experiencing anxiety and mood problems after beginning statin drugs. Yet another study from the University of California, San Diego, reported that statin use was associated with severe irritability.[58] A study of

121 women aged eighteen to twenty-seven found that women with low cholesterol are twice as likely to have depression and anxiety.[59] Supplementing one's diet with the right type of omega-3-rich fats often helps this problem dramatically. So does getting off statins.

~ *Cancer.* Statin drugs have been found to suppress the immune system (which is why they are sometimes prescribed for those with inflammatory conditions such as arthritis). And that also explains why they've had some effect on decreasing cardiovascular events such as stroke, which results from inflammation in blood vessel walls. In fact, any benefit from statins may be from this anti-inflammatory effect. Unfortunately, it is well documented that drugs that suppress the immune system increase the risk of cancer. That is why statin drugs have been found to cause cancer in rodent studies.[60] The most likely reason that we haven't yet seen this effect in studies on humans is that clinical trials haven't lasted more than two to five years. It would take longer to see this effect. Not surprisingly, CoQ_{10} is effective at lowering the risk of many cancers, including colon, rectum, breast, lung, prostate, and pancreas.[61]

I'm also very concerned about the increased risk of breast cancer in women on statins.[62] In fact, the CARE (Cholesterol and Recurrent Events) trial at Brigham and Women's Hospital in Boston found twelve new cases of breast cancer in the 250 women taking Lipitor, while there was only one new case in the placebo group.[63] While not proving a cause and effect relationship, it's certainly worrisome. Though other studies have failed to show this effect, they have not been double-blind, placebo-controlled.[64]

There is also a statistic everyone should know about: the NNT, the number needed to treat. This is the number of people who need to be on a given drug in order for one person to benefit from the treatment (so the smaller the number, the better). When it comes to statins, in those without known heart disease the number needed to treat is 104 in order for one person to prevent heart attack and 154 in order for one person to prevent stroke.[65] Even for those with known heart disease, the NNT with statins to save one life is 83 and to prevent one person from having a stroke is 125.[66] That means ninety-nine people out of a hundred (even among those diagnosed with heart disease) will get no benefit from statins. This comes into even sharper focus when you consider that one in eighteen people who already had one heart attack can prevent a second heart attack by simply adhering to the Mediterranean diet, meaning there is far more benefit from this dietary change than from taking statins.[67]

The other statistic everyone should know about is the NNH, the number needed to harm. This is the number of people who would have to be treated by a drug for one person to show some harm from it (so the larger the number, the better). For statins that number is 10, since one out of every ten people taking high-dose statins suffers from muscle pain (myopathy).[68]

A Word About the Pharmaceutical Industry

It's important to your health that you realize the degree to which the pharmaceutical industry influences medical research, medical reporting (in both medical and mainstream media), and medical prescribing. The overuse of statins is a stellar example of this influence. Marcia Angell, M.D., the former editor in chief of the prestigious *New England Journal of Medicine,* documented the way in which drug companies influence medical research, prescribing, and reporting very strongly and effectively in her book *The Truth About the Drug Companies: How They Deceive Us and What to Do About It* (Random House, 2004). (For more information on the statin debate, read *Lipitor: Thief of Memory, Statin Drugs and the Misguided War on Cholesterol* [Infinity Publishing, 2004] by Duane Graveline, M.D., a former astronaut and aerospace medical research scientist who twice developed global amnesia after taking Lipitor on his doctor's recommendation.)

The current situation with the pharmaceutical industry can be likened to the influence of the tobacco industry on the medical profession back in the 1940s and '50s when doctors and the AMA espoused the "benefits" of smoking to their patients and were paid handsomely by Big Tobacco. Eventually the truth won. And it will again.

High Blood Pressure

Blood pressure fluctuates all the time, hour by hour, day by day, and there has been extensive overdiagnosis and unnecessary treatment of millions of people because of this. It's not uncommon for blood pressure to rise simply in response to a doctor's visit! This is called "white coat syndrome," and I've seen it repeatedly. On the other hand, bona fide hypertension is a well-known risk factor for heart attack, kidney disease, and stroke.

In the past, normal blood pressure was considered to be anything below 130/85, with optimal blood pressure deemed to be 120/80. High blood pressure was diagnosed at 140/90. In 2003, the guidelines changed, and normal blood pressure was then defined as being less than 120/80 (with optimal blood pressure being 115/75). At that point, a blood pressure of 120/80 (what used to be considered optimal) was reclassified as "prehypertension." The threshold for high blood pressure remained at 140/90, which was defined as stage 1 hypertension.

But all that changed in 2017, thanks to pressure from the pharmaceutical industry. Now the definition of high blood pressure begins at 130/80, considered stage 1 hypertension. Blood pressure of 140/90 (the old stage 1) is now classified as stage 2 hypertension. When these new guidelines went into effect, 31 million Americans were immediately reclassified as having high blood pressure, bringing the revised total to 103 million. This also meant that the percentage of Americans with hypertension jumped from 32 percent to 46 percent—almost half the U.S. population. The result was that doctors put even more people on medication, with all the associated risks. Normal blood pressure is now defined as being less than 120/80, with an intermediate category called elevated blood pressure that's defined as 120–129/80.

Blood pressure can be significantly lowered by any one of the following lifestyle changes: regular exercise (such as brisk walking), biofeedback, dietary improvement, or weight loss. Even in very overweight women, losing only ten to twenty pounds will often lower blood pressure significantly. If these measures fail, then it's advisable to use blood-pressure-lowering medication, even though these medications can have side effects such as dizziness, headaches, and fatigue.

Be sure to get your lipid profile and blood pressure checked again within three to six months. *Note:* If you follow the insulin-normalizing diet I recommend at perimenopause, you can expect substantial improvements in your lipid profile, your blood sugar, and your blood pressure within two to four weeks.

Homocysteine

Elevated blood levels of the amino acid homocysteine, which is found in high amounts in animal protein, constitutes a strong risk factor for cardiovascular disease. At least 10 percent or more of the population has a genetic tendency for elevated levels of homocysteine, but there are other factors besides genetics that elevate it. When high homocysteine levels are reduced, the incidence of heart attack is cut by 20 percent, the risk of blood-clot-related strokes decreases by 40 percent, and the risk of venous blood clots elsewhere in the body plunges by an impressive 60 percent. Studies have shown that dietary intake of vitamins B_{12}, B_6, and folate can help combat an elevated homocysteine level, as can cutting back on the amount of animal-based protein in your diet. Ask your healthcare provider to determine your homocysteine level. (It should be below 7.) If it's too high, you need to add folic acid, vitamin B_{12}, and vitamin B_6 to your diet. You may also need folate supplements of 1,000–2,000 mcg for three months or so, after which point you can decrease the supplements to a maintenance amount. (As one of those with a genetic tendency toward high homocysteine, I was able to lower my levels to normal by taking extra folic acid.) You may also need methylated folate and B_{12} (see below).

Periodontal Disease and Cardiac Risk

Periodontal disease (inflammation and infection of the gums) is present in a significant percentage of adults in the United States. A number of compelling studies have shown that gum disease is a risk factor for coronary artery disease and stroke. Although no one can say that periodontal disease directly causes cardiovascular disease, research has clearly shown that periodontal disease is more prevalent in patients with acute and chronic heart disease. This association may be due, in part, to the fact that inflammation plays a central role both in gum disease and in hardening of the arteries. It has also been shown that the inflammation seen in periodontal disease is associated with narrowing of the carotid arteries, a risk factor for stroke.[69]

Periodontal disease is easily preventable (and often treatable) from the outside through proper brushing, flossing, and regular visits to the dentist for professional evaluation and cleaning. Dietary improvement and supplementation help treat it from the inside. Caring for your teeth and gums is a practical and easy way to decrease at least one risk factor for cardiovascular disease or stroke.

Smoking

Smoking is responsible for 55 percent of the cardiovascular deaths in women less than sixty-five years old because smoking increases oxidative stress enormously in every cell of the body. The Nurses' Health Study followed more than 117,000 female nurses ages thirty to fifty-five. In that study the relative risk of total coronary artery disease among smokers was four times higher than that of women who never smoked. But in women who stopped smoking, the relative risk of coronary artery disease immediately decreased to 1.5. Two years after stopping smoking, the risk dropped to that of a woman who has never smoked. Smoking is also responsible for approximately 29 percent of all cancers. Since 1987 lung cancer has been the leading cause of cancer deaths among women.[70]

At least thirteen studies have shown that smokers cease menstruation one to two years earlier than nonsmokers. The effect is dose-dependent, and the difference persists after controlling for weight. Female smokers sixty years and older also have significantly reduced bone mineral density of the hip compared with nonsmokers.[71]

HOW TO QUIT

You have to want to quit to be successful. With each subsequent attempt, however, the chances for successfully staying off tobacco increase. The biggest problem women have with successfully quitting smoking is that they often have to change their friendships and behavior patterns and begin to think of themselves as nonsmokers.

Acupuncture can help people quit, because it's helpful for detoxing addictions. Some women also do well with Smokers Anonymous programs or with one of the nicotine patches.

I recommend calling your local hospital to see what is available. Or discuss stopping smoking with your doctor.

Age

The only reason that age is a risk factor for heart disease is that by the time you reach fifty or so, the processes that clog arteries are often well established. Coronary artery disease starts in many by the teenage years. It's the result of your day-to-day decisions on all levels: emotional, physical, and psychological. To treat it, reverse it, or prevent it, you need to change those day-to-day actions that led to it in the first place.

A large study of coronary risk factors in fifteen-year-olds and young adults, for example, showed that of 197 males and 197 females, 31 percent of the males and 10 percent of the females had calcification of their coronary arteries by age fifteen. We know that these calcifications are closely associated with heart attack, stroke, and aneurysm in later life. To further figure out which individuals were more likely to have these lesions, the investigators found that the following factors were most predictive of coronary artery pathology: high body mass index and low HDL ("good") cholesterol.[72] All roads lead back to glycemic stress!

Powerful Versus Powerless

If you perceive that you are valuable and powerful in the world and have choices, then your heart will be more apt to work optimally. The opposite is also true. At least two studies have shown a relationship between a woman's job and her health. One study found that women who are employed and married have the best health, with or without children. If their husbands are supportive, so much the better. Good health is also associated with more complex and challenging jobs characterized by autonomy.

But if you feel that you have no autonomy, the risk for heart disease goes up. Clerical workers whose supervisors are demanding and whose job situations do not allow them to express anger are at increased risk for developing heart disease. Time pressure is also a risk factor that has been associated with poor health.[73]

If a woman's heart isn't in her work, she cannot express her anger about this, and she perceives that she can't leave, this conflict hits her right in the heart, an organ that is exquisitely sensitive to the effects of excessive catecholamines over time. A woman in a stressful job in which she feels she doesn't have a say is also more likely to smoke, which results in higher blood pressure and cholesterol—both additional risk factors for heart disease.

Studies suggest that low educational standing is consistently associated with higher risk of coronary artery disease in women. This isn't necessarily related to formal education, however; rather, it is tied more to the fact that those who are better educated tend to take better care of themselves and to know that they have choices. Also, body mass index and cigarette smoking are inversely related to educational attainment. Vigorous leisure-time activity is also related to educational attainment. Fitness levels assessed by treadmill have been directly related to educational attainment in women but not in men.[74] The good news is that you don't need to go back to school for an advanced degree to change your perception and take charge of your lifestyle.

The number and diversity of your friends and associates also contributes to heart health or lack of it. Women with greater numbers of children and too many demands on their time combined with a lack of emotional support have been shown to be at greater risk for heart disease. But women who perceive that their families are supportive are at lower risk.

SHARON: *Dying for Her Benefits*

Sharon had been a patient of mine for years. Though she was about twenty pounds overweight, she walked regularly and was in a very happy, supportive relationship. Her blood pressure and cholesterol were normal, and she was in good health. She was also on Premarin and Provera—two hormones that had been prescribed for her at the beginning of her menopause, for hot flashes. She had done well with this approach and there was no reason to change the prescription. (At the time, we didn't have the data on alternatives that are now available.) At the age of fifty-four Sharon developed chest pain, and a cardiac workup showed that she had narrowing of her coronary arteries. She underwent bypass surgery. When I asked Sharon if she was going through any unusual stresses around the time of her chest pain, she told me that she had been hoping she could take early retirement from her job as a university professor. She and her husband had bought a house in Florida, where they spent as much time as possible. But she discovered that if she took early retirement, she wouldn't be eligible for her full pension benefits. So she halfheartedly decided that she had no choice but to stay another ten years. It was shortly after she made this decision that she developed her chest pain.

As I did her annual pelvic and breast exam, I asked her if she really felt it was worth it to stay another ten years in a job that was literally shutting off the joy to her heart. And I was reminded that people who stay in jobs they hate strictly for their benefits rarely get to use them.

Hidden Emotions Lead to Hypertension

There is no question that factors such as obesity, salt intake, and a sedentary lifestyle are associated with hypertension. And so is stress. But not in the way we've been led to believe. Samuel J. Mann, M.D., professor of clinical medicine at the Hypertension Center of the New York–Presbyterian Hospital Weill Cornell Medical Center in New York City, has seen thousands of people with all varieties of high blood pressure. Over the years, he began to notice a pattern that didn't fit with the common view of hypertension. In his book *Healing Hypertension: A Revolutionary New Approach* (Wiley, 1999), he notes, "Even patients with severe hypertension did not seem more emotionally distressed than others. If anything, they seemed less distressed. Their high blood pressure appeared to be more related to what they did *not* seem to be feeling than to what they *were* feeling."[75] He began to see that old, unhealed, repressed trauma seemed to be a major culprit in his patients. After all, anger and stress can elevate blood pressure, but they do this temporarily and aren't the root cause of hypertension. Instead, it is our hidden emotions, says Dr. Mann, the emotions we do not feel, that lead to hypertension and many other unexplained physical disorders. To deal with hypertension at its core (or anything else, for that matter), it is necessary to bring those hidden emotions to the light, to consciousness, and to deal with them.

The late Annemarie Colbin, Ph.D., my friend and colleague and the founder of the Natural Gourmet Institute for Health and Culinary Arts in Manhattan, shared her personal experience with hypertension after she was diagnosed with it despite her very healthy lifestyle.

> I can testify to the validity of this approach. In the summer of 2000, I read about Dr. Mann in a little free newspaper that covers my New York neighborhood. At the time this seemed a surprising synchronicity, as I had suddenly found myself grappling with some episodes of extremely high blood pressure—as high as 220/120. I was unable to sleep at night, or at most slept two

to three hours, a completely new development for me. I also had trouble concentrating. Although I am very opposed to taking pharmaceutical drugs, I did consult a physician and took some anyway. I also went to my usual alternative medicine practitioners, such as my chiropractor, homeopath, and acupuncturist, which helped a little, but I knew it wasn't enough.

After reading the article about Dr. Mann, I bought his book and read more on his unique perspective. Then I went to see him, and with his encouragement started looking at what kind of hidden emotions I could be harboring. It didn't take long to figure out that the place to look would be in my repressed, or perhaps pre-verbal, memories of the three years I spent during World War II in Budapest, Hungary, when I was two to five years old. I was there with my mother (my father, I found out years later, was in a forced labor camp), and we spent many nights in cellars and basements with thirty to forty strangers, hiding from the bombs and grenades. In terms of emotions, I knew there was something there, but I had no memory of it.

One day in August, after a weekend of sleeping one night out of three, I found myself again with high blood pressure, 200/100, and I went for a walk in the park, barefoot in the grass. (I had taken this up as a de-stressor.) Thinking about the war years, and also about how I felt the sleepless night before, I realized that my night wakefulness was quiet and watchful. I did not think, worry, toss, or turn. I was just on high alert. It felt as if I was just waiting. What, I wondered, was I waiting for?

Then I remembered my mother telling me about one time when we were staying in a basement, and she was summoned upstairs by the occupying soldiers for a party, together with another young woman there. Thus, she had to leave me alone in the dark cellar with all the strangers, none of whom cared about me. I suddenly got in touch with a profound terror that a three- or four-year-old would feel—the fear that my mother might not come back. I remembered knowing that I would die if she didn't return. I had no home, no family, no friends around, nothing—it was just the two of us, and without her I had no chance of survival. I think I must have stayed awake all that night waiting for my mother, and now, in my sleepless nights, I was reliving it. I lay in the grass, on the safe ground, and shook and cried, feeling and releasing that old terror.

After a while of shaking and crying, I calmed down, got up, and went home, feeling strangely relieved. Then I checked my blood pressure. It had gone down to 137/82—in one hour! I knew I was on the right track. Since then, it still has gone up and down, and I had to do quite a lot more spiritual work, but at the time of this writing, four months later, my blood pressure seems to be keeping itself normal with no medication. It's been a harrowing four months, and I'm not finished yet, but I am certainly on the path to cleaning out that old emotional baggage, thanks to Dr. Mann's revolutionary insights.

Depression

Depression is consistently related to a high risk for heart disease in both men and women. In a survey of women in my wisdom community back in the early 2000s, 46 percent listed their biggest health concern as depression and anxiety. In contrast, only 18 percent indicated that heart disease was their greatest concern. What these and most other women don't realize is that the emotions associated with sadness or grief, anger or depression, and fear or anxiety are very much connected to heart disease (as well as bone health).

Women's blood vessels are smaller than men's and are extremely sensitive to the biochemical changes that occur in response to the emotions of daily life. These biochemical changes result in either constricted or dilated blood vessels. When your blood vessels constrict in response to emotions such as anger, grief, and fear, they do so because of an outpouring of chemicals from the sympathetic nervous system; blood flow is reduced, and tissue damage and high blood pressure are the result.

Because at least 25 percent of women suffer from depressive episodes at some point in their lives, and because women are more apt to suffer from depression than men, depression emerges as a very important and modifiable risk factor for women. Though it is well documented that both men and women often suffer from depression after a heart attack, newer data conclude that depression is an important independent risk factor for heart disease. A study from the Ohio State University College of Medicine and Public Health showed just how profoundly depression affects coronary artery disease in women. Even after adjusting for other factors such as smoking, obesity, and lack of exercise, the risk for nonfatal coronary artery disease was 73 percent higher in depressed women compared with a control group.[76] In their research, depressed women were also shown to be twice as likely to develop coronary artery disease as were normal, nondepressed women.

Similarly, profound grief and emotional distress can also stress your heart. Stress cardiomyopathy, commonly called "broken heart syndrome," is a term for sudden weakening of the heart muscle brought on by emotional trauma, such as grief, fear, extreme anger, or surprise. It can happen after experiencing the unexpected death of a loved one, a close brush with death, or being the victim of domestic abuse. While much about the physiology of broken heart syndrome remains unclear, we do know that a surge of catecholamines (stress hormones, such as adrenaline and noradrenaline) stuns the heart. This condition, which affects midlife women more than any other demographic, mimics a classic heart attack, with symptoms such as chest discomfort, shortness of breath, and a feeling of impending doom.

Cardiologist Stephen T. Sinatra, M.D., author of *Heartbreak and Heart Disease* (Keats, 1996) notes, "The person's EKG reading will be normal, as will the level of cardiac muscle enzymes in the blood and the function of the coronary arteries on angiography. The only problem is an echocardiogram pattern that shows the apex of the heart—the part that sits on the diaphragm—is ballooning outward."[77]

Although the heart isn't permanently damaged and the weakness reverses itself, Dr. Sinatra notes that "heartbreak is a real component in 'matters of the heart,' from hypertension and arrhythmia to heart attacks and heart failure." It can be a warning sign that you need to heed your heart's messages and take better care of it before more serious and irreversible damage occurs further down the line.

AS ABOVE, SO BELOW: CALLING ON THE ANGELS FOR HELP

Belinda Womack, a former cell biologist who has worked with the twelve archangels for twenty-six years or so, teaches a spiritual principle that I, and hundreds of others, have found very useful and practical. The principle is this: as above, so below. It means that what happens on one level of reality also happens on every other level of reality, whether macroscopic or microscopic. It also means that when we change something on one level, it changes all the other realms as well. In quantum physics, there is a related concept called the "butterfly effect," which posits that something as small as a butterfly flapping its wings in one place can result in a typhoon halfway across the world.

Belinda teaches us that the "below" in the equation is our subconscious thoughts and beliefs—the 85 percent of our consciousness of which we are not aware but which continuously creates our experiences. If we want to change our outer reality—and our health—we need to ask spiritual forces (in this case, the angels) to assist us in taking the heaviness of our pain or lack of health (or anything else) and handing it back to the central Sun (or the heart of the Creator; you get to determine what language you prefer to use). Belinda teaches that when we unburden ourselves in this way with the help of the angels, we bring more and more light and a higher vibration into our experience.

Here's how it is done:

> Sit quietly with your feet on the ground or the floor. Close your eyes. Take several deep breaths in and out through your nose.
>
> Now ask your guardian angels (and any angels of your choice) to please be with you. Tell them you'd like to feel their presence. Sit quietly and use your imagination to feel them.
>
> Now allow a burden to rise in your mind. It might be high cholesterol, a broken heart, grief, fear about finances, or something else.
>
> Ask the angels to help you release that pain and take it to the central Sun, where it will be dissolved.
>
> Thank the angels for their help. They're always standing by, and they delight in helping you.
>
> Then open your eyes.

Do this daily—it takes almost no time. As you release the heaviness and burdens from your "below," then more "above" can flow into your life. Watch for it. This works. And it will help immeasurably to unburden your heart so it can be joyful and healthy. For more information, check out www.belindawomack.com.

REFINED CARBOHYDRATES, SUGAR, AND HEART HEALTH: WHAT EVERY WOMAN SHOULD KNOW

By now you know that overconsumption of refined carbohydrates plays a role in developing type 2 or adult-onset diabetes, a disease whose incidence is rapidly increasing as our population grows fatter and fatter. But what most women don't know is that the same carbohydrate consumption pattern that results in obesity, poor skin, and hormone imbalance is also a potent risk factor for heart disease, hypertension, and stroke. The diet most commonly prescribed for treatment and prevention of heart disease in both men and women is a high-carbohydrate, low-fat approach. Unfortunately, this diet may have exactly the opposite effect. When compared with a higher-protein, higher-fat diet with exactly the same number of calories, the high-carbohydrate diet has been shown to increase risk factors for ischemic heart disease, such as high triglycerides and insulin, in healthy postmenopausal women. It also lowers HDL cholesterol.[78] Eating a high-carbohydrate meal has also been shown to trigger angina sooner and reduce exercise tolerance in patients with known heart disease. This is because high insulin levels can cause constriction of arteriosclerotic coronary arteries.[79] (Ironically, a diet high in refined carbohydrates was first implicated in heart attacks back in the 1950s with the book *How to Prevent Heart Attacks* [Lee Foundation for Nutritional Research, 1958], written by Benjamin Sandler, M.D. In the book, Dr. Sandler shared his phenomenal success preventing fatal heart attacks in his angina patients by prescribing a no-sugar, no-starch food plan that kept blood sugar levels stable.)[80]

The experience of many women whose husbands go on high-carbohydrate, low-fat diets following heart attacks is that the men lose weight and lower their total cholesterol while their wives gain weight and may lose some of their HDL ("good" cholesterol) on exactly the same food plan. In fact, an Italian study that followed more than 47,000 men and women for eight years showed that women who ate a high-carbohydrate diet (especially a high-glycemic-index diet) were nearly twice as likely to develop coronary artery disease than women who ate a low-carbohydrate diet.[81] Yet these findings were not true for the men in the study. To prevent this increased risk, women need to be sure to eat only those carbohydrates that don't raise insulin levels too high or too quickly.[82] (See chapter 7.)

To understand how excessive carbohydrate intake can contribute to heart disease, we have to return to the subject of insulin. When you eat carbohydrates that are converted into sugar rapidly, your body pours insulin into your blood from your pancreas. Insulin is necessary to move the sugar from your bloodstream into your cells, where it is used for energy. But insulin doesn't simply regulate your blood sugar; it also helps control the storage of fat in your body. And heart disease is basically a disease associated with too much fat in our arteries.

Here's how it happens. Insulin directs amino acids, fatty acids, and carbohydrate breakdown products into our body tissues. It also regulates the body's production of cholesterol. Insulin tells the liver to begin making LDL ("bad" cholesterol), which at high enough levels—and under the right circumstances—actually sticks to blood vessel walls that have already been damaged by glycemic stress (blood sugar that's too high) and forms a plaque. And that is the essence of coronary artery disease and also cerebrovascular disease—the kind of arterial disease that affects brain function and enhances your risk for stroke and also dementia.

If you eat a lot of sugar or a lot of high-glycemic-index carbohydrates, such as pasta, bread, candy, cookies, and potatoes (and/or alcohol), and you are prone to high blood sugar or insulin resistance (as about 75 percent of us are), your liver may well increase its synthesis of LDL and develop fatty deposits, which in turn tend to stick to your inflamed blood vessels, forming plaques and subsequently causing arteriosclerosis, or hardening of the arteries.

Insulin also drives your kidneys to retain fluid, in a way that is similar to the kind of fluid overload that is seen in coronary artery disease and congestive heart failure. Excess insulin therefore poses a significant risk for hypertension, coronary artery disease, obesity, and high cholesterol levels, not just diabetes. Fluid retention from insulin is the reason why susceptible individuals can easily put on three or four pounds after a single large carbohydrate-rich meal. (I call these "liquid" pounds.) When you greatly decrease the sugar content of your diet, this problem takes care of itself—something that can begin to happen in a matter of days. (See chapters 6 and 7.)

Insulin and Blood Vessel Wall Thickening

In addition to all its other important roles, insulin is also a growth factor in the body: excess insulin and high blood sugar result in inflammation in the lining of blood vessels throughout the body. Over time, this process promotes smooth muscle growth in your blood vessel walls, which contributes to the formation of plaque, causing your artery walls to thicken and become rigid. Excess blood sugar from chronic carbohydrate consumption irreversibly attaches to the LDL cholesterol molecules that are already stuck to the blood vessel walls. This disease process in blood vessels also includes free-radical damage, a type of cellular damage that is akin to rust on a car.[83]

Here's the bottom line: if you eat too many high-glycemic-index carbohydrates and don't exercise, then your body will convert those carbs into excess blood sugar, fat, and LDL cholesterol. In addition, the higher your intake of refined carbohydrates, the more cellular inflammation, which is the final common pathway for heart disease.[84]

Follow a diet that keeps insulin levels low—the same diet that also prevents middle-age spread, balances your hormones, and improves your skin. For some, this is a ketogenic approach. For others, a low-fat vegan approach will work best. To help you decide which one to follow, just look at the food types in each choice and go with the one that feels right. Alternatively, pick one approach and stay with it for at least a week (two weeks is even better), then see how you feel. I personally find that a low-fat vegan diet is simply not for me. I've tried this approach repeatedly, and it just never feels right. I do far better by simply focusing on decreasing all refined carbohydrates, especially sugars.

Some women are able to keep their weight and cholesterol levels normal by eating a lot of complex carbohydrates, including whole-grain breads, while others—like me and millions of others—are not. You can't go wrong, however, if your diet consists mostly of lean protein, healthy fats, and lots of fruits and vegetables. Choose the most colorful ones, such as blueberries, strawberries, collard greens, squash, and kale. These are the highest in antioxidants. Hundreds of studies have confirmed that foods rich in flavonoids, carotenoids, and other antioxidants can reduce your risk for cardiovascular disease. Women who routinely eat four to five servings of fruits and vegetables per day (particularly the green, leafy, cruciferous, and citrus varieties) have a 28 to 35 percent decreased risk of stroke—an estimated 7 percent decrease in risk for each serving, which certainly adds up over time.[85] Last but not least, avoid trans fats.

CARDIOPROTECTIVE SUPPLEMENTS

The following is a list of some of the best-studied cardioprotective foods and supplements. You don't need to take all of them. Many will be present in a good comprehensive formulation for women. But others, like a higher dose of vitamin C, a cup of green tea daily, or a clove of garlic, are easy to add to your day.

Magnesium

Among its many roles in the body, magnesium helps stabilize electrical conduction in the cardiac muscle. It also helps relax the smooth muscle in blood vessels,[86] contributing to maintenance of normal blood pressure and vascular tone, and assists insulin in transporting glucose into cells, fighting glycemic stress. Because it helps all muscles (including coronary artery muscles) relax, it's very effective in helping prevent cardiac damage and even death after a heart attack. (In fact, up to 40 to 60 percent of sudden deaths from heart attack are caused by spasm in the arteries—not blockage from clots or arrhythmias!)[87] Another reason magnesium is helpful for heart health is that it's been shown to reduce cellular inflammation,[88] which plays a huge role in cardiovascular disease. Higher magnesium intake is further associated with lower incidence of diabetes,[89] yet another major risk factor.

Magnesium deficiency is relatively common. In fact, magnesium expert Carolyn Dean, M.D., N.D., says that 80 percent of the population is deficient. Because commercial agriculture today relies heavily on inorganic fertilizers, our food supply tends to be poor in this mineral. Food processing results in decreased magnesium as well. Chronic emotional and mental stress is also associated with magnesium deficiency because the stress hormones cortisol and adrenaline release magnesium from the cells; eventually it is excreted in the urine.

Diuretics result in the loss of magnesium in the urine, too, which is why the chronic use of diuretics has been associated with sudden cardiac death. If you're on diuretics for high blood pressure or any other reason, make sure that you take additional magnesium, potassium, and zinc. Excessive use of the stomach acid inhibitor cimetidine (Tagamet) can result in magnesium deficiency as well. (This was also true of the heartburn drug ranitidine, sold as Zantac, although it's now been recalled and is no longer being prescribed.) In general, organically grown whole grains (including wheat germ and wheat bran) and vegetables are rich sources of magnesium, as are good quality sea salt and sea vegetables (such as kelp). Other good sources include almonds, peanuts, and tofu. You can even get magnesium by adding

Epsom salts (which are magnesium sulfate) to your bath, which allows the magnesium to be absorbed through the skin.

Magnesium supplements come in several forms, including magnesium oxide, magnesium chloride, magnesium threonate, and various others. Most women need at least 800 mg per day. I recommend taking 400–1,000 mg per day in divided doses with meals. Because many magnesium supplements result in loose stools (think milk of magnesia) and often are not well absorbed, I highly recommend the liquid supplements ReMag and ReMyte. Use according to directions and increase as needed (see www.rnareset.com). For more information, read *The Magnesium Miracle* (Ballantine Books, 2003, most recently updated in 2017) by Carolyn Dean, M.D., N.D.

Calcium

Calcium is needed by every cell in your body, including the electrical system of the heart. Adequate calcium intake also helps keep blood pressure normal. This mineral works in tandem with magnesium, and therefore it's important to get both. In general, you want to be sure that your calcium is balanced with magnesium. A 1:1 or 2:1 ratio is ideal. Most women get enough calcium but not nearly enough magnesium. And when calcium intake is not balanced, it can lead to tissue calcification. So you want to make sure you get enough vitamin D, vitamin K_2, and magnesium along with your calcium. Take 500–1,200 mg of calcium per day with meals, depending upon how much calcium is present in your diet.

Antioxidants

Thousands of studies have documented the ability of antioxidants to help your heart, blood vessels, and every other tissue in your body resist free-radical damage and thus stay healthy. Here's an overview of my favorites—though there are others.[90]

COENZYME Q_{10}: This nutrient is concentrated in organ foods such as liver, kidney, and heart. It helps produce ATP, the basic energy molecule in every cell of the body. It is also a powerful antioxidant. Numerous studies have documented its beneficial effects on the heart, both in maintaining health and in healing from disease. (High doses have even been found to reverse some types of cardiomyopathy.)[91]

Coenzyme Q_{10} improves the ability of the heart to pump effectively and has also been shown to help reduce high blood pressure and congestive heart failure in those who already have heart disease. It is also very important for breast health. CoQ_{10} levels in heart muscles can be ten times greater than in other tissues because the heart functions continuously, without resting. That's why any condition that impairs the ability of the heart to do its work leaves this organ more susceptible to free-radical damage.

As already noted, coenzyme Q_{10} can be depleted in women who take statin drugs, including lovastatin (Mevacor), pravastatin (Pravachol), and atorvastatin (Lipitor), to lower their cholesterol.[92] Studies have shown that almost half of patients with hypertension have coenzyme Q_{10} deficiencies. Taking 50 mg twice a day for ten weeks has been shown to significantly lower blood pressure.[93] For those individuals already on medication for elevated blood pressure, the need for antihypertensive medication declined gradually in about four and a half months in half the patients who took CoQ_{10} (225 mg per day); some were able to stop taking blood pressure medication altogether.[94] A randomized, placebo-controlled study of people taking coenzyme Q_{10} supplements with or without statin drugs found that CoQ_{10} supplementation reduced the risk of heart attack and death by 50 percent, whether the subjects were on the statin drug or not.[95]

The minimum dose of coenzyme Q_{10} I recommend is 30 mg/day. For anyone with any family history of heart disease, I'd recommend 60–90 mg/day to help prevent the disease from developing. The dose can go up to 300–400 mg per day for those with advanced heart disease.[96] (For more information, read *The Coenzyme Q10 Phenomenon,* by cardiologist Stephen Sinatra, M.D. [Keats Publishing, 1998].)

CAROTENOIDS: There are dozens of studies that show that individuals who consume high amounts of pigment-rich foods are at lower risk for heart disease. These foods are loaded with carotenoids such as beta-carotene, which has been shown to decrease risk of free-radical damage to the heart and blood vessels. In one study of individuals who already had unstable angina and had undergone coronary artery bypass, the addition of beta-carotene to their diets decreased subsequent major cardiovascular events such as heart attack, stroke, need for additional bypass procedures, and cardiac death by 50 percent.[97] Beta-carotene prevents the lipoprotein LDL ("bad" cholesterol) from becoming oxidized. The usual dose of beta-carotene is 25,000 IU per day in supplement form.

However, a mix of the carotenoids is better than taking just one.

For example, lutein is present in HDL ("good" cholesterol) and may help prevent LDL cholesterol from oxidizing. The best way to get lutein is in fruits and vegetables, but it is also available in health food stores as a supplement; take 3–6 mg per day. Lycopene is another good antioxidant; eating tomatoes a couple of times a week will give you all the lycopene you need.

VITAMIN E: This antioxidant has been shown to keep blood platelets "slippery," thus decreasing the risk of blood clots. Vitamin E is an anti-inflammatory in the heart muscle. It may also inhibit arrhythmia and cardiomyopathy. In the Nurses' Health Study, participants taking 400–800 IU of vitamin E per day reduced their risk of heart attack by 30 percent.[98] The Cambridge Heart Study, which looked at the effects of vitamin E on 2,000 patients with documented heart disease, found that those who took between 400 and 800 IU of vitamin E per day had a 77 percent decrease in cardiovascular disease over a year's time.[99] And a 2009 study of more than 77,000 midlife residents of Washington state showed that taking vitamin E supplements may reduce the risk of dying from cardiovascular disease by 28 percent.[100] (The same study showed that taking multivitamins may reduce the risk of dying from heart disease by 16 percent.)

A 2005 meta-analysis of previous studies by Edgar Miller III, M.D., Ph.D., created quite a stir when it suggested that high-dose vitamin E supplementation may increase mortality in adults.[101] Yet Dr. Miller's analysis excluded many of the larger studies with thousands of subjects because the total mortality rates were low. None of those studies showed that vitamin E increased mortality. On the other hand, many of the studies Dr. Miller did include were smaller (with less than one thousand people), and it's only the smaller studies that showed significant adverse effects from taking vitamin E. Quite a few of those studies looked at abnormal populations, i.e., older adults who already had advanced chronic degenerative disease. Also telling is that the researchers' secondary analysis showed that differences in death rates were statistically insignificant; at the highest dose of vitamin E, the risk of death was actually lower! The bottom line: not only is there solid evidence like that from the Nurses' Health Study and the Cambridge Heart Study showing vitamin E boosts cardiovascular health, but other studies show that vitamin E is associated with a significant reduction in bowel cancer,[102] reduces the risk of dementia,[103] and even slows the development of cataracts.[104] Vitamin E should definitely be part of a comprehensive supplementation program.

Dosage is 200–800 IU per day of d-alpha-tocopherol (natural vitamin E; check the label) or mixed tocopherols.

TOCOTRIENOLS: Tocotrienols are part of the vitamin E family of compounds. But compared with regular vitamin E, they are 40 to 60 times more powerful as antioxidants. Tocotrienols have a positive effect on all three of the major physical risk factors for coronary artery disease: total cholesterol levels, oxidation of low-density lipoprotein (LDL, or "bad" cholesterol), and the clumping of red blood cells that makes stroke more likely.[105] Free-radical damage (oxidative stress from poor diet, psychological stress, smoking, etc.) that accompanies LDL oxidation is particularly dangerous because it can cause serious injury to artery and vein walls.

Tocotrienols lower cholesterol by promoting the natural degradation of an enzyme (HMG-CoA reductase) that controls your liver's breakdown of LDL cholesterol. This is the same enzyme that statin drugs affect, except that tocotrienols work through a different mechanism. For that reason, you can often lower your cholesterol with tocotrienols instead of statins.

Most multivitamins don't have significant amounts of tocotrienols, so you have to add them. If you plan to use tocotrienols to lower cholesterol, take about 50 mg daily for a month, and then lower the dose to about 30 mg thereafter. (If you're already on a statin drug, add tocotrienols, because they work synergistically with statin drugs, thus enhancing their effectiveness; use about 30–55 mg per day.) Sometimes tocotrienols are included in a vitamin supplement and sometimes they are available separately. Fresh fruits, dark green leafy vegetables, almonds, peanuts, and wheat germ also contain tocotrienols and the other types of vitamin E.

SELENIUM: This antioxidant has been shown to decrease the risk of free-radical damage to blood vessel walls. The usual dose is 50–200 mcg per day.

OLIGOMERIC PROANTHOCYANIDINS (OPCS): The proanthocyanidins are in the class of foods known as the flavonoids. Cardiovascular disease risk is inversely proportional to flavonoid intake.[106] OPCs are derived from grape seeds or pine bark (one brand is Pycnogenol). This is a supplement I wouldn't live without because of its many benefits. OPCs are quickly absorbed into the bloodstream, help to regenerate the body's levels of vitamin E, and also prevent the oxidation of LDL cholesterol by free radicals. In addition, they improve blood vessel and skin elasticity by helping prevent free-radical damage to collagen, reduce or eliminate the discomfort of arthritis, help prevent circulation problems, and reduce excessive blood clotting. They also help prevent all the symptoms of allergy and hay fever. The usual dose is 40–120 mg/day.

ALPHA-LIPOIC ACID (ALA): Alpha-lipoic acid is a unique antioxidant in that it is both water- and fat-soluble. That means that it can stand guard against free-radical damage in every part of the cell. It has also been shown to help preserve intracellular levels of vitamins C and E and to help regenerate another antioxidant known as glutathione. Alpha-lipoic acid is also helpful for the metabolism of insulin, and in Germany it has been approved for the treatment of diabetic neuropathy (nerve damage). It has been shown to improve blood flow both to the nerves and to the skin. The usual dose is 50–200 mg/day.

VITAMIN C: This powerful antioxidant helps protect the endothelial lining of your blood vessels and has also been found to aid the absorption of calcium and magnesium, two key minerals for heart health. A dose of 1,000 mg per day has been shown to significantly reduce systolic blood pressure, though the mechanism is not clear. I recommend taking it in the form of plain old ascorbic acid. If you have a sensitive stomach, use the ascorbate form. I recommend at least 1,000–5,000 mg per day. You can also use liposomal vitamin C, which is fat soluble.

VITAMIN D: Many studies now link vitamin D with heart health. A 2009 review of the medical literature revealed that lower vitamin D levels are associated with an increased risk of hypertension, several types of vascular diseases, and heart failure.[107]

One promising study conducted at the Intermountain Medical Center Heart Institute in Murray, Utah, and presented at the 2010 conference of the American College of Cardiology reported that treating vitamin D deficiency with supplements may help to prevent or reduce the risk of cardiovascular disease.[108] The researchers looked at more than 9,400 men and women whose blood tests revealed low vitamin D levels during a routine doctor's visit. Patients who raised their vitamin D levels to above 30 ng/ml by their next follow-up visit (about half the group) were 33 percent less likely to have a heart attack, 20 percent less likely to develop heart failure, and 30 percent less likely to die in the next year. The same research team then crunched data on more than 41,000 patients and found that those diagnosed with severe vitamin D deficiency were most likely to also have been diagnosed with heart disease or stroke. On the other hand, the data showed that those patients who increased their levels of vitamin D to 43 ng/ml had the lowest rates of heart disease and stroke.

I often recommend supplementing with 2,000–10,000 IU of vitamin D daily, although the exact amount that is right for you depends on several factors, including where you live and how much exposure to the sun you get. For a full discussion on vitamin D, including how much of this vital nutrient you need, how to safely get vitamin D from the sun, and how to design a supplement program, see chapter 12.

B Vitamins, Folic Acid, and Niacin

Over half of all women don't get the folic acid they need. This not only puts their babies at risk for neural tube defects such as spina bifida but also increases their risk for arteriosclerosis, heart disease, and cognitive decline. It has been found that the individuals with the highest homocysteine levels also have the lowest levels of folic acid, B_{12}, and B_6. A higher dose of folic acid than the RDA is associated with a lower risk of heart attack (it may inhibit platelet aggregation and prolong clotting time) and is also the antidote for high homocysteine.[109] Women with adequate B vitamin and folate levels have a definite decreased risk for heart disease.[110] They also have a decreased risk for Alzheimer's.[111]

Niacin (vitamin B_5) is a naturally occurring "statin" that helps increase HDL, reduce inflammation, and lessen arterial constrictions. Studies show that niacin may work by keeping the liver from eliminating HDL cholesterol. One such study published in 2008 compared niacin to the prescription drug Zetia (ezetimibe). Zetia is often prescribed in addition to a statin for patients who have very high cholesterol or are at high risk for heart attack or stroke. After fourteen months, according to study results, niacin significantly reduced plaque buildup, while Zetia actually *increased* it. In addition, nine people taking Zetia died during the trial (compared to two deaths for patients taking niacin). Although the time-release prescription niacin used in the study is not available over the counter, the study concluded that adding niacin to existing treatment for high cholesterol was more beneficial than adding Zetia.[112]

The usual doses of the B vitamins are: vitamin B_6, 40–80 mg per day; niacin, 20–50 mg per day; vitamin B_{12}, 20 mcg per day; and folic acid, 400–1,000 mcg per day. It's always best to take these together with the entire B complex. (See chapter 7.)

DO YOU NEED METHYLATED FOLATE AND B₁₂?

Anywhere from 30 to 60 percent of the population has a genetically inherited difficulty with a biochemical process called methylation. Methylation means the transfer of four atoms—one carbon atom and three hydrogen atoms (CH_3, a methyl group)—from one substance to another. When optimal methylation occurs, it has a positive effect on many different biochemical reactions in the body, including cardiovascular, neurological, reproductive, and detoxification pathways. Methylation and demethylation are the mechanisms that allow the gears of the body to turn off and on for a whole host of systems. CH_3 is provided to the body through a universal methyl donor called SAM-e (S-adenosylmethionine). SAM-e readily gives away its methyl group to other substances in the body, which helps the body's systems to perform their functions. The entire system that produces SAM-e relies on one switch being turned on by a critical B vitamin called 5-MTHF (also known as L-methylfolate or quatrefolic). If enough 5-MTHF is present, the methylation cycle works well. Folic acid from the diet or supplements needs to be converted to this active form before it can be used by the body in the methylation cycle. But up to 60 percent of people have a genetic mutation that makes this conversion challenging—and then they can't make enough SAM-e, which makes it difficult to make enough glutathione, melatonin, coenzyme Q_{10}, serotonin, nitric oxide, cysteine, epinephrine, and taurine.

The good news is that there is a simple genetic test to determine whether or not you have this methylation problem. Most functional medicine doctors have easy access to this test and can order it for you. The test looks at specific enzymes that are affected by your genetic makeup, including the enzyme MTHFR (methylenetetrahydrofolate reductase), which is the most important enzyme involved in creating 5-MTHF.

You can also improve your methylation cycle by eating a whole-foods, non-processed diet that includes asparagus, avocado, broccoli, Brussels sprouts, legumes (like peas, beans, and lentils), green leafy vegetables, and rice.

It is also very helpful to engage in regular exercise and to avoid excessive intake of alcohol, smoking, and excessive coffee consumption (more than five cups per day).

Nutrients that enhance methylation include 5-MTHF (active folate), methylcobalamin (active vitamin B_{12}), active vitamin B_6, active vitamin B_2, magnesium, betaine (trimethylglycine), and vitamin D.

Proper methylation influences so many systems in the body that it can get overlooked. So ask your healthcare provider to test you for it if you suspect a problem. (I have this methylation defect myself but have never had a problem with regular folic acid or B_{12} supplements—probably because of other factors in my lifestyle. There is, as with all things, a wide variation among those affected.)

CARDIO MIRACLE: WORTH KNOWING ABOUT

My book *The Secret Pleasures of Menopause* (Hay House, 2008) was, at its core, an ode to the many health-enhancing properties of nitric oxide—including how to increase your body's production of this crucial nutrient. I wrote the book in consultation with Ferid Murad, M.D., Ph.D., who won a Nobel Prize for his pioneering work on this marvelous molecule. Many people asked me if there was a supplement they could take to increase nitric oxide. At the time, I knew that a variety of different supplements and foods enhanced the production of this molecule. But there was nothing I could recommend that would guarantee the production of nitric oxide.

When I was introduced to Cardio Miracle, I knew that I had found the holy grail of nitric-oxide-producing supplements. Cardio Miracle has been formulated to include all of the heart-healthy supplements mentioned above. Studies have shown that it enhances the production of nitric oxide from the endothelial lining of all blood vessels. It has been shown to increase oxygenation of tissues, improve circulation, improve sexual health, aid in lymphatic drainage of toxins, increase muscle strength, normalize insulin response, and support oral health. I have used and recommended this supplement for several years now and find that it lives up to the claims made about it.

Full disclosure: I am an affiliate with this company. To get a 20 percent discount when ordering the product, go to www .cardiomiracle.com/drnorthrup/index.html.

FOODS FOR HEART HEALTH

FISH: The American Heart Association now recommends that all adults eat fish (preferably fatty fish) at least twice a week because the evidence that the omega-3s it contains fight heart disease is very compelling, including findings that omega-3 fatty acids decrease risk of arrhythmias, decrease triglyceride levels, slow the growth of atherosclerotic plaque, and even slightly lower blood pressure. The well-known Nurses' Health Study showed that women who ate fish once a week cut their risk of stroke by 22 percent (and those who ate fish five or more times per week cut their risk by a whopping 52 percent!)[113] Studies have shown that 3 g per day of fish oil containing both EPA and DHA is cardioprotective because it makes platelets more slippery and decreases cellular inflammation.[114] A number of recent studies also show that fish oil lowers triglyceride levels and possesses powerful anti-clotting properties.[115]

The best way to get omega-3s is by eating cold-water fish (I recommend three servings per week), such as salmon, mackerel, swordfish, or sardines. One 4-oz. serving of salmon contains about 200 mg of DHA. If you don't eat fish regularly, supplement your diet with omega-3 supplements, from either fish oil, flax oil, hemp oil, or algae-derived DHA (good for vegans). The usual dose of DHA is at least 200 mg per day, up to 2,500 mg per day; for DHA and EPA together, start with 400 mg per day and work up to as high as 5,000 mg per day as needed.

GREEN TEA: The flavonoids in green tea are known as polyphenols. These substances have powerful antioxidant effects that may be greater than or equal to that of vitamins C and E. As little as one cup of green tea per day will provide protection.[116]

GARLIC: Garlic has a long history of use in the treatment of hypertension. One pilot study showed that high doses of garlic (2,400 mg of deodorized garlic per day) significantly lowered both diastolic and systolic blood pressure. Like alpha-lipoic acid, garlic appears to increase the activity of the endothelial cells that produce nitric oxide, which is a blood vessel relaxant.

Numerous studies have also shown that regular consumption of garlic reduces cholesterol by 10 percent or more and lowers triglyceride levels by up to 13 percent. It may also inhibit platelet aggregation and blood clot formation.[117]

The German Commission E, which evaluates therapeutic claims for natural substances, recommends a dosage level equivalent to one to four cloves of fresh raw garlic a day. This is the amount estimated to provide 4,000 mcg of allicin, one of garlic's most beneficial compounds. Many good garlic supplements are on the market. Look for one with the active ingredient alliin, because this substance is relatively odorless until it is converted into allicin in the body. Products containing this substance supply all the benefits of fresh garlic but are more socially acceptable. A daily dose should be 10 mg of alliin, or a total allicin potential of 4,000 mcg.

HAWTHORN: In her inspiring book *Herbal Rituals* (St. Martin's Press, 1998), master herbalist Judith Berger points out that hawthorn leaf, blossom, or berry (*Crataegus oxyacantha*) extracted into water or spirit-based preparations is a "fierce and protective ally for those seeking to prevent heart-related conditions which are passed on from generation to generation."[118] Hawthorn berry extract can calm palpitations, help restore blood vessel elasticity, ease fluid buildup in the heart, halt fatty degeneration of the heart, help dilate coronary arteries, and also reduce blood pressure. It can be used by those already on cardiac medication and may help you decrease your dosage. I take my hawthorn as a tea. You just buy a bag of organically grown hawthorn berries at a natural food store and steep them in hot water to taste. There is nothing standardized about this method, but I see myself as creating a healthy heart by drinking a little tea, not treating heart disease. Hawthorn has not been shown to have any adverse side effects.

If you prefer to take your hawthorn as a pill, look for a standardized extract, and use a product that contains 10 percent proanthocyanidins or 1.8 percent vitexin-4"-rhamnoside. The usual dose is 100–250 mg three times per day.

Sodium-Potassium Balance

Decreasing sodium and increasing potassium in your diet can help control high blood pressure, which is an important risk factor for heart and circulatory problems.[119] For the 60 percent of individuals whose hypertension is related to sodium intake, the effect of sodium on blood pressure can be relieved by increasing intake of potassium. Dietary potassium deficiency is caused by a diet that is low in fresh fruits and vegetables and high in sodium. This is your basic fast-food diet! A diet rich in fruits, vegetables, and whole grains can supply you with 4,000–6,000 mg of potassium a day. Drugs such as diuretics, caffeine, laxatives, aspirin, and others can also deplete your potassium. Prolonged exercise is associated with loss of potassium as well—up to 3,000 mg of potassium can be lost in one day by sweating. A diet high in potassium and low in sodium protects against high blood pressure, stroke, and heart disease. Potassium supplements have been shown to significantly lower both systolic and diastolic blood pressure, but these have side effects, including nausea, vomiting, diarrhea, and ulcers, when given in pill form at high doses. This won't happen if you increase your levels through diet alone.

Most Americans have a potassium-to-sodium dietary ratio of 1:2, but researchers recommend a 5:1 ratio. One trip to a fried-chicken joint or pizza place will mess up this ratio. Because fruits and vegetables like potatoes, bananas, and apples are such rich sources of potassium, don't get too hung up on their high glycemic indexes. Because they are whole foods, they will not raise your insulin levels high enough to really cause damage unless they are highly processed into something, such as french fries. It is the simple carbohydrates in white-flour products that really mess things up as far as both insulin and potassium-to-sodium ratios are concerned. This is yet another reason why you want to try for five servings of fruits and vegetables per day in your diet.

Because magnesium and potassium work together at the level of the cell, they are often low at the same time.

FOODS TO IMPROVE YOUR POTASSIUM-SODIUM RATIO

Potatoes	110:1 (ratio of potassium to sodium)
Carrots	75:1
Apples	90:1
Bananas	440:1
Oranges	260:1

WHAT ABOUT ASPIRIN?

In 1982 John Vane, Ph.D., won the Nobel Prize by showing that aspirin can inhibit the clumping of platelets in blood vessels. This led to the widespread recommendation to take aspirin to decrease the risk of heart attack and stroke by preventing clots from forming in arteries that have been narrowed by arteriosclerosis. Studies strongly suggest that those who have evidence of ischemia of the heart muscles (decreased oxygenation of the heart) can definitely benefit from taking aspirin.[120]

When the 2005 Women's Health Study showed that taking the equivalent of a baby aspirin every other day reduced the risk of stroke by 17 percent (but not heart attack),[121] many women began taking low-dose aspirin as a preventive measure. However, the study also highlighted the risk of gastrointestinal bleeding. Recent research has shed much more light on this.

The ASPREE (Aspirin in Reducing Events in the Elderly) study, completed in 2018, followed more than 19,000 people in the United States and Australia age sixty-five and older for just under five years. The researchers found that for healthy people in this age group, not only does aspirin therapy have no discernible benefit in terms of prolonging independent, healthy living,[122] but it also increases the risk for serious, potentially life-threatening bleeding.[123]

The bottom line: if you have had a heart attack or stroke, your doctor may want you to take a daily low dose of aspirin to help prevent another such event. But if you've never had a heart attack or stroke, aspirin therapy could very well do more harm than good.

Fortunately, there are other, far more effective and healthful ways to decrease cellular inflammation and subsequent platelet "stickiness" without any possible side effects. Here are several:

> *Eat fruits and vegetables:* Studies have shown that women who eat five to six servings of fruits and vegetables per day lower their risk of stroke by 31 percent. The strongest effect comes from the cruciferous vegetables, such as broccoli, cauliflower, Brussels sprouts, and cabbage, followed by green leafy vegetables and citrus fruit and juice.[124]
>
> *Eat carrots:* JoAnn Manson, M.D., Dr.P.H., and her colleagues at Harvard Medical School tracked 87,000 nurses for eight years in the Nurses' Health Study and found that women who ate just five large carrots per week lowered their risk of

stroke by 68 percent compared to those who ate only one carrot per week.[125] This should be front-page news!

Drink tea: Both black and green tea consumption have been shown to have beneficial effects on the endothelial lining of blood vessels, which helps decrease the risk of stroke.[126] The Zutphen Elderly Study in the Netherlands found that foods rich in an antioxidant known as quercetin (such as apples, tea, and onions) also decreased the risk of stroke. Black tea consumption (five or more cups per day) decreased the risk of stroke by 69 percent.[127]

Take tocotrienols: Tocotrienols do the same thing as aspirin without the risks of gastrointestinal bleeding. They decrease blood clotting or "stickiness" the same way aspirin does, by inhibiting the production of a potent coagulation factor known as thromboxane. As thinner, more freely flowing blood is associated with the lower risk of stroke, heart attack, and transient ischemic attack, tocotrienols have also been shown to decrease platelet aggregation by as much as 15 to 30 percent, an effect equivalent to that of baby aspirin.[128] (If you're already on aspirin, you can still take tocotrienols because they don't enhance the effect of aspirin significantly, if at all.)

Eat fish: Eating fish or taking fish oil (or another source of omega-3 fats) has consistently been shown to decrease the risk of stroke.[129]

BIOIDENTICAL PROGESTERONE: GROUNDBREAKING WEAPON AGAINST HEART DISEASE

Dimera, Inc., a tiny cardiovascular research and development company in Portland, Oregon, has hit on a giant idea. With research funded in part by grants from the National Institutes of Health, Dimera developed the first heart drug specifically for women—a form of low-dose, slow-release natural progesterone in a transdermal cream that uses gene expression to optimize its delivery method.

Dimera has shown in research using monkeys as subjects that the lower levels of progesterone common in menopause can cause abnormal coronary artery constriction. Restricted blood flow can lead to chest pain and, eventually, heart disease. But progesterone therapy can decrease the magnitude and duration of this vasoconstriction, thus keeping the heart healthy.

Because this abnormal vasoconstriction occurs intermittently, the only way it can show up in an angiogram is if the subject is experiencing angina at the time of the test. And even then, the affected blood vessels are so small that magnetic resonance (MR) or positron emission tomography (PET) scans must be used to detect it, making diagnosis of the problem difficult at best.

A 2008 study conducted by the company reviewed the cardiovascular effects of synthetic progesterone (progestin) compared to natural progesterone and found that there is in fact a minimum level of progesterone necessary for normal cardiovascular function in women.[130] Dimera believes that using natural progesterone (which does not have the unpleasant side effects that synthetic progestins cause) could keep the blood vessels healthy, thus preventing abnormal vasoconstriction. My past clinical experience also shows that natural progesterone can be helpful in treating chest pain, which is caused by prolonged vasoconstriction. More research is still needed on this subject, but small studies have already shown that as little as 20 mg of natural progesterone applied to the skin of the chest, hands, or abdomen once or twice per day can effectively treat angina. Taking progesterone orally has not proven to be as effective.

When I wrote the last edition of this book, Dimera was in the midst of clinical trials in the hope of bringing its transdermal progesterone to market. I don't believe that this has happened yet, which is most unfortunate—but also far too common when it comes to natural solutions. Still, the research has been done and it's important to know about it. (For more information, visit Dimera's website at www.dimera .net.) In the meantime, using natural progesterone cream available over the counter (PhytoGest and Pro-Gest are good brands) might well confer at least some benefits. Your doctor can also prescribe more concentrated progesterone creams or gels (available from a formulary pharmacy) that may work even better.

GET MOVING!

It should come as no surprise that maintaining a healthful lifestyle—including staying active—will go a long way toward living a longer, healthier life. The results of a 2009 study suggest that being physically active, achieving a normal weight, and never smoking are ways to effectively prevent cardiovascular disease and to extend your total life expectancy.[131] A study published the following year gives a good picture of the flip side: the collective effects of smoking, lack of physical activity, poor diet, and alcohol consumption are associated with a substantially increased risk for death.[132] According to this research, those who partake in all four unhealthy behaviors had about three times the risk of dying from cardiovascular disease or cancer, four times the risk of dying from other causes, and an overall death risk equivalent to being twelve years older than people with none of these behaviors.

Exercise provides enormous cardiovascular benefits and has been shown repeatedly to significantly reduce the risk of heart disease, hypertension, and stroke.[133] Exercise training after diagnosed coronary artery disease has also been shown to improve blood flow to the heart by improving the ability of the blood vessel lining (endothelium) to keep vessels open and also by recruiting collateral vessels in the heart muscle that help bypass vessels that have been blocked.[134] A study done at Boston's Brigham and Women's Hospital showed that women who walk two or more hours a week, especially at a brisk pace, are significantly less likely to experience any type of stroke than women who do not walk. The data for this study came from the long-term follow-up findings for the Women's Health Study, which looked at more than 39,000 healthy women age forty-five and up.[135] The benefits of exercise to help your heart even after a heart attack are evidence of just how forgiving the heart and blood vessels are when we care for them.

Your goal should be to exercise five or six days per week for at least thirty minutes. Walking is fine, but remember that true fitness includes strength, flexibility, and endurance, so activities should promote all three. Weight training, for example, builds lean muscle mass that not only increases strength but also increases your metabolic rate. Yoga is great for flexibility. Aerobic activities increase endurance. Pilates builds lean muscle mass and increases flexibility. Exercise also decreases insulin and blood sugar levels and will give you a bit more leeway with your diet.

The Role of Lymph

One of the main reasons why exercise has such healing power is that it vastly increases the lymph circulation in your body. Lymph is the clear fluid that drains from around your body's cells into the lymphatic system, a network of thin-walled vessels found throughout every organ and tissue in your body. Lymph vessels contain small valves to keep the lymph from flowing backward. Bean-shaped structures known as lymph nodes are found at frequent intervals along lymph vessels, with major centers occurring in the groin, neck, and armpits and alongside the aorta and the inferior vena cava in the chest and the abdomen. The function of the lymph nodes is threefold: (1) to filter out and destroy foreign substances, such as bacteria and dust; (2) to produce some of the white cells called lymphocytes that help fight tumors and other invaders; and (3) to produce antibodies that help in the body's immune surveillance system. All lymph eventually gets emptied into a large central vessel in our chest cavities, known as the thoracic duct, which eventually empties into our hearts, so that the lymph and blood get mixed together once again after our lymph nodes have removed the waste, bacteria, and other flotsam and jetsam from it.

In addition to its role in helping keep bacteria and other invaders in check, the lymphatic system is essential to the mechanism by which fats are processed by the body. Lymph vessels that drain the small intestine collect the digested fat from the foods we eat and pass it directly into the main blood circulation, bypassing the liver. Once fats are in the blood, they may or may not get laid down in the blood vessels of the heart, forming fatty streaks that eventually lead to hardening of the arteries and the beginning of cardiovascular disease. Whether or not this happens depends upon our diet, our exercise habits, and our emotional and psychological state.

I interviewed Jerry Lemole, M.D., a leading cardiovascular surgeon from Philadelphia, many of whose patients suffer from end-stage heart disease. His research on the role of the lymph system is both intriguing and motivating.

The HDL-Lymph Connection

The lymphatic system in the heart is intimately involved with the process that leads to coronary artery disease. LDL, the "bad" cholesterol, is a large, fluffy fat molecule that can get into blood vessel walls through breaks in the intimal tissue that forms the blood vessel lining. This is especially apt to happen when LDL cholesterol becomes oxidized. Once LDL gets stuck here, it tends to break down and leave cholesterol deposits behind.

HDL cholesterol, the "good" cholesterol, is a smooth football-shaped molecule that is small enough to actually get into the tissue around the blood vessel wall and vacuum up the cholesterol deposits left behind by LDL.

In order for HDL to do its job of vacuuming up cholesterol deposits, it needs to get to where the cholesterol is located. It does this through lymph circulation. Dr. Lemole likens HDL molecules that pick up cholesterol in the artery walls to taxicabs in New York City. If you view Manhattan from a helicopter, you'll see a certain number of cabs. At any given time, because traffic in New York is so often backed up in the tunnels that lead to and from the city, you'll have many cabs unavailable to passengers in the street who need to be picked up. If you could speed up the passage of the cabs through the tunnels, there would be more cabs available on the streets.

The same is true with the cholesterol-carrying capacity of HDL. When lymph flow is sluggish, HDL molecules simply are not available to pick up excess cholesterol deposits. If you speed up the circulation time of lymph, you'll also improve the efficiency of HDL to scavenge excess fat from your arteries.[136]

How to Speed Up Lymph Flow

1. DON'T SIT FOR LONG PERIODS OF TIME. Women who sit for long periods of time at sedentary jobs are more likely to get heart disease because the lymphatic flow through their thoracic cavity is limited.

2. BREATHE DEEPLY AND REGULARLY. Breathing fully in through your nose and inhaling air down into the lower lobes of your lungs followed by a brisk exhalation massages the thoracic duct and all the lymph vessels and nodes in your chest cavity, which helps HDL get to the places it needs to go to do its work.

3. MOVE. Lymph flow depends upon the muscles in the body to move it along. Every time you walk, do yoga, breathe deeply, run, or move your muscles briskly, you are helping jostle the lymph along.

Dr. Lemole reports that the average turnover time for proteins in lymph is once to twice per day. But when you exercise regularly, you can increase this figure to three to five times per day. So exercising gives your body three to five times more opportunity to get rid of excess cholesterol deposits in the blood vessels around your heart.

Rebounding on a mini-trampoline is particularly effective at keeping lymph moving. Anyone can do this, especially if you get a rebounder with a railing. Start with just five minutes three times a week, and add a minute a week until you get up to twenty minutes three times a week. You can do this while watching television if you like. You don't even have to jump high—just bouncing a bit is very effective.

4. AVOID OVEREXERCISE. When we exercise, we actually increase the oxidative stress in our bodies, which results in the production of free radicals in our bodies. Over time this can do more damage than good. That's why so many endurance athletes have impaired immune function, which makes them more susceptible to infections and illness. This needn't be the case if you always breathe in and out fully through your nose as you exercise and never exert yourself beyond what is comfortable with this way of breathing. (For further information about this, read *Body, Mind, and Sport* [Three Rivers Press, 2001], by John Douillard.)

Dr. Lemole recommends that you walk at a pace of about 3.6–4.0 miles per hour, which means that it should take you about thirty to forty minutes to cover two miles. Any faster than that and you will incur a lot of oxidative stress in your body that will require you to take additional antioxidant vitamins to cover the potential damage. Remember that if you exercise so that you're breathing comfortably in and out through your nose, your body will also be operating at a pace that decreases free-radical damage, because comfortable nose breathing results in a balance between your sympathetic and parasympathetic nervous systems.

Exercise lowers many cardiovascular risks, including high blood pressure. In one study, those who did not engage in vigorous exercise regularly had a 35 percent greater risk of hypertension than those who did. Though it helps to have been active in high school and college, you will not be protected unless you continue regular vigorous exercise throughout your life.

Here are three tips that will help you stick with healthy lifestyle changes (based on a 2010 study published in the journal *Circulation*):[137]

- Set specific goals that are realistically attainable within a set time limit, like committing to attend one water aerobics class a week at the local Y for at least six weeks. Goals are also best when they focus on a *behavior* (such as committing to start a walking program or promising yourself you will eat three servings of fish a week) rather than a physiologic number (such as a target cholesterol level or weight).

- Monitor your progress (by keeping a chart or a log, for example).

- Integrate more than one lifestyle change at a time (such as an exercise program and a change in your diet), because one will reinforce the other.

THE HEART-ESTROGEN LINK: WHAT'S REALLY GOING ON?

Because the incidence of heart disease in women rises at about the age of fifty, the same time that estrogen levels start to decrease, scientists assumed that heart disease after menopause must be related to an estrogen deficiency. And because studies have demonstrated that estrogen lowers LDL cholesterol, raises HDL cholesterol, and helps support blood vessel walls, scientists naturally assumed that giving everyone estrogen would solve the problem of heart disease. But the original WHI study was halted when researchers found that Prempro (Premarin plus Provera) actually increased the risk of blood clots, heart attack, and stroke in healthy women. In addition, the Heart and Estrogen/Progestin Replacement Study (HERS), the Estrogen Replacement and Atherosclerosis (ERA) study, and the WHI study all showed that estrogen replacement did *not* decrease the incidence of heart attack in women who already have heart disease, and in fact even increased the risk for a while. These results certainly decreased the unbridled enthusiasm for prescribing Premarin that had characterized the medical profession during the 1990s.[138]

But then a new wrinkle in the estrogen-heart connection appeared. In 2006, an analysis of the data from the Nurses' Health Study co-written by researcher JoAnn Manson, M.D., Dr.P.H., who was also one of the lead researchers in the WHI study, found that nurses who began taking hormone therapy near menopause did indeed have about a 30 percent lower risk for heart disease than women who didn't use hormones.[139] In comparison, nurses who started HT ten years or more after menopause showed no benefit. The study showed no difference between those who took estrogen alone and those who took it combined with synthetic progestin. The study also reanalyzed data from the WHI study and confirmed that the risk of heart problems increased in women who began taking HT ten years or more after menopause. (There was a 22 percent increase in those who started HT from ten to nineteen years after menopause.) But those who started it within a couple of years after their last menstrual period experienced an 11 percent lower risk of heart disease. Even more striking, in the estrogen-only branch of the WHI, published in 2006, women who started HT between ages fifty and fifty-nine had a 44 percent lower risk of heart disease.

This latest study makes sense given the large body of research showing that estrogen has a beneficial effect on the heart and blood vessels (at least in younger women). Here's a summary of the documented beneficial effects of estrogen on the heart and blood vessels.

~ Estrogen exerts a cardioprotective effect on blood vessels and helps coronary arteries dilate (not constrict inappropriately).[140] It directly modifies and normalizes the function of the endothelium and vascular smooth muscle.

~ It has a favorable impact on lipoproteins, cholesterol, and fibrinogen levels and reverses some adverse effects of lipid metabolism.

~ It decreases endothelium retention of LDL by coronary arteries.[141]

~ Estrogen has been used as an alternative to cholesterol-lowering drugs such as lovastatin and pravastatin. There may even be an additive effect on cholesterol and lipoproteins by combining ERT and pravastatin.[142]

Particularly intriguing have been the results of two studies that were designed specifically to look at the effects of bioidentical HT on risk for heart disease. The Kronos Longevity Research Institute conducted a placebo-controlled study called the Kronos Early Estrogen Prevention Study (KEEPS), which compared the use of bioidentical hormone therapy (using a natural estrogen patch) to conjugated estrogen therapy (Premarin) in decreasing the risk of heart disease and preventing cognitive decline in women who have reached menopause within the previous three years or so. Those women who still had a uterus were also given oral natural progesterone (Prometrium). The study followed 727 healthy women ages forty-two to fifty-eight for four years, starting in 2005. The results were reported at the annual meeting of the North American Menopause Society in October 2012.[143] The researchers found that hormone therapy had no effect on hardening of the arteries or blood pressure, although limited evidence showed it might be cardioprotective.[144] Premarin was shown to lower LDL cholesterol (the so-called bad cholesterol) and increase HDL cholesterol (the "good" cholesterol), although it also increased harmful triglycerides. The natural estrogen patch didn't change blood lipid levels, but it did improve insulin resistance. Both the group on Premarin and the group on the natural estrogen patch substantially reduced hot flashes and night sweats, experienced small gains in bone mineral density, and improved their sexual function (with those on natural hormones also seeing improvements in libido). KEEPS further showed that these therapies had no adverse effects on cognitive function (as the earlier WHI study on older women claimed). A subsequent study beginning thirteen years after the start of the original KEEPS study is now following the same women for a longer period of time. The Kronos Early Estrogen Prevention Study (KEEPS) Continuation is looking at the effects of hormone therapy and normal aging on brain structure, cognitive performance, and markers for Alzheimer's disease.

More data on natural hormones came from the Early Versus Late Intervention Trial with Estradiol (ELITE). This double-blind, placebo-controlled study sponsored by the National Institute on Aging was designed to look at whether natural estrogen therapy started soon after menopause reduced the progression of early atherosclerosis. Researchers from the Keck School of Medicine at the University of Southern California divided 643 healthy women into two groups—those who had started menopause less than six years earlier and those who had started menopause ten or more years earlier. Within each group, they compared those taking natural hormones (an estradiol pill and, if the women still had a uterus, progesterone gel applied vaginally) to a control group taking a placebo. Natural estrogen therapy was found to reduce the progression of early atherosclerosis if it was started soon after menopause, but it had no effect when it was begun ten or more years after menopause.[145] The researchers then conducted a follow-up study with the same women to see if natural hormone therapy had any cognitive effects. They concluded that estradiol neither benefited nor harmed cognitive abilities, regardless of time since menopause.[146]

Despite the promise of much of this research, I wouldn't prescribe HT to anyone just to prevent heart disease. There are too many other factors to consider, including breast cancer and stroke risk. As always, women and their physicians need to make the HT decision in partnership with their own intuition and body wisdom.

HOW TO LOVE AND RESPECT YOUR MIDLIFE HEART

The energies of love, enthusiasm, joy, and passion actually enliven your heart. To promote a healthy heart, you must have a goal, a passion, a reason for living.

Many women get heart disease when, for any number of reasons, their heart is no longer in their work or their life. A very healthy eighty-five-year-old patient without any signs of heart disease recently told me that she didn't think she'd be around much longer. Her ninety-year-old husband had been hospitalized with heart disease and wasn't back to his usual state of health. She said, "We've been married for sixty years. I couldn't go on living without him." It is well known that elderly spouses often die within weeks of each other. Even in the medical profession this is known as "dying from a broken heart."

At midlife, more than ever, our hearts are calling us home. We must remember that for every behavior—whether health-enhancing or health-destroying—there are emotions that are processed by the heart and the entire cardiovascular system. And behind every emotion, there is a belief—a perception about reality. Thoughts and beliefs that support self-love and self-worth enhance health and well-being and the lifestyle behaviors that support them. The more women truly care for themselves, the better their health is.

Emotions that we can't deal with directly and elegantly go into our bodies and drive our behaviors, pure and simple. The truth of this comes down the track like a freight train at midlife. This is the time when the dictates of our very souls cry out to be heard—a time when we must grow or risk slow (or sometimes rapid) decline and disease.

Though it has been said that "home is where the heart is," in my experience home is also where the heart most easily gets broken. And that's because we unerringly choose close relationships that re-create the dynamics of early childhood. For example, I recently had a reading with a very skilled astrologer who pointed out that I shut down my "desire nature" (the part of me that loved beautiful things, back rubs, cookies, soft fabrics, and so on) at about the age of four and a half—a time when I decided that I needed to hide some of who I really was, and also some of my personal power, in order to win the love of a parent or sibling. There are endless variations on this story. And we generally peel off these layers one by one as time goes on. The good news is that at midlife and beyond, we invariably revisit the unconscious agreements we made in childhood because we now have adult skills and the perspective necessary to update them.

All of life is a birth canal. Midlife is a particularly powerful and important one. One of the greatest challenges of midlife is to come home to ourselves. We can do this only when we allow ourselves to get to the heart of the matter—and to tell the truth about what we really want and need. Our emotions will always lead us to the right place. The famous writer and feminist Gloria Steinem once said, "The truth will set you free. But first it will piss you off." How true! Almost always, having the courage to name our needs and desires is associated with feeling and releasing childhood shame and guilt. And though this shame and guilt have many different names, I can guarantee that they always boil down to some version of "I am not lovable." This belief is so painful that far too many women use addictions—to food, alcohol, smoking, too much or too little exercise, or recreational drugs—as a way to avoid the feelings that will lead them home. It is only through naming our needs, desires, and dreams and releasing our guilt, sorrow, and shame that we will truly reach the feeling of being at home within ourselves. Self-acceptance and self-love result from being true to ourselves and to our dreams and desires. And once we begin to truly feel good about ourselves, we find we are eager to support our hearts and bodies with a healthful diet, exercise, and supplement program. Though I suggest that you follow the dietary and exercise guidelines I've outlined, I believe that it is even more important to learn what it is to love and accept yourself and to have the courage to open your heart to the possibility of living joyfully. This journey home is always poignant and often painful, but inevitably always worth it, too.

One of my perimenopausal friends whose mother had been mentally ill, and who knew that she had always used food as a way to cope with the craziness of having to care for both her mother and her younger siblings, told me that when she turned forty-three she finally was able to allow herself to really feel the pain of all those childhood years and let it go. She said, "I remember the first time I sat in my therapist's office and actually allowed myself to feel the absolute panic and terror within that was the result of fear that I'd become just like my mother. And in that moment I knew why people with severe weight problems often don't lose weight—or why they put it right back on. They prefer overeating and obesity to allowing themselves to feel the depth of despair and pain within them." Luckily my friend has a very strong faith, and with the help of God she allowed herself to finally get all those old feelings out in the open, a process that took several months and a lot of tears.

She credits this to the fact that she sailed through menopause with nary a symptom. She no longer uses food to quell her emotions and has kept her weight stable for over ten years. The only way out was through!

Whether or not you have midlife heart symptoms such as palpitations, hypertension, high cholesterol, chest pain, jaw pain, arm pain, or any other evidence of heart disease, or if you simply want to prevent heart disease in the future, you owe it to yourself to learn the language of your heart.

THE HEART-OPENING EFFECT OF PETS

One of the first things I did after my husband moved out was to go down to the animal shelter and get two cats, something I'd wanted to do for a long time—my husband had been allergic to them. I was shocked by how much love, companionship, and joy these two furry creatures brought into my life. The first cat I got, Buddy, was a real hunk of burning love. He adored being held and petted, and was a great cuddler. During those early years when I had no male companionship, Buddy was a godsend. Francine, a much smaller and daintier female, taught me a lot about being a desirable woman. She sashayed about the house with incredible style and cheekiness, as if to say, "I might allow you to pet me, but it will have to be on my terms." Though both have since died, I still feel their spirits around me. Both were powerful healers. In fact, they both died of cancer. I'm certain that they "took on" my own grief and loneliness, absorbing those difficult emotions into their own bodies for me so that I didn't have to experience that disease myself.

One of my midlife friends from New York City, a professional woman with a high-powered job, recently got a dog. She told me, "It's really true that happiness is a warm puppy. What a wonderful thing to wake up each morning to such unconditional love! Everyone in my building loves him. And when I take him for a walk, I make all kinds of new friends!" Scientific literature on the health benefits of pets proves beyond the shadow of a doubt that our hearts are touched and healed, quite literally, by the unconditional love that animals can bring to our lives.

Though animals can't offer all the different types of support that we humans need, they still provide companionship, security, and a feeling of being needed. They also help connect us to the world around us and give us a focus outside ourselves—which is very helpful for those who suffer from depression. Larry Dossey, M.D., an internist who has extensively researched the healing power of prayer, refers to companion animals as "four-legged prayer."

The presence of a pet is associated with decreased cardiovascular reactivity—which means that the influence of a pet helps us stabilize our blood vessels and heart rhythm. People have been found to have lower heart rates and lower blood pressure when they are with their pets. This translates into thousands of fewer heartbeats over months and years, which can slow the development of arteriosclerosis. Research at Brooklyn College has shown that pets slow heart rate even among highly stressed, high-intensity type A personalities.[147]

Pets of all kinds lower blood pressure. Petting a dog has been shown to decrease the blood pressure of healthy college students, hospitalized elderly people, and adults with hypertension. When bird owners talk to their birds, their blood pressure drops an average of ten points. And watching fish in an aquarium has been shown to bring blood pressure below resting levels. Research has also shown that when children are sitting quietly and reading, their blood pressure is lower when a dog is in the room.[148]

Cat owners are 30 percent less likely to have a heart attack and 40 percent less likely to suffer a stroke than those without a cat, according to a study following more than 2,400 cat owners for twenty years.[149] In those who already have heart disease, support from animal companions has been linked to increased survival, even independent of marital status and living situation. University of Pennsylvania researchers Aaron Katcher, M.D., and Erika Friedmann, Ph.D., found that people with pets lived longer after experiencing heart attacks than those without pets.[150] Subsequent research has shown that among people who have heart attacks, pet owners have one-fifth the death rate of those who do not have pets.[151] A 2019 study of Swedish data showed that those who had survived a heart attack or a stroke lived longer if they owned a dog; the risk of early death was 33 percent lower for heart attack survivors and 27 percent lower for stroke survivors, especially for those who lived alone.[152] A 2017 study from China showed that risk of coronary artery disease decreased the lon ger the subjects had owned pets, as well as the more time they spent playing with their pet.[153] If you can't own a pet yourself, volunteer at an animal shelter or visit other people's pets. They're a cardiac tonic with no side effects.

THE INTELLECT IS CERTAIN IT KNOWS, BUT THE HEART ALWAYS WINS

It has taken me more than half a lifetime to know one thing for sure: the intellect exists to serve the wisdom of the heart. Our intellect-driven society, however, leads us to believe that it's the other way around. And so we wait for the next drug or technological break-through, thinking it will save us. But in the end, the wisdom of the heart always wins.

All the drugs and technology in the world can't mend a broken heart or heal someone whose heart is no longer in the game of life. The EKG signal coming from the heart is 5,000 times stronger than the EEG signal from brain waves. So when there's a conflict between the intellect and the heart, the heart always wins. And the only way to heal the true discomforts of the heart is to feel them fully, heed their message, and have faith that your heart's desires can come to you in many different ways. It's also enormously helpful to have faith in a power greater than yourself, and then live your life robustly.

My Prescription for Preventing and Healing Heart Disease

~ Understand that each heart is self-healing if given the space and permission to feel what it needs to feel.

~ Be willing to bravely and compassionately enter the unhealed places in your heart. When you are on intimate terms with your own pain and suffering and have made a commitment to heal them, you will eventually come to the joy that is your natural state. And you will also find that you have far less difficulty keeping your heart open to others. Your very presence becomes part of the heal-ing as everyone around you realizes that they are not alone and are also worthy of openhearted acceptance, too.

~ Know that it's part of the Great Mystery why some people open their hearts to themselves and do the work of healing and others do not. Still, maintain hope and compassion, no matter how dim they may seem.

~ Rather than take on the impossible burden of thinking it is our job to fix others, we must also remember that the biggest gift we can give to another is a healed, joyful, and compassionate heart. That is, and always will be, an inside job. Besides, as much as we'd like to, we cannot heal someone who doesn't want to be healed. Nor can we convince them that we know what's best for them. This is a particularly difficult lesson for those of us who are empaths and healers.

Whether or not you get a new pet, a new job, or a new mate, midlife is a time of rebirth. The newly opening midlife heart is tender, green, and new. Don't allow it to be stepped on. Learn how to protect yourself; ask for help and allow yourself to receive it. Take heart. Have heart. Open your heart and let its wisdom lead you home. And remember, it is truly a new beginning. You're just getting started.

Epilogue
The Calm After the Storm

One day during the winter after my divorce, I awoke at six to go to my regular morning exercise class in Portland. Though the weather report said it was raining, I opened the door and walked out into a snowstorm that was dumping about two inches an hour all around me. Nevertheless, I set out. After all, I'm a veteran of snowbelt winters in western New York. As I headed south, however, I could scarcely see, and I briefly considered turning around. But in my characteristically stoic fashion I continued, certain that the weather would lighten up momentarily. Suddenly my car started fish-tailing. I was spinning in a circle, wildly out of control and heading for the guardrails. I braced myself for the crash, wondering simultaneously whether I would survive being broadsided by the oncoming traffic. After my car slammed to a halt against guardrails cushioned by snow, I braced for further collisions. Miraculously, the cars behind me were able to stop in time. Not sure what to do next, I hesitantly put my car into gear. I was able to pull out onto the highway, and I slowly continued my drive into Portland. As I entered the city the weather did indeed clear, and I ended up going to my class. Though I was shaken, the damage to my car was mostly cosmetic—I had shattered my left rear bumper, nothing else. I felt very lucky. I knew that I could have been killed.

My accident seemed like a swift energetic reenactment of my peri-menopause, complete with the shattering of my marriage and of the parts of my personality that now needed to die if I was to stay healthy and grow. The accident happened almost one year to the day from the time when my husband and I had separated and started divorce proceedings. For the past year my old life and personality had, like my vehicle on that icy road, been seized by a force beyond my control. Despite my worst fears, I had ended up able to move forward under my own power. And though at the time the impact of the breakup had felt as though it might destroy some essential part of me, the damage, like the damage to my car, turned out to be largely cosmetic. My life no longer looked as picture-perfect as it once had. Yet I discovered that the only thing of true significance that had been shattered was the closely guarded and comforting illusion that something or someone outside of myself could and should save me from living the life that I was destined to live. After twenty-four years of marriage, I had managed to spend a year without a man. I had survived a great deal of grief and pain, found that I was able to support my children and myself, and, though shaken, had emerged more fear-less than ever before.

FROM KARMA INTO GRACE

As I write this now, it has been more than twenty years since my divorce. If you had asked me a decade ago if I was over the breakup of my marriage, I'd have replied with a resounding yes. On the night that I taped my PBS show *Women's Bodies, Women's Wisdom,* I was entertaining a houseful of women ranging in age from twenty-seven to sixty. As we were digesting the eventful evening of making a TV show, one of the women asked to see a picture of my former husband. I retrieved from a drawer one in which my husband was sailing and looked particularly handsome and daring—shirtless, to reveal his six-pack abs, his glorious hair blowing, taking a godlike stance at the helm. One of the women said, "Oh my goodness!" I said, "Yeah, I didn't stand a chance." And then, rather than simply taking in the compliments about how good he had looked, I felt compelled to drag out the parts of the divorce story that painted me as the victim and him as the perpetrator.

The next morning, one of my friends, whom I'll call Patricia, told me that she had been unable to sleep the night before, and that she had decided to take a big risk and tell me how much anger she felt was still in me around my former husband. "If you ever expect to be truly happy with a man," she said, "you're going to have to find the perfection in how your marriage ended."

I knew in a heartbeat that she was absolutely correct. I had thought that my anger was a thing of the past. Yet it had arisen, unbidden, as I had run for the victim position in talking about him, wanting to justify how I had been wronged. Patricia suggested that I write him a letter outlining the perfection of the entire relationship, including its ending—and then read the letter out loud. So that very night, on the full Wolf Moon of January, I sat down with Amy Sky's song "Love Never Fails" playing, propped up my husband's beefcake picture in front of me, lit a candle, and started to write him a love letter.

I wrote about how swept away I had been by him, the handsome surgical intern I'd met when I was finishing medical school. How supportive he had been about me going into OB-GYN. How he'd taught me to tie surgical knots on my big toe. I waxed eloquent about how romantic and magical our courtship in the hospital had been, how wonderful it had felt to enter my internship happily married to someone I adored coming home to at night, and how he had made a home possible because he had enough money for a down payment.

And as I continued writing, the most amazing thing happened. All the love that I had ever felt for this man came roaring back. To my amazement, it was all still there. It hadn't gone anywhere! What a revelation! As I kept writing, I realized with great clarity that his behavior toward me had, in fact, been perfect. It was this behavior that had freed me to become the happy, healthy, successful woman I am now. I knew, deep inside, that if he had behaved any other way, I never would have had the courage or impetus to learn about business, finance, and truly taking care of myself in the world. There are no mistakes. The health of the second chakra is secured by our relationship to money, sex, and power, and I'd had some big lessons to learn about money. He had helped me learn them.

When I was finished with the letter and had cried myself out, I called Patricia. She suggested that I read the letter out loud to my daughters and to the same women who had been at my house the evening before. I arranged a conference call, lit a candle, and read the letter. I was in tears the whole time. And so was everyone else on the call, including my daughters. They had never heard the entire story of our courtship before—something that surprised me. And hearing about it in detail healed something deep within them. They realized that they had been conceived and brought up with love—that their mom and dad's relationship was not a mistake, and neither were they. My deep forgiveness of and love for their father—all expressed in that letter—gave them their father back completely.

Then Patricia suggested, "How about you take it even higher? Read it to him."

I gulped, but then I thought, *Well, why not?* I had nothing to lose. So I emailed him (he was living in London with his wife and young child) and requested that he allow me to read him a letter. It took him a while to respond. When he did, he asked me to give him some details. I told him that I had realized that I was still holding some anger about the divorce and had written a letter to him to help me forgive and release. I said that it would be an honor for me if he'd allow me to read the letter to him. He agreed, and we set up a time.

There I was, sitting in Maine in the candlelight, while he was in London, sitting comfortably in a chair, undisturbed and willing to receive what I had to say. I read him the letter, tears flowing. When I was finished, I started to get off the phone. "It's okay," he said. "Don't go." And then he said, "I know that you believe in parallel universes more than I do. But I believe that there's a place in the universe where we're still going on." And then he told me that he hoped with all his heart that I would find someone who truly deserved me. We talked about our daughters for a bit, then parted. The sweetness of that moment brings me to tears once again as I write this.

A couple of days later, he sent me an email, thanking me for his early Valentine's Day present. We didn't speak for many years after that. We didn't need to. But on that day, my divorce was truly final. I had finally moved on. And today there's not a cell in my body that feels anything but happiness and completion about the whole thing.

I was relating this story to a good friend, also a doctor, who at the time was in her eighties. (She is now approaching a hundred!) She herself went through an awful divorce when she was seventy and found out that her husband had been having an affair with the office manager. I won't go into the details except to say that I had always thought she and her husband had the ideal marriage. They had traveled together, practiced medicine together, and had six wonderful children—many of whom also became doctors. And so her divorce was a true shock to me. That was many years ago, and he has since died.

But when I told her my story, she shared the following: "One morning I awakened and felt Jim with me. And for one year, we were together again. I relived all the wonderful adventures we had had—climbing the pyramids, skiing, traveling around the world, playing with our children. It was wonderful. And then, on what would have been our sixty-fifth wedding anniversary, he left and went back into spirit. I feel complete and at peace around the whole thing. We have moved from karma into grace."

As we round the corner into midlife, we can be sure that with each ensuing year our unfinished business will keep rearing its head until we deal with it once and for all. By dealing with the final pieces of anger and resentment against my former husband, I changed both my daughters' and my own legacy around men. So did my old friend. She, too, told me that her children (midlife individuals themselves) were similarly healed by what happened between their parents. It is never too late.

AWAKENING TO OUR POWER, AWAKENING TO BEAUTY AND PLEASURE

We women are waking up all over the world. And perimenopause is a huge portal for this. Don't let anyone tell you that the passions that are now shaking you to the core are simply a hormonal storm. Don't let anyone tell you that you're asking too much or that you should be more "realistic." Your passions are real, and they are calling out to you to be acted upon. But don't panic if you feel some pain. Whenever we give birth to anything important, like the new relationship with our souls that is possible at midlife, there are going to be labor pains. You don't have to make this transition overnight. You have months, even years.

Never forget that the big wisdom of life comes at menopause. There is enormous power here. Though the mainstream media has tried to make midlife women all but invisible, we're at a turning point. There is a critical mass of us, and our power is changing the world. When we start out, we don't suspect how much we can accomplish when we go into our businesses, churches, clubs, and families and, quietly and peacefully, like the stealth missiles we are, set about changing everything for the better.

What happens when each of us, in her own unique way, starts refusing to say the lines that have been handed to us, refuses to play the roles that we've inherited from the women before us—women who did the best they could but whose roles are now as obsolete as the role I chose to play in my marriage back in the 1970s?

By the year 2008, women between the ages of fifty and sixty-five had become the largest demographic group in the United States. And for the first time in recorded history, the money we have and use is money we have earned ourselves. This changes everything! Many young women today are shocked to learn that women could not even get a credit card in their own names until the Equal Credit Opportunity Act was passed in 1974—that's less than fifty years ago. What happens when we wake up to the power that had always been there but that our mothers and grandmothers had been talked out of? What happens when, because of our sheer numbers and the circumstances of our formative years, we wake up and realize that the people we've been waiting for are us? As we flex our economic, mental, physical, and, yes, romantic muscles and put our resources where our ideals are, the world begins to change in ways that reflect our inherent women's wisdom, wisdom that has the potential to benefit every woman, man, child, and living being on this planet.

Let me end on a provocative note. Midlife women are rapidly changing the outdated archetype of the crone who lives alone in the woods. We are sexier, happier, and healthier than ever. In fact, years after menopause, I am enjoying more male attention than I ever have before. But to get to this place of truly enjoying and co-creating with men, I first had to make the sacred marriage within myself—the wedding of the inner masculine and feminine and the wedding of the Divine and the human within me. I had to become the man I always wanted to marry. This wasn't easy, and I resisted at every turn. But I did it—and nothing is more empowering. I will never again need to ask permission to spend money, nor do I need a man to provide it for me. This is true not only for me, but for millions of other women.

This fact frees us to have real relationships and full lives that are authentically our own, crafted by the dictates of our souls. This includes relationships based not on control and economic need, but instead on pleasure, freedom, beauty, joy, uplifting service, co-creation, and companionship. In every cell of my body, I know that the best is yet to come and that everything that has happened up until this point has been but a preview of the productive and delightful years ahead. Trust me—it gets better. And if you allow your soul to take the lead, it will work out better than you could ever have imagined.

Resources

Note: The phone numbers and websites listed in this section were current as of the publication date of the book.

General Resources

Women's Health Resources from Christiane Northrup, M.D.

Christiane Northrup, M.D., F.A.C.O.G., P.O. Box 199, Yarmouth, ME 04096; www.drnorthrup.com.

Dr. Northrup's website (www.drnorthrup.com) is the best place to find regularly updated blogs, articles, videos, podcasts, and other content, as well as information about her lectures and other resources, including her many books, courses, and products. Answers to many of her readers' most frequently asked questions can also be found here.

In addition, Dr. Northrup stays in touch with her large and growing community worldwide through Facebook (@DrChristianeNorthrup), Instagram (@DrChristianeNorthrup), Twitter (@DrChrisNorthrup), and her bi-weekly e-newsletter (to subscribe, sign up at www.drnorthrup.com).

BOOKS

Women's Bodies, Women's Wisdom: Creating Physical and Emotional Health and Healing (Bantam, 2020)

When it was first published in 1994, *Women's Bodies, Women's Wisdom* quickly became an international bestseller and has remained the veritable bible of women's health ever since. Now, in this completely revised and updated edition, Dr. Northrup shares the latest developments and advances for maximizing our potential for living well in our bodies today. With more than 2 million copies in print and translated into twenty languages, this groundbreaking book addresses the entire range of women's health concerns and how to transform them. It's been described as contemporary medicine at its best, combining new technologies with natural remedies and the miraculous healing powers within the body, mind, and spirit themselves.

Dodging Energy Vampires: An Empath's Guide to Evading Relationships That Drain You and Restoring Your Health and Power (Hay House, 2018)

In this book, Dr. Northrup explores the phenomenon of energy vampires (also known as personality-disordered individuals) and shows how to spot them, dodge their tactics, and take back your own energy. She draws on the latest research, along with stories from her global community as well as her own life. She delves into the dynamics of vampire-empath relationships to discover how vampires use others' energy to fuel their own dysfunctional lives. Once you recognize the patterns of behavior that mark these relationships, you'll be empowered to identify the vampires in your life, too.

A Daily Dose of Women's Wisdom (Hay House, 2017)

For decades, Dr. Northrup has been helping women navigate their lives with grace and joy. This elegant, compact volume offers her trademark wisdom in a fresh form, filled with pointed reminders "to help you develop a deeper respect for, and connection to, your own body and its exquisite guidance system to create a vibrantly healthy body, mind, and spirit." Each beautifully designed black-and-white page carries a quote that touches on a topic of deep significance, including heart-listening, epigenetics, and the importance of knowing that your decisions about medical treatment are not irreversible.

Making Life Easy (Hay House, 2016)

In this joyfully encouraging book—as useful for men as it is for women—Dr. Northrup explores the essential truth that has guided her ever since medical school: our bodies, minds, and souls are profoundly intertwined. Making life flow with ease, and truly feeling your best, is about far more than physical health; it's also about having a healthy emotional life and a robust spiritual life. When you view your physical well-being in isolation, life can become a constant battle to make your body "behave." When you acknowledge the deep connection between your beliefs and your biology and start to tune in to the Divine part of yourself, it's a whole new ballgame—and the first step in truly making your life easy.

Goddesses Never Age: The Secret Prescription for Radiance, Vitality, and Well-Being (Hay House, 2015)

Though we talk about wanting to "age gracefully," the truth is that when it comes to getting older, we're programmed to dread an inevitable decline: in our health, our looks, our sexual relationships, and even the pleasure we take in living life. But as Dr. Northrup shows us in this profoundly empowering book, we have it in us to make growing older an entirely different experience, for both our bodies and our souls.

In chapters that blend personal stories and practical exercises with the latest research on health and aging, Dr. Northrup lays out the principles of ageless living, including rejecting processed foods, releasing stuck emotions, embracing our sensuality, and connecting deeply with our Divine Source. She brings it all together in a fourteen-day Ageless Goddess Program, offering tools and inspiration for creating a healthful and soulful new way of being at any stage of life.

Beautiful Girl: Celebrating the Wonders of Your Body (Hay House, 2013)

For years, Dr. Northrup has taught women about health, wellness, and the miracle of their bodies. Now, in her first children's book, she presents these ideas to the youngest of girls. *Beautiful Girl* presents this simple but important message: that to be born female is a very special thing and carries with it magical gifts and powers that must be recognized and nurtured. Dr. Northrup believes that helping girls learn at a young age to value the wonder and uniqueness of their bodies can have positive benefits that will last throughout their lives. By reading this lovely book, little girls will learn how their bodies are perfect just the way they are, the importance of treating themselves with gentle care, and how changes are just a part of growing up.

The Secret Pleasures of Menopause (Hay House, 2008)

This book delivers a breakthrough message that will help perimenopausal and menopausal women understand that at menopause, life has just begun. It's the beginning of a very exciting and fulfilling time, full of pleasure beyond your wildest dreams. A key concept outlined in the book is the science of nitric oxide, which has been called the molecule of life force.

The Secret Pleasures of Menopause Playbook (Hay House, 2009)

This companion volume to *The Secret Pleasures of Menopause* serves as a personal guide to the territory of life-giving pleasure and provides useful exercises to help you commit to your own personal pleasure plan.

The Wisdom of Menopause Journal (Hay House, 2007)

This companion book to *The Wisdom of Menopause* helps you focus on the "me" in menopause. Designed to help you both navigate and document this important transitional time, the journal is packed with action-oriented, practical advice for your mind and body.

This journal gives you everything you need to create vibrant health in midlife on all levels—not just in your heart, bones, pelvic organs, breasts, and brain, but also in your sex life, your relationships, and even your beauty regimen! It enables you to record your current health and concerns, as well as the steps you want to take to achieve your goals in each area. You'll also find powerful affirmations, inspiring quotes, and plenty of blank pages for journaling, so you can create a record of your thoughts and feelings during this important time.

Mother-Daughter Wisdom: Understanding the Crucial Link Between Mothers, Daughters, and Health (Bantam, 2005)

Dr. Northrup explains how the mother-daughter relationship sets the stage for our state of health and well-being for our entire lives. Because our mothers are our first and most powerful female role models, our most deeply ingrained beliefs about ourselves as women come from them. And our behavior in relationships—with food, with our children, with our mates, and with ourselves—is a reflection of those beliefs. In this book, Dr. Northrup shows how once we understand our mother-daughter bonds, we can rebuild our own health, whatever our age, and create a lasting positive legacy for the next generation.

ONLINE RESOURCES

The Dr. Christiane Northrup E-Newsletter

Dr. Northrup's free biweekly newsletter is sent directly to subscribers' email addresses. It contains the most updated information on a wide variety of topics guaranteed to enhance your health on all levels. With links to take readers directly to the most up-to-date and relevant content and resources, the e-newsletter is one of the best ways to stay on track with your health. Available at www.drnorthrup.com.

DrNorthrup.com

Dr. Northrup's website houses a wealth of information, designed to both inform and uplift users. With content covering the latest medical research and trends as well as hundreds of archived health-related articles, blog posts, online seminars, inspirational audio downloads, videos, and podcasts, this is the perfect go-to resource for anyone wanting to be healthy in mind, body, and spirit.

AUDIO/VIDEO PROGRAMS

Dr. Northrup's audio and video programs are all available through www.drnorthrup.com.

Women's Bodies, Women's Wisdom, audiobook

The audiobook version of Dr. Northrup's newly updated *Women's Bodies, Women's Wisdom* addresses the entire range of women's health—from first menstrual period through menopause—and includes the latest information on all of the most important health concerns facing women today. Discover new material on why vitamin D is crucial for breast, cardiovascular, and immune system health as well as on preventing cellular inflammation (the root cause of all chronic degenerative diseases)—and so much more.

Women's Bodies, Women's Wisdom, online video

In this companion lecture to the bestselling book *Women's Bodies, Women's Wisdom,* Dr. Northrup approaches some of the most common complaints that keep women from enjoying optimal health and offers cutting-edge, holistic solutions. With her guidance, you'll discover how to access and use the most powerful inner tool you possess for beauty and overall well-being: your innate women's wisdom. This program will forever change your thinking about what is possible for your health—inside and out!

Divine Feminine Meditations, audio download

This set of three guided meditations narrated by Dr. Northrup includes:

Your Body, Your Temple: An ethereal meditation that guides you in cleansing your body temple with light, which will help you remain healthy and vibrant.

Your Breasts Are Divine: A soothing meditation that helps you bring light, love, and health to your breasts and increase your ability to give and receive.

Pelvic Bowl: A unique meditation to put you in touch with the creativity that rests within your pelvic bowl, the center of your creative self.

Dodging Energy Vampires: An Empath's Guide to Evading Relationships That Drain You and Restoring Your Health and Power, audio download

In this program, Dr. Northrup explores the phenomenon of energy vampires and shows how to spot them, dodge their tactics, and take back your own energy. She draws on the latest research, along with stories from her global community as well as her own life. She delves into the dynamics of vampire-empath relationships to discover how vampires use others' energy to fuel their own dysfunctional lives. Once you recognize the patterns of behavior that mark these relationships, you'll be empowered to identify the vampires in your life, too.

Making Life Easy, audio download

In this program, Dr. Northrup explores the essential truth that has guided her ever since medical school: our bodies, minds, and souls are profoundly intertwined. Making life flow with ease, and truly feeling your best, is about far more than physical health; it's also about having a healthy emotional life and a robust spiritual life. When you view your physical well-being in isolation, life can become a constant battle to make your body "behave." When you acknowledge the deep connection between your beliefs and your biology and start to tune in to the Divine part of yourself, it's a whole new ballgame—and the first step in truly making your life easy. Drawing on fields as diverse as epigenetics, past-life regression, and standard Western medicine, Dr. Northrup distills a brilliant career's worth of wisdom into one comprehensive user's guide to a healthy, happy, radiant life.

Goddesses Never Age: The Secret Prescription for Radiance, Vitality, and Well-Being, audio download

Though we talk about wanting to "age gracefully," the truth is that when it comes to getting older, we're programmed to dread an inevitable decline—in our health, our looks, our sexual relationships, and even the pleasure we take in living life. But as Dr. Northrup shows us in this profoundly empowering audio program, we have it in us to make growing older an entirely different experience, for both our bodies and our souls.

Inside-Out Wellness: The Wisdom of Mind-Body Healing, audio download of a program by Christiane Northrup, M.D., and Dr. Wayne W. Dyer

Dr. Northrup and Dr. Dyer team up for this inspirational and informative program that discusses how to transform the old habits, traditional beliefs, and everyday thoughts that keep you from becoming all that you can be. Topics include how to rewire your thought patterns and let go of your past so you can cultivate pleasure instead of stress, reawaken your passions, follow your bliss, and create the life you want.

Menopause and Beyond, online video and audio download

With cutting-edge medical information and guidance, Dr. Northrup invites midlife women to embrace their inner wisdom and transform the second half of their lives in this program, based on her bestselling book, *The Wisdom of Menopause.* The program focuses on heart health, hormone therapy, diet, and sexuality. Dr. Northrup also presents a five-step program that guarantees weight loss.

The Power of Joy, audio download

Life is meant to be joyous! We are pleasure-seeking creatures by nature. Joy makes you younger, smarter, more intuitive, and healthier, with better hormonal balance and immune-system functioning. Joy even positively affects your metabolism. On this audio program, Dr. Northrup prescribes a ten-step process for overcoming habitual patterns of negative thinking, guilt, and pain in order to evoke the power of joy in your life every day.

The Secret Pleasures of Menopause, audio download

Dr. Northrup believes that it's about time menopausal women came out of the closet and learned to enjoy the best years of their lives! Even though studies show that menopause does not decrease libido, ease of reaching orgasm, or sexual satisfaction, the majority of menopausal women are not experiencing the pleasure and sexual satisfaction that are their birthright. In this audio program, Dr. Northrup delivers a breakthrough message that will help millions of perimenopausal and menopausal women throughout the world understand that at menopause . . . life has just begun! It is the beginning of a very exciting and fulfilling time, full of pleasure beyond your wildest dreams!

Mother-Daughter Wisdom, audio and online video
In the course of this journey to self-realization, Dr. Northrup covers a rich range of topics that are designed to bring mothers and daughters to greater consciousness, including the five facets of feminine power, how to end the mother-daughter "chain of pain," the power of forgiveness, and how to deal with a difficult mother or daughter.

The Empowering Women Gift Collection, audio download
This program includes inspiration and knowledge for women of all ages from Dr. Northrup, Louise L. Hay, Caroline Myss, and Susan Jeffers, Ph.D.

Women's Bodies, Women's Wisdom, online course
This online course is the distillation of the wisdom Dr. Northrup gained from forty years on the front lines of women's health. It is designed to teach women everything that can go right with their bodies and how to make that their daily experience. The course is loaded with practical information, exercises, and insights to help women everywhere trust the wisdom of their bodies and their innate ability to heal.

For ages, women have been shamed and misinformed about their bodies—and this legacy has been handed down to us for millennia. This permeates not only our culture at large but also the entire medical system, where normal functions of the female body have become pathologized and medicalized. We have been alienated from understanding our bodies, and our beliefs about our worthiness have taken a plunge. Dr. Northrup is here to change that and to help you radically transform your health. "I walked a very fine line for many years," she says about her medical career, before breaking from mainstream medicine to speak the truth about women's wellness. And in this online course, she pulls no punches. She dives straight into the truth about women's health and everything you need to know to not only maintain your physical body, but also to flourish throughout your life. In these comprehensive and mesmerizing lessons, Dr. Northrup will discuss everything you ever wanted to know—and absolutely need to learn—about your body.

Dodging Energy Vampires, online course
In six powerful, jam-packed lessons, Dr. Northrup teaches you how to recognize and rid yourself of energy-vampire relationships so that you can quickly separate from people who are using your energy to fuel their dys-

functional lives. Along the way, she interviews top experts from the field of personality disorders and offers simple, clear strategies and healing practices so that you can address the wounds that are keeping you stuck.

Ageless Goddess, online course

Growing older is inevitable, but making the decision to stay fully active and engaged in life is a choice. In this online course, Dr. Northrup incorporates women's health and wellness that expand well beyond emotional, mental, and physical well-being. This innovative course teaches you a new way to view growing older that brings excitement and joy to your life, no matter your chronological age or your current quality of life. When you have the right information and guidance, youthful living can be yours and you can continue to thrive, create, and engage in your life for years to come.

Embodied Wisdom, online course

In this three-part online course, Dr. Northrup will guide you through the seven major energy centers of the body and the processes and organs they govern. And then, in real-life, practical ways, she will show you exactly how to access this vital life force in your day-to-day life to achieve vibrant health in mind, body, and spirit. Once you understand the exquisitely accurate wisdom of your body, the mystery of remaining (or becoming) vibrantly healthy is at your fingertips.

OTHER

Amata Life by Dr. Christiane Northrup

After extensive research and development, Dr. Northrup formulated an array of drug-free products—including a vaginal moisturizer, skin care, and supplements containing the herb *Pueraria mirifica*—all designed to relieve symptoms related to hormonal imbalance, especially around perimenopause and after menopause. *Pueraria mirifica* has been used for more than 700 years by both men and women in Thailand for its benefits. The products are distributed via www.amatalife.com.

Chapter 2: The Brain Catches Fire at Menopause

Toxic Emotions/Forgiveness

SUGGESTED READING

Cohen, D. (2008). *Repetition: Past Lives, Life and Rebirth*. Carlsbad, CA: Hay House, Inc. (Also see Dr. Cohen's website at www.healingrepetition .com.)

Hay, L. L. (1998). *Heal Your Body A–Z: The Mental Causes for Physical Illness and the Metaphysical Way to Overcome Them*. Carlsbad, CA: Hay House, Inc.

Holden, R. (2009). *Be Happy: Release the Power of Happiness in You.* Carlsbad, CA: Hay House, Inc.

Levine, S. (1989). *Healing into Life and Death.* New York: Doubleday and Co., Inc.

Luskin, F. (2002). *Forgive for Good: A Proven Prescription for Health and Happiness.* San Francisco: HarperSanFrancisco.

Mellin, L. (2010). *Wired for Joy: A Revolutionary Method for Creating Happiness from Within.* Carlsbad, CA: Hay House, Inc.

Northrup, C. (2020; fifth edition). *Women's Bodies, Women's Wisdom.* New York: Bantam Books.

Chapter 3: Coming Home to Yourself

Deliberate Creating

Esther and Jerry Hicks
(830-755-2299; www.abraham-hicks.com)

Esther Hicks and her late husband, Jerry, have published many books and online resources that teach the most basic law of the universe: the Law of Attraction. Their work is profoundly helpful and practical, and I have enjoyed it, learned from it, and recommended it for decades.

Feng Shui

SUGGESTED READING

Collins, T. K. (1996). *The Western Guide to Feng Shui: Creating Balance, Harmony, and Prosperity in Your Environment.* Carlsbad, CA: Hay House.

Collins, T. K. (1999). *The Western Guide to Feng Shui: Room by Room.* Carlsbad, CA: Hay House.

Kingston, K. (1999). *Clear Your Clutter with Feng Shui.* New York: Broadway Books.

Proprioceptive Writing

Proprioceptive Writing Center
(www.pwriting.org)

Proprioceptive writing (PW) is a practice that uses writing to explore the psyche, using the intellect, intuition, and imagination simultaneously. PW was first developed in the 1970s by Linda Trichter Metcalf, Ph.D., and Tobin Simon, Ph.D., after their decade of teaching writing to college students. Dr. Metcalf discovered a method of writing that uses the intellect, imagination, and intuition simultaneously to tap into one's authentic voice. I personally worked with them privately and in group settings for seven years—and that work gave me the foundation I needed to write my first book, *Women's Bodies, Women's Wisdom*. Drs. Metcalf and Simon are also the authors of *Writing the Mind Alive: The Proprioceptive Method for Finding Your Authentic Voice* (Ballantine, 2002).

Chapter 4: This Can't Be Menopause, Can It?

Holistically Oriented Physicians

Academy of Integrative Health and Medicine
(www.aihm.org)
Founded in 1978 as the American Holistic Medical Association, this organization merged with the American Board of Integrative Holistic Medicine in 2013 to become AIHM. It is an organization of licensed medical doctors (M.D.s), doctors of osteopathic medicine (D.O.s), and medical students studying for those degrees. Physicians from every specialty are represented. AIHM also has a specialty board to certify holistically trained physicians using the same rigorous criteria that other specialties have employed. The AIHM website contains both an online physician referral directory as well as a guide to choosing a holistic practitioner.

Foundation for Alternative and Integrative Medicine
(www.faim.org)
The Foundation for Alternative and Integrative Medicine (FAIM) was founded in 1998 to identify breakthrough complementary and alternative therapies and to research and report on their effectiveness. FAIM's mission also stresses the affordability of treatments, supporting the idea that cost-effective solutions are what's needed to bring health to the greatest number of people. Until 2009, the organization was known as the National Foundation for Alternative Medicine.

American Association of Colleges of Osteopathic Medicine (301-968-4100; www.aacom.org)

American Association of Naturopathic Physicians (202-237-8150; www.naturopathic.org)

American College for Advancement in Medicine (800-532-3688; www.acam.org)

Citizens for Health (www.citizens.org)

Institute for Functional Medicine (253-661-3010; www.functionalmedicine.org/findfmphysician/index.asp)

Alliance for Pharmacy Compounding (formerly known as the International Academy of Compounding Pharmacists) (281-933-8400; www.a4pc.org)

Planetree (203-732-1365; www.planetree.org)

Women in Balance Institute (503-522-1555; www.womeninbalance.org)

Hormone Testing for Adrenal and Ovarian Function

The DUTCH Test
(www.dutchtest.com)
This is the gold standard for urinary and salivary hormone testing, and it can be done in your own home. The original DUTCH (dried urine test for comprehensive hormones) test measures urinary hormones, including cortisol and sex steroids, over a twenty-four-hour period. The DUTCH Plus test adds a salivary evaluation of how your cortisol levels change throughout the day. The tests are available from Precision Analytical Lab.

My Med Lab
(888-696-3352; www.mymedlab.com)
My Med Lab is a direct-to-consumer lab service that allows you to order any of various medical tests (including salivary hormone testing) without having to see your doctor just to get the test ordered. After you order your test online or over the phone, an in-house physician in your state reviews and approves the order. Then the company uploads a digital lab order to your My Med Lab account and notifies you via email. You log on to your account, print the order, and take it to any of 2,000 patient service centers (the website includes a directory, so you can see which are closest to you). At the service center, you'll have your samples taken—and you don't need a prior appointment. Usually within a day or two, you will receive an email notifying you that your results have been posted to your online My Med Lab account.

The results include a brief explanation and a direct link to the National Library of Medicine for more detailed result information. Schedule an appointment with your doctor to discuss any abnormal findings. (Note: Your test results are kept private and will not show up on your permanent medical record unless you share them with your doctor.) Health insurance usually doesn't cover this service, although prices are extremely reasonable.

Formulary Pharmacies

See Chapter 5 Resources.

DHEA (dehydroepiandrosterone)

Pharmaceutical-grade DHEA is available from formulary pharmacies and many other locations, including Emerson Ecologics (800-654-4432 or 603-656-9778; www.emersonecologics.com).

I recommend 5 mg DHEA sublingual. Suggested dose: ½ to 1 tablet daily, or as directed.

Migraines/Headaches

Bioidentical progesterone

A few drops of concentrated bioidentical progesterone (6,000 mg progesterone/30 ml propylene glycol) applied to the skin can sometimes halt a migraine. This concentrated preparation can be obtained by prescription from any formulary pharmacy. (See also Chapter 5 Resources.) Two percent progesterone cream is also effective if used daily one to two weeks prior to one's menstrual period.

Feverfew

Tanacetum parthenium works like aspirin to inhibit prostoglandins, preventing the blood vessel spasms that trigger migraines. Mygrafew, manufactured by Nature's Way, contains dried feverfew extract (leaf) 12 mg, delivering 600 mcg parthenolides (standardized to 5 percent parthenolides). Recommended dose is 1 tablet daily. Available from Emerson Ecologics (800-654-4432 or 603-656-9778; www.emersonecologics.com).

Chapter 5: Hormone Therapy

See Chapter 4 Resources for information on hormone testing.

Individualized Hormone Therapy

Many physicians and formulary pharmacists work in partnership with their patients to provide individualized hormone-replacement solutions. Ask your physician about this kind of customized care; he or she can call a local formulary pharmacy to consult with a knowledgeable pharmacist. To locate a pharmacy that provides individualized prescriptions, contact:

Alliance for Pharmacy Compounding

(281-933-8400; www.a4pc.org)

The Alliance for Pharmacy Compounding (formerly known as the International Academy of Compounding Pharmacists, or IACP) is a nonprofit organization made up of more than 150,000 patients and compounding practitioners (including physicians, veterinarians, and nurse practitioners) nationwide. The organization's website has a locator feature that can help you find a compounding pharmacy in your area.

BodyLogicMD
(www.bodylogicmd.com)
Body Logic offers a network of physicians who specialize in bioidentical hormones, fitness, and nutrition. These doctors design a personalized program for each patient, including customized compounded bioidentical hormones, other pharmacy-grade supplements, and fitness and nutrition advice. The Body Logic website offers a directory so you can find a Body Logic physician in your area.

Progesterone Cream

Progesterone cream (2 percent strength) is available from a number of different sources. I have personally used the following preparations and find them comparable in quality and effectiveness.

Pro-Gest Cream, by Emerita. This is the first brand I ever used or recommended. Available from Emerson Ecologics (800-654-4432 or 603-656-9778; www.emersonecologics.com).

Bioidentical progesterone in capsule, suppository, or transdermal form is available through any formulary pharmacy. It is also available in regular pharmacies under the brand name Prometrium (capsules) or Crinone or Prochieve (vaginal gel).

Chapter 6: Foods and Supplements to Support the Change

Herbs

Pueraria mirifica. The Thai herb *Pueraria mirifica* contains a powerful phytoestrogen known as miroestrol that works very well for many women who prefer a safe and effective alternative to prescription hormones. Dr. Northrup has formulated a range of products (including a vaginal moisturizer, facial creams, and supplements) that contain the highest-quality *Pueraria mirifica* and effectively quell menopausal symptoms and restore moisture and a sense of well-being. They are available through Amata Life (www.amatalife.com).

PhytoEstrin. This all-natural botanical formulation contains phytoestrogens from five different sources. Ingredients include soy isoflavones, black cohosh, vitex (chasteberry), licorice root, and dong quai. Available through USANA (888-950-9595 or 905-264-9863; www.usana.com).

Black cohosh. The rhizome of *Cimicifuga racemosa* has been used by Native Americans for centuries in much the same way as the Chinese have used dong quai. It is used for the treatment of menopausal ailments due to increasing ovarian insufficiency, mild postoperative functional deficits after ovariectomy or hysterectomy, PMS, and adolescent menstrual disorders. Many different preparations are available. I recommend Menopret (formerly known as Klimadynon) and MenoFem, both of which contain a form of black cohosh called BNO 1055 that has been shown to be very effective. I also recommend the black cohosh standardized extract from Nature's Way (40 mg twice a day), available from Emerson Ecologics (800-654-4432 or 603-656-9778; www.emersonecologics.com). Remifemin is another widely used brand available in many natural food stores and pharmacies, as well as from Emerson Ecologics. Start with 1 tablet (20 mg per tablet) twice per day, or take as directed.

Maca. The herb maca has been used for centuries by many women to help balance hormones. I highly recommend the Mighty Maca and Keto-Green weight-loss products formulated by my colleague Anna Cabeca, D.O. (www.drannacabeca.com).

Chasteberry (also called vitex). There are many different brands of chasteberry or vitex. Femaprin is one, manufactured by Nature's Way from dried chasteberry. Best results are obtained with continuous use. Available from Emerson Ecologics (800-654-4432 or 603-656-9778; www.emersonecologics.com). This herb is also available in tincture form from many natural food stores.

Women's Phase II (Vitanica) is a combination of dong quai, licorice root, burdock, motherwort, and wild yam. This formula was developed by Tori Hudson, N.D., a naturopathic physician and adjunct clinical professor at Bastyr University of Natural Health Sciences. It has been tested clinically and found to help relieve many common menopausal symptoms. Available from vitanica.com.

NutraMedix Hormonal Balance for Women is a proprietary blend of seven plant extracts, including *Eustephia coccinea*, *Muira puama*, maca, tribulus, epimedium, *Eurycoma longifolia*, and *Jatropha macrantha*. Recommended dosage is 20 drops twice a day, under the tongue or in 2–4 oz. of water. Available at www.nutramedix.com.

SUPPLIERS

Avena Botanicals
(866-282-8362 or 207-594-0694; www.avenabotanicals.com)
For a variety of herbal products, including dried organic herbs, liquid extracts, oils, creams, and teas. These products are all wildcrafted and of the highest quality.

DHA/Raw Chia Seed

See Chapter 7 Resources.

Flax

The Flax Council of Canada (204-982-2115; www.flaxcouncil.ca) endeavors to provide general flax facts of interest to consumers, as well as more specialized information for nutritionists, dietitians, food producers, manufacturers, and flax growers.

Dakota Flax Gold. This is an organic flaxseed grown at Heintzman Farms (800-333-5813; www.heintzmanfarms.com) in South Dakota. A "starter kit" is available that consists of three 1-pound bags of flaxseed and an electric grinder.

Traditional Chinese Medicine

Acupuncture, used alone or in conjunction with herbs, is very effective for relieving hot flashes, insomnia, night sweats, anxiety, restlessness, emotional instability, moodiness, menstrual cramps, and excessive bleeding. It's ideal to get a referral for an acupuncturist from your healthcare practitioner, but if you can't find one this way, contact the American Association of Acupuncture and Oriental Medicine (www.aaaomonline.org).

Chapter 7: The Menopause Food Plan

Dietary Supplements

COENZYME Q_{10}

Recommended dose: 10–300 mg/day. USANA's **CoQuinone 30** contains 30 mg coenzyme Q_{10} and 12.5 mg alpha-lipoic acid per capsule. The company also offers CoQ_{10} in 100 mg capsules, available only through a customized HealthPak. Note that USANA's CoQuinone is about three times the strength of other brands' CoQ_{10}, so you don't need as much. Available through USANA (888-950-9595 or 905-264-9863; www.usana.com). I also recommend Carotec's CocoQ10, which comes in 200 mg capsules (carotec.com).

OMEGA-3 FATS

Recommended dose: There is a wide individual dosage range, so start with 400 mg per day of DHA and EPA combined and work up to as high as 5,000 mg per day if needed. Made from algae, Neuromins is my first choice for taking this oil in supplement form (see below).

Neuromins, manufactured by Nature's Way, is available from Emerson Ecologics (800-654-4432 or 603-656-9778; www.emersonecologics.com).

life'sDHA (www.lifesdha.com) makes all-vegetarian DHA capsules that come in both 100 mg and 200 mg strengths. They are available on Amazon and other online sources.

BiOmega contains both DHA and EPA derived from cold-water fish. Available through USANA (888-950-9595 or 905-264-9863; www.usana.com).

Vital Choice Alaskan Sockeye Salmon Oil (800-608-4825; www.vitalchoice .com). Wild salmon is preferable to farmed fish because it's much healthier and safer. Vital Choice is a particularly good source of wild salmon and wild salmon oil (in 1,000 mg softgels that provide 600 mg of total omega-3 fatty acids, including 240 mg of EPA and 220 mg of DHA in a three-capsule serving).

Raw Chia Seed

Chia (*Salvia hispanica L.*) has a higher concentration of omega-3 fats (in the healthiest ratio to omega-6 fats, 3:1) than any other botanical source. It's also high in fiber, antioxidants, and phytonutrients. The omega-3 fats it contains are alpha-linolenic acid (ALA), which the body converts to DHA and EPA. One of the advantages of chia over flaxseed is that it doesn't have to be ground, and the antioxidants in it prevent it from going rancid. I recommend Mila brand, a proprietary blend of chia, from Lifemax (which is available from numerous distributors you can find on the internet). For additional information about chia from University of Arizona researcher and chia expert Wayne Coates, Ph.D., visit waynecoates.com/AZchiaInfo /chia-seed-information-azchia.

MULTIVITAMINS/MINERALS

My top pick in multivitamins is the **USANA HealthPak** or **USANA CellSentials,** manufactured by USANA Health Sciences, Inc. (888-950-9595 or 905-264-9863; www.usana.com). There are many, many other good brands available as well.

PROANTHOCYANIDINS

These powerful antioxidants are found in grape seeds and pine bark. Recommendations: start with 1 mg per pound of body weight per day, divided into three doses. After two weeks, cut back to 40–80 mg per day. I recommend Proflavanol C100, available from USANA (888-950-9595 or 905-264-9863; www.usana.com).

Many other excellent brands of OPCs are also available at pharmacies and natural food stores.

PROBIOTICS

Probiotic supplements provide gastrointestinal nutritional support by augmenting naturally occurring intestinal bacteria. The intestinal microecosystem typically carries up to 400 strains of bacteria. From the point of view of intestinal health, a product that provides bacteria for multiple probiotic "niches" makes sense. These flora may become depleted in a number of ways, including antibiotic therapy, poor diet, and disease. Probiotics are useful for individuals bothered by intestinal gas and bloating, and may also be used when taking an antibiotic to prevent yeast infection. Be sure to take a probiotic whenever you're on antibiotics, but take them at different times of the day, so the antibiotic won't kill off the new friendly bacteria. Continue to take the probiotic for a week or so after you've finished your course of antibiotics. That way you'll be much less likely to get a yeast infection or GI upset from the antibiotic.

I recommend the following:

PB 8 Probiotic. Manufactured by Nutrition Now, PB 8 does not contain sugar or fructooligosaccharides (FOS). It also does not require refrigeration to maintain its potency, as most probiotics do. Take as directed on the bottle. PB 8 is available at health food stores.

Flora ReVive. These probiotic capsules contain *Saccharomyces boulardi*, a type of yeast that keeps *Candida albicans* and gut bacteria in balance. It also contains humic-fulvic acid, which is derived from high-carbon humus found in ancient compacted plant material that is broken down by soil bacteria. Inulin, a prebiotic that stimulates the growth of beneficial bacteria, is also included. Available from www.rnareset.com.

VITAMIN C

Vitamin C is vital to many body systems and processes, especially immune health, skin health, and cardiovascular function. It is not produced in the body and must be supplemented. It is a master antioxidant that kills bacteria and viruses. Most people do best with 1,000–5,000 mg per day. Increase the dosage if you feel a cold coming on or if you have any infection.

Many different types of vitamin C are available, including plain ascorbic acid, liposomal vitamin C (which is fat soluble and well absorbed), and Ester-C (which is buffered). There is a wide variability in an individual's tolerance to vitamin C doses. Tissue saturation is reached when stools become loose, so start slowly and work up. I recommend the following:

Dr. Mercola Liposomal Vitamin C. Available from www.mercola.com.

Whole C ReSet. This product contains the entire vitamin C complex and is easy on the digestive system. Available from www.rnareset.com.

Pure ascorbic acid. This product by Pure Encapsulations comes in 1,000 mg capsules and is widely available online.

Digestive Aids

ENTERIC-COATED PEPPERMINT OIL

Most of the studies performed have utilized enteric-coated peppermint oil at a dosage of 0.2 ml twice daily between meals.

Pepogest, manufactured by Nature's Way, is available from Emerson Ecologics (800-654-4432 or 603-656-9778; www.emersonecologics.com).

Peppermint Soothe, manufactured by Nature's Way, was formerly sold as Peppermint Plus by Enzymatic Therapy (which was acquired by Nature's Way). Available from Emerson Ecologics (800-654-4432 or 603-656-9778; www.emersonecologics.com), as well as at many health food stores and online.

DEGLYCYRRHIZINATED LICORICE (*Glycyrrhiza glabra*) (DGL)

Please note that the cortisol-like activity of this herb may cause a problem in people prone to hypertension. If you are taking licorice root, your blood pressure should be monitored to ensure that it stays stable.

Gaia Herbs Licorice Root Alcohol-Free (also called **Licorice Root Glycerite**) is a tincture available from Emerson Ecologics (800-654-4432 or 603-656-9778; www.emersonecologics.com). **Wise Woman Herbals Licorice Solid Extract** is also available from Emerson Ecologics. Recommended dose for the solid extract is ¼ to ½ teaspoon, two to three times a day.

Licorice root capsules are manufactured by Nature's Way to provide 450 mg deglycyrrhizinated licorice with a guaranteed natural potency of not more than 6.5 percent glycyrrhizin. Recommended dose is one to two capsules three times daily with water at mealtimes. Available from Emerson Ecologics (800-654-4432 or 603-656-9778; www.emersonecologics.com).

ADDITIONAL DIGESTIVE SUPPORT

Seacure. Manufactured by Proper Nutrition, SeaCure is a concentrated fish protein that is gaining increasing recognition for its nutritional benefits in a wide range of disease conditions. Recommended for all digestive dysfunctions, e.g., Crohn's disease, irritable bowel syndrome, and ulcerative colitis. Also helpful after chemotherapy for nutritional support and immune system support. It is certified to be free of mercury and other heavy metals. Recommended dose is 3 capsules in the morning and 3 capsules in the afternoon. Available through Emerson Ecologics (800-654-4432 or 603-656-9778; www.emersonecologics.com).

Swedish Bitters. This tonic, which is excellent for stomach upset, is widely available in health food stores in liquid or capsule form. Swedish Bitters Elixir by Gaia Herbs is available from Emerson Ecologics (800-654-4432 or 603-656-9778; www.emersonecologics.com).

Digestive enzyme. This product from USANA (888-950-9595 or 905-264-9863; www.usana.com) encourages more complete digestion and absorption of nutrients. This particular formulation also contains spirulina, a nutrient-rich blue-green algae that supports the body's natural detoxification processes.

JOINT SUPPORT

Procosa. This product from USANA (888-950-9595 or 905-264-9863; www.usana.com) contains a higher amount of glucosamine HCI as well as curcumin, a compound that comes from turmeric (a natural form of COX-2 inhibitor)—a combination not found in any other joint health products.

Chapter 8: Creating Pelvic Health and Power

See Chapter 5 Resources for information on progesterone.

Pelvic Pain

(www.pelvicpainrelief.com)
Women's pelvic health physical therapist Isa Herrera has dedicated her life to helping women recover from pelvic and sexual pain—and also avoid it in the first place. She offers books, seminars, and online training aimed at educating women about the health of their pelvic floor and sexual organs.

Fibroids

EDUCATIONAL RESOURCES

Fibroid Network
(www.fibroid.network)
The mission of the United Kingdom–based Fibroid Network is to promote education, information, support services, and research on fibroids. They maintain an international database of current research on fibroids and recommended doctors, hospitals, and natural health practitioners providing treatment for fibroids.

Fibroid Treatment Collective
(866-479-1523; www.fibroids.com)
A medical group of fibroid experts dedicated to curing fibroids with minimally invasive therapy, the Fibroid Treatment Collective in Los Angeles performed the very first uterine fibroid embolization in the United States. The organization's website has a wealth of information about fibroids and their treatment.

Cleveland Clinic's Center for Menstrual Disorders, Fibroids, and Hysteroscopic Services
(800-223-2273, ext. 46601, or 216-444-6601; http://my.clevelandclinic.org/departments/obgyn-womens-health/depts/menstrual-disorders)
This arm of the famed Cleveland Clinic was designed to give women minimally invasive options to treat menstrual aberrations and alternatives to hysterectomy. The center also gives patients access to groundbreaking clinical trials, clinical research opportunities, and education programs.

Johns Hopkins Fibroid Center
(443-997-0400; www.hopkinsmedicine.org/gynecology_obstetrics/specialty_areas/gynecological_services/treatments_services/fibroid_treatment.html)
This fibroid treatment center specializes in state-of-the-art therapies and the rapid application of new research (such as magnetic resonance imaging and guided high-intensity ultrasound), with an emphasis on minimally invasive techniques.

Center for Fibroid Biology and Therapy at Duke University Medical Center
(919-634-6654; www.dukehealth.org/treatments/obstetrics-and-gynecology/fibroids)
Duke's cutting-edge fibroid center explores all nonsurgical and medical treatment options. Treatments offered include minimally invasive surgical options, drug therapies, and noninvasive MRI-guided focused ultrasound treatment.

Menstrual Pain

Bupleurum (Xiao Yao Wan, also known as Hsiao Yao Wan). Xiao Yao Wan Plus is a Chinese nutritional supplement that helps women with PMS, menstrual cramps, and perimenopausal symptoms. It is widely available, but it's always best to consult with a trained practitioner of Traditional Chinese Medicine.

Menastil. Menastil's active ingredient is calendula oil. The U.S. Food and Drug Administration and the Homeopathic Pharmacopoeia U.S. recognize this pure grade of calendula oil for the temporary relief of menstrual pain, as a nonprescription, over-the-counter, topically applied homeopathic product. Available from Claire Ellen Products (508-366-6411; www.bestpainrelief .com).

CASTOR OIL PACKS ·

A castor oil pack consists of castor oil and wool flannel. Directions: Saturate a piece of flannel with castor oil and apply directly to area to be treated. On the side opposite the skin, lay a sheet of plastic, then apply a hot-water bottle. Use for thirty to sixty minutes five times weekly, or as directed by a practitioner. Area can be wiped clean with a dilute solution of warm water and baking soda.

Cold-pressed castor oil and wool flannel, as well as disposable castor oil packs, by Baar Products, are available from Emerson Ecologics (800-654-4432 or 603-656-9778; www.emersonecologics.com).

Heavy Bleeding/Iron Deficiency

Iron drops. Manufactured by Evolving Nutrition, La Santé Iron Drops is a nonconstipating, impressively bioavailable form of iron. Recommended dose: 1 ml daily with meals. Available from Emerson Ecologics (800-654-4432 or 603-656-9778; www.emersonecologics.com).

Yunnan Bai Yao. This herbal combination is superb for stopping bleeding without causing clotting or disrupting circulation. Available wherever Chinese herbs are sold.
See Chapter 5 Resources for information on formulary pharmacies.

Prepare for Surgery

Note: Avoid taking vitamin E for two weeks preoperatively and one week postoperatively. It may enhance bleeding.

Successful Surgery. Guided-imagery audio program by Belleruth Naparstek. Available from Health Journeys (800-800-8661 or 216-675-0496; www .healthjourneys.com).
The MP3s developed by Belleruth were designed to help the listener imagine a successful surgery experience, surrounded by protection and support, with the body cooperating fully by slowing down blood flow and speeding up its mending capacity. One recording has affirmations, while the other has continuous music to be taken into the operating room (the same music that underscores the imagery). Belleruth's work on imagery has been

studied successfully at the Cleveland Clinic, Kaiser Permanente, and University of California at Davis Medical Center.

Prepare for Surgery, Heal Faster. Book and MP3 recording by Peggy Huddleston (800-726-4173 or 781-864-2668; www.healfaster.com). I found Peggy Huddleston's book very beneficial in my own recovery from surgery. Her work has helped thousands of others as well.

Urological Problems

Estriol vaginal cream is available by prescription from any formulary pharmacy that carries bioidentical hormones. If your doctor isn't familiar with one of these, have her or him call a formulary pharmacy where the pharmacists specialize in individualized hormone replacement. Usual strength is 0.5 mg/g.

Probiotics. To treat recurrent vaginal yeast infections, I recommend Jarrow Formulas' **Fem-Dophilus** (see www.jarrow.com) and **RepHresh Pro-B** (see www.rephresh.com), which contain the two probiotic strains (*Lactobacillus rhamnosus* GR-1 and *Lactobacillus reuteri* RC-14—formerly known as *Lactobacillus fermentum* RC-14) shown in numerous studies to be helpful in both preventing and treating bacterial vaginosis and also yeast infections. (See Chapter 7 Resources for more information.)

URINARY INCONTINENCE
The book *The Bathroom Key: Put an End to Incontinence* (Demos Health, 2012) by physical therapist Kathryn Kassai and Kim Perelli contains a wide range of practical and effective approaches to treating incontinence.

Biomechanics expert Katy Bowman (www.nutritiousmovement.com) also has a wide range of resources that can help incontinence and a variety of other issues.

PELVIC FLOOR REHAB AND TRAINING
Perifit. Perifit (www.perifit.co) is a unique type of Kegel exerciser that comes with an app for your smartphone. It allows you to strengthen your pelvic muscles and track your progress the same as using a Fitbit.

Yoni egg practice. Crystal yoni egg practice is an ancient technique for vaginal and sexual fitness. I highly recommend the work of Kim Anami (www.kimanami.com) on this practice. Two good sources for yoni eggs to use in your practice are **Keggel** (https://keggel.org) and **Jade Eggs Global** (http://jadeeggsglobal.com).

Chapter 9: Sex and Menopause

See Chapter 4 Resources for information on hormone testing laboratories.

The School of Womanly Arts Global Online Community
(www.mamagenas.com)

Regena Thomashauer (a.k.a. Mama Gena) is an expert at teaching women how to deliberately cultivate pleasure as a pathway toward health and fulfillment. I highly recommend her books (*Mama Gena's School of Womanly Arts* [Simon & Schuster, 2002], *Mama Gena's Owner's and Operator's Guide to Men* [Simon & Schuster, 2003], and *Pussy: A Reclamation* [Hay House, 2016]) as well as her website (www.mamagenas.com) and her online workshops.

Chapter 10: Nurturing Your Brain

See Chapter 3 Resources for information on feng shui and Chapter 6 Resources for information on herbs.

Insomnia

To help eliminate electrical pollution (or electropollution), a major cause of insomnia, keep your cellphone turned off as much as possible, and before you go to bed, unplug TVs and other electrical appliances—even lamps! There is an increasing amount of information now available about this. I suggest you read *The Earth Prescription: Discover the Healing Power of Nature with Grounding Practices for Every Season* (Reveal Press, 2020) by Laura Koniver, M.D., as well as *Earthing: The Most Important Health Discovery Ever!* by Clinton Ober, Stephen T. Sinatra, M.D., and Martin Zucker (Basic Health Publications, 2010). And *The Non-Tinfoil Guide to EMFs: How to Fix Our Stupid Use of Technology* (N&G Media, 2019) by Nicolas Pineault.

Melatonin regulates sleep/wake cycles, and supplements can help the body adjust to different time zones. It also helps with the function of the pineal gland. Usual dosage: 0.5–3 mg. Melatonin is available from many online sources.

Valerian (*Valeriana officinalis*) root is available in tinctures, liquids, and capsules. Recommended dosage is 150–300 mg (standardized to 0.8 percent valerenic acid) at bedtime. I recommend the valerian products made by Avena Botanicals (www.avenabotanicals.com).

Passionflower (*Passiflora incarnata*) has a calming influence that makes it helpful for both insomnia and anxiety. I recommend the passionflower products made by Avena Botanicals (www.avenabotanicals.com).

Amantilla and Babuna are natural medicines that originate from the valerian plant (*Valeriana officinalis*) and the flower of the manzanilla plant (*Matricaria recutita*, commonly known as chamomile), respectively. Both are available as tinctures made by NutriMedix, which is available through Natural Healthy Concepts (www.nhc.com).

Pueraria mirifica has helped many women who report sleep improvement when they start this herb. Available through Amata Life (www.amatalife.com).

Seasonal Affective Disorder/Light Therapy

Women with SAD are often helped by light therapy. Full-spectrum lighting can also help PMS, perimenopausal symptoms, and ovulatory and other menstrual cycle disturbances. It can also increase serotonin levels.

Sunshine Sciences
(800-468-1104 or 303-834-9161; www.sunshinesciences.com)
Sunshine Sciences manufactures high-quality full-spectrum lighting in the form of energy-saving compact fluorescent lights, fluorescent tubes, and UL-approved light boxes for SAD (seasonal affective disorder). The company's Indoor Sunshine lights are made with the highest-quality blend of rare-earth phosphors to produce light with the beneficial red, orange, yellow, green, blue, and violet wavelengths and balanced amounts of the essential ultraviolet A and B wavelengths. The result is a true white light like natural sunshine. Preliminary studies show that Indoor Sunshine lights boost immune system function and vitamin D. Full-spectrum light is also known to raise serotonin levels.

Supplements for Brain Support

5-HTP is a precursor to serotonin, a neurohormone needed for melatonin production, appetite regulation, and mood regulation. 5-HTP is a natural product extracted from the seeds of *Griffonia simplicifolia*, unlike tryptophan supplements, which are produced synthetically or through bacterial fermentation. Recommended dose is 100–200 mg three times per day. Nature's Way enteric-coated 5-HTP is available from Emerson Ecologics (800-654-4432 or 603-656-9778; www.emersonecologics.com). 5-HTP is also available from Solgar (877-765-4274 or 201-944-2311; www.solgar.com).

DHA (docosahexaenoic acid). See Chapter 7 Resources for more information.

Ginkgo biloba is widely used to enhance memory and concentration, as well as to treat peripheral artery narrowing. I recommend **Ginkgo-PS** from

USANA (888-950-9595 or 905-264-9863; www.usana.com) and **Nature's Way Ginkgold,** available through natural food stores or Emerson Ecologics (800-654-4432 or 603-656-9778; www.emersonecologics.com). Recommended dosage is 40 mg three times per day.

St. John's wort (0.3 percent hypericin). More than twenty double-blind clinical studies have shown that St. John's wort is as effective as standard antidepressants at relieving symptoms of depression, but is much better tolerated and has fewer side effects. The herb's active ingredients are hypericin and hyperforin, which increase levels of brain neurotransmitters that maintain normal mood and emotional stability. **Hi Potency St. John's Wort** by Verified Quality is standardized to 0.3 percent hypericin and 3 percent hyperforin. Available from Emerson Ecologics (800-654-4432 or 603-656-9778; www.emersonecologics.com), and in health food stores. Take 300 mg three times per day, or as directed.

Inositol. Many studies indicate a therapeutic dose of 12 g per day. It's best to take it with food. I recommend **inositol powder** manufactured by Verified Quality, a mildly sweet substance that dissolves instantly in water. Available from Emerson Ecologics (800-654-4432 or 603-656-9778; www.emerson ecologics.com).

Pregnenolone is a precursor to DHEA and also to progesterone. Recommended starting dose is 10–50 mg per day, but it has been safely used in doses as high as 100–200 mg per day. Start low and gradually increase if needed. Douglas Laboratories' pregnenolone (sublingual 25 mg tablets) is available from Emerson Ecologics (800-654-4432 or 603-656-9778; www.emersonecologics.com).

Proanthocyanidins. See Chapter 7 Resources for more information.

SAM-e (S-adenosyl-L-methionine) is indicated for mood and emotional well-being, as well as joint health, mobility, and comfort. It also boosts antioxidant activity and supports immune function. The best dose for most people and conditions is 800–1,600 mg per day. Proper dosage is essential for optimal results. SAM-e by Nutricology is available from Emerson Ecologics (800-654-4432 or 603-656-9778; www.emersonecologics.com). Also widely available at natural food stores and in pharmacies.

Mercury-Free Fish Oil Supplements

BiOmega contains both DHA and EPA derived from cold-water fish. Available through USANA (888-950-9595 or 905-264-9863; www.usana.com).

Coromega Omega-3 Squeeze fish oil (877-275-3725; www.coromega.com) is available in flavored single-serving squeeze packs that even children will love.

Vital Choice Alaskan Sockeye Salmon Oil (800-608-4825; www.vitalchoice .com). Wild salmon is preferable to farmed fish because it's much healthier and safer. Vital Choice is a particularly good source of wild salmon and wild salmon oil (in 1,000 mg softgels that provide 600 mg of total omega-3 fatty acids, including 460 mg of EPA and DHA in a three-capsule serving).

Chapter 11: From Rosebud to Rose Hip

Internal Hair and Skin Care

Good skin starts within. So be sure you're on a good multivitamin at the very least. There are many on the market. I recommend the **USANA HealthPak** or **USANA CellSentails** (www.usana.com). Another excellent supplement is the herb *Pueraria mirifica,* which halts the loss of collagen and has a lovely effect when applied to the skin; available from Amata Life (www.amatalife.com).

Surgery

See Chapter 8 Resources for information on preparing for surgery.

Chapter 12: Standing Tall for Life

Urine Bone Density Testing

Bone Resorption Assessment from Genova Diagnostics (800-522-4762 or 828-253-0621; www.gdx.net) determines the rate at which you are excreting bone breakdown products and, hence, losing bone (available with a doctor's prescription).

Osteomark is marketed directly to doctors and is available through their offices.

Supplements for Bone Health

CALCIUM/MAGNESIUM SUPPLEMENTS

The best magnesium and calcium supplements on the market have been formulated by Carolyn Dean, M.D., N.D. (www.rnareset.com). She makes both ReMag and ReMyte, which are used together, and she also offers a very effective magnesium lotion that is quickly absorbed into the skin.

HERBAL INFUSIONS

Avena Botanicals
(866-282-8362 or 207-594-0694; www.avenabotanicals.com)
For a variety of herbal products, including dried organic herbs, liquid extracts, oils, creams, and teas.

VITAMIN D WITH VITAMIN K$_2$

Vitamin D supplementation, along with taking enough vitamin K$_2$, is crucial for those who spend little time outdoors, those with darker skin, and those who live in northern latitudes.

Vitamin D from USANA (888-950-9595 or 905-264-9863; www.usana.com) contains 2,000 IU of vitamin D$_3$ per tablet, as well as 30 mg of vitamin K$_2$, which is also good for bone health. Another good option is vitamin D$_3$ in Omega-3 Therapy + Vitamin D$_3$ softgels from Vital Choice (800-608-4825; www.vitalchoice.com), which contain 2,000 IU of vitamin D per softgel. Quality vitamin K$_2$ is available from Mercola (www.mercola.com).

Cod liver oil contains vitamins A and D, EPA (eicosaspentaenoic acid), and DHA (docosahexaenoic acid). Its cardiovascular benefits include lowering blood pressure, decreasing triglycerides, and reducing angina.

Genestra Cod Liver Oil DHA/EPA Forte softgels provide 720 IU vitamin A, 500 IU vitamin D, 102 mg EPA, and 126 mg DHA per gelcap. Order on Amazon through iServe, Genestra's recommended distributor.

My Med Lab (for checking levels of vitamin D). See Chapter 4 Resources.

ADDITIONAL MUSCULOSKELETAL SUPPORT

Procosa. This product from USANA (888-950-9595 or 905-264-9863; www.usana.com) contains 1,500 mg glucosamine HCI and 260 mg curcumin (turmeric extract) per tablet, as well as vitamin C, magnesium, manganese, and potassium. Usual dose: 3 tablets daily, preferably with food.

OsteoKing is a 100 percent natural formula derived from Traditional Chinese Medicine that is designed to optimize bone health. It comes in liquid form and includes a combination of six herbs. Available from Yunnan Crystal Natural Pharmaceutical Co. (www.osteoking.com).

Proanthocyanidins. See Chapter 7 Resources for more information.

Strength Training

Strong Women series

Strong Women is a series of books and programs by Miriam Nelson, Ph.D. (www.strongwomen.com).

Katy Bowman's Nutritious Movement

(www.nutritiousmovement.com)

The work of Katy Bowman is unparalleled when it comes to lifelong fitness. I recommend her book *Dynamic Aging: Simple Exercises for Whole-*

Body Mobility (Propriometrics Press, 2017). She helps women engage balance and muscular patterns that have lain dormant for years. Katy also has a podcast and good social media content.

Pilates

Pilates has been, hands down, the most effective exercise program I have ever done. I credit Pilates with the mobility, strength, and flexibility that I enjoy daily. I have done two Pilates sessions per week for twenty-plus years. There is nothing that compares to the authentic method developed by Joe Pilates. My teacher is Hope Matthews (www.thecenterforimh.com), who has also incorporated a unique system for working with the emotions and the fascia. For more information on finding a certified instructor or a training program in your area, or on obtaining Pilates method materials, visit the Pilates website at www.pilates-studio.com.

Esther Gokhale's Primal Posture

(www.thegokhalemethod.com)

Esther Gokhale has studied cultures from all over the world and found that those who don't have "modern" lifestyles do not have back pain or the other ailments that are so common to our industrialized societies. Her work on posture improvement is life changing and very often completely eliminates back pain. Her book *8 Steps to a Pain-Free Back* (Pendo Press, 2008), co-authored with Susan Adams, is very helpful. Those trained in her system work all over the world.

Chapter 13: Creating Breast Health

See Chapter 8 Resources for more information on where to obtain supplies for castor oil packs.

Mammograms Versus Thermograms

Mammogram Scam: A Breast Exposé

This award-winning documentary is a very well-researched and accuate assessment of thermography versus mammography as a breast screening modality. All women should have access to this information. Among the doctors and other experts interviewed are Joseph Mercola, D.O.; the late Ben Johnson, M.D., D.O., N.M.D.; David Marquis, D.O.; Veronique Desaulniers, D.C.; Carolyn Dean, M.D., N.D.; Julie Taguchi, M.D.; Judith Steinberg Dean, M.D.; Duncan Turner, M.D.; Christine Horner, M.D.; Philip Getson, D.O.; G. Edward Griffin; Jonathan Emord, Esq.; and Gaea Powell. You can view the hour-long film for free on YouTube at https://youtu.be/NKl-PXnZlFo.

Breast Cancer Information and Treatment

Voell, J., and Chatfield, C. (2005). *The Cancer Report: The Latest Research (How Thousands Are Achieving Permanent Recoveries)*. Naples, FL: Change Your World Press.

Information on breast cancer—including a holistic approach—has skyrocketed since the last edition of this book. Simply search online.

Cancer Treatment Centers of America

(855-993-4029; www.cancercenter.com)

Cancer Treatment Centers of America (CTCA) is a national network of hospitals that offers advanced cancer patients a comprehensive, fully integrative approach to their disease that combines conventional clinical treatments and technologies with scientifically supported complementary therapies. CTCA facilities are located in Chicago, Philadelphia, Tulsa, Phoenix, and Atlanta, and they serve patients from all over the United States. Each patient is assigned a core "empowerment team" that includes a medical oncologist, a naturopathic oncology provider, a registered dietitian, a nurse care manager, and a clinic nurse (among others) who work together to provide coordinated care throughout a patient's treatment. CTCA's goal is to present patients with clear and thorough information about their condition to empower them to make educated decisions about their care and treatment, leading to improved results and a greater quality of life.

Sanoviv Medical Institute

(800-726-6848; www.sanoviv.com)

Sanoviv is a fully accredited hospital and health center in Rosarita, Mexico (on the Baja California peninsula). This facility offers a beautiful setting with pure water, all organic food, a spa, and world-class functional medicine doctors. I have been to Sanoviv a number of times for their health assessment and detox programs. I highly recommend this place for anyone who wants to improve her health or be treated for a disease such as cancer, heart disease, or other conditions.

Lymphedema

National Lymphedema Network

(800-541-3259; www.lymphnet.org)

An internationally recognized, nonprofit information and networking organization to help those with lymphedema, either primary (the kind one is born with) or secondary (the kind one gets after an operation or injury, notably mastectomy and lymph node dissection). They provide referrals and educational courses for healthcare professionals and patients, publish a very helpful quarterly newsletter, host a biennial national conference on lymph-edema, and maintain an extensive computer database.

Supplements for Breast Health

Coenzyme Q$_{10}$. See Chapter 7 Resources for more information.

Flaxseed/chia seed. See Chapter 6 Resources for more information.

Chapter 14: Living with Heart, Passion, and Joy

SUGGESTED READING

Buckberg, G. D. (2018). *Solving the Mysteries of Heart Disease: Life-Saving Answers Ignored by the Medical Establishment.* Los Angeles: Health House Press.

Menolascino, M. (2019). *Heart Solution for Women: A Proven Program to Prevent and Reverse Heart Disease.* New York: HarperOne.

Depression

See Chapter 10 Resources for more information.

Forgiveness

See Chapter 2 Resources for more information.

Supplements for Heart Health

Many of the sources for dietary supplements recommended for heart health are detailed in Chapter 7 Resources.

Cod liver oil. See Chapter 12 Resources for more information.

Vitamin D. See Chapter 12 Resources for more information.

Vitamin K$_2$. See chapter 12 Resources for more information.

Magnesium. See Chapter 12 Resources for more information on calcium/magnesium supplements.

Hawthorn (*Crataegus oxyacantha*). Widely available in health food stores as berries for tea infusions. Also available in pill form. If you prefer to take this in pill form, look for a standardized extract, a product that contains

10 percent proanthocyanidins or 1.8 percent vitexin-4"-rhamnoside. Take 100–250 mg three times per day. **HeartCare,** manufactured by Nature's Way, is available from Emerson Ecologics (800-654-4432 or 603-656-9778; www.emersonecologics.com).

Proanthocyanidins. See Chapter 7 Resources for more information.

Vitamin C. See Chapter 7 Resources for more information.

Notes

Introduction: The Journey Begins

1. Introduction
   American Congress of Obstetricians and Gynecologists, *2011 Women's Health Statistics,* p. 33; available at www.acog.org/-/media/NewsRoom /MediaKit.pdf.

Chapter 1: Menopause Puts Your Life Under a Microscope

1. DeWolf, M. (March 1, 2017). 12 stats about working women. U.S. Department of Labor Blog, https://blog.dol.gov/2017/03/01/12-stats-about -working-women.
2. Bianchi, S. M., Sayer, L. C., Milkie, M. A., & Robinson, J. P. (2012). Housework: who did, does or will do it, and how much does it matter? *Social Forces, 91* (1), 55–63.
3. DeSilver, D. (April 30, 2018). Women scarce at top of U.S. business—and in the jobs that lead there. Pew Research Center (April 30, 2018); https:// www.pewresearch.org/fact-tank/2018/04/30/women-scarce-at-top-of-u-s -business-and-in-the-jobs-that-lead-there.
4. Zillman, C. (June 14, 2018). With first woman CFO Dhivya Suryadevara, GM enters rare Fortune 500 territory. *Fortune,* https://fortune.com/2018 /06/14/dhivya-suryadevara-gm-cfo.

5. Zarya, V. (May 21, 2018). The share of female CEOs in the Fortune 500 dropped by 25% in 2018. *Fortune,* https://fortune.com/2018/05/21 /women-fortune-500-2018.

6. Women's Media Center (2015). *The Status of Women in the U.S. Media 2015;* http://www.womensmediacenter.com/bsdimg/statusreport/2015/Status .of.Women.2015.pdf.

7. Trent, T. (2017). *The Awakened Woman: Remembering and Reigniting Our Sacred Dreams,* 66. New York: Atria/Enliven.

8. Sams, J., & Carson, D. (1988). *Medicine Cards,* 150. Santa Fe: Bear & Co.

Chapter 2: The Brain Catches Fire at Menopause

1. Seymour, L. J. (ed.) (Apr. 1999). News from Redbook. *Redbook,* 16.

2. Oren, D. A., et al. (2002). An open trial of morning light therapy for treatment of antepartum depression. *Am J Psychiatry, 159* (4), 666–669.

3. Van Middendorp, H., et al. (2010). The effects of anger and sadness on clinical pain reports and experimentally-induced pain thresholds in women with and without fibromyalgia. *Arthritis Care Res, 62,* 1370–1376.

4. Larsson, C., & Hallman, J. (1997). Is severity of premenstrual symptoms related to illness in the climacteric? *J Psychosom Obstet Gynecol, 18,* 234–243; Novaes, C., & Almeida, O. P. (1999). Premenstrual syndrome and psychiatric morbidity at the menopause. *J Psychosom Obstet Gynecol, 20,* 56–57; Arpels, J. C. (1996). The female brain hypoestrogenic continuum from PMS to menopause: A hypothesis and review of supporting data. *J Reprod Med, 41* (9), 633–639.

5. Schmidt, P., et al. (1998). Differential behavioral effects of gonadal steroids in women with and in those without premenstrual syndrome. *N Engl J Med, 338* (4), 209–216.

6. Larsson, C., & Hallman, J. (1997). Is severity of premenstrual symptoms related to illness in the climacteric? *J Psychosom Obstet Gynecol, 18,* 234–243; Novaes, C., & Almeida, O. P. (1999). Premenstrual syndrome and psychiatric morbidity at the menopause. *J Psychosom Obstet Gynecol, 20,* 56–57.

7. Benedek, T., & Rubenstein, B. (1939). Correlations between ovarian activity and psychodynamic processes: The ovulatory phase. *Psychosom Med, 1* (2), 245–270.

8. Weitoft, G. R., et al. (2000). Mortality among lone mothers in Sweden: A population study. *Lancet, 355,* 1215–1219.

9. Taylor, S. E., et al. (2002). Biobehavioral responses to stress in females: Tend-and-befriend, not fight-or-flight. *Psychol Rev, 109* (4), 745–750.

10. Trent, T. (2017). *The Awakened Woman: A Guide for Remembering & Igniting Your Sacred Dreams,* 4. New York: Simon & Schuster.

11. Herzog, A. (1997). Neuroendocrinology of epilepsy. In S. C. Schacter & O. Devinsky (eds.), *Behavioral Neurology and the Legacy of Norman Geschwind,* 235–236. Philadelphia: Lippincott, Williams & Wilkins; Moyer, K. E. (1976). *The Psychology of Aggression.* New York: Harper &

Row; Albert, I., et al. (1987). Inter-male social aggression in rats: Suppression by medical hypothalamic lesions independently of enhanced defensiveness of decreased testicular testosterone. *Physiol Behav, 39*, 693–698; Post, R. M. (1992). Transduction of psychosocial stress into the neurobiology of recurrent affective disorder. *Am J Psychiatry, 149*, 999–1010.

12. Linehan, M. (1993). *Skills Training Manual for Treating Borderline Personality Disorder*, p. 143. New York: Guilford Press.

13. Herzog, A. G. (1989). Perimenopausal depression: Possible role of anomalous brain substrates. *Brain Dysfunction, 2*, 146–154.

14. Ledoux, J. E. (1986). Sensory systems and emotions: A model of affective processing. *Integrative Psychiatry, 4*, 237–243.

15. Musante, L., et al. (1989). Potential for hostility and dimensions of anger. *Health Psychology, 8*, 343; Mittleman, M. A., et al. (1995). Triggering of acute MI onset of episodes of anger. *Circulation, 92*, 1720–1725. For an exhaustive listing of the scientific studies documenting the emotional risk factors for heart attack, see Schulz, M. L., (1998). Awakening Intuition, chapter 9, 216–250. New York: Harmony.

16. Porges, S., et al. (1996). Infant regulation of the vagal "brake" predicts child behavior problems: A psychobiological model of social behavior. *Dev Psychobiol, 29* (8), 697–712; Porges, S. (1992). Vagal tone: A physiological marker of stress vulnerability. *Pediatrics, 90*, 498–504; Donchin, Y., et al. (1992). Cardiac vagal tone predicts outcome in neurosurgical patients. *Crit Care Med, 20*, 941–949.

17. Heim, C., et al. (2000). Pituitary-adrenal and autonomic responses to stress in women after sexual and physical abuse in childhood. *JAMA, 284* (5), 592–596.

18. Lipton, B. (2005). *The Biology of Belief*. Santa Rosa, CA: Elite Books.

19. Langer, E. (2009). *Counterclockwise: Mindful Health and the Power of Possibility*, 14–117. New York: Ballantine Books.

20. Schulz, M. L., M.D., Ph.D., behavioral neuroscientist and neuropsychiatrist (Mar. 20, 2000). Personal communication.

21. Van der Kolk, B. A. (1996). The body keeps the score: Approaches to the psychobiology of posttraumatic stress disorder. In B. A. van der Kolk, A. C. McFarlane, & L. Weisaeth (eds.), *Traumatic Stress: The Effects of Overwhelming Experience on Mind, Body, and Society*, 214–241. New York: Guilford Press.

22. Clow, B. H. (1996). *The Liquid Light of Sex: Kundalini Rising at Mid-Life Crisis*. Berkeley, CA: Bear & Co. This book comes complete with charts that allow readers to determine exactly when their key life passages will or have happened, thus allowing one to take full advantage of what might otherwise be considered a crisis without meaning.

Chapter 3: Coming Home to Yourself

1. I originally learned to do this through a process called proprioceptive writing, taught by Linda Metcalf and Tobin Simon. (See Resources.)

2. Brody, E. M. (1989). *Family at Risk in Alzheimer's Disease,* 2–49. DHHS Publication no. 89-1569. Bethesda, MD: National Institute of Mental Health.
3. Richardson, C. (2009). *The Art of Extreme Self-Care,* xii. Carlsbad, CA: Hay House.
4. Current Population Survey, 2019 Annual Social and Economic Supplement. Washington, DC: U.S. Census Bureau, 2019.
5. Bertrand, M., Kamenica, E., & Pan, J. (2015). Gender identity and relative income within households. *Quarterly J Econ, 130* (2), 571–614.
6. Joy, L., Carter, N. M., Wagner, H. M., & Narayanan, S. (2007). The bottom line: Corporate performance and women's representation on boards. Catalyst; https://www.catalyst.org/wp-content/uploads/2019/01/The_Bottom _Line_Corporate_Performance_and_Womens_Representation_on _Boards.pdf.
7. Kristof, N., & WuDunn, S. (2009). *Half the Sky: Turning Oppression into Opportunity for Women Worldwide.* New York: Alfred A. Knopf.

Chapter 4: This Can't Be Menopause, Can It?

1. Randolph, J., & Sowers, M. F. (1999). Research on perimenopausal changes in 500 Michigan women, reported in *Midlife Women's Health Sourcebook.* Atlanta, GA: American Health Consultants.
2. McKinlay, S. M., et al. (1992). The normal menopause transition. *Maturitas, 14,* 103; Treloar, A. E., et al. (1981). Menstrual cyclicity and the perimenopause. *Maturitas, 3,* 249.
3. Hamilton, B. et al. (2019). Births: Provisional data for 2018. U.S. Department of Health and Human Services, Centers for Disease Control and Prevention, National Center for Health Statistics. Report No. 007, p. 3.
4. Munster, K., et al. (1992). Length and variation in the menstrual cycle— a cross-sectional study from a Danish county. *Br J Obstet Gynecol, 99* (5), 422; Collett, M. E., et al. (1954). The effect of age upon the pattern of the menstrual cycle. *Fertil Steril, 5,* 437.
5. Rannevik, G. (1995). A longitudinal study of the perimenopausal transition: Altered profiles of steroid and pituitary hormones, SHBG and bone mineral density. *Maturitas, 21,* 103.
6. Coulam, C. B., Adamson, S. C., & Annegers, J. F. (1986). Incidence of premature ovarian failure. *Am J Obstet Gynecol, 67* (4), 604–606; Miyake, T., et al. (1988). Acute oocyte loss in experimental autoimmune oophoritis as a possible model of premature ovarian failure. *Am J Obstet Gynecol, 158* (1), 186–192; Coulam, C. B. (1982). Premature gonadal failure. *Fertil Steril, 38,* 645; Gloor, H. J. (1984). Autoimmune oophoritis. *Am J Clin Pathol, 81,* 105–109; Leer, M., Patel, B., Innes, M., et al. (1980). Secondary amenorrhea due to autoimmune ovarian failure. *Aust N Z J Obstet Gynecol, 20,* 177–179; International Medical News Service (Nov.

1985). Evidence of autoimmune etiology in some premature menopause. *OB-GYN News, 20* (21), 1, 30.

7. Sumiala, S., et al. (1996). Salivary progesterone concentrations after tubal sterilization. *Obstet Gynecol, 88,* 792–796.

8. Aksel, S., et al. (1976). Vasomotor symptoms, serum estrogens and gonadotropin levels in surgical menopause. *Am J Obstet Gynecol, 126,* 165–169; Judd, H. L., & Meldrum, D. R. (1981). Physiology and pathophysiology of menstruation and menopause. In S. L. Romney, M. J. Gray, A. B. Little, et al. (eds.), *Gynecology and Obstetrics: The Health Care of Women* (2nd ed.), 885–907. New York: McGraw-Hill.

9. Saliva as a diagnostic fluid (1993). *Ann N Y Acad Sci, 694,* 1–348; Lawrence, H. P. (2002). Salivary markers of systemic disease: Noninvasive diagnosis of disease and monitoring of general health. *J Can Dent Assoc, 68* (3), 170–174; Vining, R. F., & McGinley, R. A. (1987). The measurement of hormones in saliva: Possibilities and pitfalls. *J Steroid Biochem, 27* (1–3), 81–94; Boothby, L. A., Doering, P. L., & Kipersztok, S. (2004). Bioidentical hormone therapy: A review. *Menopause, 11* (3), 356–367; Rakel, D. (ed.) (2003). *Integrative Medicine.* Philadelphia: Saunders.

10. Tai, P. L. (2008). Serum vs. saliva testing: Which one is more accurate for measuring hormones in the body? *Healthy Aging, 4* (2), 67.

11. Khan-Dawood, F. S., Choe, J. K., & Dawood, M. Y. (1984). Salivary and plasma bound and "free" testosterone in men and women. *Am J Obstet Gynecol, 148* (4), 441–445.

12. Massoudi, M. S., et al. (1995). Prevalence of thyroid antibodies among healthy middle-aged women. Findings from the thyroid study in healthy women. *Ann Epidemiol, 5* (3), 229–233.

13. AACE medical guidelines for clinical practice for the evaluation and treatment of hyperthyroidism and hypothyroidism. (2002). *Endocrine Practice, 8* (6).

14. Friedman, M., Miranda-Massari, J. R., & Gonzalez, M. J. (2006). Supraphysiological cyclic dosing of sustained release T3 in order to reset low basal body temperature. *P R Health Sci J, 1,* 23–29.

15. Caldwell, K. L., Jones, R., & Hollowell, J. G. (2005). Urinary iodine concentration: United States National Health and Nutrition Examination Survey 2001–2002. *Thyroid, 15,* 692–699; Hollowell, J. G., et al. (1998). Iodine excretion data from NHANES I and NHANES III. *J Clin Endocrinol Metab, 88,* 3401–3410.

16. Jefferies, W. McK. (1996). *The Safe Uses of Cortisone.* Springfield, IL: Charles C. Thomas.

17. Guthrie, J., et al. (1996). Hot flushes, menstrual status, and hormone levels in a population-based sample of midlife women. *Obstet Gynecol, 88,* 437–442.

18. Gold, E. B., Sternfeld, B., Kelsey, J. L., et al. (2000). Relation of demographic and lifestyle factors to symptoms in a multi-racial/ethnic population of women 40–55 years of age. *Am J Epidemiol, 152,* 463–473; Whiteman, M. K., Staropoli, C. A., Lengenberg, P. W., McCarter, R. J.,

Kjerulff, K. H., & Flaws, J. H. (2003). Smoking, body mass, and hot flashes in midlife women. *Obstet Gynecol, 101,* 264–272.

19. Leonetti, H., et al. (1999). Transdermal progesterone cream for vasomotor symptoms and postmenopausal bone loss. *Obstet Gynecol, 94,* 227–228.

20. Stearns, V., Beebe, K. L., Iyengar, M., & Dube, E. (2003). Paroxetine controlled release in the treatment of menopausal hot flashes: A randomized controlled trial. *JAMA, 289,* 2827–2834; Loprinzi, C. L., Sloan, J. A., Perez, E. A., et al. (2002). Phase III evaluation of fluoxetine for treatment of hot flashes. *J Clin Oncol, 20,* 1578–1583; Loprinzi, C. L., Kugler, J. W., Sloan, J. A., et al. (2000). Venlafaxine in management of hot flashes in survivors of breast cancer: A randomized controlled trial. *Lancet, 356,* 2059–2063.

21. Goldberg, R. M., Loprinzi, C. L., O'Fallon, J. R., et al. (1994). Transdermal clonidine for ameliorating tamoxifen-induced hot flashes. *J Clin Oncol, 12,* 155–158.

22. Irvin, J. H., Domar, A. D., Clark, C., Zuttermeister, P. C., & Friedman, R. (1996). The effects of relaxation response training on menopausal symptoms. *J Psychosom Obstet Gynecol, 17,* 202–207; Wijima, K., Melin, A., Nedstrand, E., & Hammar, M. (1997). Treatment of menopausal symptoms with applied relaxation: A pilot study. *J Behav Ther Exp Psychiatry, 28,* 251–261.

23. Freedman, R. R., & Woodward, S. (1992). Behavioral treatment of menopausal hot flashes: Evaluation by ambulatory monitoring. *Am J Obstet Gynecol, 167,* 436–439; Stevenson, D. W., & Delprato, D. J. (1983). Multiple component self-control program for menopausal hot flashes. *J Behav Ther Exp Psychiatry, 14* (2), 137–140; Domar, A. D., & Dreher, H. (1997). *Healing Mind, Healthy Woman,* 291–292. New York: Delta.

24. Ghent, W. (1993). Iodine replacement in fibrocystic disease of the breast. *Can J Surg, 36,* 453–460; Kessler, J. H. (2004). The effect of supraphysiologic levels of iodine on patients with cyclic mastalgia. *Breast J, 10* (4), 328–336.

Chapter 5: Hormone Therapy

1. Writing Group for the Women's Health Initiative Investigators (2002). Risks and benefits of estrogen plus progestin in healthy postmenopausal women: Principal result from the Women's Health Initiative randomized controlled trial. *JAMA, 288,* 327–333.

2. Lacey, J. V., et al. (2002). Menopausal hormone replacement therapy and risk of ovarian cancer. *JAMA, 288,* 334–341.

3. Grodstein, F., Manson, J. E., & Stampfer, M. J. (2006). Hormone therapy and coronary heart disease: The role of time since menopause and age at hormone initiation. *J Womens Health (Larchmt), 15* (1), 35–44.

4. Toh, S., et al. (2010). Coronary heart disease in postmenopausal recipients of estrogen plus progestin therapy: Does the increased risk ever disappear? A randomized trial. *Ann Intern Med, 152* (4), 211–217.

5. North American Menopause Society. (2010). Estrogen and progestogen use in postmenopausal women: 2010 position statement of the North American Menopause Society. *Menopause, 17,* 242–255.

6. Hodis, H. N., Mack, W. J., Henderson, V. W., Shoupe, D., Budoff, M. J., Hwang-Levine, J., Li, Y., Feng, M., Dustin, L., Kono, N., Stanczyk, F. Z., Selzer, R. H., & Azen, S. P. (2016). Vascular effects of early versus late postmenopausal treatment with estradiol. *NEJM, 374* (13), 1221–1231.

7. Santoro, N., Allshouse, A., Neal-Perry, G., Pal, L., Lobo, R. A., Naftolin, F., Black, D. M., Brinton, E. A., Budoff, M. J., Cedars, M. I., Dowling, N. M., Dunn, M., Gleason, C. E., Hodis, H. N., Isaac, B., Magnani, M., Manson, J. E., Miller, V. M., Taylor, H. S., Wharton, W., Wolff, E., Zepeda, V., & Harman, S. M. (2017). Longitudinal changes in menopausal symptoms comparing women randomized to low-dose oral conjugated estrogens or transdermal estradiol plus micronized progesterone versus placebo: the Kronos Early Estrogen Prevention Study. *Menopause, 24* (3), 238–246.

8. Miller, V. M., Naftolin, F., Asthana, S., Black, D. M., Brinton, E. A., Budoff, M. J., Cedars, M. I., Dowling, N. M. Gleason, C. E, Hodis, H. N., Jayachandran, M., Kantarci, K., Lobo, R. A., Manson, J. E., Pal, L., Santoro, N. F., Taylor, H.S., & Harman, S. M. (2019). The Kronos Early Estrogen Prevention Study (KEEPS): What have we learned? *Menopause 26* (9), 1071–1084.

9. Miller, V. M., Hodis, H. N., Lahr, B. D., Bailey, K. R, and Jayachandran, M. (2019). Changes in carotid artery intima-media thickness 3 years after cessation of menopausal hormone therapy: Follow-up from the Kronos Early Estrogen Prevention Study. *Menopause, 26* (1), 24–31.

10. Hargrove, J. T., Maxson, W. S., Wentz, A. C., & Burnett, L. S. (1989). Menopausal hormone replacement therapy with continuous daily oral micronized estradiol and progesterone. *Obstet Gynecol, 73* (4), 606–612.

11. Shen, L., Qiu, S., Chen, Y., Zhang, F., van Breemen, R. B., Nikolic, D., & Bolton, J. L. (1998). Alkylation of 2'-deoxynucleosides and DNA by the Premarin metabolite 4-hydroxyequilenin semiquinone radical. *Chem Res Toxicol, 11,* 94–101; Bhavnani, B. (1998). Pharmacokinetics and pharmacodynamics of conjugated equine estrogens: Chemistry and metabolism. *Proc Soc Biol Med, 217* (1), 6–16; Zhang, F., et al. (1999). The major metabolite of equilin, 4-hydroxyequilin, autoxidizes to an σ-quinone which isomerizes to the potent cytotoxin 4-hydroxyequilenin-σ-quinone. *Chem Res Toxicol, 12,* 204–213.

12. Cole, W., et al. (June 26, 1995). The estrogen dilemma. *Time,* 46–53 (cover story).

13. Brody, J. (Sept. 3, 2002). Sorting through the confusion about hormone replacement therapy. *New York Times.*

14. Loucks, T. L., & Berga, S. L. (2009). Does postmenopausal estrogen use confer neuroprotection? *Semin Reprod Med, 27* (3), 260–274.

15. Yan, H., Yang, W., Zhou, F., et al. (2019). Estrogen improves insulin sensitivity and suppresses gluconeogenesis via the transcription factor foxo1. *Diabetes, 68* (2), 291–304.

16. Collaborative Group on Hormonal Factors in Breast Cancer. (2019). Type

and timing of menopausal hormone therapy and breast cancer risk: Individual participant meta-analysis of the worldwide epidemiological evidence. *Lancet, 394* (10204), 1159–1168.

17. Chebowski, R. T., et al. (2019). Long-term influence of estrogen plus progestin and estrogen alone use on breast cancer incidence: The Women's Health Initiative randomized trials. San Antonio Breast Cancer Symposium, December 10–14, 2019, San Antonio, Texas. Abstract GS5-00.

18. Fournier, A., Berrino, F., & Clavel-Chapelon, F. (2008). Unequal risks for breast cancer associated with different hormone replacement therapies: Results from the E3N Cohort Study. *Breast Cancer Res Treat, 107,* 103–111.

19. Ninth Annual American Association for Cancer Research Frontiers in Cancer Prevention Research Conference, Philadelphia, Nov. 7–10, 2010.

20. Shaak, C. Personal communication about Dr. Shaak's fifteen years of ongoing clinical research on the restoration of early luteal phase hormone levels in menopausal women by transdermal application of progesterone, estradiol, and testosterone. Dr. Shaak suggests that a woman's exact dosage be determined by the combination of her symptoms, a physical exam, and lab tests. (For further information, contact Dr. Shaak at WomanWell, 405 Great Plain Avenue, Needham, MA 02492; 508-833-9957; www .womanwell.net); Hargrove, J., et al. (1998). Absorption of estradiol and progesterone delivered via Jergens lotion used as hormone replacement therapy. Poster session presented at the annual meeting of the North American Menopause Society, Philadelphia.

21. Follingstad, A. (1978). Estriol, the forgotten hormone. *JAMA, 239* (1), 29–39; Lemon, H. (1977). Clinical and experimental aspects of the anti-mammary carcinogenic activity of estriol. *Front Horm Res, 5* (1), 155–173; Lemon, H. (1975). Estriol prevention of mammary carcinoma induced by 7, 12-dimethylbenzathracene and procarbazine. *Cancer Res, 35,* 1341–1353; Lemon, H. (1973). Oestriol and prevention of breast cancer. *Lancet, 1* (802), 546–547; Lemon, H. (1980). Pathophysiologic considerations in the treatment of menopausal patients with oestrogens: The role of oestriol in the prevention of mammary cancer. *Acta Endocrinol Suppl (Copenh), 233,* 17–27; Lemon, H., Wotiz, H., Parsons, L., et al. (1966). Reduced estriol excretion in patients with breast cancer prior to endocrine therapy. *JAMA, 196,* 1128–1136.

22. Carroll, N., et al. (May 2009). Postmenopausal restoration of the estradiol/estrone ratio reduces severity of vasomotor symptoms. Paper presented at the annual meeting of the American College of Obstetricians and Gynecologists, Chicago, IL; Heimer, G. M., & Englund, D. E. (1992). Effects of vaginally administered oestriol on postmenopausal urogenital disorders: A cytohormonal study. *Maturitas, 3,* 171–179; Iosif, C. S. (1992). Effects of protracted administration of estriol on the lower urinary tract in postmenopausal women. *Arch Gynecol Obstet, 3* (251), 115–120; Kirkengen, A. L., Andersen, P., Gjersoe, E., et al. (June 1992). Oestriol in the prophylactic treatment of recurrent urinary tract infections in postmenopausal women. *Scand J Prim Health Care,* 139–142; Raz, K., & Stamm, W. (1993). A controlled trial of intravaginal estriol in postmeno-

pausal women with recurrent urinary tract infections. *N Engl J Med, 329,* 753–756.

23. Savolainen-Peltonen, H., Rahkola-Soisalo, P., Hoti, F., Vattulainen, P., Gissler, M., Ylikorkala, O., & Mikkola, T. S. (2019). Use of postmenopausal hormone therapy and risk of Alzheimer's disease in Finland: Nationwide case-control study. *BMJ, 364,* 1665.

24. Speroff, L., et al. (1999). *Clinical Gynecologic Endocrinology and Infertility* (6th ed.), 56–64. Philadelphia: Lippincott, Williams & Wilkins.

25. Speroff, L. (Sept. 1999). Commentary: Postmenopausal therapy reduces the risk of colorectal cancer. *OB/GYN Clinical Alert, 35.*

26. Love, R. R., Cameron, L., & Connell, B. L. (1991). Symptoms associated with tamoxifen treatment in postmenopausal women. *Arch Intern Med 151,* 1842–1847.

27. Li, C. I., et al. (2009). Adjuvant hormonal therapy for breast cancer and risk of hormone receptor–specific subtypes of contralateral breast cancer. *Cancer Res, 69,* 6865–6870.

28. Koenig, H., et al. (1995). Progesterone synthesis and myelin formation by Schwann cells. *Science, 268,* 1500–1503.

29. When I was a resident in OB-GYN at St. Margaret's Hospital in Boston in the mid-1970s, I routinely saw women in their late thirties and forties who had a number of children and continued to get pregnant year after year, until they welcomed a hysterectomy as a way to avoid further pregnancies. Their lives, beliefs, and biologies stand in sharp contrast to today's thirty-six-year-old professional woman who started worrying as soon as she turned thirty-five that she wouldn't be able to get pregnant. Our beliefs have subtle yet powerful effects on our biologies—effects that are confirmed by research. Brant Secunda is an American-born shaman who was trained by the Huichol Indians, who live in a remote region of Mexico. Brant reports that Huichol women routinely get pregnant in their fifties and some even in their sixties. The work of Alice Domar, Ph.D., of the Beth Israel Deaconess Medical Center and the Mind/Body Medical Institute, reports a 50 percent increase in pregnancy rates in previously infertile women, most of whom are professionals in their thirties and forties, when they participate in programs characterized by group support, deep relaxation, and attention to self-care. These pregnancies become possible because of the ability of the mind and beliefs to effect hormonal levels that better favor conception.

30. Beral, V., et al. (2011). Breast cancer risk in relation to the interval between menopause and starting hormone therapy. *J Nat Cancer Inst, 103,* 296–305.

31. Fournier, A., Berrino, F., & Clavel-Chapelon, F. (2008). Unequal risks for breast cancer associated with different hormone replacement therapies: Results from the E3N Cohort Study. *Breast Cancer Res Treat, 107,* 103–111.

32. Fournier, A., et al. (2009). Estrogen-progestogen menopausal hormone therapy and breast cancer: Does delay from menopause onset to treatment initiation influence risks? *J Clin Oncol, 27,* 5138–5143.

33. Hermsmeyer, K., et al. (2008). Cardiovascular effects of medroxyproges-

terone acetate and progesterone: A case of mistaken identity? *Nat Clin Prac Cardiovasc Med, 5*, 387–395.

34. Stanczyk, F. Z., Paulson, R. J., & Roy, S. (2005). Percutaneous administration of progesterone: Blood levels and endometrial protection. *Menopause, 12* (2), 232–237.

35. Hully, S., et al. (1998). Randomized trial of estrogen plus progestin for secondary prevention of coronary heart disease in postmenopausal women. *JAMA, 280,* 605–618; Sullivan, J. M., et al. (1995). Progestin enhances vasoconstrictor responses in postmenopausal women receiving estrogen replacement therapy. *Menopause, 4,* 193–197; Williame, J. K., et al. (1994). Effects of hormone replacement therapy on reactivity of atherosclerotic coronary arteries in cynomologous monkeys. *J Am Coll Cardiol, 24,* 1757–1761; Sarrel, P. (1999). The differential effects of oestrogens and progestins on vascular tone. *Human Reproduction Update, 5* (3), 205–209.

36. Toh, S., et al. (2010). Coronary heart disease in postmenopausal recipients of estrogen plus progestin therapy: Does the increased risk ever disappear? A randomized trial. *Ann Intern Med, 152* (4), 211–217.

37. Tang, G. W. K. (1994). The climacteric of Chinese factory workers. *Maturitas, 19,* 177–182.

38. Hammond, C. B. (1994). Women's concerns with hormone replacement therapy—compliance issues. *Fertil Steril, 62* (suppl. 2), 157S–160S.

39. Pinkerton, J. V., & Santoro, N. (2015). Compounded bioidentical hormone therapy: Identifying use trends and knowledge gaps among U.S. women. *Menopause, 22* (9), 926–936.

40. Stagnitti, M. N., & Lefkowitz, D. (Nov. 2011). Trends in hormone replacement therapy drugs utilization and expenditures for adult women in the U.S. civilian noninstitutionalized population, 2001–2008. Medical Expenditure Panel Survey, Agency for Healthcare Research and Quality, Statistical Brief #347.

41. Green, S. M., Donegan, E., Frey, B. N., Fedorkow, D. M., Key, B. L., Streiner, D. L., & McCabe, R. E. (2019). Cognitive behavior therapy for menopausal symptoms (CBT-Meno): A randomized controlled trial. *Menopause, 26* (9), 972–980; Hardy, C., Griffiths, A., Norton, S., & Hunter, M. S. (2018). Self-help cognitive behavior therapy for working women with problematic hot flushes and night sweats (MENOS@Work): A multicenter randomized controlled trial. *Menopause, 25* (5), 508–519.

42. Prague, J. K., Roberts, R. E., Comninos, A. N., Clarke, S., Jayasena, C. N., Nash, Z., Doyle, C., Papadopoulou, D. A., Bloom, S. R., Mohideen, P., Panay, N., Hunter, M. S., Veldhuis, J. D., Webber, L. C., Huson, L., & Dhillo, W. S. (2017). Neurokinin 3 receptor antagonism as a novel treatment for menopausal hot flushes: A phase 2, randomized, double-blind, placebo-controlled trial. *Lancet, 389* (10081), 1809–1820.

43. Hermsmeyer, R. K., Thompson, T. L., Pohost, G. M., & Kaski, J. C. (2008). Cardiovascular effects of medroxyprogesterone acetate and progesterone: A case of mistaken identity? *Nat Clin Prac Cardiovasc Med, 5,* 387–395.

44. Postmenopausal Estrogen/Progestin Intervention (PEPI) Trial (1995). Effects of estrogen or estrogen/progestin regimens on heart disease risk factors in postmenopausal women. *JAMA, 273,* 199–206.

45. American College of Obstetricians and Gynecologists (2004). Coronary heart disease. *Obstet Gynecol, 104* (suppl. 4), 415–485.

46. Yaffe, K., Lui, L.-Y., Grady, D., Cauley, J., Kramer, J., & Cummings, S. R. (2000). Cognitive decline in women in relation to non-protein-bound estradiol concentrations. *Lancet, 356* (9231), 708–712.

47. Ramnarine, S., MacCallum, J., & Ritchie, M. (2009). Phyto-oestrogens: Do they have a role in breast cancer therapy? *Proc Nutr Soc, 68* (OCE2), E93.

48. Grodstein, F., Newcomb, P. A., & Stampfer, M. J. (1999). Postmenopausal hormone therapy and the risk of colorectal cancer: A review and meta-analysis. *Am J Med, 106* (5), 574–582.

49. The NAMS 2017 Hormone Therapy Position Statement Advisory Panel (2017). The 2017 hormone therapy position statement of the North American Menopause Society. *Menopause, 24* (7), 728–753.

50. Hedrick, R. E., et al. (2009). Transdermal estradiol gel 0.1% for the treatment of vasomotor symptoms in postmenopausal women. *Menopause, 16,* 132–140.

51. Kolata, G. (July 9, 2002). Citing risks, U.S. will halt study of drugs for hormones. *New York Times.*

Chapter 6: Foods and Supplements to Support the Change

1. Hudson, T. (1994). A pilot study using botanical medicine in the treatment of menopausal symptoms. Portland, Oregon, National College of Naturopathic Medicine and the Bastyr University of Natural Health Sciences.

2. Tyler, V. E. (1993). *The Honest Herbal: A Sensible Guide to the Use of Herbs and Related Remedies* (3rd ed.). Binghamton, NY: Haworth Press.

3. Subcharoen P. (2004). Thai traditional medicine in the new millennium. *J Med Assoc Thai, 87* (Suppl 4), S52–S57; Malaivijitnond S. (2012). Medical applications of phytoestrogens from the Thai herb *Pueraria mirifica*. *Front Med, 6* (1), 8–21; Shimokawa, S., Kumamoto, T., Ishikawa, T., Takashi, M., Higuchi, Y., Chaichantipyuth, C., & Chansakaow, S. (2013). Quantitative analysis of miroestrol and kwakhurin for standardisation of Thai miracle herb "Kwao Keur" (*Pueraria mirifica*) and establishment of simple isolation procedure for highly estrogenic miroestrol and deoxymiroestrol. *Nat Prod Res, 27* (4–5), 371–378.

4. Elghamry, M. I., & Shihata, I. M. (1965). Biological activity of phytoestrogens. *Planta Med, 13,* 352–357.

5. Knight, D. C., & Eden, J. A. (1996). A review of the clinical effects of phytoestrogens. Part 2. *Obstet Gynecol, 87* (5, part 2), 897–904; Kaldas, R. S., & Hughes, C. L. (1989). Reproductive and general metabolic effects of phytoestrogens in mammals. *Reprod Toxicol, 3* (2), 81–89; Treeck, O.,

Lattrich, C., Springwald, A., & Ortmann, O. (2010). Estrogen receptor beta exerts growth-inhibitory effects on human mammary epithelial cells. *Breast Cancer Res Treat, 120* (3), 557–565; Jeon, G. C., Park, M. S., Yoon, D. Y., Shin, C. H., Sin, H. S., & Um, S. J. (2005). Antitumor activity of spinasterol isolated from *Pueraria* roots. *Exp Mol Med, 37* (2), 111–120; Boonchird, C., Mahapanichkul, T., & Cherdshewasart, W. (2010). Differential binding with ERalpha and ERbeta of the phytoestrogen-rich plant *Pueraria mirifica*. *Braz J Med Biol Res, 43* (2), 195–200; Ramnarine, S., MacCallum, J., & Ritchie, M. (2009). Phyto-oestrogens: Do they have a role in breast cancer therapy? *Proc Nutr Soc, 68* (OCE2), E93.

6. Rose, D. P. (1992). Dietary fiber, phytoestrogens, and breast cancer. *Nutrition, 8,* 47–51.

7. Tamaya, T., et al. (1986). Inhibition by plant herb extracts of steroid bindings in uterus, liver, and serum of the rabbit. *Acta Obstet Gynecol Scand, 65,* 839–842.

8. Manonai, J., et al. (2008). Effects and safety of *Pueraria mirifica* on lipid profiles and biochemical markers of bone turnover rates in healthy postmenopausal women. *Menopause, 15* (3), 530–535; Urasopon, N., et al. (2007). *Pueraria mirifica*, a phytoestrogen-rich herb, prevents bone loss in orchidectomized rats. *Maturitas, 56,* 3, 322–331.

9. Chandeying, V., & Sangthawan, M. (2007). Efficacy comparison of *Pueraria mirifica* (PM) against conjugated equine estrogen (CEE) with/without medroxyprogesterone acetate (MPA) in the treatment of climacteric symptoms in perimenopausal women: Phase III study. *J Med Assoc Thai, 90, 9,* 1720–1726.

10. Personal correspondence with C. Deachapunya, Department of Physiology, Faculty of Medicine, Srinakharinwirot University, Bangkok, Thailand; Poonyachoti, S. et al. (2008). Effects of *Pueraria mirifica*, phytoestrogens and 17b-estradiol on growth and expression of ERA in primary culture of porcine endometrial epithelial cells. *Acta Horticulturae (ISHS), 786,* 67–72.

11. Ramnarine, S., MacCallum, J., & Ritchie, M. (2009). Phyto-oestrogens: Do they have a role in breast cancer therapy? *Proc Nutr Soc, 68,* E93.

12. Yoshiro, K. (1985). The physiological actions of tan-kwei and cnidium. *Bull Oriental Healing Arts Institute USA, 10,* 269–278; Harada, M., Suzuki, M., & Ozaki, Y. (1984). Effects of Japanese *Angelica* root and peony root on uterine contraction in the rabbit *in situ. J Pharmacol Dynam, 7,* 304–311; Zhu, D. P. O. (1987). Dong quai. *Am J Chinese Med, 15,* 117–125.

13. Bohnert, K.-J. (Spring 1997). The use of *Vitex agnus-castus* for hyperprolactinemia. *Q Rev Natural Med,* 19–20; American Botanical Council (1992). *Kommission E monograph: Agnus casti fructus (chaste tree fruits).* Fort Worth, TX.

14. Duker, E. M., et al. (1991). Effects of extracts from *Cimicifuga racemosa* on gonadotropin release in menopausal women and ovariectomized rats. *Planta Med, 57,* 420–424.

15. Geller, S. E., et al. (2009). Safety and efficacy of black cohosh and red

clover for the management of vasomotor symptoms: A randomized controlled trial. *Menopause, 16* (6), 1156–1166.

16. Wuttke, W., et al. (2003). The *Cimicifuga* preparation BNO 1055 vs. conjugated estrogens in a double-blind placebo-controlled study: Effects on menopause symptoms and bone markers. *Maturitas, 44,* S67–S77; Hernandez Munoz, G., & Pluchino, S. (2003). *Cimicifuga racemosa* for the treatment of hot flushes in women surviving breast cancer, *Maturitas, 44,* S59–S65.

17. Hudson, T. (2008–2009). Maca: New insights on an ancient plant. *Integr Med, 7* (6), 54–57.

18. Council for Responsible Nutrition (June 17, 2009). International researchers convene meeting on isoflavones. Press release.

19. Margaret Ritchie, Ph.D. (June 2009). Personal communication.

20. Jeon, G. C., Park, M. S., Yoon, D. Y., Shin, C. H., Sin, H. S., & Um, S. J. (2005). Antitumor activity of spinasterol isolated from *Pueraria* roots. *Exp Mol Med, 37* (2), 111–120; Boonchird, C., Mahapanichkul, T., & Cherdshewasart, W. (2010). Differential binding with ERalpha and ERbeta of the phytoestrogen-rich plant *Pueraria mirifica. Braz J Med Biol Res, 43* (2), 195–200; Ramnarine, S., MacCallum, J., & Ritchie, M. (2009). Phyto-oestrogens: Do they have a role in breast cancer therapy? *Proc Nutr Soc, 68* (OCE2), E93.

21. Aldercreutz, H., et al. (1986). Determination of urinary lignans and phytoestrogen metabolites, potential antiestrogens and anticarcinogens in urine of women on various habitual diets. *J Steroid Biochem, 25* (5B), 791–797.

22. Aldercreutz, H. (1984). Does fiber-rich food containing animal lignan precursors protect against both colon and breast cancer? An extension of the "fiber hypothesis." *Gastroenterology, 86* (4), 761–764; Jenab, M., et al. (1996). The influence of flaxseed and lignans on colon carcinogenesis and beta-glucuronidase activity. *Carcinogenesis, 17* (6), 1343–1348; Johnstone, P. V. (1995). Flaxseed oil and cancer: Alpha-linolenic acid and carcinogenesis. In S. C. Cunnane & L. U. Thompson (eds.), *Flaxseed in Human Nutrition.* Champaign, IL: AOCS Press; Serraino, M., et al. (1991). The effect of flaxseed supplementation on early risk markers for mammary carcinogenesis. *Cancer Lett, 60,* 135–142; Serraino, M., et al. (1992). The effect of flaxseed supplementation on the initiation and promotional stages of mammary tumorigenesis. *Nutr Cancer, 17,* 153–159.

23. Lampe, J. W., et al. (1994). Urinary lignan and isoflavonoid excretion in premenopausal women consuming flaxseed powder. *Am J Clin Nutr, 60,* 122–128; Mousavi, Y., et al. (1992). Enterolactone and estradiol inhibit each other's proliferative effect on MCF and breast cancer cells in culture. *J Steroid Biochem Mol Biol, 41,* 615–619.

24. Bierenbaum, M. L., et al. (1993). Reducing atherogenic risk in hyperlipemic humans with flaxseed supplementation: A preliminary report. *J Am College Nutr, 12* (5), 501–504.

25. Micallef, M., et al. (2009). Plasma n-3 polyunsaturated fatty acids are negatively associated with obesity. *Br J Nutr, 102* (9), 1370–1374.

26. Parra, D., et al. (2008). A diet rich in long chain omega-3 fatty acids modulates satiety in overweight and obese volunteers during weight loss. *Appetite, 51* (3), 676–680.

27. Maes, M., et al. (2000). In humans, serum polyunsaturated fatty acid levels predict the response of proinflammatory cytokines to psychologic stress. *Biol Psychiatry, 47* (10), 910–920.

28. Bougnoux, P., et al. (2009). Improving outcome of chemotherapy of metastatic breast cancer by docosahexaenoic acid: A phase II trial. *Br J Cancer, 101* (12), 1978–1985.

29. Manson, J. E., Cook, N. R., Lee, I. M., Christen, W., Bassuk, S. S., Mora, S., Gibson, H., Gordon, D., Copeland, T., D'Agostino, D., Friedenberg, G., Ridge, C., Bubes, V., Giovannucci, E. L., Willett, W. C., Buring, J. E., & VITAL Research Group (2019). Vitamin D supplements and prevention of cancer and cardiovascular disease. *N Engl J Med, 380* (1), 33–44.

30. Yalagala, P., Sugasini, D., Dasarathi, S., Pahan, K., & Subbaiah, P. V. (2019). Dietary lysophosphatidylcholine-EPA enriches both EPA and DHA in the brain: Potential treatment for depression. *J Lipid R, 60* (3), 566–578.

31. Middleton, E., & Kandaswami, C. (Nov. 1994). Potential health-promoting properties of citrus bioflavonoids. *Food Technology,* 115–119.

32. I am indebted to Maureen Tsao, M.Ac., and her mother, Fern Tsao, for their assistance in preparing this section on Traditional Chinese Medicine and menopause.

33. Vernejoul, P., et al. (1985). Étude des meridiens d'acupuncture par les traceurs radioactifs [The study of acupuncture meridians using radioactive tracers]. *Bull Acad Natl Méd, 169* (7), 1071–1075.

Chapter 7: The Menopause Food Plan

1. Huang, I. C., Frangakis, C., & Wu, A. W. (2006). The relationship of excess body weight and health-related quality of life: Evidence from a population study in Taiwan. *Int J Obesity, 30* (8), 1250–1259; Pan, A., Kawachi, I., Luo, N., Manson, J. E., Willett, W. C., Hu, F. B., & Okereke, O. I. (2014). Changes in body weight and health-related quality of life: 2 cohorts of U.S. women. *Am J Epidemiol, 180* (3), 254–262; Hayes, M., Baxter, H., Müller-Nordhorn, J., Hohls, J. K., & Muckelbauer, R. (2017). The longitudinal association between weight change and health-related quality of life in adults and children: A systematic review. *Obes Rev, 18* (12), 1398–1411; Fine, J. T., Colditz, G. A., Coakley, E. H., Moseley, G., Manson, J. E., Willett, W. C., & Kawachi, I. (1999). A prospective study of weight change and health-related quality of life in women. *JAMA, 282,* 2136–2142.

2. Ward, Z. J., Bleich, S. N., Cradock, A. L., Barrett, J. L., Giles, C. M., Flax, C., Long, M. W., & Gortmaker, S. L. (2019). Projected U.S. state-level prevalence of adult obesity and severe obesity. *N Engl J Med, 381* (25), 2440–2450.

3. Baillie-Hamilton, P. F. (2002). Chemical toxins: A hypothesis to explain the global obesity epidemic. *J Altern Complement Med, 8* (2), 185–192.

4. *Atkins' New Diet Revolution* was the number-one bestselling diet book of the late 1990s. The research supporting the book is sound, though controversial.

5. A clinical study of the Atkins diet presented at the Southern Society of General Internal Medicine in New Orleans (1999) by lead researcher Eric Charles Westman, M.D., of Duke University in Durham, North Carolina, failed to show any adverse effects on kidney and liver function in the forty-one mildly obese study subjects who limited their carbohydrate intake to less than 20 g per day. They also took a multivitamin-mineral and fish oil supplement and exercised three times per week. The Durham study lasted for four months and test subjects dropped an average of twenty-one pounds each. Cholesterol levels dropped 6.1 percent and triglycerides dropped by 40 percent, while protective HDL cholesterol levels increased by about 7 percent. Blood pressure and body composition also underwent favorable changes. The results of the Durham study were supported in a second, larger study of 319 overweight or obese patients conducted over a period of one year at the Atkins Center for Complementary Medicine in New York City. Results were similar, laying to rest any safety concerns. Under many perimenopausal conditions, however, even the Atkins diet may not be as effective as it is during other life stages, nor as it is for men.

6. Koithan, M. (2009). Mind-body solutions for obesity. *J Nurse Pract, 5* (7), 536–537.

7. Koliada, A., Syzenko, G., Moseiko, V., Budovska, L., Puchkov, K., Perederiy, V., Gavalko, Y., Dorofeyev, A., Romanenko, M., Tkach, S., Sineok, L., Lushchak, O., & Vaiserman, A. (2017). Association between body mass index and Firmicutes/Bacteroidetes ratio in an adult Ukrainian population. *BMC Microbiol, 17* (1), 120.

8. Ségurel, L., & Bon, C. (2017). On the evolution of lactase persistence in humans. Annual Review of Genomics and Human Genetics, 18, 297–319.

9. de Wit, W., & Bigaud, N. (2019). *No Plastic in Nature: Assessing Plastic Ingestion from Nature to People.* Gland, Switzerland: WWF.

10. Donley, N. (2019). The USA lags behind other agricultural nations in banning harmful pesticides. *Environ Health, 18* (1), 44.

11. Dunneram, Y., Greenwood, D. C., Burley, V. J., & Cade, J. E. (2018). Dietary intake and age at natural menopause: Results from the UK Women's Cohort Study. *J Epidemiol Commun H, 72* (8), 733–740.

12. Fukagawa, N. K., et al. (1990). Effect of age on body composition and resting metabolic rate. *Am J Physiol, 259,* E233; Ganesan, R. (1995). Aversive and hypophagic effects of estradiol. *Physiol Behav, 55* (2), 279–285.

13. Sieri, S., et al. (2010). Dietary glycemic load and index and risk of coronary heart disease in a large Italian cohort: The EPICOR study. *Arch Intern Med, 170,* 640–647.

14. Welsh, J. A., et al. (2010). Caloric sweetener consumption and dyslipidemia among US adults. *JAMA, 303,* 1490–1497.

15. Groff, J. L., & Gropper, S. (2000). *Advanced Nutrition and Human Metabolism,* 147, 252, 447. Belmont, CA: Wadsworth.

16. Zhao, N., Liu, C. C., Van Ingelgom, A. J., Martens, Y. A., Linares, C., Knight, J. A., Painter, M. M., Sullivan, P. M., & Bu, G. (2017). Apolipoprotein E4 impairs neuronal insulin signaling by trapping insulin receptor in the endosomes. *Neuron, 96* (1), 115–129.e5.

17. Tobias, D. K., Chen, M., Manson, J. E., Ludwig, D. S., Willett, W., & Hu, F. B. (2015). Effect of low-fat diet interventions versus other diet interventions on long-term weight change in adults: a systematic review and meta-analysis. *Lancet Diabetes Endo, 3* (12), 968–979.

18. Reaven, G. M. (2000). *Syndrome X: Overcoming the Silent Killer That Can Give You a Heart Attack.* New York: Simon & Schuster.

19. Eriksson, J., et al. (1989). Early metabolic defects in persons at increased risk for non-insulin-dependent diabetes mellitus. *N Engl J Med, 321,* 337–343; Lillioja, S., et al. (1993). Insulin resistance and insulin secretory dysfunction as precursors of non-insulin-dependent diabetes mellitus: Prospective studies of the Pima Indians. *N Engl J Med, 329,* 1988–1992.

20. Reaven, G. M. (1988). Role of insulin resistance in human disease. *Diabetes, 37,* 1595–1607; Zavaroni, I., et al. (1989). Risk factors for coronary artery disease in healthy persons with hyperinsulinemia and normal glucose tolerance. *N Engl J Med, 320,* 702–706.

21. Fuh, M. M., et al. (1987). Abnormalities of carbohydrate and lipid metabolism in patients with hypertension. *Arch Intern Med, 147,* 1035–1038; Zavaroni, I., et al. (1987). Evidence that multiple risk factors for coronary artery disease exist in persons with abnormal glucose tolerance. *Am J Med, 83,* 609–612.

22. Nestler, J., et al. (1999). Ovulatory and metabolic effects of D-chiro-inositol in the polycystic ovary syndrome. *N Engl J Med, 340,* 1314–1320.

23. Kazer, R. (1995). Insulin resistance, insulin-like growth factor 1 and breast cancer: A hypothesis. *Int J Cancer, 62* (4), 403–406.

24. Bruning, P. F., Bonfrer, J. M., van Noord, P. A., Hart, A. A., de Jong-Bakker, M., & Nooijen, W. J. (1992). Insulin resistance and breast-cancer risk. *Int J Cancer, 52* (4), 511–516; Seely, S. (1983). Diet and breast cancer: The possible connection with sugar consumption. *Med Hypotheses, 11,* 319–327.

25. Bruning, P. F., Bonfrer, J. M., van Noord, P. A., Hart, A. A., de Jong-Bakker, M., & Nooijen, W. J. (1992). Insulin resistance and breast-cancer risk. *Int J Cancer, 52* (4), 511–516.

26. Kazer, R. (1995). Insulin resistance, insulin-like growth factor 1 and breast cancer: A hypothesis. *Int J Cancer, 62* (4), 403–406.

27. Samsel, A., & Seneff, S. (2013). Glyphosate's suppression of cytochrome P450 enzymes and amino acid biosynthesis by the gut microbiome: Pathways to modern diseases. *Entropy, 15,* 1416–1463.

28. Micha, R., et al. (2010). Red and processed meat consumption and risk of incident coronary heart disease, stroke, and diabetes mellitus: A systematic review and meta-analysis. *Circulation, 121,* 2271–2283.

29. Huang, Z., Willett, W. C., Colditz, G. A., Hunter, D. J., Manson, J. E.,

Rosner, B., Speizer, F. E., & Hankinson, S. E. (1999). Waist circumference, waist:hip ratio, and risk of breast cancer in the Nurses' Health Study. *Am J Epidemiol, 150* (12), 1316–1324. Dr. Zhi-ping Huang from the Harvard School of Public Health and his colleagues examined the association between waist circumference and waist-to-hip ratio with subsequent risk for breast cancer. Those with a waist circumference between 32 and 35.9 inches had a breast cancer risk 1.5 times greater than normal, while those with a waist circumference between 36 and 55 inches had a risk that was almost twice that of women whose waists were between 15 and 27.9 inches. Abdominal adiposity is associated with an excess of androgen and increased conversion of androgen to estrogen in fatty tissue. The research also concluded that "all postmenopausal hormone users were at increased risk of breast cancer regardless of central obesity."

30. Wild, R. D., et al. (1985). Lipoprotein lipid concentrations and cardiovascular risk in women with polycystic ovarian syndrome. *J Clin Endocrinol Metab, 61,* 946; Rexrode, K., et al. (1998). Abdominal adiposity and coronary heart disease in women. *JAMA, 280,* 1843–1848; Gillespie, L. (1999). *The Menopause Diet: Lose Weight and Boost Your Energy,* 18. Beverly Hills, CA: Healthy Life Publications.

31. Adams, K. F., et al. (2006). Overweight, obesity, and mortality in a large prospective cohort of persons age 50 to 71 years old. *N Engl J Med, 355* (8), 763–778.

32. Jia, H., & Lubetkin, E. I. (2010). Trends in quality-adjusted life-years lost contributed by smoking and obesity. *Am J Prev Med, 38,* 138–144.

33. Huang, Z., Willett, W. C., Colditz, G. A., Hunter, D. J., Manson, J. E., Rosner, B., Speizer, F. E., & Hankinson, S. E. (1999). Waist circumference, waist:hip ratio, and risk of breast cancer in the Nurses' Health Study. *Am J Epidemiol, 150* (12), 1316–1324.

34. Onstad, M. A., Schmandt, R. E., & Lu, K. H. (2016). Addressing the role of obesity in endometrial cancer risk, prevention, and treatment. *J Clin Oncol, 34* (35), 4225–4230.

35. Setiawan, V. W., Yang, H. P., Pike, M. C., McCann, S. E., Yu, H., Xiang, Y. B., Wolk, A., Wentzensen, N., Weiss, N. S., Webb, P. M., van den Brandt, P. A., van de Vijver, K., Thompson, P. J., Australian National Endometrial Cancer Study Group, Strom, B. L., Spurdle, A. B., Soslow, R. A., Shu, X. O., Schairer, C., Sacerdote, C., . . . & Horn-Ross, P. L. (2013). Type I and II endometrial cancers: Have they different risk factors?. *J Clin Oncol, 31* (20), 2607–2618.

36. Moriyama, C. K., et al. (2008). A randomized, placebo-controlled trial of the effects of physical exercises and estrogen therapy on health-related quality of life in postmenopausal women. *Menopause, 15,* 613–618.

37. Physical Activity Guidelines Advisory Committee (2008). *Physical Activity Guidelines Advisory Committee Report, 2008.* Washington, DC: U.S. Department of Health and Human Services, 2008. www.health.gov /paguidelines/Report/pdf/CommitteeReport.pdf.

38. Lee, I. M., et al. (2010). Physical activity and weight gain prevention. *JAMA, 303,* 1173–1179.

39. Arsenis, N. C., You, T., Ogawa, E. F., Tinsley, G. M., & Zuo, L. (2017). Physical activity and telomere length: Impact of aging and potential mechanisms of action. *Oncotarget, 8* (27), 45008–45019.

40. Duggal, N. A., Pollock, R. D., Lazarus, N. R., Harridge S., & Lord, J. M. (2018). Major features of immunesenescence, including reduced thymic output, are ameliorated by high levels of physical activity in adulthood. *Aging Cell, 17* (2), e12750.

41. Campbell, T., et al. (2009). A yearlong exercise intervention decreases CRP among obese postmenopausal women. *Med Sci Sports Exerc, 41* (8), 1533–1539.

42. Hackney, M. E., et al. (2007). Effects of tango on functional mobility in Parkinson's disease: A preliminary study. *J Neurol Phys Ther, 31,* 173–179.

43. Hackney, M. E., et al. (2009). Health-related quality of life and alternative forms of exercise in Parkinson disease. *Parkinsonism Relat Disord, 15,* 644–648.

44. Duncan, R. P., & Earhart, G. M. (2012). Randomized controlled trial of community-based dancing to modify disease progression in Parkinson disease. *Neurorehabil Neural Repair, 26* (2), 132–143.

45. Verghese, J., Lipton, R. B., Katz, M. J., Hall, C. B., Derby, C. A., Kuslansky, G., Ambrose, A. F., Sliwinski, M., & Buschke, H. (2003). Leisure activities and the risk of dementia in the elderly. *N Engl J Med, 348* (25), 2508–2516.

46. Larsen, T. M., et al. (2010). Diets with high or low protein content and glycemic index for weight-loss maintenance. *N Engl J Med, 363,* 2101–2113.

47. Carmen, M., Safer, D. L., Saslow, L. R., Kalayjian, T., Mason, A. E., Westman, E. C., & Sethi Dalai, S. (2020). Treating binge eating and food addiction symptoms with low-carbohydrate Ketogenic diets: A case series. *J Eat Disord, 8,* 2.

48. Ludvigsson, J. F., et al. (2009). Small-intestinal histopathology and mortality risk in celiac disease. *JAMA, 302,* 1171–1178.

49. Cutler, R. G. (1984). Carotenoids and retinol: Their possible importance in determining longevity of primate species. *Proc Natl Acad Sci, 81,* 7627–7631.

50. Murakoshi, M., et al. (1992). Potent preventive action of alpha-carotene against carcinogenesis. *Cancer Res, 52,* 6583–6587.

51. Franceschi, S., et al. (1994). Tomatoes and risk of digestive-tract cancers. *Int J Cancer, 59,* 181–184.

52. Park, J. E., et al. (2010). Stevia rebaudiana Bertoni extract supplementation improves lipid and carnitine profiles in C57BL/6J mice fed a high-fat diet. *J Sci Food Agric, 90,* 1099–1105.

53. Mozaffarian, D., et al. (2010). Effects on coronary heart disease of increasing polyunsaturated fat in place of saturated fat: A systematic review and meta-analysis of randomized controlled trials. *PLoS Med, 7,* e1000252.

54. Wang, D. D., Li, Y., Chiuve, S. E., Stampfer, M. J., Manson, J. E., Rimm, E. B., Willett, W. C., & Hu, F. B. (2016). Association of specific dietary

fats with total and cause-specific mortality. *JAMA Intern Med, 176* (8), 1134–1145.

55. Hornstra, G. (2000). Essential fatty acids in mothers and their neonates. *Am J Clin Nutr, 71* (suppl.), 1262S–1269S.

56. Hwang, J. H., et al. (2010). Dietary supplements reduce the risk of cervical intraepithelial neoplasia. *Int J Gynecol Cancer, 20,* 398–403.

57. Ianoli, P., et al. (1998). Glucocorticoids upregulate intestinal nutrient transport in a time-dependent substrate-specific fashion. *J Gastrointest Surg, 2* (5), 449–457.

58. McGuigan, J. E. (1994). Peptic ulcer and gastritis. In K. Isselbacher et al. (eds.), *Harrison's Principles of Internal Medicine, vol. 2* (13th ed.), 1369. New York: McGraw-Hill.

59. Murray, M., & Pizzorno, J. (1998). *Encyclopedia of Natural Medicine,* 134–137. Rocklin, CA: Prima Publishing; van Marle, J., et al. (1981). Deglycyrrhizinised licorice (DGL) and renewal of the rat stomach epithelium. *Eur J Pharmacol, 72,* 219–275.

Chapter 8: Creating Pelvic Health and Power

1. Lukes, A. S., et al. (2010). Tranexamic acid treatment for heavy menstrual bleeding: A randomized controlled trial. *Obstet Gynecol, 116* 865–875.

2. Stewart, E. A., Cookson, C. L., Gandolfo, R. A., & Schulze-Rath, R. (2017). Epidemiology of uterine fibroids: A systematic review. *BJOG, 124* (10), 1501–1512.

3. Lepine, L. A., et al. (1997). Hysterectomy surveillance—United States, 1980–1993. *MMWR, 46,* 1–15.

4. Society of Interventional Radiology. (March 6, 2017). Minimally invasive, less expensive treatment for uterine fibroids underutilized: national study suggests many women are not aware of benefits of uterine fibroid embolization. *Science Daily;* www.sciencedaily.com/releases/2017/03/17030609 2746.htm.

5. Bradley, L., & Newman, J. (2000). Uterine artery embolization for treatment of fibroids: From scalpel to catheter. *The Female Patient, 25,* 71–78.

6. Domingo, S., & Pellicer, A. (2009). Overview of current trends in hysterectomy. *Expert Rev Obstet Gynecol, 4* (6), 673–685.

7. West, S. (1994). *The Hysterectomy Hoax.* New York: Doubleday.

8. Garcia, C. R., & Cutler, W. B. (1984). Preservation of the ovary: A reevaluation. *Fertil Steril, 42* (4), 510–514.

9. Cutler, W. B. (1999). Human sex-attractant pheromones: Discovery, research, development, and application in sex therapy. *Psychiat Ann, 29,* 54–59.

10. Hasson, H. (1993). Cervical removal at hysterectomy for benign disease: Risks and benefits. *J Reprod Med, 58* (10), 781–789.

11. Parker, W. H. (2010). Bilateral oophorectomy versus ovarian conservation: Effects on long-term women's health. *J Minim Invasive Gynecol, 17,* 161–166.

12. Parker, W. H., et al. (2009). Ovarian conservation at the time of hysterectomy and long-term health outcomes in the Nurses' Health Study. *Obstet Gynecol, 113,* 1027–1037.

13. Koushik, A., et al. (2009). Characteristics of menstruation and pregnancy and the risk of lung cancer in women. *Int J Cancer, 125,* 2428–2433.

14. Parker, W. H., et al. (2009). Ovarian conservation at the time of hysterectomy and long-term health outcomes in the Nurses' Health Study. *Obstet Gynecol, 113,* 1027–1037.

15. Ibid.

16. Rivera, C. M., et al. (2009). Increased mortality for neurological and mental diseases following early bilateral oophorectomy. *Neuroepidemiology, 33,* 32–40.

17. Parker, W. H. (2010). Bilateral oophorectomy versus ovarian conservation: Effects on long-term women's health. *J Minim Invasive Gynecol, 17,* 161–166.

18. Ibid.

19. Ibid.

20. Ibid.

21. Speroff, T., et al. (1991). A risk-benefit analysis of elective bilateral oophorectomy: Effect of changes in compliance with estrogen therapy on outcome. *Am J Obstet Gynecol, 164,* 65–174.

22. Carlson, K., Miller, B., & Fowler, F. (1994). The Maine Women's Health Study. I. Outcomes of hysterectomy. *Obstet Gynecol, 83,* 556–565.

23. Rogo-Gupta, L., Rodriguez, L. V., Litwin, M. S., Herzog, T. J., Neugut, A. I., Lu, Y. S., Raz, S., Hershman, D. L., & Wright, J. D. (2012). Trends in surgical mesh use for pelvic organ prolapse from 2000 to 2010. *Obstet Gynecol, 120* (5), 1105–1115; Food and Drug Administration. (July 2011). Urogynecologic surgical mesh: Update on the safety and effectiveness of transvaginal placement for pelvic organ prolapse. Washington, DC: U.S. Food and Drug Administration, Centers for Devices and Radiological Health; see www.fda.gov/downloads/MedicalDevices/Safety/Alerts andNotices/UCM262760.pdf.

24. Kaplan, S., & Goldstein, M. (April 17, 2019). F.D.A. orders pelvic mesh, tied to injuries, off market. *New York Times,* www.nytimes.com/2019/04 /16/health/vaginal-pelvic-mesh-fda.html.

25. Food and Drug Administration. (Oct. 2008). FDA public health notification: Serious complications associated with transvaginal placement of surgical mesh in repair of pelvic organ prolapse and stress urinary incontinence.

26. Food and Drug Administration. (July 2011). Urogynecologic surgical mesh: Update on the safety and effectiveness of transvaginal placement for pelvic organ prolapse. www.fda.gov/downloads/MedicalDevices/Safety /AlertsandNotices/UCM262760.pdf.

27. Kaplan, S., & Goldstein, M. (April 17, 2019). F.D.A. orders pelvic mesh, tied to injuries, off market. *New York Times,* www.nytimes.com/2019/04 /16/health/vaginal-pelvic-mesh-fda.html.

28. Wise, J. (2017). NICE to ban mesh for vaginal wall prolapse. *BMJ, 359,* j5523.

29. Adams, L. (December 11, 2017). Mesh risks not passed on to doctors. BBC News; www.bbc.com/news/uk-scotland-42307953.

30. *60 Minutes.* (May 13, 2018). Gynecological mesh: The medical device that has 100,000 women suing; www.cbsnews.com/news/boston-scientific -gynecological-mesh-the-medical-device-that-has-100000-women-suing -2019-04-17.

31. Food and Drug Administration. (April 16, 2019). FDA takes action to protect women's health, orders manufacturers of surgical mesh intended for transvaginal repair of pelvic organ prolapse to stop selling all devices; www.fda.gov/news-events/press-announcements/fda-takes-action -protect-womens-health-orders-manufacturers-surgical-mesh-intended -transvaginal. Food and Drug Administration. Urogynecologic surgical mesh implants; www.fda.gov/medical-devices/implants-and-prosthetics /urogynecologic-surgical-mesh-implants.

32. Llamas, M. (Nov. 2019; updated March 4, 2020). Transvaginal mesh lawsuits. *Drugwatch;* www.drugwatch.com/transvaginal-mesh/lawsuits.

33. Kaplan, S., & Goldstein, M. (April 17, 2019). F.D.A. orders pelvic mesh, tied to injuries, off market. *New York Times,* www.nytimes.com/2019/04 /16/health/vaginal-pelvic-mesh-fda.html.

34. Weston A. Price Foundation. (June 22, 2011). Government data proves raw milk safe: Raw milk risk extremely small compared to risk of other foods; https://www.westonaprice.org/government-data-proves-raw-milk -safe.

35. Badalian, S. S., & Rosenbaum, P. F. (2010). Vitamin D and pelvic floor disorders in women: Results from the National Health and Nutrition Examination Survey. *Obstet Gynecol, 115,* 795–803.

36. Reddy, P., & Edwards, L. R. (2019). Magnesium supplementation in vitamin D deficiency. *Am J Ther, 26* (1), e124–e132.

37. Martinez, R. C., et al. (2009). Effect of Lactobacillus rhamnosus GR-1 and Lactobacillus reuteri RC-14 on the ability of Candida albicans to infect cells and induce inflammation. *Microbiol Immunol, 53,* 4874–4895; Martinez, R. C., et al. (2009). Improved treatment of vulvovaginal candidiasis with fluconazole plus probiotic Lactobacillus rhamnosus GR-1 and Lactobacillus reuteri RC-14. *Lett Appl Microbiol, 48,* 269–274; Anukam, K., et al. (2006). Augmentation of antimicrobial metronidazole therapy of bacterial vaginosis with oral probiotic Lactobacillus rhamnosus GR-1 and Lactobacillus reuteri RC-14: Randomized, double-blind, placebo controlled trial. *Microbes Infect, 8,* 1450–1454; Morelli, L., et al. (2004). Utilization of the intestinal tract as a delivery system for urogenital probiotics. *J Clini Gastroenterol, 38,* S107–S110; Reid, G., et al. (2004). Nucleic acid–based diagnosis of bacterial vaginosis and improved management using probiotic lactobacilli. *J Med Food, 7,* 223–228; Reid, G., et al. (2003). Oral use of Lactobacillus rhamnosus GR-1 and L. fermentum RC-14 significantly alters vaginal flora: Randomized, placebo-controlled

trial in 64 healthy women. *FEMS Immunol Med Microbiol, 35,* 131–134; Reid, G., et al. (2003). Effect of lactobacilli oral supplement on the vaginal microflora of antibiotic treated patients: Randomized, placebo-controlled study. *Nutraceuticals & Food, 8,* 145–148; Gardiner, G., et al. (2002). Oral administration of the probiotic combination Lactobacillus rhamnosus GR-1 and L. fermentum RC-14 for human intestinal applications. *Int Dairy J, 12,* 191–196; Reid, G., et al. (2001). Probiotic lactobacillus dose required to restore and maintain a normal vaginal flora. *FEMS Immunol Med Microbiol, 32,* 37–41; Reid, G., et al. (2001). Oral probiotics can resolve urogenital infections. FEMS *Immunol Med Microbiol, 30,* 49–52.

38. Helms, J. M. (1987). Acupuncture for the management of primary dysmenorrhea. *Obstet Gynecol, 69* (1), 51–56.

39. Bhatia, N., Tchou, D. C. H., et al. (1988). Pelvic floor musculature exercises in treatment of anatomical urinary stress incontinence. *Phys Ther, 68,* 652–655; Diokno, A. (1996). The benefits of conservative management in SUI. *Contemp Urol, 8,* 36–48.

40. Singla, A. (2000). An update on the management of SUI. *Contemp Ob Gyn, 45* (1), 68–85.

41. Wu, J. M., et al. (2009). Forecasting the prevalence of pelvic floor disorders in U.S. women: 2010 to 2050. *Obstet Gynecol, 114,* 278–283.

42. Rohner T. J., Jr., & Rohner. J. F. (1997). Urinary incontinence in America: The social significance. In P. D. O'Donnel (ed.), *Urinary Incontinence.* St. Louis, MO: Mosby-Yearbook, Inc.

43. Resnick, N. (1998). Improving treatment of urinary incontinence. *JAMA, 280* (23), 2034–2035.

44. Pandit, M., et al. (2000). Quantification of intramuscular nerves within the female striated urogenital sphincter muscles. *Obstet Gynecol, 95,* 797–800.

45. Bergman, A., & Elia, G. (1995). Three surgical procedures for genuine stress incontinence. Five-year follow-up of a prospective randomized study. *Am J Obstet Gynecol, 173,* 66–71.

46. Singla, A. (2000). An update on the management of SUI. *Contemp Ob Gyn, 45* (1), 77.

47. Glazener, C. M., & Cooper, K. (2004). Bladder neck needle suspension for urinary incontinence in women. Cochrane Database Syst. Rev., CD003636.

48. Santarosa, R. P., & Blaivas, J. G. (1994). Periurethral injection of autologous fat for the treatment of sphincteric incontinence. *J Urol, 151,* 607–611; Bard, C. R. (1990). PMAA submission to U.S. Food and Drug Administration for IDE #G850010.

49. Aragón, I. M., Imbroda, B. H., & Lara, M. F. (2018). Cell therapy clinical trials for stress urinary incontinence: Current status and perspectives. *Int J Med Sci, 15* (3), 195–204; Lee, C. N., Jang, J. B., Kim, J. Y., Koh, C., Baek, J. Y., & Lee, K. J. (2010). Human cord blood stem cell therapy for treatment of stress urinary incontinence. *J Korean Med Sci, 25* (6), 813–816; Shin, J. H., Ryu, C. M., Yu, H. Y., Shin, D. M., & Choo, M. S. (2020). Current and future directions of stem cell therapy for bladder dysfunction. *Stem Cell Rev, 16* (1), 82–93.

50. Ridout, A. E., & Yoong, W. (2010). Tibial nerve stimulation for overactive bladder syndrome unresponsive to medical therapy. *J Obstet Gynaecol, 30*, 111–114.

51. Santos-Silva, A., da Silva, C. M., & Cruz, F. (2013). Botulinum toxin treatment for bladder dysfunction. *Int J Urol, 20* (10), 956–962; Anger, J. T., et al. (2010). Outcomes of intravesical botulinum toxin for idiopathic overactive bladder symptoms: A systematic review of the literature. *J Urol, 183*, 2258–2264.

52. Petrou, S. P., et al. (2009). Botulinum A toxin/dimethyl sulfoxide bladder instillations for women with refractory idiopathic detrusor overactivity: A phase ½ study. *Mayo Clin Proc, 84*, 702–706.

53. Burgio, K., et al. (1998). Behavioral vs. drug treatment for urge incontinence in older women: A randomized trial. *JAMA, 280* (23), 1995–2000.

54. Freedman, M., et al. (2009). Twice-weekly synthetic conjugated estrogens vaginal cream for the treatment of vaginal atrophy. *Menopause, 16*, 735–741.

Chapter 9: Sex and Menopause

1. Gavrilov, L. A., & Gavrilova, N. S. (Nov. 19, 2007). New findings on human longevity predictors. Paper presented at the annual meeting of the Gerontological Society of America, San Francisco, CA.

2. Solway, E., Clark, S., Singer, D., Kirch, M., & Malani, P. (May 2018). Let's talk about sex, national poll on healthy aging; Institute for Healthcare Policy and Innovation at the University of Michigan; https://deepblue .lib.umich.edu/bitstream/handle/2027.42/143212/NPHA-Sexual-Health -Report_050118_final.pdf.

3. Trompeter, S. E., Bettencourt, R., & Barrett-Connor, E. (2012). Sexual activity and satisfaction in healthy community-dwelling older women. *Am J Med, 125* (1), 37–43.e1.

4. Lindau, S. T., et al. (2007). A study of sexuality and health among older adults in the United States. *N Engl J Med, 357*, 762–774.

5. Hartmann, U., et al. (2004). Low sexual desire in midlife and older women: Personality factors, psychosocial development, present sexuality. *Menopause, 11* (6, part 2), 726–740.

6. Basson, R. (2004). Recent advances in women's sexual function and dysfunction. *Menopause, 11* (6, part 2), 714–725.

7. *NAMS Supplement—Update on Sexuality at Menopause and Beyond: Normative, Adaptive, Problematic, Dysfunctional.* North American Menopause Society, vol. 11, no. 6 (Nov. 2004), 708–786.

8. Bancroft, J., Loftus, J., & Long, J. S. (2003). Distress about sex: A national survey of women in heterosexual relationships. *Arch Sex Behav, 32* (3), 193–208.

9. Shifren, J., et al. (2008). Sexual problems and distress in United States women: Prevalence and correlates. *Obstet Gynecol, 112*, 970–978.

10. Wilson, D. (June 19, 2010). Drug for sexual desire disorder opposed by

panel. *New York Times,* www.nytimes.com/2010/06/19/business/19sexpill
.html.

11. Sarrel, P., & Whitehead, M. I. (1985). Sex and menopause: Defining the issues. *Maturitas, 7,* 217–224.

12. Van Lunsen, R. H., & Laan, E. (2004). Genital vascular responsiveness and sexual feelings in midlife women: Psychophysiologic, brain, and genital imaging studies. *Menopause, 11* (6, part 2), 741–748.

13. Harder, H., Starkings, R., Fallowfield, L. J., Menon, U., Jacobs, I. J., Jenkins, V. A., & UKCTOCS Trialists (2019). Sexual functioning in 4,418 postmenopausal women participating in UKCTOCS: A qualitative free-text analysis. *Menopause, 26* (10), 1100–1009.

14. Food and Drug Administration. (June 21, 2019). FDA approves new treatment for hypoactive sexual desire disorder in premenopausal women; https://www.fda.gov/news-events/press-announcements/fda-approves-new-treatment-hypoactive-sexual-desire-disorder-premenopausal-women.

15. Miller, K., & Cohen, M. (June 24, 2019). Does Vyleesi have side effects? Inside the new libido-boosting drug for women. *Prevention;* https://www.prevention.com/sex/a28168410/vyleesi-libido-drug-women.

16. Avis, N., et al. (2005). Correlates of sexual function among multi-ethnic middle-aged women: Results from the Study of Women's Health Across the Nation (SWAN). *Menopause, 12* (4), 385–398; Dennerstein, L., & Lehert, P. (2004). Women's sexual functioning, lifestyle, mid-age, and menopause in 12 European countries. *Menopause, 11* (6, part 2), 778–785.

17. Diamond, L. M. (2008). *Sexual Fluidity: Understanding Women's Love and Desire.* Cambridge, MA: Harvard University Press.

18. Brody, S. (2006). Blood pressure reactivity to stress is better for people who recently had penile-vaginal intercourse than for people who had other or no sexual activity. *Biol Psychol, 71,* 214–222.

19. Jankowski, M., et al. (2010). Anti-inflammatory effect of oxytocin in rat myocardial infarction. *Basic Res Cardiol, 105,* 205–218.

20. Raghunandan, C., et al. (Jan. 19, 2010; epub ahead of print). A comparative study of the effects of local estrogen with or without local testosterone on vulvovaginal and sexual dysfunction in postmenopausal women. *J Sex Med.*

21. Bergmark, K., et al. (1999). Vaginal changes and sexuality in women with a history of cervical cancer. *N Engl J Med, 340,* 1383–1389.

22. Savage, L. (1999). *Reclaiming Goddess Sexuality, 23.* Carlsbad, CA: Hay House.

23. Bodansky, S., & Bodansky, V. (2000). *Extended Massive Orgasm: How You Can Give and Receive Intense Sexual Pleasure.* Alameda, CA: Hunter House.

24. Love, P., & Robinson, J. (1994). *Hot Monogamy: Essential Steps to More Passionate, Intimate Lovemaking, 371.* New York: Dutton.

25. Hurlburth, D. F. (1991). The role of assertiveness in female sexuality: A comparative study between sexually assertive and sexually non-assertive women. *J Sex Marital Ther, 12,* 183–190; Hoch, Z., et al. (1981). An

evaluation of sexual performance comparison between sexually dysfunctional couples. *J Sex Marital Ther, 17,* 90–102.

26. Zussman L., et al. (1981). Sexual responses after hysterectomy-oophorectomy: Recent studies and reconsideration of psychogenesis. *Am J Obstet Gynecol, 40* (7), 725–729.

27. Bachman, G. A. (1985). Correlates of sexual desire in postmenopausal women. *Maturitas, 3,* 211.

28. Graziottin, A., & Basson, R. (2004). Sexual dysfunction in women with premature menopause. *Menopause, 11* (6, part 2), 766–777.

29. Alexander, J. L., et al. (2004). The effects of postmenopausal hormone therapies on female sexual functioning: A review of double-blind, randomized controlled trials. *Menopause, 11* (6, part 2), 749–765.

30. Sarrel, P. (1990). Sexuality and menopause. *Obstet Gynecol, 75* (suppl. 4), 26S–35S; Sarrel, P. (1982). Sex problems after menopause: A study of 50 married couples treated in a sex counseling programme. *Maturitas, 4* (4), 231–239.

31. Van Lunsen, R. H., & Laan, E. (2004). Genital vascular responsiveness and sexual feelings in midlife women: Psychophysiologic, brain, and genital imaging studies. *Menopause, 11* (6, part 2), 741–748.

32. Sarrel, P. (1990). Sexuality and menopause. *Obstet Gynecol, 75* (suppl. 4), 26S–35S.

33. Pitkin, J., & British Menopause Society Medical Advisory Council. (2018). BMS—Consensus statement. *Post Reprod Health, 24* (3), 133–138.

34. Crandall, C. J., Hovey, K. M., Andrews, C. A., Chlebowski, R. T., Stefanick, M. L., Lane, D. S., Shifren, J., Chen, C., Kaunitz, A. M., Cauley, J. A., & Manson, J. E. (2018). Breast cancer, endometrial cancer, and cardiovascular events in participants who used vaginal estrogen in the Women's Health Initiative Observational Study. *Menopause, 25* (1), 11–20; Constantine, G. D., Graham, S., Lapane, K., Ohleth, K., Bernick, B., Liu, J., & Mirkin, S. (2019). Endometrial safety of low-dose vaginal estrogens in menopausal women: A systematic evidence review. *Menopause, 26* (7), 800–807.

35. Mitchell, C. M., Reed, S. D., Diem, S., Larson, J. C., Newton, K. M., Ensrud, K. E., LaCroix, A. Z., Caan, B., & Guthrie, K. A. (2018). Efficacy of vaginal estradiol or vaginal moisturizer vs placebo for treating postmenopausal vulvovaginal symptoms: A randomized clinical trial. *JAMA Int Med, 178* (5), 681–690.

36. Filippini, M., Luvero, D., Salvatore, S., Pieralli, A., Montera, R., Plotti, F., Candiani, M., & Angioli, R. (2020). Efficacy of fractional CO2 laser treatment in postmenopausal women with genitourinary syndrome: A multicenter study. *Menopause, 27* (1), 43–49; Cruz, V. L., Steiner, M. L., Pompei, L. M., Strufaldi, R., Fonseca, F., Santiago, L., Wajsfeld, T., & Fernandes, C. E. (2018). Randomized, double-blind, placebo-controlled clinical trial for evaluating the efficacy of fractional CO2 laser compared with topical estriol in the treatment of vaginal atrophy in postmenopausal women. *Menopause, 25* (1), 21–28; Salvatore, S., Leone Roberti Maggiore, U.,

Athanasiou, S., Origoni, M., Candiani, M., Calligaro, A., & Zerbinati, N. (2015). Histological study on the effects of microablative fractional CO2 laser on atrophic vaginal tissue: An ex vivo study. *Menopause, 22* (8), 845–849.

37. Sarrel, P., et al. (1998). Estrogen and estrogen-androgen replacement in postmenopausal women dissatisfied with estrogen-only therapy. *J Reprod Med, 43* (10), 847–856; Sherwin, B., et al. (1985). Differential symptom response to parenteral estrogen and/or androgen administration in the surgical menopause. *Am J Obstet Gynecol, 151,* 153–160.

38. Davis, S. R., et al. (2008). Testosterone for low libido in postmenopausal women not taking estrogen. *N Engl J Med, 359,* 2005–2017.

39. Labrie, F., Archer, D. F., Koltun, W., Vachon, A., Young, D., Frenette, L., Portman, D., Montesino, M., Côté, I., Parent, J., Lavoie, L., Martel, C., Vaillancourt, M., Balser, J., Moyneur, É., & Members of the VVA Prasterone Research Group (2018). Efficacy of intravaginal dehydroepiandrosterone (DHEA) on moderate to severe dyspareunia and vaginal dryness, symptoms of vulvovaginal atrophy, and of the genitourinary syndrome of menopause. *Menopause, 25* (11), 1339–1353; Labrie, F., Derogatis, L., Archer, D. F., Koltun, W., Vachon, A., Young, D., Frenette, L., Portman, D., Montesino, M., Côté, I., Parent, J., Lavoie, L., Beauregard, A., Martel, C., Vaillancourt, M., Balser, J., Moyneur, É., & Members of the VVA Prasterone Research Group (2015). Effect of intravaginal prasterone on sexual dysfunction in postmenopausal women with vulvovaginal atrophy. *The Journal of Sexual Medicine, 12* (12), 2401–2412; Martel, C., Labrie, F., Archer, D. F., Ke, Y., Gonthier, R., Simard, J. N., Lavoie, L., Vaillancourt, M., Montesino, M., Balser, J., Moyneur, É., & Other Participating Members of the Prasterone Clinical Research Group (2016). Serum steroid concentrations remain within normal postmenopausal values in women receiving daily 6.5 mg intravaginal prasterone for 12 weeks. *J Steroid Biochem Mol Biol, 159,* 142–153.

40. Love, P., & Robinson, J. (1994). *Hot Monogamy: Essential Steps to More Passionate, Intimate Lovemaking,* 73–76. New York: Dutton; commenting on the study of Schreiner-Engel, P. (1981). Sexual arousability and the menstrual cycle. *Psychosom Med, 43,* 1999–2212.

41. Idso, C. (2009). Sexually transmitted infection prevention in newly single older women: A forgotten health promotion need. *J Nurse Practitioners, 5,* 440–446.

42. American Cancer Society. (July 21, 2020). HPV vaccines. www.cancer.org /cancer/cancer-causes/infectious-agents/hpv/hpv-vaccines.html.

43. Slade, B. A., Leidel, L., Vellozzi, C., Woo, E. J., Hua, W., Sutherland, A., Izurieta, H. S., Ball, R., Miller, N., Braun, M. M., Markowitz, L. E., & Iskander, J. (2009). Postlicensure safety surveillance for quadrivalent human papillomavirus recombinant vaccine. *JAMA, 302* (7), 750–757.

44. Australian Institute of Health and Welfare. (2020). *Cancer Data in Australia.* https://www.aihw.gov.au/reports/cancer/cancer-data-in-australia.

45. Noone, A. M., Howlader, N., Krapcho, M., Miller, D., Brest, A., Yu, M., Ruhl, J., Tatalovich, Z., Mariotto, A., Lewis, D. R., Chen, H. S., Feuer,

E. J., & Cronin, K. A. (eds.). *SEER Cancer Statistics Review, 1975–2015*. National Cancer Institute. Bethesda, MD, https://seer.cancer.gov/csr/1975 _2015, based on November 2017 SEER data submission, posted to the SEER website, April 2018; https://seer.cancer.gov/statfacts/html/cervix.html.

46. Martínez-Lavín, M., & Amezcua-Guerra, L. (2017). Serious adverse events after HPV vaccination: A critical review of randomized trials and post-marketing case series. *Clin Rheumatol, 36* (10), 2169–2178; Inbar, R., Weiss, R., Tomljenovic, L., Arango, M. T., Deri, Y., Shaw, C. A., Chapman, J., Blank, M., & Shoenfeld, Y. (2017). Behavioral abnormalities in female mice following administration of aluminum adjuvants and the human papillomavirus (HPV) vaccine Gardasil. *Immunol Res, 65* (1), 136–149; Tomljenovic, L., Spinosa, J. P., & Shaw, C. A. (2013). Human papillomavirus (HPV) vaccines as an option for preventing cervical malignancies: (How) effective and safe? *Curr Pharm Des, 19* (8), 1466–1487; Joelving, F. (December 17, 2017). What the Gardasil testing may have missed. *Slate,* https://slate.com/health-and-science/2017/12/flaws-in-the -clinical-trials-for-gardasil-made-it-harder-to-properly-assess-safety.html.

47. Wright, T. C., Jr, Stoler, M. H., Behrens, C. M., Apple, R., Derion, T., & Wright, T. L. (2012). The ATHENA human papillomavirus study: Design, methods, and baseline results. *Am J Obstet Gynecol, 206* (1), 46.e1–46.e11.

48. Guo, F., Hirth, J. M., & Berenson, A. B. (2015). Comparison of HPV prevalence between HPV-vaccinated and non-vaccinated young adult women (20–26 years). *Hum Vaccines Immunother, 11* (10), 2337–2344.

49. Harper, D. M., Vierthaler, S. L., & Santee, J. A. (2010). Review of Gardasil. *J Vaccines Vacc, 1* (107), 1000107.

50. From a documentary called *One More Girl* from ThinkExist Films that is now in postproduction; to see the clip with this information, visit https:// youtu.be/sSdCxgF0blc.

51. Love, P., & Robinson, J. (1994). *Hot Monogamy: Essential Steps to More Passionate, Intimate Lovemaking,* 234–235. New York: Dutton.

Chapter 10: Nurturing Your Brain

1. Bliwise, D. L., et al. (1992). Prevalence of self-reported poor sleep in a healthy population age 50–65. *Soc Sci Med, 34* (49), 49.

2. Walsh, J. K., et al. (1992). Insomnia. In S. Chokroverty (ed.), *Sleep Disorders Medicine: A Comprehensive Textbook* (100). Stoneham, MA: Butterworth.

3. Grandner, M., Mullington, J. M., Hashmi, S. D., Redeker, N. S., Watson, N. F., & Morgenthaler, T. I. (2018). Sleep duration and hypertension: Analysis of > 700,000 adults by age and sex. *J Clin Sleep Med, 14* (6), 1031–1039.

4. Reutrakul, S., & Van Cauter, E. (2018). Sleep influences on obesity, insulin resistance, and risk of type 2 diabetes. *Metab Clin Exp, 84,* 56–66.

5. Watson, N. F., Buchwald, D., Delrow, J. J., Altemeier, W. A., Vitiello,

M. V., Pack, A. I., Bamshad, M., Noonan, C., & Gharib, S. A. (2017). Transcriptional signatures of sleep duration discordance in monozygotic twins. *Sleep, 40* (1), zsw019.

6. Gottlieb, D. J., Somers, V. K., Punjabi, N. M., & Winkelman, J. W. (2017). Restless legs syndrome and cardiovascular disease: A research roadmap. *Sleep Med, 31,* 10–17; May, A. M., Van Wagoner, D. R., & Mehra, R. (2017). OSA and cardiac arrhythmogenesis: Mechanistic insights. *Chest, 151* (1), 225–241.

7. Lyall, L. M., Wyse, C. A., Graham, N., Ferguson, A., Lyall, D. M., Cullen, B., Celis Morales, C. A., Biello, S. M., Mackay, D., Ward, J., Strawbridge, R. J., Gill, J., Bailey, M., Pell, J. P., & Smith, D. J. (2018). Association of disrupted circadian rhythmicity with mood disorders, subjective well-being, and cognitive function: A cross-sectional study of 91,105 participants from the UK Biobank. *Lancet Psychiatry, 5* (6), 507–514.

8. Pillai, J. A., & Leverenz, J. B. (2017). Sleep and neurodegeneration: A critical appraisal. *Chest, 151* (6), 1375–1386; Sprecher, K. E., Koscik, R. L., Carlsson, C. M., Zetterberg, H., Blennow, K., Okonkwo, O. C., Sager, M. A., Asthana, S., Johnson, S. C., Benca, R. M., & Bendlin, B. B. (2017). Poor sleep is associated with CSF biomarkers of amyloid pathology in cognitively normal adults. *Neurology, 89* (5), 445–453.

9. Gangwisch, J. E., et al. (2005). Inadequate sleep as a risk factor for obesity: Analyses of the NHANES I. *Sleep, 28,* 1289–1296.

10. Wild, C. J., Nichols, E. S., Battista, M. E., Stojanoski, B., & Owen, A. M. (2018). Dissociable effects of self-reported daily sleep duration on high-level cognitive abilities. *Sleep, 41* (12), zsy182.

11. Rapkin, A., et al. (1997). Progesterone metabolite allopregnenolone in women with premenstrual syndrome. *Obstet Gynecol, 90* (5), 709–714.

12. Mousa, H. A. (2016). Health effects of alkaline diet and water, reduction of digestive-tract bacterial load, and earthing. *Altern Ther Health Med, 22* (Suppl 1), 24–33.

13. Menigoz, W., Latz, T. T., Ely, R. A., Kamei, C., Melvin, G., & Sinatra, D. (2020). Integrative and lifestyle medicine strategies should include earthing (grounding): Review of research evidence and clinical observations. *Explore (NY), 16* (3), 152–160.

14. Chevalier, G., Patel, S., Weiss, L., Chopra, D., & Mills, P. J. (2019). The effects of grounding (earthing) on bodyworkers' pain and overall quality of life: A randomized controlled trial. *Explore NY, 15* (3), 181–190.

15. Cowden, W. L., Saenz, A., & Icaza, J. (Sept. 4–Oct. 21, 2005). The treatment of insomnia in patients of 4 hospitals in Guayaquil, Ecuador, using two novel herbal extracts: A double-blind, randomized, multiple cross-over, placebo controlled, multicenter study. Unpublished study sponsored by Nutramedix LLC and Bionatus S. A. in Guayaquil, Ecuador; www.bionatus.com/nutramedix/pages/moreinfo_babuna.html.

16. Leathwood, P. D., et al. (1985). Aqueous extract of valerian root (*Valeriana officinalis* L.) reduces latency to fall asleep in man. *Planta Med, 54,* 144–148.

17. Murray, M. (1998). *5-HTP: The Natural Way to Overcome Depression, Obesity, and Insomnia.* New York: Bantam Books.

18. Holm, E., Staedt, U., Heep, J., Kortsik, C., Behne, F., Kaske, A., & Mennicke, I. (1991). *Untersuchungen zum Wirkungsprofil von D, L-Kavain: Zerebrale Angriffsorte und Schlaf-Wach-Rhythmus im Tier-experiment.* [The action profile of D, L-kavain: Cerebral sites and sleep-wakefulness rhythm in animals.] *Arzneimittelforschung, 41* (7), 673–683; ANPA Committee on Research (2000). The use of herbal alternative medicines in neuropsychiatry: A report of the ANPA Committee on Research. *J Neuropsychiatry Clin Neurosci, 12,* 177–192.

19. McKinlay, J. B., et al. (1987). The relative contribution of endocrine changes and social circumstances to depression in mid-aged women. *J Health Soc Behav, 28,* 345–363; Woods, N. F., & Mitchell, E. S. (1996). Patterns of depressed mood in midlife women: Observations from the Seattle Midlife Women's Health Study. *Res Nurs Health, 19* (2), 111–123; Martinsen, E. W. (1990). Benefits of exercise for the treatment of depression. *Sports Med, 9* (6), 380–389; Morgan, J., et al. (1970). Psychological effects of chronic physical activity. *Med Sci Sports, 2* (4), 213–217; Kessler, R. C., et al. (1993). Sex and depression in the National Comorbidity Survey. I: Lifetime prevalence, chronicity and recurrence. *J Affect Disord, 29,* 85.

20. Pratt, L. (1996). Depression, psychotropic medication and risk of myocardial infarction. *Circulation, 94* (12), 3123–3129; Michelson, D., et al. (1996). Bone mineral density in women with depression. *N Engl J Med, 335,* 1176–1181; Denollet, J., et al. (1996). Personality as independent predictor of long-term mortality in patients with coronary heart disease. *Lancet, 347,* 417–421; Frasure-Smith, N., Lesperance, F., & Talajic, M. (1995). Depression and 18-month prognosis after myocardial infarction. *Circulation, 91* (4), 999–1005.

21. Sarno, J. (1991). *Healing Back Pain: The Mind-Body Connection,* 26–27. New York: Warner Books; Shealy, N. (1995). *Miracles Do Happen* (250). Rockport, MA: Element Books.

22. Woods, N. F., Mitchell, E. S., & Adams, C. (2000). Memory functioning among midlife women: Observations from the Seattle Midlife Women's Health Study. *Menopause, 7* (4), 257–265.

23. Denollet, J., et al. (2009). Anxiety predicted premature all-cause and cardiovascular death in a 10-year follow-up of middle-aged women. *J Clin Epidemiol, 62,* 452–456.

24. Felitti, V. J., Anda, R. F., Nordenberg, D., Williamson, D. F., Spitz, A. M., Edwards, V., Koss, M. P., & Marks, J. S. (1998). Relationship of childhood abuse and household dysfunction to many of the leading causes of death in adults. The Adverse Childhood Experiences (ACE) Study. *Am J Prev Med, 14* (4), 245–258.

25. Aleem, F. A. (1985). Menopausal syndrome: Plasma levels of beta-endorphin in postmenopausal women measured by a specific radioimmunoassay. *Maturitas, 7,* 329–334; Genazzani, A. R., et al. (1988). Steroid replace-

ment treatment increases beta-endorphin and beta-lipotropin plasma levels in postmenopausal women. *Gynecol Obstet Invest, 26,* 153–159.

26. Roca, C. A., et al. (1999). Gonadal steroids and affective illness. *Neuroscientist, 5* (4), 227–237; Halbreich, U. (1997). Role of estrogen in postmenopausal depression. *Neurology, 48* (5, suppl. 7), S16–S20.

27. Garcia-Segura, L. M., et al. (1996). Effect of sex steroids on brain cells. In B. G. Wren (ed.), *Progress in the Management of the Menopause. The Proceedings of the 9th International Congress on the Menopause, Sydney, Australia,* 278–285. New York: Parthenon Publishing.

28. Smoller, J. W., et al. (2009). Antidepressant use and risk of incident cardiovascular morbidity and mortality among postmenopausal women in the women's health initiative study. *Arch Intern Med, 169,* 2128–2139.

29. Turner, E. H., et al. (2008). Selective publication of antidepressant trials and its influence on apparent efficacy. *N Engl J Med, 358,* 252–260.

30. Fournier, J. C., et al. (2010). Antidepressant drug effects and depression severity: A patient-level meta-analysis. *JAMA, 303,* 47–53.

31. Pert, C. B. (Oct. 20, 1997). Letter to the editor. *Time, 150* (16).

32. Doogan, D. P., & Caillard, V. (1992). Sertraline in the prevention of depression. *Br J Psychiatry, 160,* 217–222; Eric, L. (1991). A prospective, double-blind, comparative, multicenter study of paroxitine and placebo preventing recurrent major depressive episodes. *Biol Psychiatry, 29* (suppl. 1), 254S–255S.

33. Young, R. J. (1979). Effect of regular exercise on cognitive functioning and personality. *Br J Sports Med, 13* (3), 110–117; Gutin, B. (1966). Effect of increase in physical fitness on mental ability following physical and mental stress. *Res Q, 37* (2), 211–220.

34. Hamer, M., Stamatakis, E., & Steptoe, A. (2009). Dose response relationship between physical activity and mental health: The Scottish Health Survey. *Br J Sports Med, 43,* 14, 1111–1114.

35. Rehfeld, K., Müller, P., Aye, N., Schmicker, M., Dordevic, M., Kaufmann, J., Hökelmann, A., & Müller, N. G. (2017). Dancing or fitness sport? The effects of two training programs on hippocampal plasticity and balance abilities in healthy seniors. *Front Hum Neurosci, 11,* 305.

36. Delextrat, A. A., Warner, S., Graham, S., & Neupert, E. (2016). An 8-week exercise intervention based on Zumba improves aerobic fitness and psychological well-being in healthy women. *J Phys Act Health, 13* (2), 131–139; Norouzi, E., Hosseini, F., Vaezmosavi, M., Gerber, M., Pühse, U., & Brand, S. (2019). Zumba dancing and aerobic exercise can improve working memory, motor function, and depressive symptoms in female patients with fibromyalgia. *Eur J Sport Sci,* 1–11 (advance online publication).

37. Meeusen, R., & De Meirleir, K. (1995). Exercise and brain neurotransmission. *Sports Med, 20* (3), 160–188.

38. Crippa, J. A., Guimarães, F. S., Campos, A. C., & Zuardi, A. W. (2018). Translational investigation of the therapeutic potential of cannabidiol (CBD): Toward a new age. *Front Immunol, 9,* 2009.

39. Lesperance, F., et al. (2009). The efficacy of eicosapentaenoic acid for major depression: Results of the OMEGA-3D trial, 9th World Congress

of Biological Psychiatry, Abstract FC-25-005. Presented July 1, 2009, in Paris, France; www.wfsbp-congress.org/fileadmin/user_upload/WFSBP _Final_Programme_090625.pdf.

40. Coppen, A. (1967). The biochemistry of affective disorders. *Br J Psychiatry, 113,* 1237–1264; Stewart, J. W., et al. (1984). Low B6 levels in depressed outpatients. *Biol Psychiatry, 19* (4), 613–616; Hall, R. C. W., & Joffe, J. R. (1973). Hypomagnesemia: Physical and psychiatric symptoms. *JAMA, 224* (13), 1749–1751; Lieb, J., Karmali, R., & Horrobin, D. (1983). Elevated levels of prostaglandin E2 and thromboxane B2 in depression. *Prostaglandins Leukot Med, 10* (4), 361–367.

41. Fux, M., Levine, J., Aviv, A., & Belmaker, R. H. (1996). Inositol treatment of obsessive-compulsive disorder. *Am J Psychiatry, 153* (9), 1219–1221; Levine, J., et al. (1995). Double-blind, controlled trial of inositol treatment of depression. *Am J Psychiatry, 152,* 792–794.

42. DeVenna, M., & Rigamoni, R. (1992). Oral S-adenosyl-L-methionine in depression. *Curr Ther Res, 52,* 478–485; Di Benedetto, P., et al. (1993). Clinical evaluation of S-adenosyl-L-methionine versus transcutaneous electrical nerve stimulation in primary fibromyalgia. *Curr Ther Res, 53,* 222–229; Muskin, P. R., ed. (2000). *Complementary and Alternative Medicine and Psychiatry (Review of Psychiatry).* (Vol. 19, 8–18). Washington, DC: American Psychiatric Association Press; Shehin, V. O., et al. (1990). SAM-e in adult ADHD. *Psychopharmacol Bull, 25,* 249–253.

43. Boldrini, M., Fulmore, C. A., Tartt, A. N., Simeon, L. R., Pavlova, I., Poposka, V., Rosoklija, G. B., Stankov, A., Arango, V., Dwork, A. J., Hen, R., & Mann, J. J. (2018). Human hippocampal neurogenesis persists throughout aging. *Cell Stem Cell, 22* (4), 589–599.e5; Moreno-Jiménez, E. P., Flor-García, M., Terreros-Roncal, J., Rábano, A., Cafini, F., Pallas-Bazarra, N., Ávila, J., & Llorens-Martín, M. (2019). Adult hippocampal neurogenesis is abundant in neurologically healthy subjects and drops sharply in patients with Alzheimer's disease. *Nature Med, 25* (4), 554–560.

44. Peters R. (2006). Ageing and the brain. *Postgrad Med J, 82* (964), 84–88.

45. Maguire, E. A., Woollett, K., & Spiers, H. J. (2006). London taxi drivers and bus drivers: A structural MRI and neuropsychological analysis. *Hippocampus, 16* (12), 1091–1101; Woollett, K., Spiers, H. J., & Maguire, E. A. (2009). Talent in the taxi: A model system for exploring expertise. *Philos Trans R Soc Lond B Biol Sci, 364* (1522), 1407–1416.

46. Gould, E., et al. (1999). Learning enhances adult neurogenesis in the hippocampal formation. *Nature Neurosci, 2,* 260–265.

47. Greendale, G. A., et al. (2009). Effects of the menopause transition and hormone use on cognitive performance in midlife women. *Neurology, 72,* 1850–1857.

48. Evans, P. H. (1991). Cephaloconiosis: A free radical perspective on the proposed particulate-induced etiopathogenesis of Alzheimer's dementia and related disorders. *Med Hypotheses, 34* (3), 209–219.

49. Mittal, K., & Katare, D. P. (2016). Shared links between type 2 diabetes mellitus and Alzheimer's disease: A review. *Diabetes Metab Syndr, 10* (2, suppl. 1), S144–S149; Barbagallo, M., & Dominguez, L. J. (2014). Type 2

diabetes mellitus and Alzheimer's disease. *World J Diabetes, 5* (6), 889–893; de la Monte, S. M., & Wands, J. R. (2008); Alzheimer's disease is type 3 diabetes—evidence reviewed. *J Diabetes Sci Tech, 2* (6), 1101–1113; Kandimalla, R., Thirumala, V., & Reddy, P. H. (2017). Is Alzheimer's disease a type 3 diabetes? A critical appraisal. *Biochim Biophys Acta, 1863* (5), 1078–1089.

50. Martens, Y. A., Linares, C., Knight, J. A., Painter, M. M., Sullivan, P. M., & Bu, G. (2017). Apolipoprotein E4 impairs neuronal insulin signaling by trapping insulin receptor in the endosomes. *Neuron, 96* (1), 115–129.e5.

51. Ekblad, L. L., Johansson, J., Helin, S., Viitanen, M., Laine, H., Puukka, P., Jula, A., & Rinne, J. O. (2018). Midlife insulin resistance, *APOE* genotype, and late-life brain amyloid accumulation. *Neurology, 90* (13), e1150–e1157.

52. Freedman, M., et al. (1984). Computerized axial tomography in aging. In M. L. L. Albert (ed.), *Clinical Neurology of Aging.* New York: Oxford University Press; Lehr, J., & Schmitz-Scherzer, R. (1976). Survivors and non-survivors: Two fundamental patterns of aging. In H. Thomae (ed.), *Patterns of Aging: Findings from the Bonn Longitudinal Study of Aging.* Basel: S. Karger; Benton, M. L., et al. (1981). Normative observations on neuropsychological test performance in old age. *J Clin Neuropsychiatry, 3,* 33–42.

53. Boyle, P. A., et al. (2010). Effect of a purpose in life on risk of incident Alzheimer disease and mild cognitive impairment in community-dwelling older persons. *Arch Gen Psychiatry, 67* (3), 304–310.

54. 2020 Alzheimer's disease facts and figures. (2020). *Alzheimers Dement,* doi: 10.1002/alz.12068; www.alz.org/media/Documents/alzheimers-facts-and-figures-infographic.pdf.

55. Applewhite, A. (2019). *This Chair Rocks: A Manifesto Against Ageism,* 4. New York: Celadon Books.

56. Plassman, B. L., et al. (2007). Prevalence of dementia in the United States: The aging, demographics and memory study. *Neuroepidemiology, 29,* 125–132.

57. Nash, J. M. (July 24, 2000). The new science of Alzheimer's. *Time, 156* (4), 51.

58. Snowdon, D., et al. (1996). Linguistic ability in early life and cognitive function and Alzheimer's disease in late life: Findings from the Nun Study. *JAMA, 275* (7), 528–532; Snowdon, D., et al. (1997). Brain infarction and the clinical expression of Alzheimer's disease: The Nun Study. *JAMA, 277* (10), 813–817.

59. Wilson, R. S., et al. (2010). Cognitive activity and the cognitive morbidity of Alzheimer disease. *Neurology, 75,* 990–996.

60. Jefferson, A. L. (2010). Cardiac index is associated with brain aging: The Framingham heart study. *Circulation, 122,* 690–697; Jefferson, A. L. (2010). Cardiac output as a potential risk factor for abnormal brain aging. *Journal of Alzheimer's Disease, 20,* 813–821.

61. Baldereschi, M., et al. (1998). Estrogen replacement therapy and Alzheimer's disease in the Italian Longitudinal Study on Aging. *Neurology, 50,* 996–1002; Kawas, C., et al. (1997). A prospective study of estro-

gen replacement therapy and the risk of developing Alzheimer's disease: The Baltimore Longitudinal Study of Aging. *Neurology, 48,* 1517–1521; Paganini-Hill, A., & Henderson, V. W. (1996). Estrogen replacement therapy and risk of Alzheimer's disease. *Arch Intern Med, 156* (19), 2213–2217; Tang, M. X., et al. (1996). Effect of œstrogen during menopause on risk and age at onset of Alzheimer's disease. *Lancet, 358,* 429–432; Ohkura, V., et al. (1994). Evaluation of estrogen treatment in female patients with dementia of Alzheimer's type. *Endocrinol J, 41,* 361–371; Henderson, V., et al. (1994). Estrogen replacement therapy in older women: Comparisons between Alzheimer's disease cases and nondemented control subjects. *Arch Neurol, 51,* 896–900; Paganini-Hill, A., et al. (1994). Estrogen deficiency and risk of Alzheimer's disease in women. *Am J Epidemiol, 140,* 256–261; Brenner, D. E., et al. (1994). Postmenopausal estrogen replacement therapy on the risk of Alzheimer's disease: A population-based case control study. *Am J Epidemiol, 140,* 262–267; Honjo, H., et al. (1993). An effect of conjugated estrogen to cognitive impairment in women with senile dementia, Alzheimer's type: A placebo-controlled double-blind study. *J Jpn Menopause Soc, 1,* 167–171; Kantor, H., et al. (1973). Estrogen for older women. *Am J Obstet Gynecol, 116,* 115–118; Caldwell, B. M. (1954). An evaluation of psychological effects of sex hormone administration in aged women. *J Gerontol, 9,* 168–174.

62. McEwen, B. S., et al. (1999). Inhibition of dendritic spine induction on hippocampal ca-1 pyramidal neurons by nonsteroidal estrogen antagonists in female rats. *Endocrinol, 140,* 1044–1047.

63. Manly, J. J., et al. (2000). Endogenous estrogen levels and Alzheimer's disease among postmenopausal women. *Neurology, 54,* 833–837.

64. Baldereschi, M., et al. (1998). Estrogen replacement therapy and Alzheimer's disease in the Italian Longitudinal Study on Aging. *Neurology, 50,* 996–1002; Schneider, L. S., et al. (1996). Effects of estrogen replacement therapy on response to tacrine in patients with Alzheimer's disease. *Neurology, 46,* 1580–1584; Brinton, R. D., et al. (1997). 17-beta-estradiol increases the growth and survival of cultured cortical neurons. *Neurochem Res, 22,* 1339–1351; Brinton, R. D., et al. (1997). Equilin, a principal component of the estrogen replacement therapy Premarin, increases the growth of cortical neurons via an NMDA receptor-dependent mechanism. *Exp Neurol, 147,* 211–220; Matsumoto, A., et al. (1985). Estrogen stimulates neuronal plasticity in the deafferented hypothalamic arculate nucleus in aged female rats. *Neurosci Res, 2,* 412–418; Okhura, T., et al. (1995). Estrogen increases cerebral and cerebellar blood flow in postmenopausal women. *Menopause, 2,* 13–18; Singh, M., et al. (1994). Ovarian steroid deprivation results in a reversible learning impairment and compromised cholinergic function in female Sprague-Dawley rats. *Brain Res, 644,* 305–312; Singh, M., et al. (1996). The effect of ovariectomy and estradiol replacement on brain derived neurotrophic factor messenger hippocampal brain expression in cortical and hippocampal brain regions of female Sprague-Dawley rats. *Endocrinology, 136,* 2320–2324.

65. Rivera, C. M., et al. (2009). Increased mortality for neurological and mental diseases following early bilateral oophorectomy. *Neuroepidemiology, 33*, 32–40.

66. Sherwin, B. (1997). Estrogen effects of cognition in menopausal women. *Neurology, 48* (suppl. 7), S21–S26.

67. McEwen, B. S., & Wooley, C. S. (1994). Estradiol and progesterone regulate neuronal structure and synaptic connectivity in adult as well as developing brain. *Exp Gerontol, 29,* 431–436; Wooley, C. S., & McEwen, B. S. (1993). Roles of estradiol and progesterone in regulation of hippocampal dendritic spine density during the estrous cycle in the rat. *J Comp Neurol, 336,* 293–306.

68. Loucks, T. L., & Berga, S. L. (2009). Does postmenopausal estrogen use confer neuroprotection? *Semin Reprod Med, 27,* 260–274.

69. McLaughlin, I. J., et al. (1990). Zinc in depressive disorder. *Acta Psychiatr Scand, 82,* 451–453.

70. Shaw, D. M., et al. (1988). Senile dementia and nutrition [letter]. *BMJ, 288,* 792–793.

71. Gibson, Q. E., et al. (1988). Reduced activities of thiamine dependent enzymes in the brains and peripheral tissues of patients with Alzheimer's disease. *Arch Neurol, 45,* 836–840.

72. Strachan, R. N., & Henderson, J. G. (1967). Dementia and folate deficiency. *Q J Med, 36,* 189–204; Perkins. A. J., et al. (1999). Association of antioxidants and memory in multiethnic elderly sample using the Third National Health and Nutrition Examination Study. *Am J Epidemiol, 150,* 37–44.

73. Knekt, P., et al. (2010). Serum vitamin D and the risk of Parkinson disease. *Arch Neurol, 67,* 808–811.

74. Feart, C., Helmer, C., Merle, B., Herrmann, F. R., Annweiler, C., Dartigues, J. F., Delcourt, C., & Samieri, C. (2017). Associations of lower vitamin D concentrations with cognitive decline and long-term risk of dementia and Alzheimer's disease in older adults. *Alzheimers Dement, 13* (11), 1207–1216.

75. Chai, B., Gao, F., Wu, R., Dong, T., Gu, C., Lin, Q., & Zhang, Y. (2019). Vitamin D deficiency as a risk factor for dementia and Alzheimer's disease: An updated meta-analysis. *BMC Neurol, 19* (1), 284.

76. Rovio, S., et al. (2005). Leisure-time physical activity at midlife and the risk of dementia and Alzheimer's disease. *Lancet Neurol, 4* (11), 705–711.

77. Morris, J. K., Vidoni, E. D., Johnson, D. K., Van Sciver, A., Mahnken, J. D., Honea, R. A., Wilkins, H. M., Brooks, W. M., Billinger, S. A., Swerdlow, R. H., & Burns, J. M. (2017). Aerobic exercise for Alzheimer's disease: A randomized controlled pilot trial. *PloS One, 12* (2), e0170547; Farina, N., Rusted, J., & Tabet, N. (2014). The effect of exercise interventions on cognitive outcome in Alzheimer's disease: A systematic review. *Int Psychogeriatrics, 26* (1), 9–18; Elwood, P., Galante, J., Pickering, J., Palmer, S., Bayer, A., Ben-Shlomo, Y., Longley, M., & Gallacher, J. (2013). Healthy lifestyles reduce the incidence of chronic diseases and dementia: Evidence from the Caerphilly cohort study. *PloS One, 8* (12), e81877;

Abe K. (2012). Total daily physical activity and the risk of AD and cognitive decline in older adults. *Neurology, 79* (10), 1071; Erickson, K. I., & Kramer, A. F. (2009). Aerobic exercise effects on cognitive and neural plasticity in older adults. *Br J Sports Med, 43,* 22–24; Liu-Ambrose, T., et al. (2008). Otago home-based strength and balance retraining improves executive functioning in older fallers: A randomized controlled trial. *J Am Geriatr Soc, 56,* 1821–1830; M. Angevaren et al. (July 16, 2008). Physical activity and enhanced fitness to improve cognitive function in older people without known cognitive impairment. *Cochrane Database of System Reviews, 2,* CD005381.

78. Jia, R. X., Liang, J. H., Xu, Y., & Wang, Y. Q. (2019). Effects of physical activity and exercise on the cognitive function of patients with Alzheimer disease: A meta-analysis. *BMC Geriatrics, 19* (1), 181.

79. Petrovitch, H., & White, L. (2005). Exercise and cognitive function. *Lancet Neurol, 4* (11), 690–691.

80. McDermott, O., Crellin, N., Ridder, H. M., & Orrell, M. (2013). Music therapy in dementia: A narrative synthesis systematic review. *Int J Geriatric Psychiatry, 28* (8), 781–794.

81. van der Meer, A., & van der Weel, F. (2017). Only three fingers write, but the whole brain works: A high-density EEG study showing advantages of drawing over typing for learning. *Front Psychol, 8,* 706.

82. Hoffman and Herbert (1990). Beware of cold remedies in the elderly. *Courtlandt Forum,* 28–41.

83. Lim, S. Y., & Suzuki, H. (2000). Intakes of dietary docosahexaenoic acid ethyl ester and egg phosphatidylcholine improve maze-learning ability in young and old mice. *J Nutr, 130* (6), 1629–1632; Gamoh, S., et al. (1999). Chronic administration of docosahexaenoic acid improves reference memory-related learning ability in young rats. *Neuroscience, 93* (1), 237–241; Calon, F., et al. (2004). Docosahexaenoic acid protects from dendritic pathology in an Alzheimer's disease mouse model. *Neuron, 43* (5), 633–645.

84. Kalmijn, S., et al. (2004). Dietary intake of fatty acids and fish in relation to cognitive performance at middle age. *Neurology, 62* (2), 275–280.

85. He, F. J., et al. (2006). Fruit and vegetable consumption and stroke: Meta-analysis of cohort studies. *Lancet, 367,* 320–326.

86. Sawatsri, S., Yamkunthong, W. and Sidell, N. (2004). Development of *Pueraria mirifica* (Thai herb) for ERT and inhibits neurotoxic in Alzheimer's model in vitro. *J Med Assoc Thai, 87* (3), S272.

87. Anukulthanakorn, K., Parhar, I. S., Jaroenporn, S., Kitahashi, T., Watanbe, G., & Malaivijitnond, S. (2016). Neurotherapeutic effects of *Pueraria mirifica* extract in early- and late-stage cognitive impaired rats. *Phytother Res, 30* (6), 929–39, doi: 10.1002/ptr.5595.

88. Rubio, J., Dang, H., Gong, M., Liu, X., Chen, S. L., & Gonzales, G. F. (2007). Aqueous and hydroalcoholic extracts of black maca (*Lepidium meyenii*) improve scopolamine-induced memory impairment in mice. *Food Chem Toxicol, 45* (10), 1882–1890.

89. Wang, R., Yan, H., & Tang, X. C. (2006). Progress in studies of huperzine

A, a natural cholinesterase inhibitor from Chinese herbal medicine. *Acta Pharmacol Sin, 27* (1), 1–26.

90. Pan, Y., et al. (2000). Soy phytoestrogens improve radial arm maze performance in ovariectomized retired breeder rats and do not attenuate benefits of 17-beta-estradiol treatment. *Menopause, 7* (4), 230–235; Kim, H., et al. (2000). Attenuation of neurodegeneration-relevant modifications of brain proteins by dietary soy. *Biofactors, 12* (1–4), 243–250. Review.

91. Pan, Y., et al. (1999). Effect of estradiol and soy phytoestrogens on choline acetyltransferase and nerve growth factor mRNAs in the frontal cortex and hippocampus of female rats. *Proc Soc Exp Biol Med, 221* (2), 118–125.

92. Zeng, H., Chen, Q., & Zhao, B. (2004). Genistein ameliorates beta-amyloid peptide (25–35)-induced hippocampal neuronal apoptosis. *Free Radic Biol Med, 36* (2), 180–188; Sonee, M., Sum, T., Wang, C., & Mukherjee, S. K. (2004). The soy isoflavone, genistein, protects human cortical neuronal cells from oxidative stress. *Neurotoxicology, 25* (5), 885–891.

93. File, S. E., et al. (2001). Eating soya improves human memory. *Psychopharmacology (Berl), 157* (4), 430–436.

94. File, S. E., et al. (2005). Cognitive improvement after 6 weeks of soy supplements in postmenopausal women is limited to frontal lobe function. *Menopause, 12* (2), 193–201.

95. Kritz-Silverstein, D., Von Muhlen, D., Barrett-Connor, E., & Bressel, M. A. (2003). Isoflavones and cognitive function in older women: The Soy and Postmenopausal Health In Aging (SOPHIA) Study. *Menopause, 10* (3), 196–202.

96. Refat, S. L., et al. (1990). Effect of exposure of miners to aluminum powder. *Lancet, 336,* 1162–1165.

97. Exley C. (2020). An aluminium adjuvant in a vaccine is an acute exposure to aluminium. *J Trace Elem Med Biol, 57,* 57–59; Exley, C., Schley, L., Murray, S., Hackney, C. M., & Birchall, J. D. (1995). Aluminium, beta-amyloid and non-enzymatic glycosylation. *FEBS Lett, 364* (2), 182–184.

98. Council on Scientific Affairs (1985). Aspartame: Review on safety issues. *JAMA, 254* (3), 400–402; U.S. Department of Health and Human Services (1980). *Decision of the Public Board of Inquiry* (DHHS docket 75F-0335). Rockville, MD: Food and Drug Administration; Wurtman, R. J. (1983). Neurochemical changes following high-dose aspartame with dietary carbohydrates. *N Engl J Med, 309,* 429–430; Yokogoshi, H., et al. (1984). Effects of aspartame and glucose administration on brain and plasma levels of large neutral amino acids and brain 5-hydroxyindoles. *Am J Clin Nutr, 40* (1), 1–7; Aspartame Consumer Safety Network, P.O. Box 780634, Dallas, TX 75378. Tel: 214–352–4268.

99. McEwen, B. S., et al. (1999). Inhibition of dendritic spine induction on hippocampal ca-1 pyramidal neurons by nonsteroidal estrogen antagonists in female rats. *Endocrinol, 140,* 1044–1047.

100. Levy, B. R., Slade, M. D., Kunkel, S. R., & Kasl, S. V. (2002). Longevity increased by positive self-perceptions of aging. *J Pers Soc Psychol, 83* (2), 261–270.

101. Connor, J. R., Melone, J. H., & Yuen, A. R. (1981). Dendritic length in aged rats' occipital cortex: An environmentally induced response. *Experimental Neurology, 73* (3), 827–830; Connor, J. R., Diamond, M. C., & Johnson, R. E. (1980). Aging and environmental influences on two types of dendritic spines in the rat occipital cortex. *Exp Neurol, 70* (2), 371–379.

102. Eriksson, P., et al. (1998). Neurogenesis in the adult human hippocampus. *Nature Med, 4* (11), 1313–1317.

103. Diamond, M., et al. (1985). Plasticity in the 904-day male rat cerebral cortex. *Exp Neurol, 87,* 309–317.

104. Yaffe, K., et al. (2010). Posttraumatic stress disorder and risk of dementia among US veterans. *Arch Gen Psychiatry, 67,* 608–613.

105. Matz-Costa, C., Carr, D. C., McNamara, T. K., & James, J. B. (2016). Physical, cognitive, social, and emotional mediators of activity involvement and health in later life. *Res Aging, 38* (7), 791–815.

106. Hausdorff, J., et al. (1999). The power of ageism on physical function of older persons: Reversibility of age-related gait changes. *J Am Geriatric Soc, 47,* 1346–1349.

107. Langer, E. (1989). *Mindfulness,* 113. Reading, MA: Addison-Wesley.

Chapter 11: From Rosebud to Rose Hip

1. Serri, R., Romano, M. C., & Sparavigna, A. (2010). Quitting smoking rejuvenates the skin: Results of a pilot project on smoking cessation conducted in Milan, Italy. *Skinmed, 8* (1), 23–29.

2. Fisher, G. J., et al. (1997). Pathophysiology of premature skin aging induced by ultraviolet light. *N Engl J Med, 337* (20), 1419–1428.

3. Mosher, C. E., & Danoff-Burg, S. (2010). Addiction to indoor tanning: Relation to anxiety, depression, and substance use. *Arch Dermatol, 146,* 412–417.

4. Cosgrove, M. C., et al. (2007). Dietary nutrient intakes and skin-aging appearance among middle-aged American women. *Am J Clin Nutr, 86,* 1225–1231.

5. National Toxicology Program (2012). Technical report on the photococarcinogenesis study of retinoic acid and retinyl palmitate in skh-1 mice. NIH Publication No. 12-5910. National Institutes of Health, Public Health Service, U.S. Department of Health and Human Services; https://ntp.niehs.nih.gov/ntp/htdocs/lt_rpts/tr568_508.pdf.

6. Tolleson, W. H., Cherng, S. H., Xia, Q., Boudreau, M., Yin, J. J., Wamer, W. G., Howard, P. C., Yu, H., & Fu, P. P. (2005). Photodecomposition and phototoxicity of natural retinoids. *Int J Environ Res Public Health, 2* (1), 147–155; Yan, J., Xia, Q., Wamer, W. G., Boudreau, M. D., Warbritton, A., Howard, P. C., & Fu, P. P. (2007). Levels of retinyl palmitate and retinol in the skin of SKH-1 mice topically treated with retinyl palmitate and concomitant exposure to simulated solar light for thirteen weeks. *Toxicol Industrial Health, 23* (10), 581–589; Fu, P. P., Howard, P. C., Culp, S. G., Xia, Q., Webb, P. J., Blankenship, L. R., et al. (2002). Do topically applied

skin creams containing retinyl palmitate affect the photocarcinogenecity of simulated solar light? *J Food Drug Anal, 10,* 262–268.

7. Wang, T., Martin, S., Papadopulos, A., Harper, C. B., Mavlyutov, T. A., Niranjan, D., Glass, N. R., Cooper-White, J. J., Sibarita, J. B., Choquet, D., Davletov, B., & Meunier, F. A. (2015). Control of autophagosome axonal retrograde flux by presynaptic activity unveiled using botulinum neurotoxin type a. *J Neurosci, 35* (15), 6179–6194.

8. Hennenlotter, A., Dresel, C., Castrop, F., Ceballos-Baumann, A. O., Wohlschläger, A. M., & Haslinger, B. (2009). The link between facial feedback and neural activity within central circuitries of emotion—new insights from botulinum toxin-induced denervation of frown muscles. *Cerebral Cortex, 19* (3), 537–542; Havas, D. A., Glenberg, A. M., Gutowski, K. A., Lucarelli, M. J., & Davidson, R. J. (2010). Cosmetic use of botulinum toxin-a affects processing of emotional language. *Psychol Sci, 21* (7), 895–900; Neal, D. T., & Chartrand, T. L. (2011). Embodied emotion perception: Amplifying and dampening facial feedback modulates emotion perception accuracy. *Soc Psychol Personal Sci, 2* (6), 673–678; Kim, M. J., Neta, M., Davis, F. C., Ruberry, E. J., Dinescu, D., Heatherton, T. F., Stotland, M. A., & Whalen, P. J. (2014). Botulinum toxin-induced facial muscle paralysis affects amygdala responses to the perception of emotional expressions: Preliminary findings from an A-B-A design. *Biol Mood Anxiety Disord, 4,* 11; Haenzi, S., Stefanics, G., Lanaras, T., Calcagni, M., & Ghosh, A. (2014). Altered cortical activation from the hand after facial botulinum toxin treatment. *Ann Clin Transl Neurol, 1* (1), 64–68; Baumeister, J. C., Papa, G., & Foroni, F. (2016). Deeper than skin deep—The effect of botulinum toxin-A on emotion processing. *Toxicon, 118,* 86–90.

9. Van Scott, E. J., & Yu, R. J. (1989). Alpha hydroxy acids: Procedures for use in clinical practice. *Cutis, 43* (3), 222–228.

10. Van Scott, E. J., & Yu, R. J. (1984). Hyperkeratinization, corneocyte cohesion, and alpha hydroxy acids. *J Am Acad Dermatol, 11* (5, part 1), 867–879; Stiller, M. J., et al. (1996). Topical 8% glycolic acid and 8% L-lactic acid creams for the treatment of photodamaged skin: A double-blind vehicle-controlled clinical trial. *Arch Dermatol, 132* (6), 631–636.

11. Steenvoorden, D. P., & van Henegouwen, G. M. (1997). The use of endogenous antioxidants to improve photoprotection. *J Photochem Photobiol B, 41* (1–2), 1–10.

12. Fuchs, J., & Kern, H. (1998). Modulation of UV-light-induced skin inflammation by D-alpha-tocopherol and L-ascorbic acid: A clinical study using solar simulated radiation. *Free Radic Biol Med, 25* (9), 1006–1012; Steenvoorden, D. P., & Beijersbergen van Henegouwen, G. (1999). Protection against UV-induced systemic immunosuppression in mice by a single topical application of the antioxidant vitamins C and E. *Int J Radiat Biol, 75* (6), 747–755.

13. Cosgrove, M. C., et al. (2007). Dietary nutrient intakes and skin-aging appearance among middle-aged American women. *Am J Clin Nutr, 86,* 1225–1231.

14. Serbinova, E., et al. (1991). Free radical recycling and intermembrane mobility in the antioxidant properties of alpha-tocopherol and alphatocotrienol. *Free Radic Biol Med, 10,* 263–275.

15. Traber, M. G., et al. (1998). Penetration and distribution of alpha-tocopherol, alpha- or gamma-tocotrienols applied individually onto murine skin. *Lipids, 33* (1), 87–91.

16. Hoppe, U., et al. (1999). Coenzyme Q_{10}, a cutaneous antioxidant and energizer. *Biofactors, 9* (2–4), 371–378.

17. Sinatra, S. (1998). *The Coenzyme Q_{10} Phenomenon.* Chicago: Keats Publishing.

18. Swanson, C. L., et al. (Mar. 8, 2010). Biomarker analysis confirms the anti-oxidant and anti-inflammatory activity of a colorless turmeric extract, in vitro. Presented at the annual meeting of the American Academy of Dermatology, Miami, FL.

19. Bangha, E., Elsner, P., Kistler, G. S. (1996). Suppression of UV-induced erythema by topical treatment with melatonin (N-acetyl-5-methoxytryptamine): A dose response study. *Arch Dermatol Res, 288* (9), 522–526.

20. Zhao, J., Wang, J., Chen, Y., & Agarwal, R. (1999). Anti-tumor-promoting activity of a polyphenolic fraction isolated from grape seeds in the mouse skin two-stage initiation-promotion protocol and identification of procyanidin B5-3'-gallate as the most effective antioxidant constituent. *Carcinogenesis, 20* (9), 1737–1745; Kanda, T., et al. (1998). Inhibitory effects of apple polyphenol on induced histamine release from RBL-2H3 cells and rat mast cells. *Biosci Biotechnol Biochem, 62* (7), 1284–1289; Tomen, Inc. (1994–1999). Unpublished data.

21. Cho, S., Lee, S., Lee, M. J., Lee, D. H., Won, C. H., Kim, S. M., & Chung, J. H. (2009). Dietary aloe vera supplementation improves facial wrinkles and elasticity and it increases the type I procollagen gene expression in human skin in vivo. *Ann Dermatol, 21* (1), 6–11.

22. Cho, S., Won, C. H., Lee, D. H., Lee, M. J., Lee, S., So, S. H., Lee, S. K., Koo, B. S., Kim, N. M., & Chung, J. H. (2009). Red ginseng root extract mixed with *Torilus fructus* and *Corni fructus* improves facial wrinkles and increases type I procollagen synthesis in human skin: A randomized, double-blind, placebo-controlled study. *J Med Food, 12* (6), 1252–1259.

23. Furumura, M., Sato, N., Kusaba, N., Takagaki, K., & Nakayama, J. (2012). Oral administration of French maritime pine bark extract (Flavangenol®) improves clinical symptoms in photoaged facial skin. *Clin Interv Aging, 7,* 275–286.

24. Heinrich, U., Neukam, K., Tronnier, H., Sies, H., & Stahl, W. (2006). Long-term ingestion of high flavanol cocoa provides photoprotection against UV-induced erythema and improves skin condition in women. *J Nutr, 136* (6), 1565–1569.

25. Owen, D. R., et al. (Feb. 1999). Anti-aging technology for skincare '99. *Global Cosmetic Industry,* 38–43.

26. Katayama, K., et al. (1993). A pentapeptide from type I procollagen promotes extracellular matrix production. *J Biol Chem, 268* (14), 9941–9944.

27. Ibid.

28. Sederma, Inc. Unpublished data.

29. Wilkinson, R. E. Photoaging: The role of UV radiation in premature skin aging and a review of effective defense strategies. Article published on the Trienelle website at www.trienelle.com/research-monograph.aspx.

30. Schmidt, J., et al. (1998). Treatment of skin aging with topical estrogens. *Int J Pharm Compounding*, 2 (4), 270–274.

31. Draelos, Z. (Nov. 2005). The effect of Revival soy on the health and appearance of the skin, hair, and nails in postmenopausal women. Results of unpublished study available at www.revivalsoy.com/home/newsletter /v08n01/art2.html?flash6=yes.

32. Tiyasatkulkovit, W., Malaivijitnond, S., Charoenphandhu, N., Havill, L. M., Ford, A. L., & VandeBerg, J. L. (2014). *Pueraria mirifica* extract and puerarin enhance proliferation and expression of alkaline phosphatase and type I collagen in primary baboon osteoblasts. *Phytomed, 21* (12), 1498–1503.

33. Kim, S. Y., et al. (2004). Protective effects of dietary soy isoflavones against UV-induced skin-aging in hairless mouse model. *J Am Coll Nutr, 23* (2), 157–162; Miyazaki, K., Hanamizu, T., Iizuka, R., & Chiba, K. (2002). Genistein and daidzein stimulate hyaluronic acid production in transformed human keratinocyte culture and hairless mouse skin. *Skin Pharmacol Appl Skin Physiol, 15* (3), 175–183; DiSilvestro, R. (Sept. 2003). A diversity of soy antioxidant effects. Presented at the fifth annual International Symposium on the Role of Soy in Preventing and Treating Chronic Disease, Orlando, FL; Djuric, Z., Chen, G., Doerge, D. R., Heilbrun, L. K., & Kucuk, O. (2001). Effect of soy isoflavone supplementation on markers of oxidative stress in men and women. *Cancer Lett, 172* (1), 1–6.

34. Saliou, C., et al. (1999). French *Pinus maritima* bark extract prevents ultraviolet-induced NF-KB–dependent gene expression in a human keratinocyte cell line. Abstract of a poster presentation at the Oxygen Club of California, 1999 World Congress.

35. Eberlein-Konig, B., et al. (1998). Protective effect against sunburn of combined systemic ascorbic acid and vitamin E. *J Am Acad Dermatol, 38,* 45–48.

36. Engels, W. D. (1982). Dermatological disorders: Psychosomatic illness review (No. 4 in the series). *Psychosomatics, 23* (12), 1209–1219; Bick, E. (1968). Experience of the skin in early object relations. *Int J Psychoanal, 49,* 484–486.

37. Strauss, J. S., & Pochi, P. E. (1963). The human sebaceous gland: Its regulation by steroidal hormones, and its use as an end organ for assaying androgenicity *in vivo. Recent Prog Horm Res, 19,* 385–444.

38. Peck, G. L., et al. (1979). Prolonged remissions of cystic and conglobate acne with 13-retinoic acid. *N Engl J Med, 300,* 329–333.

39. Engels, W. D. (1982). Dermatological disorders: Psychosomatic illness review (No. 4 in the series). *Psychosomatics, 23* (12), 1209–1219; Bick, E. (1968). Experience of the skin in early object relations. *Int J Psychoanal, 49,* 484–486; Kaplan, H. I., & Sadock, B. J. (eds.) (1989). *Comprehensive*

Textbook of Psychiatry (5th ed.), 1221. Philadelphia, PA: Lippincott, Williams & Wilkins.

40. DeVille, R. L., et al. (1994). Androgenic alopecia in women: Treatment with 2% topical minoxidil solution. *Arch Dermatol, 130* (3), 303–307.

41. Lewenberg, A. (1996). Minoxidil-tretinoin combination for hair regrowth: Effects of frequency, dosage, and mode of application. *Advances in Therapy, 13* (5), 274–283.

42. Halsner, U. E., & Lucas, M. W. (1995). New aspects in hair transplantation for women. *Dermatol Surg, 21* (7), 605–610.

43. Hayden, T., et al. (Aug. 9, 1999). Our quest to be perfect. *Newsweek,* 52–59.

44. Burkitt, D. P., et al. (1974). Dietary fiber and disease. *JAMA, 229* (8), 1068–1074; Braunwald, E. (ed.) (1987). *Harrison's Principles of Internal Medicine* (11th ed.). New York: McGraw-Hill.

45. Grismond, G. L. (1981). Treatment of pregnancy-induced phlebopathies. *Minerva Ginecol, 33,* 221–230.

46. Ries, W. (1976). Prevention of venous disease from nutritional-physiologic aspect. ZFA, 31 (4), 383–388; Braunwald, E. (ed.) (1987). *Harrison's Principles of Internal Medicine* (11th ed.). New York: McGraw-Hill.

47. Ako, H., et al. (1981). Isolation of fibrinolysis enzyme activator from commercial bromelain. *Arch Int Pharmacodyn, 254,* 157–167.

Chapter 12: Standing Tall for Life

1. NIH Consensus Development Panel on Osteoporosis Prevention, Diagnosis, and Therapy. (Feb. 14, 2001). Osteoporosis prevention, diagnosis, and therapy. *JAMA, 285* (6), 785–795.

2. Harvey, N., Dennison, E., & Cooper, C. (2010). Osteoporosis: Impact on health and economics. *Nat Rev Rheumatol, 6* (2), 99–105.

3. Adeyemi, A., & Delhougne, G. (2019). Incidence and economic burden of intertrochanteric fracture: A Medicare claims database analysis. *JB JS Open Access, 4* (1), e0045.

4. Falch, J. A., Mowé, M., & Bøhmer, T. (1998). Low levels of serum ascorbic acid in elderly patients with hip fracture. *Scand J Clin Lab Invest, 58* (3), 225–228.

5. Morton, D. J., Barrett-Connor, E. L., & Schneider, D. L. (2001). Vitamin C supplement use and bone mineral density in postmenopausal women. *J Bone Miner Res, 16* (1), 135–140; Leveille, S. G., LaCroix, A. Z., Koepsell, T. D., Beresford, S. A., Van Belle, G., & Buchner, D. M. (1997). Dietary vitamin C and bone mineral density in postmenopausal women in Washington State, USA. *J Epidemiol Commun H, 51* (5), 479–485.

6. Shipman, P., et al. (1985). *The Human Skeleton.* Cambridge, MA: Harvard University Press; Brown, J. (1990). *The Science of Human Nutrition.* New York: Harcourt Brace Jovanovich.

7. Lanyon, L. E. (1993). Skeletal responses to physical loading. In G. Mundy

    & J. T. Martin (eds.), *Physiology & Pharmacology of Bone, 107,* 485–505. Berlin: Springer-Verlag.

8. Travis, J. (2000). Boning up: Turning on cells that build bone and turning off ones that destroy it. *Science News, 157,* 41–42.

9. Manolagas, S. C. (1995). Sex steroids, cytokines, and the bone marrow: New concepts on the pathogenesis of osteoporosis. *Ciba Foundation Symposium, 191,* 187–202.

10. Riggs, B., et al. (1986). In women dietary calcium intake and rates of bone loss from midradius and lumbar spine are not related. *J Bone Miner Res, 1* (suppl.), 167; Genant, H. K., et al. (1985). Osteoporosis: Assessment by quantitative computed tomography. *Orthop Clin North Am, 16* (3), 557–568.

11. Trotter, M., et al. (1974). Sequential changes in weight, density, and percentage weight of human skeletons from an early fetal period through old age. *Anat Rec, 179,* 1–8.

12. Adams, P., et al. (1970). Osteoporosis and the effects of aging on bone mass in elderly men and women. *J Medical News Series, 39,* 601–615.

13. Harris, S., et al. (1992). Rates of change in bone mineral density of the spine, heel, femoral neck and radius in healthy postmenopausal women. *J Bone Miner Res, 17* (1), 87–95; Riggs, B., et al. (1985). Rates of bone loss in the appendicular and axial skeletons of women: Evidence of substantial vertebral bone loss before menopause. *J Clin Invest, 77,* 1487–1491.

14. Fujita, T., et al. (1992). Comparison of osteoporosis and calcium intake between Japan and the United States. *Proc Soc Exp Biol Med, 200* (2), 149–152.

15. Frost, H. (1985). The pathomechanics of osteoporosis. *Clin Orthop, 200,* 198–225.

16. Chappard, D., et al. (1988). Spatial distribution of trabeculae in iliac bones from 145 osteoporotic females. *Maturitas, 10,* 353–360; Biewener, A. A. (1993). Safety factors in bone strength. *Calcif Tissue Int, 53* (suppl. 1), S68–S74.

17. Brown, S. (1996). *Better Bones, Better Body: Beyond Estrogen and Calcium.* Los Angeles: Keats Publishing.

18. Lees, B., et al. (1993). Differences in proximal femur bone density over two centuries. *Lancet, 341,* 673–675; Eaton, S., et al. (1991). Calcium in evolutionary perspective. *Am J Clin Nutr, 54* (suppl.), 281S–287S.

19. Fiatarone, M. A., Marks, E. C., Ryan, N. D., Meredith, C. N., Lipsitz, L. A., & Evans, W. J. (1990). High-intensity strength training in nonagenarians: Effects on skeletal muscle. *JAMA, 263* (22), 3029–3034.

20. Bauer, D. C., et al. (1993). Factors associated with appendicular bone mass in older women. *Ann Intern Med, 118* (9), 647–665.

21. Rigotti, N. A., et al. (1984). Osteoporosis in women with anorexia nervosa. *N Engl J Med, 311* (25), 1601–1605.

22. Prior, J., et al. (1990). Spinal bone loss and ovulatory disturbances. *N Engl J Med, 323* (18), 1221–1227; Cann, C., et al. (1984). Decreased spinal mineral content in amenorrheic women. *JAMA, 251* (5), 626–629.

23. Schuckit, M. (1994). Section 5: Alcohol and alcoholism. In K. Isselbacher

et al. (eds.), *Harrison's Principles of Internal Medicine*, vol. 2 (13th ed.), 2420. New York: McGraw-Hill.

24. Diamond, T., et al. (1989). Ethanol reduces bone formation and may cause osteoporosis. *Am J Med, 86*, 282–288; Bikler, D. D., et al. (1985). Bone disease in alcohol abuse. *Ann Intern Med, 103*, 42–48.

25. Gold, P. W., et al. (1986). Responses to corticotropin-releasing hormone in the hypercortisolism of depression and Cushing's disease: Pathophysiology and diagnostic implications. *N Engl J Med, 314*, 1329–1335; Michelson, D., et al. (1996). Bone mineral density in women with depression. *N Engl J Med, 335* (16), 1176–1181.

26. Tatemi, S., et al. (1991). Effect of experimental human magnesium depletion on parathyroid hormone secretion and 1,25-dihydroxyvitamin D metabolism. *J Clin Endocrinol Metab, 73* (5), 1067–1072; Gaby, A., & Wright, J. (1988). *Nutrients and Bone Health*. Seattle, WA: Wright/Gaby Nutrition Institute.

27. Adinoff, A. D., & Hollister, J. R. (1983). Steroid-induced fracture and bone loss in patients with asthma. *N Engl J Med, 309* (5), 265–268.

28. Hahn, T. J., et al. (1988). Altered mineral metabolism in glycocorticoidinduced osteopaenia: Effect of 25-hydroxyvitamin D administration. *J Clin Invest, 64*, 655–665.

29. Crilly, R. G., et al. (1981). Steroid hormones, ageing and bone. *Clin Endocrinol Metab, 10* (1), 115–139.

30. Johnell, O., et al. (1979). Bone morphology in epileptics. *Calcif Tissue Int, 28* (2), 93–97.

31. Briot, K., et al. (2010). Accuracy of patient-reported height loss and risk factors for height loss among postmenopausal women. *Can Med Assoc J, 182*, 558–562.

32. Franklin, J. A., et al. (1992). Long-term thyroxine treatment and bone mineral density. *Lancet, 340*, 9–13; Paul, T. L., et al. (1988). Long-term L-thyroxine therapy is associated with decreased hip bone density in premenopausal women. *JAMA, 259*, 3137–3141; Coindre, J. M., et al. (1986). Bone loss in hypothyroidism with hormone replacement: A histomorphometric study. *Arch Intern Med, 146*, 48–53.

33. Järvinen, T. L., Michaëlsson, K., Aspenberg, P., & Sievänen, H. (2015). Osteoporosis: The emperor has no clothes. *J Intern Med, 277* (6), 662–673. doi: 10.1111/joim.12366.

34. Aurégan, J. C., Bosser, C., Bensidhoum, M., Bégué, T., & Hoc, T. (2018). Correlation between skin and bone parameters in women with postmenopausal osteoporosis: A systematic review. *EFORT Open Rev, 3* (8), 449–460; Yoneda, P., Biancolin, S. E., Gomes, M. S., & Miot, H. A. (2011). Association between skin thickness and bone density in adult women. *An Bras Dermatol, 86* (5), 878–884; Brincat, M. P., et al. (1996). A screening model for osteoporosis using dermal skin thickness and bone densitometry. In B. G. Wren (ed.), *Progress in the Management of the Menopause: The Proceedings of the 8th International Congress on the Menopause*, 175–178. Sydney: Parthenon Publishing Group.

35. Robins, S. P. (1995). Collagen crosslinks in metabolic bone disease. *Acta*

Orthop Scan, 66 (266, suppl.), S171–S175; Garnero, P., et al. (1994). Comparison of new biochemical markers of bone turnover in late post-menopausal osteoporotic women in response to alendronate treatment. *J Clin Endocrinol Metab, 79,* 1693–1700; Chesnut, C., et al. (1997). Hormone replacement therapy in postmenopausal women: Urinary N-telopeptide of type I collagen monitors therapeutic effect and predicts response of bone mineral density. *Am J Med, 102,* 29–37.

36. Cummings, S. R., et al. (in press). Regression to mean in clinical practice: Women who seem to lose bone density during treatment for osteoporosis usually gain if treatment is continued. *JAMA.* Cited in B. Ettinger (2000). Sequential osteoporosis treatment for women with postmenopausal osteoporosis. *Menopausal Medicine, Newsletter of the American Society for Reproductive Medicine, 8* (2), 3.

37. Watts, N. B., et al. (1995). Comparison of oral estrogens and estrogens plus androgen on bone mineral density, menopausal symptoms, and lipid-lipoprotein profiles in surgical menopause. *Obstet Gynecol, 85,* 529–537.

38. Cummings, S., et al. (1998). Endogenous hormones and the risk of hip and vertebral fractures among older women. *N Engl J Med, 339,* 733–738.

39. Riggs, B., & Melton, L. (1986). Involutional osteoporosis. *N Engl J Med, 26,* 1676–1686. Buchanan, J. R., et al. (1988). Early vertebral trabecular bone loss in normal premenopausal women. *J Bone Miner Res, 3* (5), 583–587.

40. Carter, M. D., et al. (1991). Bone mineral content at three sites in normal perimenopausal women. *Clin Orthop, 266,* 295–300; Harris, S., & Dawson-Hughes, B. (1992). Op. cit.

41. Heaney, R. P. (1990). Estrogen-calcium interactions in the post-menopause: A quantitative description. *J Bone Miner Res, 11* (1), 67–84.

42. Speroff, L. (Oct. 1999). Treatment options for the prevention of osteoporosis. *OB/GYN Clinical Alert, 46.*

43. Lee, J. (1991). Is natural progesterone the missing link in osteoporosis prevention and treatment? *Med Hypotheses, 35,* 316–318; Prior, J. (1991). Progesterone and the prevention of osteoporosis. *Can J Ob-Gyn Women's Healthcare, 3* (4), 178–183; Lee, J. (1990). Osteoporosis reversal: The role of progesterone. *Clin Nutr Rev, 10,* 884–889; Prior, M. C., et al. (1994). Cyclic medroxyprogesterone increases bone density: A controlled trial in active women with menstrual cycle disturbances. *Am J Med, 96,* 521–530; Adachi, J. D., et al. (1997). A double-blind randomized controlled trial of the effects of medroxyprogesterone acetate on bone density of women taking oestrogen replacement therapy. *Br J Obstet Gynaecol, 104,* 64–70; Prior, J. C., et al. (1997). Premenopausal ovariectomy-related bone loss: A randomized, double-blind, one-year trial of conjugated estrogen or medroxyprogesterone acetate. *J Bone Miner Res, 12* (11), 1851–1863.

44. Rossouw, J. E., et al. (2002). Risks and benefits of estrogen plus progestin in healthy postmenopausal women: Principal results from the Women's Health Initiative randomized controlled trial. *JAMA, 288* (3), 321–333.

45. Lindsay, R., Gallagher, J. C., Kleerekoper, M., & Pickar, J. H. (2002). Effect of lower doses of conjugated equine estrogens with and without

medroxyprogesterone acetate on bone in early postmenopausal women. *JAMA, 287* (20), 2668–2676.

46. Tremollieres, F. A., Strong, D. D., Baylink, D. J., & Mohan, S. (1992). Progesterone and promegestone stimulate human bone cell proliferation and insulin-like growth factor-2 production. *Acta Endocrinol (Copenh), 26* (4), 329–337.

47. Manonai, J., Chittacharoen, A., Udomsubpayakul, U., Theppisai, H., & Theppisai, U. (2008). Effects and safety of *Pueraria mirifica* on lipid profiles and biochemical markers of bone turnover rates in healthy postmenopausal women. *Menopause, 15* (3), 530–535; Kittivanichkul, D., Charoenphandhu, N., Khemawoot, P., & Malaivijitnond, S. (2016). *Pueraria mirifica* alleviates cortical bone loss in naturally menopausal monkeys. *J Endocrinol, 231* (2), 121–133.

48. Urasopon, N., Hamada, Y., Asaoka, K., Cherdshewasart, W., & Malaivijitnond, S. (2007). *Pueraria mirifica*, a phytoestrogen-rich herb, prevents bone loss in orchidectomized rats. *Maturitas, 56* (3), 322–331; Urasopon, N., Hamada, Y., Cherdshewasart, W., & Malaivijitnond, S. (2008). Preventive effects of *Pueraria mirifica* on bone loss in ovariectomized rats. *Maturitas, 59* (2), 137–148.

49. Dawson-Hughes, G., et al. (1990). A controlled trial of the effects of calcium supplementation on bone density in postmenopausal women. *N Engl J Med, 323,* 878–883.

50. Feskanich, D., et al. (2003). Calcium, vitamin D, milk consumption, and hip fractures: A prospective study among postmenopausal women. *Am J Clin Nutr, 77,* 504–511.

51. Bischoff-Ferrari, H. A., et al. (2007). Calcium intake and hip fracture risk in men and women: A meta-analysis of prospective cohort studies and randomized controlled trials. *Am J Clin Nutr, 86,* 1780–1790.

52. Castleman, M. (2009). The calcium myth. *Natural Solutions,* 57–62; www.naturalsolutionsmag.com/articles-display/15403/The-Calcium-Myth.

53. Aiello, L., & Wheeler, P. (1995). The expensive tissue hypothesis: The brain and the digestive system in human and primate evolution. *Current Anthropology, 36* (2), 199–221; Lorenz, K., & Lee, V. A. (1997). The nutritional and physiological impact of cereal products in human nutrition. *Crit Rev Food Sci Nutr, 8,* 383–456; Cassiday, C. M. (1980). Nutrition and health in agriculturalists and hunter-gatherers: A case study of two prehistoric populations. In R. F. Kandel, G. H. Pelto, & N. W. Jerome (eds.), *Nutritional Anthropology: Contemporary Approaches to Diet and Culture,* 117–145. Pleasantville, NY: Redgrave Publishing Company; Eaton, S. B., & Nelson, D. A. (1991). Calcium in evolutionary perspective. *Am J Clin Nutr, 54* (suppl.), 281S–287S; Goodman, A. H., Dufour, D., & Pelto, G. H. (2000). *Nutritional Anthropology: Biocultural Perspectives on Food and Nutrition.* Mountain View, CA: Mayfield Publishing. See also *The Paleopathology Newsletter,* published by the Paleopathology Association. Contact: Ms. Eve Cockburn, 18655 Parkside, Detroit, MI 48221–2208.

54. Zofková, I., & Kancheva, R. L. (1995). The relationship between magnesium and calciotropic hormones. *Magne Res, 8* (1), 77–84.

55. Saggese, G., Bertelloni, S., Baroncelli, G. I., Federico, G., Calisti, L., & Fusaro, C. (1989). Bone demineralization and impaired mineral metabolism in insulin-dependent diabetes mellitus: A possible role of magnesium deficiency. *Helv Paediatr Acta, 43* (5–6), 405–414.

56. McGuigan, J. (1994). Peptic ulcer and gastritis. In K. Isselbacher, et al. (eds.), *Harrison's Principles of Internal Medicine, vol. 2* (13th ed.), 1369. New York: McGraw-Hill.

57. Odvina, C. V., et al. (2005). Severely suppressed bone turnover: A potential complication of alendronate therapy. *J Clin Endocrinol Metab, 90,* 1294–1301.

58. Bauer, D. C., et al. (2004). Change in bone turnover and hip, non-spine, and vertebral fracture in alendronate-treated women: The fracture intervention trial, *J Bone Miner Res, 19,* 1250–1258; Kwek, E. B., et al. (2008). An emerging pattern of subtrochanteric stress fractures: A long-term complication of alendronate therapy? *Injury, 39,* 224–231; Neviaser, A. S., et al. (2008). Low-energy femoral shaft fractures associated with alendronate use. *J Orthop Trauma, 22,* 346–350; Parker-Pope, T. (July 15, 2008). Drugs to build bones may weaken them. *New York Times,* www.nytimes.com/2008/07/15/health/15well.html?partne=rssnyt&emc=rss; Cheung, R. K., et al. (2007). Sequential non-traumatic femoral shaft fractures in a patient on long-term alendronate. *Hong Kong Med J, 13,* 485–489; American Association of Orthopaedic Surgeons (AAOS) 2010 Annual Meeting: Abstract 241, presented Mar. 10, 2010; Abstract 339, presented Mar. 11, 2010.

59. Guyatt, G. H., et al. (2002). Summary of meta-analyses of therapies for postmenopausal osteoporosis and the relationship between bone density and fractures. *Endocrinol Metab Clin North Am, 31* (3), 659–679, xii; Cranney, A., et al. (2002). Meta-analyses of therapies for postmenopausal osteoporosis. IX: Summary of meta-analyses of therapies for postmenopausal osteoporosis. *Endocr Rev, 23* (4), 570–578; Black, D. M., et al. (1996). Randomised trial of effect of alendronate on risk of fracture in women with existing vertebral fractures. Fracture Intervention Trial Research Group. *Lancet, 348* (9041), 1535–1541; McClung, M. R., et al. (Feb. 1, 2001). Effect of risedronate on the risk of hip fracture in elderly women. Hip Intervention Program Study Group. *N Engl J Med, 344* (5), 333–340; Harris, S. T., et al. (1999). Effects of risedronate treatment on vertebral and nonvertebral fractures in women with postmenopausal osteoporosis: A randomized controlled trial. Vertebral Efficacy with Risedronate Therapy (VERT) Study Group. *JAMA, 282* (14), 1344–1352.

60. Alonso-Coello, P., et al. (2008). Drugs for pre-osteoporosis: Prevention or disease mongering? *BMJ, 336,* 126–129.

61. DeGroen, P. C. (1996). Esophagitis associated with the use of alendronate. *N Engl J Med, 335,* 1016–1021.

62. Ruggiero, S. L., et al. (2004). Osteonecrosis of the jaws associated with the use of bisphosphonates: A review of 63 cases. *J Oral Maxillofacial Surg, 62,* 527–534.

63. Watts, N. B., & Diab, D. L. (2010). Long-term use of bisphosphonates in

osteoporosis. *J Clin Endocrinol Metab, 95,* 1555–1565; Speroff, L. (2005). Is long-term alendronate treatment a problem? *OB/GYN Clinical Alert, 22,* 9–10.

64. Lewiecki, E. M., Dinavahi, R. V., Lazaretti-Castro, M., Ebeling, P. R., Adachi, J. D., Miyauchi, A., Gielen, E., Milmont, C. E., Libanati, C., & Grauer, A. (2019). One year of romosozumab followed by two years of denosumab maintains fracture risk reductions: Results of the FRAME Extension Study. *J Bone Miner Res, 34* (3), 419–428; Saag, K. G., Petersen, J., Brandi, M. L., Karaplis, A. C., Lorentzon, M., Thomas, T., Maddox, J., Fan, M., Meisner, P. D., & Grauer, A. (2017). Romosozumab or alendronate for fracture prevention in women with osteoporosis. *N Engl J Med, 377* (15), 1417–1427.

65. Silverman, S. L., & Azria, M. (2002). The analgesic role of calcitonin following osteoporotic fracture. *Osteoporos Int, 13* (11), 858–867.

66. Phoosuwan, M., et al. (2009). The effects of weight bearing yoga training on the bone resorption markers of the postmenopausal woman. *J Med Assoc Thai, 92 (*suppl. 5), S102–S108.

67. Nelson, M., et al. (1994). Effects of high-intensity strength training on multiple risk factors for osteoporotic fractures: A randomized controlled trial. *JAMA, 272* (24), 1909–1914.

68. Nelson, M. (2000). *Strong Women Stay Young.* New York: Bantam.

69. Fiatarone, M., et al. (1994). Exercise training and nutritional supplementation for physical frailty in very elderly people. *N Engl J Med, 330* (25), 1769–1775.

70. Bischoff-Ferrari, H. (2009). Effect of extended physiotherapy and high-dose vitamin D on rate of falls and hospital re-admission after acute hip fracture: A randomized controlled trial. Presented at the 31st annual meeting of the American Society for Bone and Mineral Research (ASBMR), Denver, CO.

71. Sinaki, M., & Mikkelsen, B. A. (1984). Postmenopausal spinal osteoporosis: Flexion vs. extension. *Arch Phys Med Rehab, 65,* 593–596.

72. Rosen, C., et al. (1994). The effects of sunlight and diet on bone loss in elderly women from rural Maine. *Maine J Health Issues, 1* (2), 35–48. (Study done by Michael Holick in Bangor, Maine.)

73. Vieth, R. (1999). Vitamin D supplementation, 25-hydroxyvitamin D concentrations, and safety. *Am J Clin Nutr, 69,* 842–856. (Anyone who is serious about gathering more information on vitamin D and sunlight should read this impressive review article on the subject.)

74. Ibid.

75. Dobnig, H., et al. (2008). Independent association of low serum 25-hydroxyvitamin D and 1,25-dihydroxyvitamin D levels with all-cause and cardiovascular mortality. *Arch Intern Med, 168,* 1340–1349.

76. Neer, R. M., et al. (1971). Stimulation by artificial lighting of calcium absorption in elderly human subjects. *Nature, 229,* 255.

77. Holick, M. F. (1995). Environmental factors that influence the cutaneous production of vitamin D. *Am J Clin Nutr, 61* (suppl. 3), 638S–645S.

78. Dawson-Hughes, B., et al. (1991). Effect of vitamin D supplementation on

wintertime and overall bone loss in healthy postmenopausal women. *Ann Intern Med, 115* (7), 505–511.

79. Ibid.

80. Sanders, K. M., et al. (2010). Annual high-dose oral vitamin D and falls and fractures in older women: A randomized controlled trial. *JAMA, 303,* 1815–1822.

81. McNeil, T. (Spring 1998). The vitamin D guru: School of medicine professor sees the light and spreads the news. *Bostonia,* 34–35.

82. Vieth, R. (1999). Op. cit.

83. Berger, J. (1998), 64–72. *Herbal Rituals.* New York: St. Martin's Press.

84. Weed, S. (1989). *Healing Wise: Wise Woman's Herbal* (262). Woodstock, NY: Ashtree Publications.

85. Munger, R. G. (1999). Prospective study of dietary protein intake and risk of hip fracture in postmenopausal women. *Am J Clin Nutr, 69* (1), 147–152.

86. Abraham, G. (1991). The importance of magnesium in the management of primary postmenopausal osteoporosis: A review. *J Nutr Med, 2,* 165–178; Gaby, A., & Wright, J. (1990). Nutrients and osteoporosis: A review article. *J Nutr Med, 1,* 63–72.

87. Buckley, L. M., et al. (1996). Calcium and vitamin D_3 supplementation prevents bone loss in the spine secondary to low-dose corticosteroids in patients with rheumatoid arthritis. A randomized, double-blind, placebo-controlled trial. *Ann Intern Med, 125* (12), 961–968.

88. Nielson, B. E., et al. (1987). Effects of dietary boron on mineral, estrogen, and testosterone metabolism in postmenopausal women. *FASEB, 1,* 394–397.

89. Cauley, J. A., et al. (2008). Serum 25-hydroxyvitamin D concentrations and risk for hip fractures. *Ann Intern Med, 149,* 242–250.

90. Koshihara, Y., et al. (2003). Vitamin K stimulates osteoblastogenesis and inhibits osteoclastogenesis in human bone marrow cell culture. *J Endocrinol, 176,* 339–348; Hidaka, T., et al. (2002). Treatment for patients with postmenopausal osteoporosis who have been placed on HRT and show a decrease in bone mineral density: Effects of concomitant administration of vitamin K_2. *J Bone Miner Metab, 20,* 235–239; Hirano, J., & Ishii, Y. (2002). Effects of vitamin K_2, vitamin D, and calcium on the bone metabolism of rats in the growth phase. *J Orthop Sci, 7,* 364–369; Shiraki, M., et al. (2000). Vitamin K_2 (menatetrenone) effectively prevents fractures and sustains lumbar bone mineral density in osteoporosis. *J Bone Miner Res, 15,* 515–521; Iwamoto, J., et al. (2000). Effect of combined administration of vitamin D_3 and vitamin K_2 on bone mineral density of the lumbar spine in postmenopausal women with osteoporosis. *J Orthop Sci, 5,* 546–551.

91. Iwamoto, J., et al. (2003). Treatment with vitamin D_3 and/or vitamin K_2 for postmenopausal osteoporosis. *Keio J Med, 52,* 147–150; Iwamoto, J., et al. (2000). Effect of combined administration of vitamin D_3 and vitamin K_2 on bone mineral density of the lumbar spine in postmenopausal women with osteoporosis. *J Orthop Sci, 5,* 546–551.

92. Huang, Z. B., Wan, S. L., Lu, Y. J., Ning, L., Liu, C., & Fan, S. W. (2015). Does vitamin K_2 play a role in the prevention and treatment of osteoporosis for postmenopausal women: A meta-analysis of randomized controlled trials. *Osteoporos Int, 26* (3), 1175–1186; Knapen, M. H., Drummen, N. E., Smit, E., Vermeer, C., & Theuwissen, E. (2013). Three-year low-dose menaquinone-7 supplementation helps decrease bone loss in healthy postmenopausal women. *Osteoporos Int, 24* (9), 2499–2507; Vermeer, C., Shearer, M. J., Zittermann, A., Bolton-Smith, C., Szulc, P., Hodges, S., Walter, P., Rambeck, W., Stöcklin, E., & Weber, P. (2004). Beyond deficiency: Potential benefits of increased intakes of vitamin K for bone and vascular health. *Eur J Nutr, 43* (6), 325–335.

93. Manonai, J., et al. (2008). Effects and safety of *Pueraria mirifica* on lipid profiles and biochemical markers of bone turnover rates in healthy post-menopausal women. *Menopause, 15,* 530–535; Urasopon, N., et al. (2007). *Pueraria mirifica,* a phytoestrogen-rich herb, prevents bone loss in orchidectomized rats. *Maturitas, 56,* 322–331; Urasopon, N., et al. (2008). Preventive effects of *Pueraria mirifica* on bone loss in ovariecto-mized rats. *Maturitas, 59,* 137–148.

94. Li, Y., et al. (2010). Bone mineral content is positively correlated to n-3 fatty acids in the femur of growing rats. *Br J Nutr, 104* (5), 674–685; Griel, A. E., et al. (2007). An increase in dietary n-3 fatty acids decreases a marker of bone resorption in humans. *Nutr J, 6,* 2.

95. Potter, S. M., Baum, J. A., Teng, H., Stillman, R. J., Shay, N. F., & Erdman, J. W. (1998). Soy protein and isoflavones: Their effects on blood lipids and bone density in postmenopausal women. *Am J Clin Nutr, 68* (6, suppl.), 1375S–1379S.

96. Zhang, X., et al. (2005). Prospective cohort study of soy food consumption and risk of bone fracture among postmenopausal women. *Arch Intern Med, 165* (16), 1890–1895.

97. Lydeking-Olsen, E., et al. (2004). Soymilk or progesterone for prevention of bone loss—a 2-year randomized, placebo-controlled trial. *Eur J Nutr, 43* (4), 246–257. Epub Apr. 14, 2004.

98. Bonfield, T. (June 15, 1999). Research backs benefits of soy—post-menopausal women take note. *Cincinnati Enquirer.* This study, which was conducted by Dr. Michael Scheiber, of the Obstetrics and Gynecology Department at the University of Cincinnati, and Dr. Kenneth Setchell, director of mass spectrometry at Children's Hospital Medical Center, demonstrated that eating three servings of soy foods per day containing a total of about 70 mg of soy isoflavones had definite bone-building effects that may be as good as those of estrogen.

99. Bitto, A., Burnett, B. P., Polito, F., Marini, H., Levy, R. M., Armbruster, M. A., Minutoli, L., Di Stefano, V., Irrera, N., Antoci, S., Granese, R., Squadrito, F., & Altavilla, D. (2008). Effects of genistein aglycone in osteoporotic, ovariectomized rats: A comparison with alendronate, raloxifene and oestradiol. *Br J Pharmacol, 155* (6), 896–905.

100. Urasopon, N., et al. (2008). Preventive effects of *Pueraria mirifica* on bone loss in ovariectomized rats. *Maturitas, 59,* 137–148; Urasopon, N., et al.

(2007). *Pueraria mirifica*, a phytoestrogen-rich herb, prevents bone loss in orchidectomized rats. *Maturitas, 56,* 322–331.

101. Hegarty, V., et al. (2000). Tea drinking and bone mineral density in older women. *Am J Clin Nutr, 71,* 1003–1007.

102. Spilmont, M., Léotoing, L., Davicco, M. J., Lebecque, P., Mercier, S., Miot-Noirault, E., Pilet, P., Rios, L., Wittrant, Y., & Coxam, V. (2014). Pomegranate and its derivatives can improve bone health through decreased inflammation and oxidative stress in an animal model of postmenopausal osteoporosis. *Eur J Nutr, 53* (5), 1155–1164.

103. Mori-Okamoto, J., Otawara-Hamamoto, Y., Yamato, H., & Yoshimura, H. (2004). Pomegranate extract improves a depressive state and bone properties in menopausal syndrome model ovariectomized mice. *J Ethnopharmacol, 92* (1), 93–101.

104. Shuid, A. N., & Mohamed, I. N. (2013). Pomegranate use to attenuate bone loss in major musculoskeletal diseases: An evidence-based review. *Curr Drug Targets, 14* (13), 1565–1578.

Chapter 13: Creating Breast Health

1. Toikkanene, S., et al. (1991). Factors predicting late mortality from breast cancer. *Eur J Cancer, 27* (5), 586–591.

2. Chen, C. C., et al. (1995). Adverse life events and breast cancer: Case-control study. *BMJ, 311,* 1527–1530.

3. Dreher, Henry. (Oct. 12, 2005). Personal communication.

4. Levy, S., et al. (1987). Correlation of stress factors with sustained depression of natural killer cell activity and predicted prognosis in patients with breast cancer. *J Clin Oncol, 5,* 348–353.

5. Spiegel, D., et al. (1989). The effect of psychosocial treatment on survival of patients with metastatic breast cancer. *Lancet, 2* (8668), 888–891.

6. Prior, J. (1992). Critique of estrogen treatment for heart attack prevention: The Nurses' Health Study. *A Friend Indeed, 8* (8), 3–4; Schairer, C., et al. (2000). Menopausal estrogen and estrogen-progestin replacement therapy and breast cancer risk. *JAMA, 283* (4), 485–491.

7. Bulbrook, P. D., Swain, M. C., Wang, D. Y., et al. (1976). Breast cancer in Britain and Japan: Plasma oestradiol-17b, oestrone, and progesterone, and their urinary metabolites in normal British and Japanese women. *Eur J Cancer, 12,* 725–735.

8. Seely, S., et al. (1983). Diet and breast cancer: The possible connection with sugar consumption. *Med Hypotheses, 11,* 319–327; Kazer, R. (1995). Insulin resistance, insulin-like growth factor I and breast cancer: A hypothesis. *Int J Cancer, 62,* 403–406; Bruning, P., et al. (1992). Insulin resistance and breast-cancer risk. *Int J Cancer, 52,* 511–516.

9. Tavani, A., Giordano, L., Gallus, S., Talamini, R., Franceschi, S., Giacosa, A., Montella, M., & La Vecchia, C. (2006). Consumption of sweet foods and breast cancer risk in Italy. *Ann Oncol, 17* (2), 341–345.

10. Romieu, I., Ferrari, P., Rinaldi, S., Slimani, N., Jenab, M., Olsen, A., Tjon-

neland, A., Overvad, K., Boutron-Ruault, M. C., Lajous, M., Kaaks, R., Teucher, B., Boeing, H., Trichopoulou, A., Naska, A., Vasilopoulo, E., Sacerdote, C., Tumino, R., Masala, G., Sieri, S., . . . & Clavel-Chapelon, F. (2012). Dietary glycemic index and glycemic load and breast cancer risk in the European Prospective Investigation into Cancer and Nutrition (EPIC). *Am J Clin Nutr, 96* (2), 345–355.

11. Coleman, B. C. (Mar. 10, 1999). Fatty diet and breast cancer: No link? *Portland Press Herald.*

12. Adlercreutz, H., et al. (1982). Excretion of the lignans enterolactone and enterodiol and of equol in omnivorous and vegetarian postmenopausal women and in women with breast cancer. *Lancet, 2* (8311), 1295–1299.

13. Goldin, B. R., Adlercreutz, H., et al. (1982). Estrogen excretion patterns and plasma levels in vegetarian and omnivorous women. *N Engl J Med, 307,* 1542–1547.

14. Percival, M. (1997). Phytonutrients and detoxification. *Clinical Nutrition Insights,* 1–4. Published by the Foundation for the Advancement of Nutritional Education. Available from Metagenics North East, P.O. Box 848, Kingston, NH 03848.

15. van den Brandt, P. A., & Schulpen, M. (2017). Mediterranean diet adherence and risk of postmenopausal breast cancer: Results of a cohort study and meta-analysis. *Int J Cancer, 140* (10), 2220–2231.

16. Chlebowski, R. T., Aragaki, A. K., Anderson, G. L., Simon, M. S., Manson, J. E., Neuhouser, M. L., Pan, K., Stefanic, M. L., Rohan, T. E., Lane, D., Qi, L., Snetselaar, L., & Prentice, R. L. (2018). Association of low-fat dietary pattern with breast cancer overall survival: A secondary analysis of the Women's Health Initiative Randomized Clinical Trial. *JAMA Oncol, 4* (10), e181212.

17. Zava, D., & Duwe, G. (1997). Estrogenic and antiproliferative properties of genistein and other flavonoids in human breast cancer cells in vitro. *Nutr Cancer, 27* (1), 31–40.

18. Shu, X. O., et al. (2009). Soy food intake and breast cancer survival. *JAMA, 302,* 2437–2443.

19. Kang, X., et al. (Oct. 18, 2010). Effect of soy isoflavones on breast cancer recurrence and death for patients receiving adjuvant endocrine therapy. *Can Med Assoc J, 182* (17), 1857–1862.

20. Wayne, S. J., Neuhouser, M. L., Koprowski, C., Ulrich, C. M., Wiggins, C., Gilliland, F., Baumgartner, K. B., Baumgartner, R. N., McTiernan, A., Bernstein, L., & Ballard-Barbash, R. (2009). Breast cancer survivors who use estrogenic botanical supplements have lower serum estrogen levels than non users. *Breast Cancer Res Treat, 117* (1), 111–119.

21. Ramnarine, S., et al. (2009). Phyto-oestrogens: Do they have a role in breast cancer therapy? *Proc Nutr Soc, 68 (OCE),* E93.

22. Jeon, G. C., Park, M. S., Yoon, D. Y., Shin, C. H., Sin, H. S., & Um, S. J. (2005). Antitumor activity of spinasterol isolated from *Pueraria* roots. *Exp Mol Med, 37* (2), 111–120; Boonchird, C., Mahapanichkul, T., & Cherdshewasart, W. (2010). Differential binding with ERalpha and ER-beta of the phytoestrogen-rich plant *Pueraria mirifica. Braz J Med Biol*

Res, 43 (2), 195–200; Ramnarine, S., MacCallum, J., & Ritchie, M. (2009). Phyto-oestrogens: Do they have a role in breast cancer therapy? *Proc Nutr Soc, 68* (OCE2), E93.

23. Bagga, D., et al. (1997). Dietary modulation of omega-3/omega-6 polyun-saturated fatty acid ratios in patients with breast cancer. *J Nat Cancer Inst, 89* (15), 1123–1131.

24. Brasky, T. M., et al. (2010). Specialty supplements and breast cancer risk in the Vitamins and Lifestyle (VITAL) Cohort. *Cancer Epidemiol Biomarkers Prev, 19,* 1696–1708.

25. Bougnoux, P., et al. (2009). Improving outcome of chemotherapy of metastatic breast cancer by docosahexaenoic acid: A phase II trial. *Br J Cancer, 101* (12), 1978–1985.

26. Garland, C. F., et al. (2009). Vitamin D for cancer prevention: Global perspective. *Ann Epidemiol, 19,* 468–483.

27. Garland, C. F., et al. (2007). Vitamin D and prevention of breast cancer: Pooled analysis. *J Steroid Biochem Mol Biol, 103,* 708–711.

28. McDonnell, S. L., Baggerly, C. A., French, C. B., Baggerly, L. L., Garland, C. F., Gorham, E. D., Hollis, B. W., Trump, D. L., & Lappe, J. M. (2018). Breast cancer risk markedly lower with serum 25-hydroxyvitamin D concentrations ≥ 60 vs < 20 ng/ml (150 vs 50 nmol/L): Pooled analysis of two randomized trials and a prospective cohort. *PloS One, 13* (6), e0199265.

29. McDonnell, S. L., Baggerly, C., French, C. B., Baggerly, L. L., Garland, C. F., Gorham, E. D., Lappe, J. M., & Heaney, R. P. (2016). Serum 25-hydroxyvitamin D concentrations ≥ 40 ng/ml are associated with > 65% lower cancer risk: Pooled analysis of randomized trial and prospective cohort study. *PloS One, 11* (4), e0152441.

30. American Society of Clinical Oncology 2008 Annual Meeting: Abstract 511. Preview presscast, May 15, 2008.

31. Goodwin, P. J., et al. (2009). Prognostic effects of 25-hydroxyvitamin D levels in early breast cancer. *J Clin Oncol, 27,* 3757–3763.

32. Kessler, J. H. (2004). The effect of supraphysiologic levels of iodine on patients with cyclic mastalgia. *Breast J, 10,* 328–336.

33. Ghent, W. R., et al. (1993). Iodine replacement in fibrocystic disease of the breast. *Can J Surg, 35,* 453–460.

34. Fitzgibbons, P. L., et al. (1998). Benign breast changes and the risk for subsequent breast cancer: An update of the 1985 consensus statement. Cancer Committee of the College of American Pathologists. *Arch Pathol Lab Med, 122,* 1053–1055; Hartmann, L. C., et al. (2005). Benign breast disease and the risk of breast cancer. *N Engl J Med, 353,* 229–237.

35. Garcia-Solis, P., et al. (2005). Inhibition of N-methyl-N-nitrosourea-induced mammary carcinogenesis by molecular iodine (I2) but not by iodide (I-) treatment. Evidence that I2 prevents cancer promotion. *Mol Cell Endocrinol, 236,* 49–57.

36. Shrivastava, A. (2006). Molecular iodine induces caspase-independent apoptosis in human breast carcinoma cells involving the mitochondria-mediated pathway. *J Biol Chem, 281,* 19762–19771.

37. Aceves, C., et al. (2005). Is iodine a gatekeeper of the integrity of the mammary gland? *J Mammary Gland Biol Neoplasia, 10,* 189–196.
38. Eskin, B. A., et al. (1967). Mammary gland dysplasia in iodine deficiency. *JAMA, 200,* 115–119.
39. Stadel, B. V. (1976). Dietary iodine and risk of breast, endometrial, and ovarian cancer. *Lancet, 1* (7965), 890–891.
40. Lockwood, K., et al. (1994). Partial and complete regression of breast cancer in patients in relation to dosage of coenzyme Q_{10}. *Biochem Biophys Res Comm, 199* (3), 1504–1508.
41. Pierce, B. L., et al. (2009). Elevated biomarkers of inflammation are associated with reduced survival among breast cancer patients. *J Clin Oncol, 27,* 3437–3444.
42. Guo, L., Liu, S., Zhang, S., Chen, Q., Zhang, M., Quan, P., Lu, J., & Sun, X. (May 22, 2015). C-reactive protein and risk of breast cancer: A systematic review and meta-analysis. *Sci Rep, 5,* 10508.
43. Li, C. I., et al. (2010). Alcohol consumption risk of postmenopausal breast cancer by subtype: The women's health initiative observational study. *J Natl Cancer Inst, 102,* 1422–1431.
44. Willett, W. C., et al. (1987). Moderate alcohol consumption and the risk of breast cancer. *N Engl J Med, 316,* 1174–1180.
45. Li, C. I., et al. (2009). Relationship between potentially modifiable lifestyle factors and risk of second primary contralateral breast cancer among women diagnosed with estrogen receptor–positive invasive breast cancer. *J Clin Oncol, 27,* 5312–5318.
46. Ginsburg, E. (1996). Effects of alcohol ingestion on estrogens in postmenopausal women. *JAMA, 276* (21), 1747–1751.
47. Zhang, S., et al. (1989). A prospective study of folate intake and the risk of breast cancer. *JAMA, 281* (17), 1632–1637.
48. Ambrosone, C., et al. (1996). Cigarette smoking, N-acetyltransferase 2 genetic polymorphisms, and breast cancer risk. *JAMA, 276* (18), 1494–1501.
49. Bernstein, L., et al. (2005). Lifetime recreational exercise activity and breast cancer risk among black women and white women. *J Natl Cancer Inst., 97* (22), 1671–1679.
50. Thune, I., et al. (1997). Physical activity and the risk of breast cancer. *N Engl J Med, 336,* 1269–1275.
51. Peters, T. M., et al. (2009). Intensity and timing of physical activity in relation to postmenopausal breast cancer risk: The prospective NIH-AARP diet and health study. *BMC Cancer, 9,* 349.
52. Verkasalo, P. K., et al. (2005). Sleep duration and breast cancer: A prospective cohort study. *Cancer Res, 65* (20), 9595–9600.
53. Blask, D. E., et al. (2005). Melatonin-depleted blood from premenopausal women exposed to light at night stimulates growth of human breast cancer xenografts in nude rats. *Cancer Res, 65* (23), 11174–11184.
54. Schernhammer, E. S., & Hankinson, S. E. (2005). Urinary melatonin levels and breast cancer risk. *J Natl Cancer Inst, 97* (14), 1084–1087.
55. Schernhammer, E. S., et al. (2001). Rotating night shifts and risk of breast

cancer in women participating in the Nurses' Health Study. *J Natl Cancer Inst, 93* (20), 1563–1568.

56. Carlson, L. E., Beattie, T. L., Giese-Davis, J., Faris, P., Tamagawa, R., Fick, L. J., Degelman, E. S., & Speca, M. (2015). Mindfulness-based cancer recovery and supportive-expressive therapy maintain telomere length relative to controls in distressed breast cancer survivors. *Cancer, 121* (3), 476–484.

57. Biegler, K. A., Anderson, A. K., Wenzel, L. B., Osann, K., & Nelson, E. L. (2012). Longitudinal change in telomere length and the chronic stress response in a randomized pilot biobehavioral clinical study: Implications for cancer prevention. *Cancer Prev Res, 5* (10), 1173–1182.

58. Glass, A. G., et al. (2007). Breast cancer incidence, 1980–2006: Combined roles of menopausal hormone therapy, screening mammography, and estrogen receptor status. *J Natl Cancer Inst, 99,* 1152–1161; Ravdin, P. M., et al. (2007). The decrease in breast-cancer incidence in 2003 in the United States. *N Engl J Med, 356,* 1670–1674; Clarke, C. A., et al. (2006). Recent declines in hormone therapy utilization and breast cancer incidence: Clinical and population-based evidence. *J Clin Oncol, 24,* e49–e50.

59. Welch, H. G., & Black, W. C. (1997). Using autopsy series to estimate the disease "reservoir" for ductal carcinoma in situ of the breast: How much more breast cancer can we find? *Ann Intern Med, 127* (11), 1023–1028; Nielsen, M., et al. (1987). Breast cancer and atypia among young and middle-aged women: A study of 110 medicolegal autopsies. *Br J Cancer, 56* (6), 814–819.

60. Welch, H. G., & Black, W. C. (1997). Using autopsy series to estimate the disease "reservoir" for ductal carcinoma in situ of the breast: How much more breast cancer can we find? *Ann Intern Med, 127* (11), 1023–1028.

61. Zahl, P., Maehlen, J., & Welch, H. G. (2008). The natural history of invasive breast cancers detected by screening mammography. *Arch Intern Med, 168,* 21, 2311–2316.

62. Parker-Pope, T. (Oct. 22, 2009). Benefits and risks of cancer screening are not always clear, experts say. *New York Times,* http://www.nytimes.com /2009/10/22/health/22screen.html#; Esserman, L., et al. (2009). Rethinking screening for breast cancer and prostate cancer. *JAMA, 302,* 1685–1692; Kolata, G. (Oct. 21, 2009). Cancer society, in shift, has concerns on screenings. *New York Times,* www.nytimes.com/2009/10/21/health /21cancer.html#.

63. Parker-Pope, T. (Oct. 22, 2009). Benefits and risks of cancer screening are not always clear, experts say. *New York Times,* http://www.nytimes.com /2009/10/22/health/22screen.html#.

64. Moody-Ayers, S., et al. (2000). "Benign" tumors and "early detection" in mammography-screened patients of a natural cohort with breast cancer. *Arch Intern Med, 160* (8), 1109–1115.

65. National Institutes of Health Consensus Development Panel. (1997). National Institutes of Health Consensus Development Conference Statement: Breast cancer screening for women ages 40–49. *J Natl Cancer Inst, 89* (14), 1015–1026.

66. Prager, K. (1996). Outrage over mammogram screening unwarranted. *Medical Tribune.* Quoted by Gina Kolata in the *New York Times* (Jan. 28, 1997).

67. Baines, C. (2005). Rethinking breast screening—again. *BMJ, 331,* 1031.

68. Van Netten, J. P., et al. (1994). Physical trauma and breast cancer. *Lancet, 343* (8903), 978–979.

69. Christiansen, C. L., et al. (2000). Predicting the cumulative risk of false-positive mammograms. *J Natl Cancer Inst, 92* (20), 1657–1666.

70. Elmore, J. G., et al. (1998). Ten-year risk of false positive screening mammograms and clinical breast exams. *N Engl J Med, 338* (16), 1089–1096.

71. Brodersen, J., & Siersma, V. D. (2013). Long-term psychosocial consequences of false-positive screening mammography. *Ann Fam Med, 11* (2), 106–115.

72. Gotzsche, P. C., & Olsen, O. (2001). Is screening for breast cancer with mammography justifiable? *Lancet, 355,* 129–134; Gotzsche, P. C., & Olsen, O. (2001). Cochrane review on screening for breast cancer with mammography. *Lancet, 358,* 1340–1342.

73. Bleyer, A., & Welch, H. G. (2012). Effect of three decades of screening mammography on breast-cancer incidence. *N Engl J Med, 367* (21), 1998–2005.

74. Gøtzsche, P. C., & Jørgensen, K. J. (2013). Screening for breast cancer with mammography. *Cochrane Database Syst Rev, 2013* (6), CD001877.

75. Kerlikowske, K., et al. (1999). Continuing screening mammography in women aged 70 to 79 years: Impact on life expectancy and cost-effectiveness. *JAMA, 282,* 22, 2156–2163.

76. Narod, S. A., Iqbal, J., Giannakeas, V., Sopik, V., & Sun, P. (2015). Breast cancer mortality after a diagnosis of ductal carcinoma in situ. *JAMA Oncol, 1* (7), 888–896.

77. Esserman, L., & Yau, C. (2015). Rethinking the standard for ductal carcinoma in situ treatment. *JAMA Oncol, 1* (7), 881–883.

78. Kolata, G. (August 21, 2015). Doubt is raised on quick surgery on breast lesion. *New York Times,* A1.

79. Esserman, L. J., Thompson, I. M., Jr, & Reid, B. (2013). Overdiagnosis and overtreatment in cancer: An opportunity for improvement. *JAMA, 310* (8), 797–798.

80. Esserman, L. J., & WISDOM Study and Athena Investigators (2017). The WISDOM Study: Breaking the deadlock in the breast cancer screening debate. *NPJ Breast Cancer, 3,* 34.

81. Shieh, Y., Eklund, M., Madlensky, L., Sawyer, S. D., Thompson, C. K., Stover Fiscalini, A., Ziv, E., Van't Veer, L. J., Esserman, L. J., Tice, J. A., & Athena Breast Health Network Investigators (2017). Breast cancer screening in the precision medicine era: Risk-based screening in a population-based trial. *J Natl Cancer Inst, 109* (5), 10.1093/jnci/djw290.

82. Hwang, S. and Miller, K. D. (January 17, 2018). "Cultural change": Dialing back the discussion and treatment of DCIS. *Medscape;* www.medscape.com/viewarticle/891198.

83. Marzouk, K., Assel, M., Ehdaie, B., & Vickers, A. (2018). Long-term can-

cer specific anxiety in men undergoing active surveillance of prostate cancer: Findings from a large prospective cohort. *J Urol, 200* (6), 1250–1255.

84. Bleicher, R. J., et al. (2009). Association of routine pretreatment magnetic resonance imaging with time to surgery, mastectomy rate, and margin status. *J Am Coll Surg, 209,* 180–187.

85. Parisky, Y. R., et al. (2003). Efficacy of computerized infrared imaging analysis to evaluate mammographically suspicious lesions. *Am J Roentgenol, 180,* 263–269.

86. Amalric, R., Giraud, D., Altschuler, C., Amalric, F., Spitalier, J. M., Brandone, J. M., Ayme, Y., & Gardiol, A. A. (1982). Does infrared thermography truly have a role in present-day breast cancer management? *Prog Clin Biol Res, 107,* 269–278.

87. Bronzino, J. D. (ed.) (2006). *Medical Devices and Systems (The Biomedical Engineering Handbook).* Boca Raton: CRC Press/Taylor & Francis Group.

88. Gautherie, M., & Gros, C. M. (1980). Breast thermography and cancer risk prediction. *Cancer, 45,* 51–56.

89. Arora, N., et al. (2008). Effectiveness of a noninvasive digital infrared thermal imaging system in the detection of breast cancer. *Am J Surg, 196,* 523–526.

90. Cong, W., Intes, X., & Wang, G. (2017). Optical tomographic imaging for breast cancer detection. *J Biomed Optics, 22* (9), 1–6.

91. Lee, K. (2011). Optical mammography: Diffuse optical imaging of breast cancer. *World J Clin Oncol, 2* (1), 64–72.

92. Moore, F. (1978). Breast self-examination. *N Engl J Med, 299* (6), 304–305.

93. Thomas, D. B., et al. (2002). Randomized trial of breast self-examination in Shanghai: Final results. *J Natl Cancer Inst, 94,* 1445–1457.

94. Semiglazov, V. F., et al. (1999). Interim results of a prospective randomized study of self-examination for early detection of breast cancer (Russia/St. Petersburg/WHO). *Voprosy Onkologii, 45* (3), 265–271.

95. U.S. Preventive Services Task Force (Nov. 17, 2009). Screening for breast cancer: U.S. Preventive Services Task Force recommendation statement. *Ann Intern Med, 151,* 716–726; www.annals.org/content/151/10/716.full.

96. Siu, A. L., & U.S. Preventive Services Task Force (2016). Screening for breast cancer: U.S. Preventive Services Task Force recommendation statement. *Ann Intern Med, 164* (4), 279–296.

97. Wyrick, D. (2005). Personal communication. Dana Wyrick is a registered massage therapist who developed this self-massage routine for breast health after studying with lymphedema therapy specialists in Europe and Australia, where the technique is far more common.

98. U.S. Preventive Services Task Force (Nov. 17, 2009). Screening for breast cancer: U.S. Preventive Services Task Force recommendation statement. *Ann Intern Med, 151,* 716–726; www.annals.org/content/151/10/716.full.

99. Mandelblatt, J. S., et al. (2009). Effects of mammography screening under different screening schedules: Model estimates of potential benefits and harms. *Ann Intern Med, 151* (10), 738–747; www.annals.org/content/151/10/738.full.

100. Kerlikowske, K., et al. (1993). Positive predictive value of screening mammography by age and family history of breast cancer. *JAMA, 270* (2), 444.

101. Sparano, J. A., Gray, R. J., Makower, D. F., Pritchard, K. I., Albain, K. S., Hayes, D. F., Geyer, C. E., Jr, Dees, E. C., Goetz, M. P., Olson, J. A., Jr, Lively, T., Badve, S. S., Saphner, T. J., Wagner, L. I., Whelan, T. J., Ellis, M. J., Paik, S., Wood, W. C., Ravdin, P. M., Keane, M. M., . . . & Sledge, G. W., Jr. (2018). Adjuvant chemotherapy guided by a 21-gene expression assay in breast cancer. *N Engl J Med, 379* (2), 111–121.

102. National Council on Aging (1997). *Myths and Perceptions About Aging and Women's Health.* Washington, DC: National Council on Aging; Assessing the odds (editorial). *Lancet, 350* (9091), 1563.

103. Love, S. (2005). *Dr. Susan Love's Breast Book* (145). Cambridge, MA: Da Capo Lifelong Books.

104. Ries, L. A. G., Eisner, M. P., Kosary, C. L., Hankey, B. F., Miller, B. A., Kleg, L., & Edwards, B. K. (eds.) (2000). *SEER Cancer Statistics Review, 1973–1993.* Bethesda, MD: National Cancer Institute; Black, W. C., et al. (1995). Perceptions of breast cancer risk and screening effectiveness in women younger than 50 years old. *J Nat Cancer Inst, 87,* 720–731.

105. www.cancer.gov/types/breast/risk-fact-sheet.

106. Phillips, K. A. (1999). Putting the risk of breast cancer in perspective. *N Engl J Med, 340* (2), 141–144.

107. Cutler, W., et al. (2020). Long term absence of invasive breast cancer diagnosis in 2,402,672 pre and postmenopausal women: A systematic review and meta-analysis. *PLoS One, 15* (9), e0237925.

108. Kuchenbaecker, K. B., Hopper, J. L., Barnes, D. R., Phillips, K. A., Mooij, T. M., Roos-Blom, M. J., Jervis, S., van Leeuwen, F. E., Milne, R. L., Andrieu, N., Goldgar, D. E., Terry, M. B., Rookus, M. A., Easton, D. F., Antoniou, A. C., BRCA1 and BRCA2 Cohort Consortium, McGuffog, L., Evans, D. G., Barrowdale, D., Frost, D., . . . & Olsson, H. (2017). Risks of breast, ovarian, and contralateral breast cancer for BRCA1 and BRCA2 mutation carriers. *JAMA, 317* (23), 2402–2416.

109. Hirshaut, Y., & Pressman, P. (2000). *Breast Cancer: The Complete Guide,* 256. New York: Bantam.

110. American College of Obstetrics & Gynecology, Committee on Genetics (Oct. 1996). *Breast-Ovarian Cancer Screening* (Committee Opinion no. 176). Washington, DC.

111. Collins, F. S. (1986). BRCA1—lots of mutations, lots of dilemmas. *N Engl J Med, 334* (3), 186–188.

112. Copson, E. R., Maishman, T. C., Tapper, W. J., Cutress, R. I., Greville-Heygate, S., Altman, D. G., Eccles, B., Gerty, S., Durcan, L. T., Jones, L., Evans, D. G., Thompson, A. M., Pharoah, P., Easton, D. F., Dunning, A. M., Hanby, A., Lakhani, S., Eeles, R., Gilbert, F. J., Hamed, H., Hodgson, S., Simmonds, P., Stanton, L., & Eccles, D. M. (2018). Germline BRCA mutation and outcome in young-onset breast cancer (POSH): A prospective cohort study. *Lancet Oncol, 19* (2), 169–180.

113. Kesaniemi, Y. A. (unpublished data). Cited in Viitanen, A. (1996), A new estrogen gel: Clinical benefits. In Wren, B. G. (ed.), *Progress in the Man-*

agement of the Menopause: The Proceedings of the 8th International Congress on the Menopause (168). Sydney, Australia: Parthenon.

114. LaVecchia, C., Negri, E., Franceschi, S., et al. (1995). Hormone replacement therapy and breast cancer risk: A cooperative Italian study. *Br J Cancer, 72,* 244–248.

115. Beral, V., et al. (2010). Breast cancer risk in relation to the interval between menopause and starting hormone therapy. *J Nat Cancer Inst, 103,* 296–305.

116. Campagnoli, C., et al. (1999). HRT and breast cancer risk: A clue for interpreting the available data. *Maturitas, 33,* 185–190; Collaborative Group on Hormonal Factors in Breast Cancer (1997). Breast cancer and hormone replacement therapy: Collaborative reanalysis of data from 51 epidemiological studies of 52,705 women with breast cancer and 108,411 without breast cancer. *Lancet, 350,* 1047–1059.

117. Chlebowski, R. T., et al. (2010). Estrogen plus progestin and breast cancer incidence and mortality in postmenopausal women. *JAMA, 304,* 1684–1692.

118. Bhavani, B. R., et al. (1994). Pharmacokinetics of 17 beta-dihydroequilin sulfate and 17 beta-dihydroequilin in normal postmenopausal women. *J Clin Endocrinol Metab, 78,* 197–204.

119. Hargrove, J., & Eisenberg, E. (1995). Menopause. *Med Clin North Am, 79* (6), 1337–1363.

120. Campagnoli, C., et al. (1999). HRT and breast cancer risk: A clue for interpreting the available data. *Maturitas, 33,* 185–190; Collaborative Group on Hormonal Factors in Breast Cancer (1997). Breast cancer and hormone replacement therapy: Collaborative reanalysis of data from 51 epidemiological studies of 52,705 women with breast cancer and 108,411 without breast cancer. *Lancet, 350,* 1047–1059.

121. Beral V., Million Women Study Collaborators (2003). Breast cancer and hormone-replacement therapy in the Million Women Study. *Lancet, 362* (9382), 419–427.

122. Coombs, N. J., et al. (2005). Hormone replacement therapy and breast cancer: Estimate of risk. *BMJ, 331* (7512), 347–349.

123. Coombs, N. J., et al. (2005). Hormone replacement therapy and breast cancer risk in California. *Breast J, 11* (6), 410–415.

124. Campagnoli, C., et al. (1999). HRT and breast cancer risk: A clue for interpreting the available data. *Maturitas, 33,* 185–190. Given the results of the WHI study on Prempro and the financial losses suffered by Wyeth Ayerst as a result, it's doubtful that we'll ever have the data needed to prove this!

125. Eden J. (2017). The endometrial and breast safety of menopausal hormone therapy containing micronised progesterone: A short review. *Aust NZ J Obstet Gyn, 57* (1), 12–15.

126. Fournier, A., et al. (2008). Unequal risks for breast cancer associated with different hormone replacement therapies: Results from the e3n cohort study. *Breast Cancer Res Treat, 107,* 103–111.

127. Fournier, A., et al. (2009). Estrogen-progestogen menopausal hormone

therapy and breast cancer; does delay from menopause onset to treatment initiation influence risks? *Journal of Clinical Oncology, 27,* 5138–5143.

128. Holtorf, K. (2009). The bioidentical hormone debate: Are bioidentical hormones (estradiol, estriol, and progesterone) safer or more efficacious than commonly used synthetic versions in hormone replacement therapy? *Postgrad Med, 121* (1), 73–85.

129. Huang, Z., Willett, W. C., Colditz, G. A., Hunter, D. J., Manson, J. E., Rosner, B., Speizer, F. E., & Hankinson, S. E. (1999). Waist circumference, waist:hip ratio, and risk of breast cancer in the Nurses' Health Study. *Am J Epidemiol, 150* (12) 1316–1324. "Furthermore," they write, "it has been proposed that abdominal adiposity is associated with an excess of androgen and increased conversion of androgen to estrogen in adipose tissue." They also point out that hormone use by postmenopausal women likely raises hormone levels in all those women. "[A]s a result, all post-menopausal hormone users were at increased risk of breast cancer regardless of central obesity," they reason.

130. Melamed, M., et al. (1997). Molecular and kinetic basis for the mixed agonist/antagonist activity of estriol. *Mol Endocrinol, 11,* 12, 1868–1878.

131. Rajkumar, L., et al. (2004). Prevention of mammary carcinogenesis by short-term estrogen and progestin treatments. *Breast Cancer Res, 6,* 1, R31–7.

132. Chlebowski, R., et al. (2009). Breast cancer after use of estrogen plus progestin in postmenopausal women. *N Engl J Med, 360* (6), 573–587.

133. Henrich, J. B. (1992). The postmenopausal estrogen/breast cancer controversy. *JAMA, 268,* 1900–1902; Wotiz, H. H., Beebe, D. R., & Muller, E. (1984). Effect of estrogen on DMBA-induced breast tumors. *J Steroid Biochem, 20,* 1067–1075.

134. Drife, J. O. (1986). Breast development in puberty. *Ann N Y Acad Sci, 464,* 58–65; Dulbecco, R., et al. (1982). Cell types and morphogenesis in the mammary gland. *Proc Natl Acad Sci U S A, 79,* 7346–7350; Longacre, T., & Bartow, S. (1986). A correlative morphologic study of human breast and endometrium in the menstrual cycle. *Am J Surgical Path, 10* (6), 382–393; Weinberg, R. A. (Sept. 1996). How cancer arises. *Scientific American,* 62–70.

135. Lemon, H. (1973). Oestriol and prevention of breast cancer. *Lancet, 1* (802), 546; Lemon, H. (1975). Estriol prevention of mammary carcinoma induced by 7,12-dimethyl-benzanthracene and procarbazine. *Cancer Res, 35,* 1341–1353; Lemon, H. (1980). Pathophysiologic considerations in the treatment of menopausal patients with oestrogens: The role of oestriol in the prevention of mammary cancer. *Acta Endocrinol, 1,* 17–27; Lemon, H., Wotiz, H., Parsons, L., et al. (1966). Reduced estriol excretion in patients with breast cancer prior to endocrine therapy. *JAMA, 196,* 1128–1136.

136. Bu, S. Z., et al. (1997). Progesterone induces apoptosis and upregulation of p53 expression in human ovarian carcinoma cell lines. *Cancer, 79* (10), 1944–1950.

137. Zava, D. T., & Duwe, G. (1997). Estrogen and antiproliferative properties

of genistein and other flavonoids in human breast cancer cells *in vivo*. *Nutr Cancer, 27* (1), 31–40.

138. Cowan, A. D., et al. (1961). Breast cancer incidence in women with a history of progesterone deficiency. *Am J Epidemiol, 114* (2), 209.

139. Chang, K. J., et al. (1995). Influences of percutaneous administration of estradiol and progesterone on human breast epithelial cell cycle *in vivo*. *Fertil Steril, 63,* 785–791.

140. Badwe, R. A., et al. (1991). Timing of surgery during menstrual cycle and survival of premenopausal women with operable breast cancer. *Lancet, 337,* 1261–1264.

141. Hrushesky, W. (1996). Breast cancer, timing of surgery, and the menstrual cycle: Call for prospective trial. *J Womens Health, 5* (6), 555–566.

142. Wren, B., & Eden, J. A. (1996). Do progestogens reduce the risk of breast cancer? A review of the evidence. *Menopause, 3* (1), 4–12.

143. Ibid.

144. McEwen, B. S., et al. (1999). Inhibition of dendritic spine induction on hippocampal ca-1 pyramidal neurons by nonsteroidal estrogen antagonist in female rats. *Endocrinology, 140,* 1044–1047; McEwen, B. S., & Wooley, C. S. (1994). Estradiol and progesterone regulate neuronal structure and synaptic connectivity in adult as well as developing brain. *Exper Gerontol, 29,* 431–436; Wooley, C. S., & McEwen, B. S. (1993). Roles of estradiol and progesterone in regulation of hippocampal dendritic spine density during the estrous cycle in the rat. *J Comp Neurol, 336,* 293–306.

145. Timmerman, D., et al. (1998). A randomized trial on the use of ultrasonography or office hysteroscopy for endometrial assessment in postmenopausal patients with breast cancer who were treated with tamoxifen. *Am J Obstet Gynecol, 179,* 62–70; Franchi, M., et al. (1999). Endometrial thickness in tamoxifen-treated patients: An independent predictor of endometrial disease. *Obstet Gynecol, 93,* 1004–1008; Ramonetta, L. M., et al. (1999). Endometrial cancer in polyps associated with tamoxifen use. *Am J Obstet Gynecol, 180,* 340–341.

146. Osborne, C. K. (1999). Questions and answers about tamoxifen. In *Tamoxifen for the Treatment and Prevention of Breast Cancer.* V. Craig, (ed.). Melville, NY. (1995). NSABP halts B-14 trial: No benefit seen beyond 5 years of tamoxifen use. *J Nat Cancer Inst, 87,* 1829.

147. Bramwell, V. H., Pritchard, K. I., Tu, D., Tonkin, K., Vachhrajani, H., Vandenberg, T. A., Robert, J., Arnold, A., O'Reilly, S. E., Graham, B., & Shepherd, L. (2010). A randomized placebo-controlled study of tamoxifen after adjuvant chemotherapy in premenopausal women with early breast cancer (National Cancer Institute of Canada—Clinical Trials Group Trial, MA.12). *Ann Oncol, 21* (2), 283–290.

148. Fisher, B. (1998). Tamoxifen for prevention of breast cancer: Report of the National Surgical Adjuvant Breast and Bowel Project P-1 Study. *J Nat Cancer Inst, 90* (18), 1371–1388.

149. Gail, M. H., et al. (1989). Projecting individualized probabilities of devel-

oping breast cancer for white females who are being examined annually. *J Nat Cancer Inst, 81* (24), 1879–1886.

150. Melnikow, J., et al. (July 24, 2006; epub ahead of print). Chemoprevention: Drug pricing and mortality: The case of tamoxifen. *Cancer*.

151. Gandey, A. (2006). Tamoxifen fails to reduce breast cancer risk in most women. *Medscape Medical News,* July 26, 2006; http://www.medscape .com/viewarticle/54157.

152. Li, C. I., et al. (2009). Adjuvant hormonal therapy for breast cancer and risk of hormone receptor-specific subtypes of contralateral breast cancer. *Cancer Res, 69,* 6865–6870.

153. Nestoriuc, Y., von Blanckenburg, P., Schuricht, F., Barsky, A. J., Hadji, P., Albert, U. S., & Rief, W. (2016). Is it best to expect the worst? Influence of patients' side-effect expectations on endocrine treatment outcome in a 2-year prospective clinical cohort study. *Ann Oncol, 27* (10), 1909–1915.

154. Ninth Annual American Association for Cancer Research (AACR) International Conference on Frontiers in Cancer Prevention Research: Abstract B10. Presented Nov. 11, 2010.

155. Cuzick, J., et al. (2008). Treatment-emergent endocrine symptoms and the risk of breast cancer recurrence: A retrospective analysis of the ATAC trial. *Lancet Oncol, 9,* 1143–1148.

Chapter 14: Living with Heart, Passion, and Joy

1. Jefferson, A. L., et al. (2010). Cardiac index is associated with brain aging. The Framingham Heart Study. *Circulation, 122,* 690–697.

2. Svendsen, N. A. (Oct. 1999). Personal letter, excerpted in *Health Wisdom for Women,* 6 (10), 8. Used here with permission from the author.

3. Tremollieres, F. A., et al. (1999). Coronary heart disease risk factors and menopause: A study in 1,684 French women. *Atherosclerosis, 142* (2), 415–423.

4. Ridker, P. M., et al. (2002). Comparison of C-reactive protein and low-density lipoprotein cholesterol levels in the prediction of first cardiovascular events. *N Engl J Med, 347,* 1557–1565.

5. Agin, D. (2010). *More Than Genes,* 87. New York: Oxford University Press; Barker, D. J. (1981). Geographical variations in disease in Britain. *BMJ (Clin Res Ed), 283,* 398–400; Barker, D. J., et al. (June 1982). Incidence of diabetes amongst people aged 18–50 years in nine British towns: A collaborative study. *Diabetologia, 22,* 421–425; Barker, D. J., & Osmond, C. (1987). Inequalities in health in Britain: Specific explanations in three Lancashire towns. *BMJ (Clin Res Ed), 294,* 749–752; Bateson, P., et al. (2004). Developmental plasticity and human health. *Nature, 430,* 419–421.

6. Webber, L. S., et al. (1979). Occurrence in children of multiple risk factors for coronary artery disease: The Bogalusa Heart Study. *Prev Med, 8,* 407–418; Khoury, P., et al. (1980). Clustering and interrelationships of coro-

nary heart disease risk factors in schoolchildren, ages 6–19. *Am J Epidemiol, 112*, 524–538.

7. Clow, B. H. (1996). *Liquid Light of Sex: Kundalini Rising at Mid-Life Crisis* (103–104). Santa Fe, NM: Bear & Co.

8. National Center for Health Statistics (2018). Health Data Interactive; Centers for Disease Control and Prevention. WISQARS leading causes of death reports.

9. Benjamin, E. J., Blaha, M. J., Chiuve, S. E., Cushman, M., Das, S. R., Deo, R., de Ferranti, S. D., Floyd, J., Fornage, M., Gillespie, C., Isasi, C. R., Jiménez, M. C., Jordan, L. C., Judd, S. E., Lackland, D., Lichtman, J. H., Lisabeth, L., Liu, S., Longenecker, C. T., Mackey, R. H., . . . & American Heart Association Statistics Committee and Stroke Statistics Subcommittee (2017). Heart disease and stroke statistics—2017 update: A report from the American Heart Association. *Circulation, 135* (10), e146–e603.

10. Benjamin, E. J., Muntner, P., Alonso, A., Bittencourt, M. S., Callaway, C. W., Carson, A. P., Chamberlain, A. M., Chang, A. R., Cheng, S., Das, S. R., Delling, F. N., Djousse, L., Elkind, M., Ferguson, J. F., Fornage, M., Jordan, L. C., Khan, S. S., Kissela, B. M., Knutson, K. L., Kwan, T. W., . . . & American Heart Association Council on Epidemiology and Prevention Statistics Committee and Stroke Statistics Subcommittee (2019). Heart disease and stroke statistics—2019 update: A report from the American Heart Association. *Circulation, 139* (10), e56–e528.

11. Childre, D., & Martin, H. (1999). *The HeartMath Solution* (foreword). San Francisco: HarperSanFrancisco.

12. Skinner, J. (1993). Neurocardiology: Brain mechanisms underlying fatal cardiac arrhythmias. *Neurologic Clinics, 11* (2), 325–351.

13. HeartMath LLC (May 2009). Return on investment. White paper.

14. McCraty, R., et al. (1998). The impact of a new emotional self-management program on stress, emotions, heart rate variability, DHEA and cortisol. *Integr Physiol Behav Sci, 33*, 151–170.

15. Kudenchuk, P. J., et al. (1996). Comparison of presentation, treatment and outcome of acute myocardial infarction in men vs. women (The Myocardial Infarction Triage and Intervention Registry). *Am J Cardiology, 78* (1), 9–14.

16. Mackay, M. H., et al. (2009). Gender differences in reported symptoms of acute coronary syndromes. *Can J Cardiol, 25*, 115b.

17. Cooper, G. S. (1999). Menstrual and reproductive risk factors for ischemic heart disease. *Epidemiology, 10* (3), 255–259; Hazeltine, F. P., & Jacobson, B. (1997). *Women's Health Research: A Medical and Policy Primer* (173). Washington, DC: APA Press.

18. Alabas, O. A., Gale, C. P., Hall, M., Rutherford, M. J., Szummer, K., Lawesson, S. S., Alfredsson, J., Lindahl, B., & Jernberg, T. (2017). Sex differences in treatments, relative survival, and excess mortality following acute myocardial infarction: National Cohort Study using the SWEDEHEART registry. *J Am Heart Assoc, 6* (12), e007123.

19. Li, S., Fonarow, G. C., Mukamal, K. J., Liang, L., Schulte, P. J., Smith,

E. E., DeVore, A., Hernandez, A. F., Peterson, E. D., & Bhatt, D. L. (2016). Sex and race/ethnicity-related disparities in care and outcomes after hospitalization for coronary artery disease among older adults. *Circulation, 9* (2, suppl. 1), S36–S44.

20. Mehta, L. S., Beckie, T. M., DeVon, H. A., Grines, C. L., Krumholz, H. M., Johnson, M. N., Lindley, K. J., Vaccarino, V., Wang, T. Y., Watson, K. E., Wenger, N. K., & American Heart Association Cardiovascular Disease in Women and Special Populations Committee of the Council on Clinical Cardiology, Council on Epidemiology and Prevention, Council on Cardiovascular and Stroke Nursing, and Council on Quality of Care and Outcomes Research (2016). Acute myocardial infarction in women: A scientific statement from the American Heart Association. *Circulation, 133* (9), 916–947.

21. Iribarren, C., et al. (2000). Association of hostility with coronary artery calcification in young adults: The CARDIA Study. *JAMA, 283* (19), 2546–2551.

22. Friedman, M., & Rosenman, R. (1974). *Type A Behavior and Your Heart.* New York: Alfred A. Knopf.

23. Nasir, K., Bittencourt, M. S., Blaha, M. J., Blankstein, R., Agatson, A. S., Rivera, J. J., Miedema, M. D., Sibley, C. T., Shaw, L. J., Blumenthal, R. S., Budoff, M. J., & Krumholz, H. M. (2015). Implications of coronary artery calcium testing among statin candidates according to American College of Cardiology/American Heart Association Cholesterol Management Guidelines: MESA (Multi-Ethnic Study of Atherosclerosis). *J Am Coll Cardiol, 66* (15), 1657–1668.

24. Stampfer, M., et al. (2000). Primary prevention of coronary heart disease in women through diet and lifestyle. *N Engl J Med, 343,* 16–22.

25. Arsenault, B. J., et al. (July 2010; epub ahead of print). The hypertriglyceridemic-waist phenotype and the risk of coronary artery disease: Results from the EPIC-Norfolk Prospective Population Study. *Can Med Assoc J.*

26. Mo-Suwan, L., & Lebel, L. (1996). Risk factors for cardiovascular disease in obese and normal school-age children: Association of insulin with other cardiovascular risk factors. *Biomed Environ Sci, 9* (2–3), 269–275; Wing, R. R., & Jeffery, R. W. (1995). Effect of modest weight loss on changes in cardiovascular risk factors: Are there differences between men and women between weight loss and maintenance? *Int J Obes Relat Metab Disord, 19* (1), 67–73.

27. Virani, S. S., Alonso, A., Benjamin, E. J., Bittencourt, M. S., Callaway, C. W., Carson, A. P., Chamberlain, A. M., Chang, A. R., Cheng, S., Delling, F. N., Djousse, L., Elkind, M., Ferguson, J. F., Fornage, M., Khan, S. S., Kissela, B. M., Knutson, K. L., Kwan, T. W., Lackland, D. T., Lewis, T. T., . . . & American Heart Association Council on Epidemiology and Prevention Statistics Committee and Stroke Statistics Subcommittee (2020). Heart disease and stroke statistics—2020 update: A report from the American Heart Association. *Circulation, 141* (9), e139–e596.

28. Brunzell, J. D., et al. (2008). Lipoprotein management in patients with

cardiometabolic risk: Consensus statement from the American Diabetes Association and the American College of Cardiology Foundation. *Diabetes Care, 31,* 811–822.

29. Kones, R. (2009). The Jupiter study, CRP screening, and aggressive statin therapy—implications for the primary prevention of cardiovascular disease. *Ther Adv Cardiovasc Dis, 3,* 309–315.

30. Grundy, S. M., et al. (2004). Implications of recent clinical trials for the National Cholesterol Education Program Adult Treatment Panel III guidelines. *Circulation, 110* (2), 227–239.

31. Ravnskov, U., Diamond, D. M., Hama, R., Hamazaki, T., Hammarskjöld, B., Hynes, N., Kendrick, M., Langsjoen, P. H., Malhotra, A., Mascitelli, L., McCully, K. S., Ogushi, Y., Okuyama, H., Rosch, P. J., Schersten, T., Sultan, S., & Sundberg, R. (2016). Lack of an association or an inverse association between low-density-lipoprotein cholesterol and mortality in the elderly: A systematic review. *BMJ Open, 6* (6), e010401.

32. Vancheri, F., Backlund, L., Strender, L. E., Godman, B., & Wettermark, B. (2016). Time trends in statin utilisation and coronary mortality in Western European countries. *BMJ Open, 6* (3), e010500.

33. Kristensen, M. L., Christensen, P. M., & Hallas, J. (2015). The effect of statins on average survival in randomised trials, an analysis of end point postponement. *BMJ Open, 5* (9), e007118.

34. ALLHAT Officers and Coordinators for the ALLHAT Collaborative Research Group (2002). Major outcomes in moderately hypercholesterolemic, hypertensive patients randomized to pravastatin vs. usual care: The Antihypertensive and Lipid-Lowering Treatment to Prevent Heart Attack Trial (ALLHAT-LLT). *JAMA, 288* (23), 2998–3007.

35. Heart Protection Study Collaborative Group (2002), MRC/BHF Heart Protection Study of cholesterol lowering with simvastatin in 20,536 high-risk individuals: A randomised placebo-controlled trial. *Lancet, 360* (9326), 7–22.

36. Matsuzaki, M., et al. (2002). Large-scale cohort study of the relationship between serum cholesterol concentration and coronary events with low-dose simvastatin therapy in Japanese patients with hypercholesterolemia. *Circ J, 66* (12), 1087–1095.

37. Newman, C. B., et al. (2003). Safety of atorvastatin derived from analysis of 44 completed trials in 9,416 patients. *Am J Cardio, 92* (6), 670–676.

38. Sever, P. S., et al. (2003). Prevention of coronary and stroke events with atorvastatin in hypertensive patients who have average or lower-than-average cholesterol concentrations, in the Anglo-Scandinavian Cardiac Outcomes Trial—Lipid Lowering Arm (ASCOT-LLA): A multicentre randomised controlled trial. *Lancet, 361* (9364), 1149–1158.

39. Jenkins, A. J. (2003). Might money spent on statins be better spent? *BMJ, 327* (7420), 933.

40. Manuel, D. G., et al. (2006). Effectiveness and efficiency of different guidelines on statin treatment for preventing deaths from coronary heart disease: Modelling study. *BMJ, 332,* 1419.

41. Randomised trial of cholesterol lowering in 4,444 patients with coronary

heart disease: The Scandinavian Simvastatin Survival Study (4S). (1994). *Lancet, 344,* 1383–1389; Prevention of cardiovascular events and death with pravastatin in patients with coronary heart disease and a broad range of initial cholesterol levels: The Long-Term Intervention with Pravastatin in Ischaemic Disease (LIPID) Study Group (1998). *N Engl J Med, 339,* 1349–1357; Downs, J. R., et al. (1998). Primary prevention of acute coronary events with lovastatin in men and women with average cholesterol levels: Results of AFCAPS/TexCAPS. Air Force/Texas Coronary Atherosclerosis Prevention Study. *JAMA, 279,* 1615–1622; Dale, K. M., et al. (2007). Impact of gender on statin efficacy. *Curr Med Res Opin, 23,* 565–574.

42. Walsh, J. M., & Pignone, M. (2004). Drug treatment of hyperlipidemia in women. *JAMA, 291,* 2243–2252.

43. Ulmer, H., et al. (2004). Why Eve is not Adam: Prospective follow-up in 149,650 women and men of cholesterol and other risk factors related to cardiovascular and all-cause mortality. *J Womens Health, 13,* 41–53.

44. Tikhonoff, V., et al. (2005). Low-density lipoprotein cholesterol and mortality in older people. *J Am Geriatr Soc, 53,* 2159–2164.

45. Harris, J. I., et al. (2004). Statin treatment alters serum n-3 and n-6 fatty acids in hypercholesterolemic patients. *Prostaglandins Leukot Essent Fatty Acids, 71,* 263–269.

46. Maki, K. C., et al. (2010). Baseline lipoprotein lipids and low-density lipoprotein cholesterol response to prescription omega-3 acid ethyl ester added to simvastatin therapy. *Am J Cardiol, 105,* 1409–1412; Bays, H. E., et al. (2010). Long-term up to 24-month efficacy and safety of concomitant prescription omega-3-acid ethyl esters and simvastatin in hypertriglyceridemic patients. *Curr Med Res Opin, 26,* 907–915; Bays, H. E., et al. (2010). Effects of prescription omega-3-acid ethyl esters on non-high-density lipoprotein cholesterol when coadministered with escalating doses of atorvastatin. *Mayo Clin Proc, 85,* 122–128; Maki, K. C., et al. (2008); Effects of adding prescription omega-3 acid ethyl esters to simvastatin (20 mg/day) on lipids and lipoprotein particles in men and women with mixed dyslipidemia. *Am J Cardiol, 102,* 429–433; Davidson, M. H., et al. (2007). Efficacy and tolerability of adding prescription omega-3 fatty acids 4 g/d to simvastatin 40 mg/d in hypertriglyceridemic patients: An 8-week, randomized, double-blind, placebo-controlled study. *Clin Ther, 29,* 1354–1367; Hong, H., et al. (2004). Effects of simvastatin combined with omega-3 fatty acids on high sensitive C-reactive protein, lipidemia, and fibrinolysis in patients with mixed dyslipidemia. *Chin Med Sci J, 19,* 145–149; Durrington, P. N., et al. (2001). An omega-3 polyunsaturated fatty acid concentrate administered for one year decreased triglycerides in simvastatin treated patients with coronary heart disease and persisting hypertriglyceridaemia. *Heart, 85,* 544–548.

47. Scott, R. S., et al. (1991). Simvastatin and side effects. *N Z Med J, 104,* 493–495; Wierzbicki, A. S., et al. (1999). Atorvastatin compared with simvastatin-based therapies in the management of severe familial hyperlipidaemias. *QJM, 92,* 387–394.

48. Laise, E. (Nov. 2003). The Lipitor dilemma. *Smart Money: The Wall Street Journal Magazine of Personal Business, 12* (11), 90–96.

49. Hamilton-Craig, I. (2001). Statin-associated myopathy. *Med J Aust, 175* (9), 486–489.

50. Golomb, B. A., et al. (2007). Physician response to patient reports of adverse drug effects: Implications for patient-targeted adverse effect surveillance. *Drug Safety, 30,* 669–675.

51. Gaist, D., et al. (2002). Statins and risk of polyneuropathy: A case-control study. *Neurology, 58* (9), 1333–1337.

52. Schwartz, G. G., et al. (2001). Effects of atorvastatin on early recurrent ischemic events in acute coronary syndromes: The MIRACL study: A randomized controlled trial. *JAMA, 285* (13), 1711–1718.

53. King, D. S., et al. (2003). Cognitive impairment associated with atorvastatin and simvastatin. *Pharmacotherapy, 23,* 1663–1667.

54. Evans, M. A., & Golomb, B. A. (2009). Statin-associated adverse cognitive effects: Survey results from 171 patients. *Pharmacotherapy, 29,* 800–811.

55. Langsjoen, P. H., & Langsjoen, A. M. (2003). The clinical use of HMG CoA-reductase inhibitors and the associated depletion of coenzyme Q_{10}. A review of animal and human publications. *Biofactors, 18* (1–4), 101–111.

56. Tatley, M., & Savage, R. (2007). Psychiatric adverse reactions with statins, fibrates and ezetimibe: Implications for the use of lipid-lowering agents. *Drug Safety, 30,* 195–201.

57. Buajordet, I., et al. (1997). Statins—the pattern of adverse effects with emphasis on mental reactions: Data from a national and an international database. *Tidsskr Nor Laegeforen, 117,* 3210–3213.

58. Golomb, B. A., et al. (2004). Severe irritability associated with statin cholesterol-lowering drugs. *QJM, 97,* 229–235.

59. Suarez, E. C. (1999). Relations of trait depression and anxiety to low lipid and lipoprotein concentrations in healthy young adult women. *Psychosom Med, 61* (3), 273–279.

60. Newman, T. B., & Hulley, S. B. (1996). Carcinogenicity of lipid-lowering drugs. *JAMA, 275* (1), 55–60.

61. Folkers, K., et al. (1997). Activities of vitamin Q_{10} in animal models and a serious deficiency in patients with cancer. *Biochem Biophys Res Commun, 234* (2), 296–299; Lockwood, K., et al. (1995). Progress on therapy of breast cancer with vitamin Q_{10} and the regression of metastases. *Biochem Biophys Res Commun, 212* (1), 172–177.

62. Sinatra, S. (2000). *Heart Sense for Women,* 108. Washington, DC: Lifeline.

63. Sacks, F. M., et al. (1996). The effect of pravastatin on coronary events after myocardial infarction in patients with average cholesterol levels. Cholesterol and Recurrent Events Trial investigators. *N Engl J Med, 335* (14), 1001–1009.

64. Boudreau, D. M., et al. (2004). The association between 3-hydroxy-3-methylglutaryl coenzyme A inhibitor use and breast carcinoma risk among postmenopausal women: A case-control study. *Cancer, 100* (11), 2308–2316.

65. Ray, K. K., Seshasai, S. R., Erqou, S., Sever, P., Jukema, J. W., Ford, I., &

Sattar, N. (2010). Statins and all-cause mortality in high-risk primary prevention: A meta-analysis of 11 randomized controlled trials involving 65,229 participants. *Arch Intern Med, 170* (12), 1024–1031.

66. Thavendiranathan, P., Bagai, A., Brookhart, M. A., & Choudhry, N. K. (2006). Primary prevention of cardiovascular diseases with statin therapy: A meta-analysis of randomized controlled trials. *Arch Intern Medicine, 166* (21), 2307–2313; Baigent, C., Keech, A., Kearney, P. M., Blackwell, L., Buck, G., Pollicino, C., Kirby, A., Sourjina, T., Peto, R., Collins, R., Simes, R., & Cholesterol Treatment Trialists' (CTT) Collaborators (2005). Efficacy and safety of cholesterol-lowering treatment: Prospective meta-analysis of data from 90,056 participants in 14 randomised trials of statins. *Lancet, 366* (9493), 1267–1278; Ridker, P. M., Danielson, E., Fonseca, F. A., Genest, J., Gotto, A. M., Jr, Kastelein, J. J., Koenig, W., Libby, P., Lorenzatti, A. J., MacFadyen, J. G., Nordestgaard, B. G., Shepherd, J., Willerson, J. T., Glynn, R. J., & JUPITER Study Group (2008). Rosuvastatin to prevent vascular events in men and women with elevated C-reactive protein. *N Engl J Med, 359* (21), 2195–2207; Sattar, N., Preiss, D., Murray, H. M., Welsh, P., Buckley, B. M., de Craen, A. J., Seshasai, S. R., McMurray, J. J., Freeman, D. J., Jukema, J. W., Macfarlane, P. W., Packard, C. J., Stott, D. J., Westendorp, R. G., Shepherd, J., Davis, B. R., Pressel, S. L., Marchioli, R., Marfisi, R. M., Maggioni, A. P., . . . & Ford, I. (2010). Statins and risk of incident diabetes: A collaborative meta-analysis of randomised statin trials. *Lancet, 375* (9716), 735–742.

67. de Lorgeril, M., Salen, P., Martin, J. L., Monjaud, I., Boucher, P., & Mamelle, N. (1998). Mediterranean dietary pattern in a randomized trial: Prolonged survival and possible reduced cancer rate. *Arch Intern Med, 158* (11), 1181–1187; de Lorgeril, M., Renaud, S., Mamelle, N., Salen, P., Martin, J. L., Monjaud, I., Guidollet, J., Touboul, P., & Delaye, J. (1994). Mediterranean alpha-linolenic acid-rich diet in secondary prevention of coronary heart disease. *Lancet, 343* (8911), 1454–1459.

68. Bruckert, E., Hayem, G., Dejager, S., Yau, C., & Bégaud, B. (2005). Mild to moderate muscular symptoms with high-dosage statin therapy in hyperlipidemic patients—the PRIMO study. *Cardiovasc Drugs Ther, 19* (6), 403–414.

69. Wu, T., et al. (2000). Periodontal disease and risk of cerebrovascular disease: The first national health and nutrition examination survey and its follow-up study. *Arch Intern Med, 160* (18), 2749–2755; Hujoel, P. P., et al. (2000). Periodontal disease and coronary heart disease risk. *JAMA, 284* (11), 1406–1410.

70. Siegel, R. L., Miller, K. D., & Jemal, A. (2020). Cancer statistics, 2020. *CA, 70* (1), 7–30.

71. Hollenbach, K. A., et al. (1993). Cigarette smoking and bone mineral density in older men and women. *Am J Public Health, 83,* 1265–1270.

72. Berenson, G. S., et al. (1998). Association between multiple cardiovascular risk factors and atherosclerosis in children and young adults. *N Engl J Med, 338,* 1650–1656.

73. Mann, D. (May 2, 1996). Job stress can cause fatal MI. *Medical Tribune,*

Primary Care Edition, 21; Suadicani, P., Hein, H. O., & Gyntelberg, F. (1993). Are social inequalities as associated with the risk of ischaemic heart disease a result of psychosocial working conditions? *Atherosclerosis, 101* (2), 165–175; Legault, S. E., et al. (1995). Pathophysiology and time course of silent myocardial ischemia during mental stress: Clinical, anatomical, and physiological correlates. *Br Heart J, 73,* 242–249; Kaplan, G. A., & Keil, J. E. (1993). Socioeconomic factors and cardiovascular disease: A review of the literature. *Circulation, 88,* 1973–1998.

74. Castelli, W. P. (1988). Cardiovascular disease in women. *Am J Obstet Gynecol, 158* (6), 1553–1560, 1566–1567; Lacroix, A. Z. (1994). Psychosocial factors in risk of coronary heart disease in women: An epidemiologic perspective. *Fertil Steril, 62* (suppl. 2), 133S–139S; Mahoney, L. T., et al. (1996). Coronary risk factors measured in childhood and young adult life are associated with coronary artery calcification in young adults: The Muscatine Study. *J Am Coll Cardiol, 27* (2), 277–284; Schaefer, E. J., et al. (1994). Factors associated with low and elevated plasma HDL cholesterol and apolipoprotein A-I levels in the Framingham Offspring Study. *J Lipid Research, 35* (5), 871–872; Garrison, R. J., et al. (1993). Educational attainment and coronary heart disease risk: The Framingham Offspring Study. *Prev Med, 22* (1), 54–64.

75. Mann, S. J. (1999). *Healing Hypertension: A Revolutionary New Approach* (2). New York: John Wiley.

76. Ferketich, A. K., et al. (2000). Depression as an antecedent to heart disease among women and men in the NHANES I Study. *Arch Intern Med, 160,* 1261–1268.

77. Sinatra, S. (Aug. 26, 2010). Heart failure in women: A serious and insidious condition. Guest author on www.drnorthrup.com.

78. Jeppesen, J. (1997). Effects of low-fat high-carbohydrate diets on risk for ischemic heart disease in postmenopausal women. *Am J Clin Nutr, 65* (4), 1027–1033.

79. Kearney, M. T., et al. (1997). William Heberden revisited: Postprandial angina—interval between food and exercise and meal composition are important determinants of time to onset of ischemia and maximal exercise tolerance. *J Am Coll Cardiol, 29* (2), 302–307.

80. To read this book online, see www.seleneriverpress.com/media/pdf_docs /0_How_to_Prevent_Heart_Attacks_BEN_SANDLER_MD_1958.pdf.

81. Sieri, S., et al. (2010). Dietary glycemic load and index and risk of coronary heart disease in a large Italian cohort: The EPICOR study. *Arch Intern Med, 170,* 640–647.

82. Crapo, P. A., et al. (1976). Plasma glucose and insulin responses to orally administered simple and complex carbohydrates. *Diabetes, 25* (9), 741–747; Crapo, P. A. (1977). Postprandial plasma-glucose and -insulin responses to different complex carbohydrates. *Diabetes, 26* (12), 1178–1183.

83. Modan, M., et al. (1985). Hyperinsulinemia: A link between hypertension, obesity and glucose intolerance. *J Clin Invest, 75,* 809–817.

84. Ridker, P. M., et al. (2000). C-reactive protein and other markers of inflammation in the prediction of cardiovascular disease in women. *N Engl*

J Med, 342 (12), 836–843; Black, H. R. (1990). Coronary artery disease paradox: The role of hyperinsulinemia and insulin resistance and its implications for therapy. *J Cardiovasc Pharmacol,* 15 (suppl. 5), 26S–38S; Brindley, D. M., & Rolland, Y. (1989). Possible connections between stress, diabetes, obesity, hypertension, and altered lipoprotein metabolism that may result in arteriosclerosis. *Clin Sci,* 77 (5), 453–461; DeFronzo, R., & Ferrannini, E. (1991). Insulin resistance: A multifaceted syndrome responsible for NIDDM, obesity, hypertension, dyslipidemia, and atherosclerotic cardiovascular disease. *Diabetes Care,* 14 (3), 173–194; Eades, M., & Eades, M. D. (1996). *Protein Power.* New York: Bantam; Kazer, R. (1995). Insulin resistance, insulin-like growth factor I and breast cancer: A hypothesis. *Int J Cancer,* 62, 403–406; Lehninger, A. L. (1993). *Principles of Biochemistry.* New York: Worth; Jeppesen, J. (1997). Effects of low-fat high-carbohydrate diets on risk for ischemic heart disease in postmenopausal women. *Am J Clin Nutr,* 65 (4), 1027–1033.

85. Tribble, D. L. (1999). AHA science advisory. Antioxidant consumption and risk of coronary heart disease: Emphasis on vitamin C, vitamin E, and beta-carotene: A statement for health care professionals from the American Heart Association. *Circulation,* 99 (4), 591–595.

86. Witteman, J. C., et al. (1994). Reduction of blood pressure with oral magnesium supplementation in women with mild to moderate hypertension. *Am J Clin Nutr,* 60 (1), 129–135.

87. Eisenberg, M. J. (1992). Magnesium deficiency and sudden death. *Am Heart J,* 124, 2, 544–549; Turlapaty, P. D., & Altura, B. M. (1980). Magnesium deficiency produces spasms in coronary arteries: Relationship to etiology of sudden death ischemic heart disease. *Science,* 208 (4440), 198–200; Altura, B. M. (1979). Sudden death ischemic heart disease and dietary magnesium intake: Is the target site coronary vascular smooth muscle? *Med Hypotheses,* 5, 8, 843–848.

88. Simental-Mendia, L. E., Sahebkar, A., Rodriguez-Moran, M., Zambrano-Galvan, G., & Guerrero-Romero, F. (2017). Effect of magnesium supplementation on plasma C-reactive protein concentrations: A systematic review and meta-analysis of randomized controlled trials. *Curr Pharm Des,* 23 (31), 4678–4686.

89. Dong, J. Y., Xun, P., He, K., & Qin, L. Q. (2011). Magnesium intake and risk of type 2 diabetes: Meta-analysis of prospective cohort studies. *Diabetes Dare,* 34 (9), 2116–2122.

90. Altura, B. M., et al. (1991). Cardiovascular risk factors and magensium: Relationships to atherosclerosis, ischemic heart disease, and hypertension. *Magnes Trace Elem,* 10, 182–192; Bostick, R. M. (1999). Relation of Ca+, vitamin D, and dairy food intake to ischemic heart disease mortality among postmenopausal women. *Am J Epidemiol,* 149 (2), 151–161; Morrison, H., et al. (1996). Serum folate and risk of fatal coronary heart disease. *JAMA,* 275 (24), 1893–1896; Stampfer, M. J., et al. (1993). Vitamin E consumption and the risk of coronary disease in women. *N Engl J Med,* 328, 1444–1449; Yochum, L., et al. (1999). Dietary flavonoid intake and risk of cardiovascular disease in postmenopausal women. *Am J*

Epidemiol, 149 (10), 943–949; Kushi, L. H., et al. (1996). Dietary antioxidant vitamins and death from coronary heart disease in postmenopausal women. *N Engl J Med, 334,* 1156–1162.

91. Digiesi, V., et al. (1990). Effect of coenzyme Q_{10} on essential hypertension. *Curr Ther Res, 47,* 841–845.

92. Ghirlanda, G., et al. (1993). Evidence of plasma CoQ_{10}-lowering effects by HMG-CoA reductase inhibitors: A double-blind, placebo-controlled study. *J Clin Pharmacol, 33,* 226–229.

93. Singh, R. B., et al. (1999). Effect of hydrosoluble coenzyme Q_{10} on blood pressures and insulin resistance in hypertensive patients with coronary artery disease. *J Human Hypertension, 13* (3), 203–208.

94. Yamagami, T., et al. (1977). Study of coenzyme Q_{10} in essential hypertension. In K. Folkers & Y. Yamamura (eds.), *Biochemical and Clinical Aspects of Coenzyme Q_{10}, vol. 1* (231–242). Amsterdam: Elsevier.

95. Singh, R. B., et al. (2003). Effect of coenzyme Q_{10} on risk of atherosclerosis in patients with recent myocardial infarction. *Mol Cell Biochem, 246* (1–2), 75–82.

96. Sinatra, S. (1998). *The Coenzyme Q_{10} Phenomenon.* Los Angeles: Keats Publishing.

97. Howard, A. N., et al. (1996). Do hydroxycarotenoids prevent coronary heart disease? A comparison between Belfast and Toulouse. *Int J Vitamin Nutr Res, 66,* 113–118.

98. Stampfer, M. J., et al. (1993). Vitamin E consumption and the risk of coronary disease in women. *N Engl J Med, 328* (20), 1444–1449.

99. Stephens, N. G., et al. (1996). Randomized controlled trial of vitamin E in patients with coronary disease. Cambridge Heart Antioxidant Study (CHAOS). *Lancet, 347,* 781–786.

100. Pocobelli, G., et al. (2009). Use of supplements of multivitamins, vitamin C, and vitamin E in relation to mortality. *Am J Epidemiol, 170,* 472–483.

101. Miller, E. R. (2005). Meta-analysis: High-dosage vitamin E supplementation may increase all-cause mortality. *Ann Intern Med, 142* (1), 37–46.

102. Bostick, R. M., et al. (1993). Reduced risk of colon cancer with high intakes of vitamin E: The Iowa women's health study. *Cancer Res, 53* (18), 4230–4237.

103. Zandi, P. P. (2004). Reduced risk of Alzheimer disease in users of antioxidant vitamin supplements: The Cache County study. *Arch Neurol, 61* (1), 82–88.

104. Lu, M. (2005). Prospective study of dietary fat and risk of cataract extraction among U.S. women. *Am J Epidemiol, 161* (10), 948–959.

105. Newaz, M. A., & Nawal, N. N. (1999). Effect of gamma-tocotrienol on blood pressure, lipid peroxidation and total antioxidant status in spontaneously hypertensive rats (SHR). *Clin Exp Hyperens, 21* (8), 1297–1313; Qureshi, A. A., & Peterson, D. M. (2001). The combined effects of novel tocotrienols and lovastatin on lipid metabolism in chickens. *Atherosclerosis, 156* (1), 39–47; Sen, C. K., Khanna, S., Roy, S., & Packer, L. (2000). Molecular basis of vitamin E action. Tocotrienol potently inhibits glutamate-induced pp60(c-Src) kinase activation and death of HT4 neuro-

nal cells. *J Biol Chem, 275* (17), 13049–13055; Theriault, A., et al. (1999). Tocotrienol: A review of its therapeutic potential. *Clin Biochem, 32* (5), 309–319.

106. Janson, M. (1997). Drug free management of hypertension. *Am J Nat Med, 4* (8), 14–17.

107. Nemerovski, C. W., et al. (2009). Vitamin D and cardiovascular disease. *Pharmacotherapy, 29,* 691–708.

108. Anderson, J. L., et al. (2010). Relation of vitamin D deficiency to cardiovascular risk factors, disease status, and incident events in a general healthcare population. *Am J Cardiol, 106,* 963–968.

109. Gaziano, J. M. (1994). Antioxidant vitamins and coronary artery disease risk. *Am J Med, 97* (suppl.), 3S–21S; Nenseter, M. S., Volden, V., Berg, T., et al. (1995). No effect of beta-carotene supplementation on the susceptibility of low-density lipoprotein to *in vitro* oxidation among hypercholesterolaemic postmenopausal women. *Scan J Clin Lab Invest, 55,* 477–485; Riemersma, R. A., et al. (1991). Risk of angina pectoris and plasma concentrations of vitamin A, E, C, and carotene. *Lancet, 337* (8732), 1–5; Stampfer, M. J., Hennekens, C. H., Manson, J. E., et al. (1993). Vitamin E consumption and the risk of coronary disease in women. *N Engl J Med, 328* (20), 1444–1449; Steinberg, E., et al. (1992). Antioxidants in the prevention of human atherosclerosis. *Circulation, 85* (6), 2238–2343; Street, D. A., Comstock, G. W., Salkeld, R. M., Schuep, W., & Klag, M. J. (1994). Serum antioxidants and myocardial infarction. Are low levels of carotenoids and alpha-tocopherol risk factors for myocardial infarction? *Circulation, 90* (3), 1154–1161.

110. Rimm, E. B. (1998). Folate and vitamin B_6 from diet and supplements in relation to risk of coronary heart disease among women. *JAMA, 279,* 359–364.

111. Douaud, G., Refsum, H., de Jager, C. A., Jacoby, R., Nichols, T. E., Smith, S. M., & Smith, A. D. (2013). Preventing Alzheimer's disease-related gray matter atrophy by B-vitamin treatment. *Proc Natl Acad Sci, 110* (23), 9523–9528; Calvaresi, E., & Bryan, J. (2001). B vitamins, cognition, and aging: A review. *J Gerontol B Psychol, 56* (6), P327–P339; Houghton, L. A., Green, T. J., Donovan, U. M., Gibson, R. S., Stephen, A. M., & O'Connor, D. L. (1997). Association between dietary fiber intake and the folate status of a group of female adolescents. *Am J Clin Nutr, 66* (6), 1414–1421; Obersby, D., Chappell, D. C., Dunnett, A., & Tsiami, A. A. (2013). Plasma total homocysteine status of vegetarians compared with omnivores: A systematic review and meta-analysis. *Br J Nutr, 109* (5), 785–794; Smith, A. D., Smith, S. M., de Jager, C. A., Whitbread, P., Johnston, C., Agacinski, G., Oulhaj, A., Bradley, K. M., Jacoby, R., & Refsum, H. (2010). Homocysteine-lowering by B vitamins slows the rate of accelerated brain atrophy in mild cognitive impairment: A randomized controlled trial. *PloS One, 5* (9), e12244.

112. Zhang, L. H., et al. (2008). Niacin inhibits surface expression of ATP synthase beta chain in HepG2 cells: Implications for raising HDL. *J Lipid Res, 49,* 1195–1201.

113. Iso, H., et al. (2001). Intake of fish and omega-3 fatty acids and risk of stroke in women. *JAMA, 285,* 304–312.

114. Leaf, A., et al. (1988). Cardiovascular effect of n-3 fatty acids. *N Engl J Med, 318* (9), 549–557; von Schaky, C., et al. (1999). The effect of dietary omega-3 fatty acids in coronary atherosclerosis: A randomized, double-blind, placebo-controlled trial. *Ann Intern Med, 130* (7), 554–562.

115. Vanschoonbeek, K., et al. (2007). Plasma triacylglycerol and coagulation factor concentrations predict the anticoagulant effect of dietary fish oil in overweight subjects. *J Nutr, 137,* 7–13; Schwellenbach, L. J., et al. (2006). The triglyceride-lowering effects of a modest dose of docosahexaenoic acid alone versus in combination with low dose eicosapentaenoic acid in patients with coronary artery disease and elevated triglycerides. *J Am Coll Nutr, 25,* 480–485; Moore, C. S., et al. (2006). Oily fish reduces plasma triacylglycerols: A primary prevention study in overweight men and women. *Nutrition, 22,* 1012–1024; Vanschoonbeek, K., et al. (2004). Variable hypocoagulant effect of fish oil intake in humans: Modulation of fibrinogen level and thrombin generation. *Arterioscler Thromb Vasc Biol, 24,* 1734–1740.

116. Hertog, M. G., et al. (1997). Antioxidant flavonols and coronary heart disease. *Lancet, 349* (9053), 699.

117. Jain, A. K., et al. (1993). Can garlic reduce levels of serum lipids? A controlled clinical study. *Am J Med, 94,* 632–635; Kleijnen, J., et al. (1989). Garlic, onions, and cardiovascular risk factors: A review of the evidence from human experiments with emphasis on commercially available preparations. *Br J Clin Pharmacol, 28,* 535–544; Mader, F. H. (1990). Treatment of hyperlipidemia with garlic powder tablets. *Arzneim-Forsch, 40,* 1111–1116; McMahon, F. G., & Vargas, R. (1993). Can garlic lower blood pressure? A pilot study. *Pharmacotherapy, 13* (4), 406–407.

118. Berger, J. (1998). *Herbal Rituals* (132–138). New York: St. Martin's Press.

119. Skrabal, F. (1981). Low sodium/high potassium diet for the prevention of hypertension: Probable mechanisms of action. *Lancet, 2* (8252), 895–900.

120. Alpers, G. W., et al. (1999). Antiplatelet therapy: New foundations for optimal treatment decisions. *Neurology, 53* (7, suppl. 4), 25S–31S; Antiplatelet Trialists' Collaboration (1994). Collaborative overview of randomised trials of antiplatelet therapy—1: Prevention of death, myocardial infarction, and stroke by prolonged antiplatelet therapy in various categories of patients. *BMJ, 308,* 81–106; DeAbago, F. J., et al. (1999). Association between SSRIs and upper GI bleeding. *BMJ, 319,* 1106–1109; Easton, J. D., et al. (1999). Antiplatelet therapy: Views from the experts. *Neurology, 53* (7, suppl. 4), 32S–37S; Rong, Y., et al. (1994). Pycnogenol protects vascular endothelial cells from induced oxidant injury. *Biotechnol Ther, 5* (3–4), 117–126.

121. Ridker, P. M., et al. (2005). A randomized trial of low-dose aspirin in the primary prevention of cardiovascular disease in women. *N Engl J Med, 352* (13), 1293–1304.

122. McNeil, J. J., Woods, R. L., Nelson, M. R., Reid, C. M., Kirpach, B., Wolfe, R., Storey, E., Shah, R. C., Lockery, J. E., Tonkin, A. M., Newman,

A. B., Williamson, J. D., Margolis, K. L., Ernst, M. E., Abhayaratna, W. P., Stocks, N., Fitzgerald, S. M., Orchard, S. G., Trevaks, R. E., Beilin, L. J., . . . & ASPREE Investigator Group (2018). Effect of aspirin on disability-free survival in the healthy elderly. *N Engl J Med, 379* (16), 1499–1508.

123. McNeil, J. J., Nelson, M. R., Woods, R. L., Lockery, J. E., Wolfe, R., Reid, C. M., Kirpach, B., Shah, R. C., Ives, D. G., Storey, E., Ryan, J., Tonkin, A. M., Newman, A. B., Williamson, J. D., Margolis, K. L., Ernst, M. E., Abhayaratna, W. P., Stocks, N., Fitzgerald, S. M., Orchard, S. G., . . . & ASPREE Investigator Group (2018). Effect of aspirin on all-cause mortality in the healthy elderly. *N Engl J Med, 379* (16), 1519–1528.

124. Joshipura, K. J., et al. (1999). Fruit and vegetable intake in relation to risk of ischemic stroke. *JAMA, 282* (13), 1233–1239.

125. Osganian, S. K., et al. (2003). Dietary carotenoids and risk of coronary artery disease in women. *Am J Clin Nutr, 77* (6), 1390–1399.

126. Duffy, S. J., et al. (2001). Short- and long-term black tea consumption reverses endothelial dysfunction in patients with coronary artery disease. *Circulation, 104* (2), 151–156.

127. Keli, S. O., et al. (1996). Dietary flavonoids, antioxidant vitamins, and incidence of stroke: The Zutphen study. *Arch Intern Med, 156* (6), 637–642.

128. Quereshi, A. A., & Quereshi, N. (1993). Tocotrienols: Novel hypocholesterolemic agents with antioxidant properties. In Packer, L., & Fuchs, J. (eds.), *Vitamin E in Health and Disease*. New York: Marcel Dekker.

129. Oh, R. (2005). Practical applications of fish oil (omega-3 fatty acids) in primary care. *J Am Board Fam Pract, 18* (1), 28–36; Mozaffarian, D., et al. (2005). Fish consumption and stroke risk in elderly individuals: The cardiovascular health study. *Arch Intern Med, 165* (2), 200–206; Iso, H., et al. (2001). Intake of fish and omega-3 fatty acids and risk of stroke in women. *JAMA, 285* (3), 304–312.

130. Hermsmeyer, R. K., et al. (2008). Cardiovascular effects of medroxyprogesterone acetate and progesterone: A case of mistaken identity? *Nat Clin Pract Cardiovasc Med, 5,* 387–395.

131. Nusselder, W. J., et al. (2009). Living healthier for longer: Comparative effects of three heart-healthy behaviors on life expectancy with and without cardiovascular disease. *BMC Public Health, 9,* 487.

132. Kvaavik, E., et al. (2010). Influence of individual and combined health behaviors on total and cause-specific mortality in men and women: The United Kingdom health and lifestyle survey. *Arch Intern Med, 170,* 711–718.

133. Hambrecht, R., et al. (2000). Effect of exercise on coronary endothelial function in patients with coronary artery disease. *N Engl J Med, 342,* 454–460; Goldman, E. (Nov. 1, 1999). Exercise equals estrogen for lowering heart risk. *Int Med News,* 16.

134. Belardinelli, R., et al. (1998). Effects of moderate exercise training on thallium uptake and contractile response to low-dose dobutamine of dysfunctional myocardium in patients with ischemic cardiomyopathy. *Circulation, 97,* 553–561.

135. Sattelmair, J. R., et al. (2010). Physical activity and risk of stroke in women. *Stroke, 41,* 1243–1250.

136. Lemole, J. (Feb. 1999). Personal interview for *Health Wisdom for Women.*

137. Artinian, N. T., et al. (2010). Interventions to promote physical activity and dietary lifestyle changes for cardiovascular risk factor reduction in adults: A scientific statement from the American Heart Association. *Circulation, 122,* 406–441.

138. Herrington, D., et al. (2000). Effects of estrogen replacement on the progression of coronary artery atherosclerosis. *N Engl J Med, 343,* 522–529; Hulley, S., et al., for the Heart and Estrogen/Progestin Replacement Study (HERS) Research Group (1998). Randomized trial of estrogen plus progestin for secondary prevention of coronary heart disease in postmenopausal women. *JAMA, 280,* 605–613; no authors listed (Mar. 13, 2000). Estrogen replacement and atherosclerosis (ERA). Presented at the 49th annual meeting of the American College of Cardiology, Anaheim, CA.

139. Grodstein, F., Manson, J. E., & Stampfer, M. J. (2006). Hormone therapy and coronary heart disease: The role of time since menopause and age at hormone initiation. *J Womens Health (Larchmt), 15* (1), 35–44.

140. Koh, K. K., Mincemoyer, R., Bui, M. N., et al. (1997). Effects of hormone replacement therapy on fibrinolysis in postmenopausal women. *N Engl J Med, 336,* 683–690; Nasr, A., & Breckwoldt, M. (1998). Estrogen replacement therapy and cardiovascular protection: Lipid mechanisms are the tip of an iceberg. *Gynecol Endocrinol, 12,* 43–59; Oparil, S. (1999). Arthur C. Corcoran Memorial Lecture: Hormones and vasoprotection. *Hypertension, 33,* 170–176; Pines, A., Mijatovic, V., van der Mooren, M. J., et al. (1997). Hormone replacement therapy and cardioprotection: Basic concepts and clinical considerations. *Eur J Gynecol Reprod Biol, 71,* 193–197; van der Mooren, M. J., Mijatovic, V., & van Baal, W. M. (1998). Hormone replacement therapy in postmenopausal women with specific risk factors for coronary artery disease. *Maturitas, 30,* 27–36; Rosano, G. (1996). 17-ß-estradiol therapy lessens angina in postmenopausal women with syndrome X. *J Am Coll Cardiol, 28,* 1500–1505.

141. Clarkson, T. B., & Anthony, M. S. (1997). Effects on the cardiovascular system: Basic aspects. In Lindsay, R., Dempster, D. W., & Jordan, V. C. (eds.). *Estrogens and Antiestrogens* (89–118). Philadelphia: Lippincott-Raven; Gerhard, M., & Ganz, P. (1995). How do we explain the clinical benefits of estrogen? From bedside to bench. *Circulation, 92,* 5–8; Reis, S. E., Gloth, S. T., Blumenthal, R. S., et al. (1994). Ethinyl estradiol acutely attenuates abnormal coronary vasomotor responses to acetylcholine in postmenopausal women. *Circulation, 89* (1), 52–60; Sullivan, J. M. (1996). Hormone replacement therapy in cardiovascular disease: The human model. *Br J Obstet Gynaecol, 103* (suppl. 13), 50S–67S.

142. Darling, G. M., Johns, J. A., McCloud, P. L., et al. (1997). Estrogen and progestin compared with simvastatin for hypercholesterolemia in postmenopausal women. *N Engl J Med, 337,* 595–601; Davidson, M. H., Testolin, L. M., Maki, K. C., et al. (1997). A comparison of estrogen replacement, pravastatin, and combined treatment for the management of

hypercholesterolemia in postmenopausal women. *Arch Intern Med, 157,* 1186–1192; Koh, K. K., Cardillo, C., Bui, M. N., et al. (1997). Vascular effects of estrogen and cholesterol-lowering therapies in hypercholesterolemic postmenopausal women. *Circulation, 99,* 354–360.

143. Twenty-third Annual Conference of the North American Menopause Society: Kronos Longevity Research Institute Plenary Symposium #1— Presidential Symposium: New Findings from the Kronos Early Prevention Study (KEEPS) Randomized Trial. Presented October 6–12, 2012.

144. Harman, S. M., Black, D. M., Naftolin, F., Brinton, E. A., Budoff, M. J., Cedars, M. I., Hopkins, P. N., Lobo, R. A., Manson, J. E., Merriam, G. R., Miller, V. M., Neal-Perry, G., Santoro, N., Taylor, H. S., Vittinghoff, E., Yan, M., & Hodis, H. N. (2014). Arterial imaging outcomes and cardiovascular risk factors in recently menopausal women: A randomized trial. *Ann Intern Med, 161* (4), 249–260.

145. Hodis, H. N., Mack, W. J., Henderson, V. W., Shoupe, D., Budoff, M. J., Hwang-Levine, J., Li, Y., Feng, M., Dustin, L., Kono, N., Stanczyk, F. Z., Selzer, R. H., Azen, S. P., & ELITE Research Group (2016). Vascular effects of early versus late postmenopausal treatment with estradiol. *N Engl J Med, 374* (13), 1221–1231.

146. Henderson, V. W., St. John, J. A., Howard, H. N., McCleary, C. A., Stanczyk, F. Z., Shoupe, D., Kono, N., Dustin, L., Allayee, H., & Mack, W. J. (2016). Cognitive effects of estradiol after menopause: A randomized trial of the timing hypothesis. *Neurol, 87* (7), 699–708.

147. Fitzgerald, F. T. (1986). The therapeutic value of pets. *West J Med, 144,* 103–105.

148. Ibid.

149. Qureshi, A. I., Memon, M. Z., Vazquez, G., & Suri, M. F. (2009). Cat ownership and the risk of fatal cardiovascular diseases: Results from the Second National Health and Nutrition Examination Study Mortality Follow-up Study. *J Vasc Interv Neurol, 2* (1), 132–135.

150. Friedmann, E., Katcher, A., Lunch, J. J., & Thomas, S. A. (1980). Animal companions and the one-year survival of patients after discharge from a coronary care unit. *Public Health Reports, 95,* 307–312.

151. Beck, A., & Katcher, A. (1983). *Between Pets and People: The Importance of Animal Companionship.* New York: Putnam; Katcher, A., & Beck, A. (1983). *New Perspectives on Our Lives with Companion Animals.* Philadelphia: University of Pennsylvania Press.

152. Mubanga, M., Byberg, L., Egenvall, A., Ingelsson, E., & Fall, T. (2019). Dog ownership and survival after a major cardiovascular event: A register-based prospective study. *Circulation, 12* (10), e005342.

153. Xie, Z. Y., Zhao, D., Chen, B. R., Wang, Y. N., Ma, Y., Shi, H. J., Yang, Y., Wang, Z. M., & Wang, L. S. (2017). Association between pet ownership and coronary artery disease in a Chinese population. *Medicine, 96* (13), e6466.

Index

Page numbers of illustrations appear in italics.

About the Author

Christiane Northrup, M.D., an OB-GYN physician, is a leading authority in the field of women's health and wellness and the *New York Times* bestselling author of *Women's Bodies, Women's Wisdom, The Wisdom of Menopause,* and *Goddesses Never Age: The Secret Prescription for Radiance, Vitality, and Well-Being.* In *Making Life Easy: A Simple Guide to a Divinely Inspired Life,* Dr. Northrup reveals her secrets to mind/body/spirit well-being. *Dodging Energy Vampires* offers radical "upstream" preventive medicine.

Internationally known for her empowering approach, Dr. Northrup embraces medicine that acknowledges the unity of mind, body, emotions, and spirit and teaches women to create health by tuning in to their inner wisdom. After spending decades transforming women's understanding of their sacred bodies and processes, Dr. Northrup now teaches women how to thrive at every stage of life.

drnorthrup.com
Facebook.com/DrChristianeNorthrup
Twitter: @DrChrisNorthrup
Instagram: @DrChristianeNorthrup